ACSM's
Resources for the
Personal Trainer

THIRD EDITION

■ SENIOR EDITOR

Walter R. Thompson, PhD, FACSM
Regents Professor
Department of Kinesiology and Health (College of Education)
Division of Nutrition (School of Health Professions, College of Health and Human Sciences)
Georgia State University
Atlanta, Georgia

■ ASSOCIATE EDITORS

Barbara A. Bushman, PhD, FACSM
Professor
Department of Health, Physical Education and Recreation
Missouri State University
Springfield, Missouri

Julie Desch, MD
Founder
New Day Wellness
Palo Alto, California

Len Kravitz, PhD
Associate Professor and Coordinator of Exercise Science
Department of Health, Exercise and Sports Sciences
University of New Mexico
Albuquerque, New Mexico

ACSM's
Resources for the
Personal Trainer

THIRD EDITION

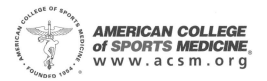

AMERICAN COLLEGE
of SPORTS MEDICINE®
www.acsm.org

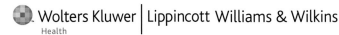

Wolters Kluwer | Lippincott Williams & Wilkins
Health

Philadelphia • Baltimore • New York • London
Buenos Aires • Hong Kong • Sydney • Tokyo

Acquisitions Editor: Emily Lupash
Product Manager: Andrea M. Klingler
Marketing Manager: Christen Murphy
Designer: Holly McLaughlin
Compositor: Aptara, Inc.

Third Edition

Copyright © 2010 Lippincott Williams & Wilkins, a Wolters Kluwer business

351 West Camden Street   530 Walnut Street
Baltimore, MD 21201   Philadelphia, PA 19106

Printed in China

9 8 7 6 5 4 3 2 1

Library of Congress Cataloging-in-Publication Data

ACSM's resources for the personal trainer. — 3rd ed.
    p. ; cm.
  Includes bibliographical references and index.
  ISBN 978-0-7817-9772-6 (alk. paper)
  1. Personal trainers. I. American College of Sports Medicine. II.
Title: Resource for the personal trainer.
  [DNLM: 1. Physical Education and Training. 2. Exercise—physiology.
QT 255 A1873 2010]
  GV428.7.A47 2010
  613.7′1—dc22

                               2009024494

DISCLAIMER

    Care has been taken to confirm the accuracy of the information present and to describe generally accepted practices. However, the authors, editors, and publisher are not responsible for errors or omissions or for any consequences from application of the information in this book and make no warranty, expressed or implied, with respect to the currency, completeness, or accuracy of the contents of the publication. Application of this information in a particular situation remains the professional responsibility of the practitioner; the clinical treatments described and recommended may not be considered absolute and universal recommendations.

    The authors, editors, and publisher have exerted every effort to ensure that drug selection and dosage set forth in this text are in accordance with the current recommendations and practice at the time of publication. However, in view of ongoing research, changes in government regulations, and the constant flow of information relating to drug therapy and drug reactions, the reader is urged to check the package insert for each drug for any change in indications and dosage and for added warnings and precautions. This is particularly important when the recommended agent is a new or infrequently employed drug.

    Some drugs and medical devices presented in this publication have Food and Drug Administration (FDA) clearance for limited use in restricted research settings. It is the responsibility of the health care provider to ascertain the FDA status of each drug or device planned for use in their clinical practice.

To purchase additional copies of this book, call our customer service department at **(800) 638-3030** or fax orders to **(301) 223-2320**. International customers should call **(301) 223-2300**.

Visit Lippincott Williams & Wilkins on the Internet: **http://www.lww.com**. Lippincott Williams & Wilkins customer service representatives are available from 8:30 am to 6:00 pm, EST.

Laura Alderman, MEd
MeritCare Medical Center
Fargo, North Dakota

William R. Barfield, PhD, FACSM
College of Charleston & Medical University of South Carolina
Charleston, South Carolina

Dan Benardot, PhD, DHC, RD, FACSM
Georgia State University
Atlanta, Georgia

Christopher Berger, PhD
University of Kentucky
Lexington, Kentucky

Barbara A. Bushman, PhD, FACSM
Missouri State University
Springfield, Missouri

Nikki Carosone, MS
Plus One Health Management, Inc.
New York, NY

Carol N. Cole, MS
Sinclair Community College
Dayton, Ohio

Richard T. Cotton, MA
American College of Sports Medicine
Indianapolis, Indiana

Lance C. Dalleck, PhD
Minnesota State University
Mankato, Minnesota

Shala E. Davis, PhD, FACSM
East Stroudsburg University of Pennsylvania
East Stroudsburg, Pennsylvania

Julie Desch, MD
New Day Wellness
Palo Alto, California

Julie J. Downing, PhD, FACSM
Central Oregon Community College
Bend, Oregon

Heidi Duskey, MA
Zest! Coaching
Medford, Massachusetts

Gregory B. Dwyer, PhD, FACSM
East Stroudsburg University of Pennsylvania
East Stroudsburg, Pennsylvania

Rebecca Ellis, PhD
Georgia State University
Atlanta, Georgia

Maren S. Fragala, MS
University of Connecticut
Storrs, Connecticut

Ellen G. Goldman, MEd
EnerG Coaching
Livingston, New Jersey

B. Sue Graves, EdD, FACSM
Florida Atlantic University
Davie, Florida

Billie Jo Hance, BS
Take Care Health Systems
Sunnyvale, California

Disa L. Hatfield, PhD
University of Rhode Island
Kingston, Rhode Island

Stanley Sai-chuen Hui, PhD, FACSM, FAAHPERD
The Chinese University of Hong Kong
Shatin, N.T., Hong Kong

Jeffrey M. Janot, PhD
University of Wisconsin–Eau Claire
Eau Claire, Wisconsin

Alexandra Jurasin, MS
Plus One Health Management, Inc.
New York, NY

William J. Kraemer, PhD, FACSM
University of Connecticut
Storrs, Connecticut

Len Kravitz, PhD
University of New Mexico
Albuquerque, New Mexico

Mike Motta, MS
Plus One Health Management, Inc.
New York, New York

Cynthia Pavell, MS
Fitness + Wellness
Springfield, Virginia

Neal I. Pire, MA, FACSM
InsPIRE Training Systems
Ridgewood, New Jersey

Kathleen Querner, MA
Sinclair Community College
Dayton, Ohio

Stacey Scarmack, MS
Retrofit_U
Lancaster, Ohio

Jan Schroeder, PhD
California State University Long Beach
Long Beach, California

Barry A. Spiering, PhD
Wyle Laboratories
Houston, Texas

Gwendolyn A. Thomas, MA
University of Connecticut
Storrs, Connecticut

Deon L. Thompson, PhD, FAACVPR
Georgia State University
Atlanta, Georgia

Walter R. Thompson, PhD, FACSM, FAACVPR
Georgia State University
Atlanta, Georgia

Jakob L. Vingren, PhD
University of North Texas
Denton, Texas

Jacquelyn Wesson, JD, RN
Wesson & Wesson, LLC
Warrior, Alabama

Christina Beaudoin, PhD
Grand Valley State University
Allendale, Michigan

Kimberly DeLeo, BS, PTA
Fitness Resource Associates, Inc.
Mattapoisett, Massachusetts

Julie J. Downing, PhD, FACSM
Central Oregon Community College
Bend, Oregon

Karen A. Edwards, MS
Auburn Regional Medical Center–Heart Care
Center
Auburn, Washington

JoAnn M. Eickhoff-Shemek, PhD, FACSM, FAWHP
University of South Florida
Tampa, Florida

Yuri Feito, MS, MPH
The University of Tennessee
Knoxville, Tennessee

Teresa C. Fitts, DPE
Westfield State College
Westfield, Massachusetts

Ellen Glickman, PhD, FACSM
Kent State University
Kent, Ohio

Dennis J. Guillot, MS
Nicholls State University
Thibodaux, Louisiana

Janet S. Hamilton, MA
Running Strong Professional Coaching
Stockbridge, Georgia

Laura Hanson, BA
Scripps Mercy Hospital
San Diego, California

Amanda Harris, BS
ACAC Fitness & Wellness Center
Keswick, Virginia

Marisa Hastie, MS
Lane Community College
Eugene, Oregon

Rachel Jarvis, MA
Edward Hospital
Naperville, Illinois

Thomas P. LaFontaine, PhD, FACSM, FAACVPR
PREVENT Consulting Services, LLC
Columbia, Missouri

Rebecca Langton, MA
Training Wheels Fitness Education Services LLC
Wake Forest, North Carolina

Matthew W. Parrott, PhD
HP Fitness, L.L.C.
Kansas City, Missouri

Neal Pire, MA, FACSM
Inspire Training Systems
Ridgewood, New Jersey

Matthew Saval, MS
Henry Ford Hospital
Detroit, Michigan

Thomas J. Spring, MS
William Beaumont Hospital
Royal Oak, Michigan

Christie L. Ward, MS
University of Rhode Island
Kingston, Rhode Island

Foreword

The personal training industry is positioned for tremendous growth. The public's interest in exercise and fitness has never been stronger. A survey commissioned by the National Coalition for Promoting Physical Activity and Health and the Centers for Disease Control and Prevention found that more than 30 million American adults are thinking about starting an exercise program. The obesity rates alone clearly indicate that our country needs us! This poses incredible opportunity for personal trainers in the United States. This interest is fueled by the demographic and aging trends our society is undergoing. Americans are now spending more money on their health and fitness including personal training, perhaps because boomers can now afford it and because it can help them stay healthy in a way that maximizes their available time.

According to the World Health Organization, by the year 2020, approximately 16% of our citizens will be over the age of 65. These trends, if our older population remains sedentary, will put an incredible strain on our society and on our medical system. As baby boomers age, it will drive the growth of the personal training industry. These individuals will embrace fitness to stay in shape physically and mentally, maintain their youth, and live longer. They are health conscious and disgruntled with the current medical system, have the money to afford our services, are noticing that their bodies are changing, and don't like the changes. They are taking their health into their own hands. They are a generation that is not going to just accept the aging process but instead will not go down without a fight.

The interest from this population will demand that a personal trainer fully understand the changes that a person experiences as he or she ages and what can be done to prevent, reverse, or manage these changes better. A trainer will need to learn how to design programs that focus on muscle strength, and integrate balance training, torso stabilization, and full body movements. Trainers will need to know which exercises and stretches will help counteract many of the postural deviations this population is experiencing. They will need to know how to explain Kegels, menopause, and osteoarthritis. Methods to manage weight gain, back pain, menopause, high cholesterol, deteriorating bone density, and joint aches will need to be addressed. This population will require programs that are effective and results-driven but yet, gentler on their bodies. Price will not be as great of a concern for this population. Fifty-year-olds used to be the poorest members of our society, but they are now the wealthiest. They have discretionary income and are willing to spend it on their health.

The opportunities in our industry are endless. Whether you want to focus on our aging population, the overweight/obese segment, kids fitness, sports-specific conditioning, pre/postnatal fitness, injury postrehabilitation or just general fitness, you can easily carve out a niche in your community. Personal Training is now considered a viable career rather than a part-time job until you get a "real" job. Reputable Personal Trainers are starting to get the respect we deserve—after all, aren't we making huge, significant differences in people's lives! For those who take the necessary steps to separate themselves apart from underqualified fitness trainers, a very prosperous, successful, and rewarding future awaits. We may not all become millionaires but we will be able to pay the mortgage, put our kids through college, and have some extra discretionary income to take vacations and maybe even hire a Personal Trainer for ourselves!

Overall, we should all be very excited. We have chosen a career that both is personally rewarding and should allow us each to make an income that can maintain a good standard of living. However, only trainers who clearly take their business seriously will reap the benefits.

Fortunately, you've taken a solid step by investing in this book. Since 1954 the American College of Sports Medicine (ACSM) has been the leading international organization in sports medicine and the exercise sciences. Now you can take advantage of their wealth of experience inside *ACSM's Resources for the Personal Trainer.*

In the pages that follow, the ACSM has orchestrated the collaboration of some of the best minds in the science of exercise physiology and the business of Personal Training. From initial client assessments to functional anatomy and biomechanics, this book combines academic insight with practical examples that have been tested in real-world personal training facilities. You will learn the well-established importance of goal setting to some cutting-edge concepts that involve lifestyle coaching and behavioral change. In addition to a wealth of practical and theoretic information integral to the success of any Personal Trainer, this manual will also provide you with critical business skills to enhance your revenues and income. The *ACSM's Resources for the Personal Trainer* is a comprehensive, how-to resource from a team of professionals who have taken great pains to provide you with their many years of experience, knowledge, successes, failures, and practical tools.

Read carefully and absorb as much as you can from the ideas and information captured in this text. A savvy Personal Trainer will capitalize on the competitive advantages that you will have at your fingertips inside *ACSM's Resources for the Personal Trainer.*

We wish you success and prosperity.

Alex and Sherri McMillan

Alex & Sherri McMillan, MSc, have been inspiring the world to adopt a fitness lifestyle for more than 30 years collectively and have received numerous industry awards including IDEA Fitness Directors of the Year, IDEA Personal Trainer of the Year, and CanFitPro Fitness Presenter of the Year. Their trainer studios, Northwest Personal Training, in Vancouver, Washington, and Portland, Oregon, were recently awarded the BBB Business of the Year award. As fitness trainers, fitness columnists, authors of five books and manuals, stars in various fitness DVDs, and international fitness presenters, they are spokespersons for Nike, Nautilus, Twist Conditioning, and PowerBar.

Preface

This third edition of *ACSM's Resources for the Personal Trainer* represents a significant revision of the successful first and second editions. Thanks to some very dedicated members of the ACSM Committee on Certification and Registry Boards (previously chaired by Dino Costanzo and now by Madeline Paternostro-Bayles) and staff of the ACSM (directed by Dick Cotton), the first edition was a compilation of edited select chapters of other ACSM resource books. They were effectively rewritten to make them applicable to the Personal Trainer. The second edition, while keeping constant the high standards established by the first edition, was a considerable revision written by the world's most respected scientists and practitioners. Many of them are pioneers in the personal training industry. This third edition of *ACSM's Resources for the Personal Trainer* carries on the tradition of excellence established by the first and second editions. One very important addition to the third edition is an entire section dedicated to behavior modification. The Personal Trainer should read, study, and perhaps get additional training in this most important area. Learning about human behavior modification could enhance the Personal Trainer's business exponentially in so many ways.

OVERVIEW

This third edition continues to recognize the Personal Trainer as a professional in the continuum of creating healthy lifestyles. It provides the Personal Trainer with all the tools and scientific evidence to bring to his or her clients safe and effective exercise programs. It also can be the basis for forming a true partnership with physicians and other referral networks. The book is divided into six distinctly different parts, ranging from an introduction to the profession of personal training (for the professional first entering the field) to how to run your own business. In between are chapters dedicated to exercise physiology, biomechanics, anatomy, behavior modification, and nutrition. Even the most experienced Personal Trainer will find the science and evidence-based approach to be perhaps a new way to incorporate knowledge transfer from the Personal Trainer to the client (making the personal training session more enjoyable for the client, who now knows why he or she is doing an exercise the proper way, which increases the compliance rate, making the Personal Trainer happier and perhaps even more wealthy). The middle chapters include establishing goals and objectives for clients and a "how to" manual for assessing strength, flexibility, and risk stratification. Other chapters have been dedicated to developing resistance, cardiorespiratory, and flexibility training programs.

Specific elements within this book that will appeal to the Personal Trainer include a list of objectives preceding each chapter. Numerous four-color tables, figures, and photographs will help the Personal Trainer understand the written material. In addition, the bibliography for each chapter is contained at the conclusion of each chapter so the reader does not have to turn to the back of the book for a reference.

ORGANIZATION

The chapters are divided into six parts designed for ease of navigation through the text. The behavior modification chapters were kept separate from the business of personal training and the more hard-core sciences. Using this approach, we believe that the text will be useful for every Personal Trainer. In addition, the current knowledge, skills, and abilities required for ACSM certification for Personal Trainers are included as an appendix for those preparing to sit for the examination. The six parts of the book include the following.

Part I: Introduction to the Field and Profession of Personal Training. Two introductory chapters are designed to introduce the new and aspiring Personal Trainer to the profession. The first chapter provides great insight into why the health and fitness professions are some of the fastest growing industries in the world and how the Personal Trainer can capitalize on this growth. The second chapter provides a career track for the Personal Trainer. Did you ever wonder why you had an interest in personal training and whether you were ever going to have a decent income? This chapter might help you answer those questions.

Part II: The Science of Personal Training. The four chapters in this part provide the scientific foundations for personal training. Every Personal Trainer, regardless of experience, will find these chapters helpful. For the Personal Trainer just starting out, these chapters introduce the scientific basis for exercise. For the advanced Personal Trainer, these chapters serve as a foundational resource for specific lifestyle modification programs. These four chapters include anatomy and kinesiology, applied biomechanics, exercise physiology, and nutrition.

Part III: Behavior Modification. The newest section of this book is dedicated to learning how and why people are either willing or unwilling to change their behavior. One of the most frustrating aspects of personal training is when a client refuses to change a deleterious habit or even "cheats" between training sessions. Chapters include the concept of "coaching"—a new way of looking at and creating your relationship with a client. After reading these chapters, you will forever change your approach to personal training.

Part IV: Initial Client Screening. This part of the book walks the Personal Trainer through a series of steps from the first client meeting through a comprehensive health-related physical fitness assessment. Capitalizing on the learning objectives of Part III, this section establishes a framework for developing client-centered goals and objectives. Though certainly not an exhaustive list of physical fitness assessments, Chapter 14 provides critical techniques to evaluate a client both in the field and in the laboratory. This section includes many tables and figures that will assist with placing clients into various fitness categories.

Part V: Developing the Exercise Program. The first chapter of this part introduces the concept of developing a client-centered exercise program. Based on the goals established by the client and the Personal Trainer, the next three chapters (resistance training, cardiorespiratory, and flexibility programs) are specific "how to" chapters. For example, a Personal Trainer who wants to develop a resistance training program can turn to Chapter 16 and learn "how to" develop a muscle group-specific program. There is an entire chapter dedicated to the proper sequencing of exercises within a given personal training session. New to this book is an entire chapter written for the Personal Trainer who encounters someone with special needs. As more people decide that exercise is a good thing, Personal Trainers will encounter these special populations. This chapter also discusses the scope of a Personal Trainer's knowledge, skills, and abilities when it comes to working with these "special populations."

Part VI: The Business of Personal Training. So, you have made the decision to start a business, which translates to "how do I make a profit in this business of personal training" (after all, we can only take altruism so far). These two chapters introduce the professional Personal Trainer to common business practices and provide information on how to avoid some of the common mistakes beginners typically make in the development of their practices. The last chapter deals specifically with legal issues. Written by a practicing attorney with years of experience litigating court cases, this chapter is last because it is somewhat of a warning to Personal Trainers. Take your responsibility seriously. Get the necessary training and experience. Stay out of court.

INSTRUCTOR RESOURCES

We understand the demand on an instructor's time, so to make the job easier, instructors will receive access to Resources upon adoption of the third edition of *ACSM's Resources for the Personal Trainer*. The Instructor's Resources are available online at http://thepoint.lww.com/ACSMpersonaltrainer and include the following:

➤ A test generator
➤ PowerPoint slides for every chapter
➤ An image bank that contains all of the figures and tables from the book
➤ Lesson plans to help in course preparation
➤ Full text online

In this constantly evolving profession and increasing need for the personal delivery of health-related services, a definitive resource must be revised constantly. The ACSM welcomes your comments and suggestions on future editions.

Dr. Walt Thompson

Acknowledgments

The editors sincerely thank the many volunteer contributors of this book and the previous editions. This was a major undertaking as we took the very best from the previous edition, added contemporary scientific evidence, and wrote a whole new section on behavior modification. The editors also thank the many reviewers who spent countless hours ensuring that the book represented the facts based on scientific evidence, as we know them today. In all, there were more than 50 editors, contributors, and reviewers—all of them volunteers. We thank the ACSM Committee on Certification and Registry Boards (formerly chaired by Dino Costanzo and now by Madeline Paternostro-Bayles), the national staff of the ACSM Certification Department (Dick Cotton, National Director of Certification, and Hope Wood, Assistant Director of Certification), the ACSM Publications Committee (chaired by Jeff Roitman) and former ACSM Assistant Executive Vice President D. Mark Robertson for having the faith in the editorial team to complete this project on time. Finally, the editors thank our good friends at Lippincott Williams & Wilkins, our publishing partners for this project. Specific thanks go out to our product manager, Andrea Klingler, who not only guided us through this process but also made many editorial suggestions making this book even better than it was before we submitted manuscript pages to her. We also thank photographer Mark Lozier for his patience and understanding during the photo shoot and acquisitions editor Emily Lupash for her constant and unwavering encouragement. Finally, this book is dedicated to the professional Personal Trainer. We remain convinced that the public health is better off today than yesterday and will be even better tomorrow because of your dedication.

Walt Thompson
Barbara Bushman
Julie Desch
Len Kravitz

Table of Contents

PART I: INTRODUCTION TO THE FIELD AND PROFESSION OF PERSONAL TRAINING

PART II: THE SCIENCE OF PERSONAL TRAINING

PART III: BEHAVIOR MODIFICATION

PART IV: INITIAL CLIENT SCREENING

PART V: DEVELOPING THE EXERCISE PROGRAM

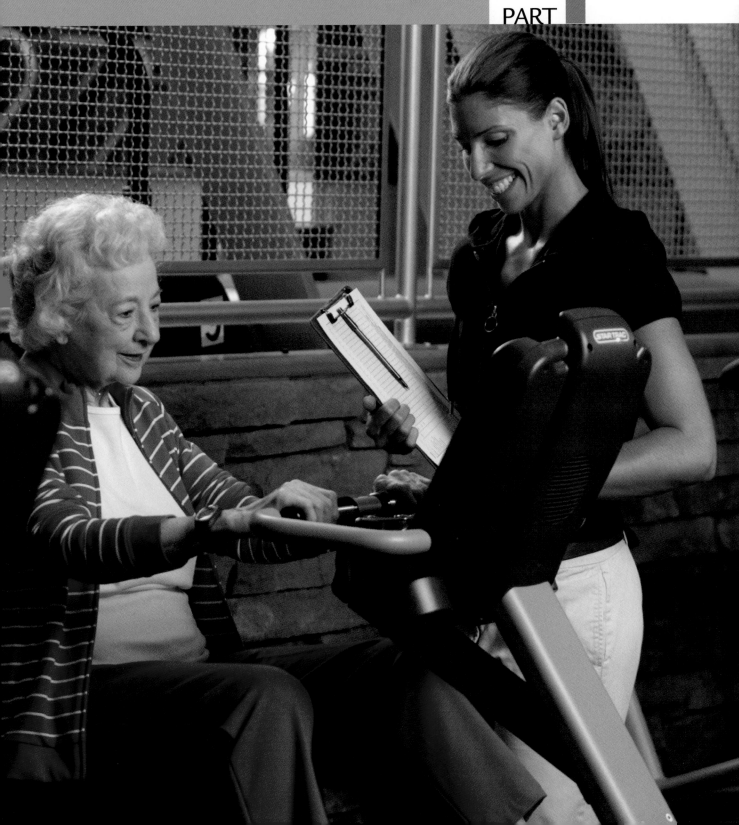

Introduction to the Field and Profession of Personal Training

PART I

CHAPTER 1

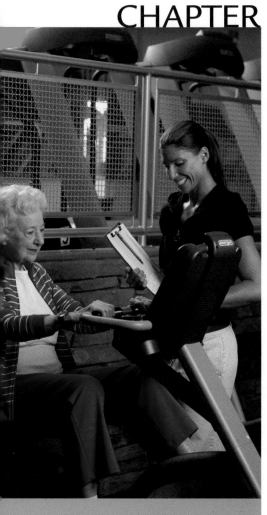

Introduction to Personal Training

OBJECTIVES

- Describe the current state of the fitness industry as it specifically applies to personal training
- Identify professional career environments and options for Personal Trainers
- Identify future trends that will affect the fitness industry and personal training

Personal Training (practiced by one referred to in this book as the "Personal Trainer" but often described as a "fitness trainer," "personal fitness trainer," "fitness professional," or "exercise professional") is emerging as one of the fastest growing professions in the United States.

According to the U.S. Department of Labor, Bureau of Labor Statistics, the job outlook for this profession is projected to "grow much faster than the average" for all occupations between 2006 and 2016, which is further defined as an increase of 27% during this time period (5). The expected increase in fitness worker job opportunities is primarily due to more people (including the many baby boomers) spending time and money on fitness, as well as an increasing number of businesses recognizing the health and fitness benefits that such programs provide for their employees (5).

> *According to the U.S. Department of Labor, Bureau of Labor Statistics, the job outlook for this profession is projected to "grow much faster than the average" for all occupations between 2006 and 2016.*

Baby boomers (approximately 78 million Americans born from 1946 to 1964) are the first generation in the United States that grew up exercising and now they are reaching retirement age; they have the time, money, and desire to begin or continue exercising in their 70s and beyond (14). The overall life expectancy at birth in the United States has increased to an average age of 78.14 years: men at 75.29 years and women at 81.13 years (8). With the U.S. population estimated to be 303,824,646 as of July 2008, there are many people who value health and fitness and will require the services of Personal Trainers (8).

Employment opportunities for Personal Trainers are available in more diverse settings than ever before and include (but are not limited to) the following:

- Commercial (for-profit) fitness centers
- Community (not-for-profit) fitness centers
- Corporate fitness/wellness centers
- University wellness/adult fitness centers
- Owner/operator (self-employed) studios, fitness centers, and in-home businesses
- Medical fitness centers (MFCs)
- Municipal/city recreation/public parks/family centers
- Governmental/military fitness centers
- Activity centers/retirement centers/assisted living communities for older adults
- Worksite health promotion (WHP) programs

Each of these employment settings is reviewed in more detail later in this chapter. Indeed, these opportunities and the diversity of work settings are predicted to increase further as the population continues to both grow and age as well as transition further to a more sedentary (i.e., physically inactive) lifestyle. It appears then that now is the best time to commit to the profession of personal training. There may be no other profession better placed to enhance the quality of life of the growing, aging, and increasingly sedentary population now and in the foreseeable future.

THE FITNESS INDUSTRY—AN OVERVIEW OF THE LANDSCAPE

Interestingly, although the population may be larger and more physically inactive than ever, the health club industry has never been in better "shape." Consider the following facts for the United States from the International Health, Racquet and Sportsclub Association (IHRSA), a trade association serving the health and fitness club industry (12):

29,636	Number of U.S. health clubs
41.5 million	Number of U.S. health club members
$18.5 billion	Total U.S. fitness industry revenues for 2007
266,000	Number of U.S. full-time fitness employees
1.0 million	Number of U.S. part-time fitness employees

TABLE 1.1	PERCENT OF PHYSICAL ACTIVITY LEVELS FOR AMERICANS: 2007		
Group	Recommended	Insufficient	Inactive
Overall	48.8	37.7	13.5
Female	47.1	38.7	14.2
Male	50.7	36.7	12.6

Adapted from Centers for Disease Control and Prevention Website [Internet]. U.S. physical activity statistics, 2007. Atlanta (GA): Centers for Disease Control and Prevention; [cited 2008 Nov 26]. Available from: http://apps.nccd.cdc.gov/PASurveillance/StateSumResultV.asp

Although these numbers may appear impressive, only 13.6% of the population are currently members of health or fitness clubs. In addition, the majority of Americans perform inadequate amounts of physical activity and exercise. According to the Centers for Disease Control and Prevention in 2007 (Table 1.1), 51.2% of Americans are either insufficiently active or totally inactive, with levels of activity decreasing with age (7). Therefore, a large proportion of the population could benefit from involvement in some type of regular physical activity as part of a healthy lifestyle, whether as a member of a health club or on their own. Personal Trainers, then, are well positioned to influence public health in this regard. First, as the health club industry continues to grow, so too will the demand for highly qualified and certified fitness professionals to serve the needs of their members. Even now, competent Personal Trainers are in high demand. Second, most people are not health club members and most likely will never become health club members. These individuals may not feel comfortable exercising in public, or perhaps a health club is not conveniently located near their home or place of work. Fortunately, these individuals can benefit just as much by in-home personal training, which is another growing segment of the Personal Trainer job market.

Despite the growth of the fitness industry and emerging opportunities for physical fitness, high inactivity rates among Americans have not really changed in the past 20 years.

Despite the growth of the fitness industry and emerging opportunities for physical fitness, high inactivity rates among Americans have not really changed in the past 20 years. Public schools continue to cut back or are eliminating physical education. In fact, Illinois is the only state that currently requires physical education every day from kindergarten through high school according to the National Association for Sport and Physical Education (13).

Healthcare costs are rising exponentially as the medical field continues to focus more on treatment than on prevention. Food portion sizes in restaurants are increasing. In 2007, only one state (Colorado) had obesity prevalence less than 20% (Fig. 1.1). Thirty states had obesity prevalence

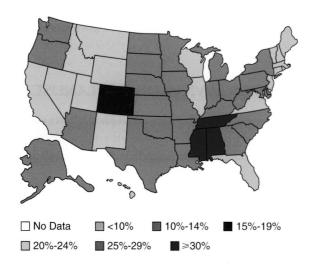

FIGURE 1.1. Prevalence of obesity in percentage (body mass index ≥ 30) in U.S. adults in 2007. The data shown in these maps were collected through the Centers for Disease Control and Prevention's (CDC's) Behavioral Risk Factor Surveillance System (BRFSS). Each year, state health departments use standard procedures to collect data through a series of monthly telephone interviews with U.S. adults. Prevalence estimates generated for the maps may vary slightly from those generated for the states by the BRFSS as slightly different analytic methods are used. From the CDC Web site [Internet]. Atlanta (GA): CDC, U.S. obesity trends 1985–2007; [cited 2008 Nov 26]. Available from: http://www.cdc.gov/nccdphp/dnpa/obesity/trend/maps

☐ No Data   ▨ <10%   ▨ 10%-14%   ■ 15%-19%
▨ 20%-24%   ▨ 25%-29%   ■ ≥30%

between 25% and 29% of the population, and three of these states had obesity prevalence greater than 30% (Alabama 30.3%, Mississippi 32.0%, and Tennessee 30.1%). When one includes overweight in addition to obesity, an astonishing 66% of American adults and 32.1% of children are overweight or obese (6). With these conditions, the time is right for highly qualified Personal Trainers (with the help of physicians) to lead the charge toward a healthier nation.

Exercise is Medicine™

On November 5, 2007, the American College of Sports Medicine (ACSM) in partnership with the American Medical Association launched Exercise is Medicine™, a program designed to encourage America's patients to incorporate physical activity and exercise into their daily routine. Exercise is Medicine™ encourages doctors to assess and review every patient's physical activity program at every visit. For those patients not already exercising, the physician is asked to prescribe exercise to their patients and to record physical activity as a vital sign during patient visits.

Exercise is Medicine™ has a Web site (www.exerciseismedicine.org) that is very user-friendly and that provides many helpful resources for physicians, health and fitness professionals, as well as the general public (Fig. 1.2). It encourages the public to do the following: Exercise and don't think of it as only for the spandex-wearing, muscle-bound crowd. Physical activity is for everyone, and not just for the sake of looking better in your favorite pair of jeans. Just 30 minutes of exercise per day can help prevent and treat numerous chronic conditions such as high blood pressure, diabetes, and joint pain. Talk with your doctor about the best exercise plan for you, and make physical activity part of your life and healthcare plan (3).

A recent survey conducted of the public by ACSM found that nearly two thirds of patients (65%) would be more interested in exercising to stay healthy if advised by their doctors and given additional resources (3). Four out of 10 physicians (41%) talk to their patients about the importance of exercise, but don't always offer suggestions on the best ways to be physically active. Patients (25%) look to their doctor first for advice on exercise and physical activity (3). It is rather uncommon for a physician to refer patients directly to Personal Trainers, although that trend is changing with the Exercise is Medicine™ initiative. Typically they simply encourage exercise by walking or do not address exercise at all. However, physicians often refer patients with known disease or a recent cardiac/pulmonary event to cardiac/pulmonary rehabilitation. For patients without established disease, many physicians could refer patients to Personal Trainers for exercise guidance if the proper referral mechanism was established.

American Fitness Index™

Another new public health initiative is the ACSM American Fitness Index™ (AFI). The AFI is a program to help cities understand how the health of their residents and community assets that support active, healthy lifestyles compares to that of other cities nationwide. The overall goal of the AFI program

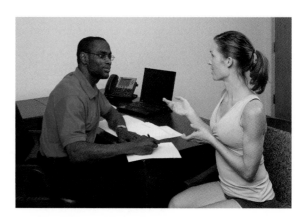

FIGURE 1.2. A trainer and a client doing an initial client consultation.

is to improve the health, fitness, and quality of life of the nation through promoting physical activity. The AFI is using three primary means to achieve their task: (a) collecting and disseminating city health data, (b) providing resources, and (c) assisting communities to connect with health promotion partners.

> *The American Fitness Index™ is a program to help cities understand how the health of their residents and community assets that support active, healthy lifestyles compares to that of other cities nationwide.*

The AFI reflects a composite of community indicators for preventive health behaviors, levels of chronic disease conditions, access to healthcare, and community supports and policies for physical activity. In addition, demographic and economic diversity and levels of violent crime are shown for each metropolitan area. Cities with the highest scores are considered to have high *community* fitness, a concept akin to an individual having high *personal* fitness.

Sixteen large metropolitan areas were included in this pilot phase of the AFI program. San Francisco, California, ranked first in the pilot study with 403 points, closely followed by Seattle, Washington, with 401 points, and Boston, Massachusetts, rounded out the top three with 370 points. While Houston, Texas, and Los Angeles, California, were low at 209 and 208 points respectively, Detroit, Michigan, had by far the lowest score at 149 points clearly revealing some much-needed improvements in that city and in others.

The results revealed the 16 metropolitan areas were diverse in their community fitness levels. Cities that ranked near the top of the index have much strength that supports healthy living and few challenges that hinder healthy choices. The opposite was found for cities near the bottom of the AFI. The cities are recognized for their strengths and encouraged to consider focusing future efforts on improving items listed as challenges for healthy, active living. It is anticipated that the index will be expanded to include the 50 largest metropolitan cities in the United States. For further information, see www.americanfitnessindex.org (4).

THE PROFESSION OF PERSONAL TRAINING

As mentioned previously, the profession of personal training is rapidly evolving and employment opportunities are wide ranging and will continue to increase. But what does a Personal Trainer do? Depending on the work setting, Personal Trainers may perform any or all of the following tasks (a noninclusive list):

➤ Screen and interview potential clients to determine their readiness for exercise and physical activity. This may involve communicating with the client's healthcare team (especially for clients with special needs): physicians, nurse practitioners, registered dieticians, physical therapists, occupational therapists, and others.

➤ Perform fitness tests or assessments (as appropriate) on clients to determine their current level of fitness.

➤ Help clients set realistic goals, modify goals as needed, and provide motivation for adherence to the program.

➤ Develop exercise regimens and programs (often referred to as an "exercise prescription") for clients to follow and modify programs as necessary, based on progression and goals.

➤ Demonstrate and instruct specific techniques to clients for the safe and effective performance of various exercise movements.

➤ Correct incorrect or dangerous exercise techniques or training programs.

➤ Supervise or "spot" (physically assisting your client with an exercise that usually involves free weights or dumbbells to minimize risk of injury) clients when they are performing exercise movements.

➤ Maintain records of clients' progress or lack thereof with respect to the exercise prescription.

➤ Be a knowledgeable resource to accurately answer clients' health and fitness questions. Educate clients about health and fitness with the ultimate goal to have clients become independent exercisers (provided they have approval from their physician to do so).

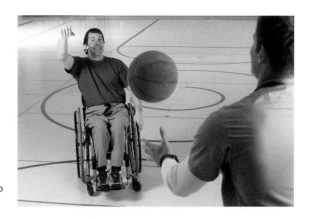

FIGURE 1.3. A trainer working with a client who has a physical disability.

Other responsibilities not directly involving a client may be assigned or performed as needed. These usually include administrative paperwork, maintenance of equipment, and cleaning of equipment and facilities as required.

> *Many Personal Trainers also obtain additional instruction or specialty certifications in areas such as kickboxing, cancer, yoga, aquatic exercise, wellness coaching, studio cycling, and disabilities.*

Many Personal Trainers also obtain additional instruction or specialty certifications in areas such as kickboxing, cancer, yoga, aquatic exercise, wellness coaching, studio cycling, and disabilities (Fig. 1.3). These specialties should not be confused with "core" or primary certifications, such as the ACSM Certified Personal Trainer. Additional specialty certifications make you more valuable and also allow you to have a wider variety of responsibilities, such as teaching group exercise classes. The ACSM has recently added two new specialty certifications.

1. *Disability Specialty Certification.* This is a joint certification between the ACSM and the National Center on Physical Activity and Disabilities (NCPAD). It is titled the ACSM/NCPAD Certified Inclusive Fitness Trainer (CIFT). A CIFT is a fitness professional involved in developing and implementing an individualized exercise program for a person who may have a physical, sensory, or cognitive disability, who is healthy or has medical clearance to perform independent physical activity.

   The minimum requirements for someone to take the CIFT examination are:
   - Any current ACSM Certification or current National Commission for Certifying Agencies (NCCA)-accredited, health/fitness-related certifications **and**
   - Current Adult CPR (with practical skills component) and AED Certification.

2. *Cancer Specialty Certification.* This certification is an industry-first for professionals working in the area of health and fitness, specifically to work with individuals who have been affected by cancer. This specialty certification was developed by a group of subject-matter experts (SMEs) representing the ACSM and the American Cancer Society. More than 10 million cancer survivors are alive today, and because living a healthy, active lifestyle is so important for these individuals, ACSM professionals have the potential to make a significant contribution by earning the specialty certification to safely and effectively work with people who have been affected by cancer.

   The minimum requirements to take the Cancer Specialty examination are as follows:
   - Any current ACSM or current NCCA-accredited certification **and**
   - Certification in adult CPR & AED **and**
   - Bachelor's degree (in any field) **and**
   - 500 hours of experience training older adults or individuals with chronic conditions **or** 10,000 hours of experience training older adults or individuals with chronic conditions.

Even though more health clubs than ever before are requiring certifications for current and future employees, some health clubs still hire Personal Trainers without certifications. This does not

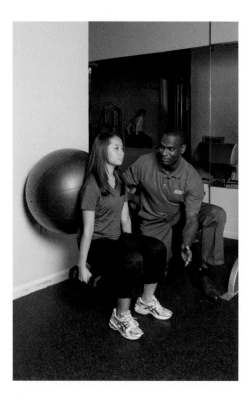

FIGURE 1.4. A trainer spotting a squat exercise of a client who is on a bosu ball (with light dumbbells in each hand).

mean that you don't need a certification! You owe it to yourself as a true professional, as well as to the clients you serve, to document your competence, and certification is the best way to accomplish this objective. Also, the health club industry is unique in that there are a large number of organizations that offer certifications in this field, and even among the health clubs that do require certifications, there is no agreement on which ones are universally accepted. One of your first tasks in pursuing a career in personal training will be to determine which certification(s) best suits your personal and professional goals.

The kinds of fitness facilities are diverse, with the most numerous being multipurpose commercial for-profit clubs, followed by community, corporate, and MFCs. Although there are many core similarities between facilities, there is also great variety in size, structure, target markets, program offerings, amenities, membership fees, contracts, staffing, and equipment. This variety is necessary to attract and serve many different populations with many different interests (Fig. 1.4).

With the member retention rate varying greatly across the industry, most clubs and centers must continually recruit new members. Because many experts agree that the majority of a club's membership base will come from within a 10- to 15-minute drive time from home to the facility, clubs that are located close to one another are typically competing for the same members. This means that Personal Trainers are vying for the same clients as well. However, Personal Trainers, just like clubs, can differentiate themselves from the competition in a number of ways, such as focusing on a specific clientele (e.g., women, children, seniors, athletes), developing expertise in a given area, offering small-group training in addition to individual sessions, offering a different price point, and using multiple locations.

The Definition of a Personal Trainer

The ACSM scope of practice for the ACSM Certified Personal Trainer is:

The ACSM Certified Personal Trainer is a fitness professional who develops and implements an individualized approach to exercise leadership in healthy populations and/or those individuals with medical clearance to exercise.

Using a variety of teaching techniques, the ACSM Certified Personal Trainer is proficient in:

➤ leading and demonstrating safe and effective methods of exercise by applying the fundamental principles of exercise science,
➤ writing appropriate exercise recommendations,
➤ leading and demonstrating safe and effective methods of exercise, and
➤ motivating individuals to begin and to continue with their healthy behaviors.

As mentioned previously, the health and fitness industry is unique in that it has a wide variety of certifications available to the potential fitness professional. Organizations that offer certifications are commercial (for-profit) as well as nonprofit. Some have services and benefits that facilitate professional development, such as publications and conferences. Before committing to a specific certification, study each one for its relevance to your situation. Ask fellow students (if applicable) or coworkers or potential employers, or talk to some professional Personal Trainers in the area for specific recommendations.

Some certification organizations recognize other certifications for the purposes of continuing education. Most legitimate certifications will require their respective certified professionals to pursue educational opportunities, commonly referred to as *continuing education units* (CEUs) or *continuing education credits* (CECs). These CEUs/CECs are required in an ongoing fashion for a certified professional to maintain his or her certification status and as one way to maintain professional competence. Some certifications are complementary to others, and again, multiple certifications could make you more valuable to a potential employer. Currently ACSM Certified Personal Trainers need to obtain 45 CEUs every 3 years. There is a nominal administrative fee associated with recertification.

> **ACSM Certified Personal Trainers need to obtain 45 CEUs every 3 years. There is a nominal administrative fee associated with recertification.**

Becoming a Personal Trainer

Because of the large number of certification organizations, the prerequisites and eligibility requirements for becoming a Personal Trainer vary widely. Some are stand-alone certifications, whereas others, such as those offered by ACSM, are part of a progressive professional development pathway in which the scope of practice increases in both depth and scope as the prerequisites and eligibility requirements increase. For example, entry into the ACSM professional development pathway for emerging professionals has minimal requirements for the ACSM Certified Personal Trainer:

➤ a high school diploma or equivalent **and**
➤ 18 years of age **and**
➤ current adult CPR certification that has a practical skills examination component (such as the American Heart Association [AHA] or the American Red Cross).

The ACSM Certified Health Fitness Specialist (formerly known as the ACSM Certified Health/Fitness Instructor®) requires minimally:

➤ an associate's degree or a bachelor's degree in a health-related field from a regionally accredited college or university (one is eligible to sit for the examination if the candidate is in the last term or semester of his or her degree program) **and**
➤ current Adult CPR certification that has a practical skills examination component (such as the AHA or the American Red Cross).

The ACSM Certified Clinical Exercise Specialist (formerly known as ACSM Certified Exercise Specialist®) requires minimally:

➤ a bachelor's degree in an allied health field from a regionally accredited college or university (one is eligible to sit for the examination if the candidate is in the last term of his or her degree program) **and**

➤ minimum of 600 hours of practical experience in a clinical exercise program **and**

➤ current certification as a Basic Life Support Provider or CPR for the Professional Rescuer (available through the AHA or the American Red Cross).

Finally, an ACSM Registered Clinical Exercise Physiologist minimally requires:

➤ a master's degree from a college or university in exercise science, movement science, exercise physiology, or kinesiology **and**

➤ current certification as a Basic Life Support Provider or CPR for the Professional Rescuer **and**

➤ one of the following: ACSM Certified Clinical Exercise Specialist certification (current or expired) or 600 hours of clinical experience.

It is important that you consider not only what you want to do now but in the next few years as well, as you determine your educational preparation and what certification(s) you may need to realize your career goals. Your background and interests will combine in determining how fast and by what process you can begin your career. One should ensure that the certifying agency is accredited by the NCCA. The NCCA is the accreditation body of the National Organization for Competency Assurance. The NCCA is a widely recognized, independent, nongovernmental agency that accredits professional certifications in a variety of professions. The NCCA comprehensively reviews the certification organization's procedures, protocols, and operations and determines if the certification properly discriminates between those who are qualified and those who are not qualified to be awarded the respective credential.

The Backgrounds of Personal Trainers

The Personal Fitness Trainer profession has evolved to the point where there is now a mandatory or standardized academic preparation model that exists for physicians, nurses, or other allied healthcare professionals. The Committee on Accreditation for the Exercise Sciences (CoAES) was established in April 2004 under the auspices of the Commission on Accreditation of Allied Health Education Programs (CAAHEP). The primary role of the CoAES is to establish standards and guidelines for academic programs that facilitate the preparation of students seeking employment in the health, fitness, and exercise industry. The secondary role of the CoAES is to establish and implement a process of self-study, review, and recommendation for all programs seeking CAAHEP accreditation.

> *The Committee on Accreditation for the Exercise Sciences (CoAES) was established in April 2004 under the auspices of the Commission on Accreditation of Allied Health Education Programs (CAAHEP).*

Programmatic accreditation through the CAAHEP is specifically intended for exercise science or related departments (physical education, kinesiology, etc.) with a professional preparation tract designed for students seeking employment opportunities in the health, fitness, and exercise industry.

The CAAHEP is the largest programmatic accreditor in the health sciences field and it reviews and accredits more than 2,000 educational programs in 20 health science occupations such as Personal Fitness Trainer. See www.coaes.org and www.caahep.org for more information or to find a CAAHEP-accredited academic institution in your state.

It is important to both obtain an exercise science degree from a CAAHEP-accredited academic program and possess a certification from a NCCA-accredited certifying agency and, because of the many different types of certifications that exist, the background of today's Personal Trainer varies significantly with respect to educational preparation and work-related experience. Some individuals commit to the profession early and pursue an appropriate course of study in college. Many of these individuals actually begin working part-time at a local health club or at the university student recreation center, gaining valuable "hands-on" practical experience to complement their studies. Other Personal Trainers enter the profession later in life as a new career, or as a second career on a part-time basis while maintaining their primary career pursuit (Fig. 1.5). Ideally, the Personal Trainer will

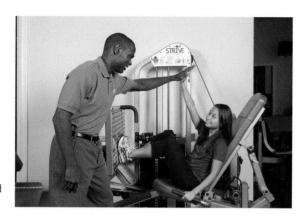

FIGURE 1.5. A trainer and a client have reached a goal.

have a good combination of education, work-related experience, and even first-person perspective experiences as either an athlete or a former client.

EDUCATIONAL BACKGROUND

As the profession of personal training continues to evolve and grow, more and more educational opportunities become available. Many certification organizations offer workshops and online examination preparation opportunities. From a formal academic training perspective, there are certificate, associate's, bachelor's, master's, and doctoral degree programs available for fitness professionals. Typically, certificate programs (both in-person and online) range from 1 year to 18 months in duration. Associate degree programs range in length from 18 months to 2 years. Bachelor's degree programs are usually 4 years in duration. Master's degree programs are typically 18 months to 2 years beyond a bachelor's degree. Finally, a doctoral degree program is usually 3 years beyond a master's degree. Also, internships, practicums, or student cooperative work experiences (typically unpaid opportunities to work under the direct supervision of an experienced fitness professional) may or may not be part of these different types of programs. Common names for these academic programs include exercise science, exercise physiology, physical education, kinesiology, sport science, personal trainer, fitness specialist, and others. Currently, the CAAHEP accredits academic programs for Personal Fitness Trainer (certificate and associate degrees), Exercise Science (bachelor's degree), and both Clinical Exercise Physiology and Applied Exercise Physiology graduate programs.

> *The CAAHEP accredits academic programs for Personal Fitness Trainer (certificate and associate degrees), Exercise Science (bachelor's degree), and both Clinical Exercise Physiology and Applied Exercise Physiology graduate programs.*

Please note that increasingly more health clubs actually require their Personal Trainers to have degrees, and long-term employment advancement may require a degree at some health clubs. Also, most fitness directors, those individuals who have management/supervisory responsibilities over the floor staff (Personal Trainers), usually have degrees.

WORK-RELATED BACKGROUND

It is possible for Personal Trainers to obtain employment without a related degree, especially if they have one or more certifications and some prior industry-related work experience. For many individuals who want a career change, pursuing a second degree or even a first degree later in life simply is not possible. Some health clubs have formal training paths and processes for their employees that may include assigning a more experienced Personal Trainer as a mentor or scheduling periodic staff training sessions, sometimes referred to as "in-services." Some health clubs may even pay for continuing education opportunities for their staff as one benefit of employment. If not, look for an experienced Personal Trainer either at your facility or elsewhere with an exemplary reputation who would consider taking on an apprentice. Many certification organizations have educational opportunities, such as workshops, that can also provide a good review of the various areas of content, especially as they relate to preparing for a certification examination. It is always advisable for all professionals working in this environment to seek a college degree whenever possible.

EXPERIENTIAL BACKGROUND

Some Personal Trainers were once college, professional, or elite athletes. Like those who are changing careers, some may not have a related academic degree, and some no college degree at all. However, their passion for a particular sport or a love of exercise in general usually motivates them sufficiently to fill in any knowledge gaps they may have as they begin their personal training career. Again, if you are one of these individuals, commit to the profession by obtaining one or more certifications from reputable organizations such as the ACSM, as well as obtaining relevant, work-related experience under the supervision of a proven, experienced (preferably degree holder) Personal Trainer.

Another type of experiential background from a first-person perspective is as a former client. These individuals usually are people who had such a significant positive or transformational experience that their lives were changed for the better. Think of an obese patient who loses hundreds of pounds and now thinks of himself or herself as healthy, or the previously sedentary individual who now competes in marathons regularly. Much like the professional athlete, these individuals feel strongly about reproducing their positive experience for others but may not have a college degree. Similarly, by being proactive from a self-study perspective, obtaining one or more certifications and combining these with work-related experience, these individuals can become competent professional Personal Trainers over time.

Regardless of your background, starting down the career path as a Personal Trainer doesn't have to be complicated. To get started, determine from where you are starting, and then where you want to be professionally in 1, 2, or 5 years. Ask yourself the following questions:

➤ Do I have a college degree related to the field and is it from a CAAHEP-accredited academic institution?
➤ If not, is it feasible for me to go back to obtain a certificate or degree on either a part-time or full-time basis?
➤ Was I ever a client of a Personal Trainer, and did I have a positive experience in achieving my goals?
➤ Do I have experience as a college, professional, or elite athlete who provides me with some first-person experiences?
➤ Which certifications and certifying agency are appropriate for me to pursue now and in the future? The certifying agency (such as ACSM) should be well-respected, provide peer-reviewed materials, and be NCCA-accredited.
➤ Which certifications have study materials and/or workshops to help me accumulate a core body of knowledge?
➤ Where can I begin obtaining the necessary skills, either by observing a more experienced Personal Trainer or by volunteering at a local health club?
➤ Which certifying organizations and, specifically, which level of certification do potential employers in my city expect to see when hiring Personal Trainers for their clubs?

PROFESSIONAL WORK ENVIRONMENTS

For-Profit

Commercial clubs dominate the fitness landscape and include independents, chains, licensed gyms, and franchises. Many opportunities for gainful employment exist within the commercial club industry. Most clubs advertise employment opportunities locally or regionally, whereas some also post them

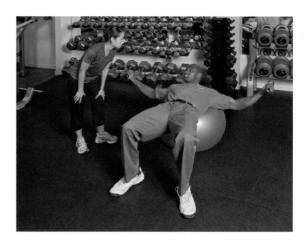

FIGURE 1.6. A trainer demonstrating a fly motion using a stability ball as a bench press.

> *Commercial clubs dominate the fitness landscape and include independents, chains, licensed gyms, and franchises.*

on their corporate Web sites. It is wise to thoroughly investigate a company's policies concerning compensation, benefits, policies, and opportunities for advancement before accepting a position.

Licensed gyms and franchises have been a popular choice for a new club (Fig. 1.6). The benefits of choosing a franchise include brand recognition, access to proven operational systems, logo usage, marketing templates, in-depth training, and ongoing support. Franchisers then retain the right to dictate most aspects of the facility, including colors, layout, décor, equipment, programs, and product sales. Initial fees for fitness franchises can range from $10,000 to more than $100,000, and equipment may or may not be included in the cost. There is also a monthly franchising fee, which is either a set amount or a percentage of gross revenue (typically about 5%). Licensed gyms operate on a much simpler model. A fee is paid to use (license) the name and logo. Licensees typically have much more flexibility in how they operate the facility than do franchisees, but they also do not receive as much operational support.

Not-for-Profit

Not-for-profit (or nonprofit) organizations with fitness centers make up a large proportion of the total market. According to the IHRSA Fair Competition Annual Report (11), approximately 38%

> *Approximately 38% of the total membership in health clubs is from the nonprofit (tax-exempt) sector.*

of the total membership in health clubs is from the nonprofit (tax-exempt) sector. Some examples of the larger nonprofit organizations in which fitness professionals can find relevant employment include the Young Men's Christian Association (YMCA), Jewish Community Centers (JCC), hospital-based clubs, municipal and military fitness facilities, as well as college/university recreation centers.

Personal Trainers may find that some nonprofits may not have rates of pay comparable with those of their for-profit counterparts but at the same time may provide better benefits. Nonprofit work (regardless of the industry) creates a strong sense of mission throughout the organization and carries a significant commitment to service with respect to their specific members or constituents. Nonprofit fitness centers fill a significant role in the fitness professional job market, and it is ultimately up to the individual to determine the most appropriate place of employment for his or her personal and professional goals.

Medical Fitness Centers

The growing relationship between the fitness industry and the healthcare field is evidenced by the steady growth of MFCs and the establishment of the Medical Fitness Association. The numbers of MFCs and the number of members they serve have seen a compounded annual growth rate of 15% since 1985. Conservative projections (assuming a growth rate of 7.5%) estimate more than 3 million members and 1150 MFCs by the year 2010. While it is true that there are a number of extremely large MFCs, approximately 30%–50% of the current 715 centers are less than 10,000–20,000 square feet, with a heavy concentration of all centers in the Southeast and upper Midwest sections of the United States. Although they offer a number of clinical and wellness services not typically found in traditional clubs, personal training tops the list of reported nonmembership fee services, with 78% of centers offering such a program. In addition, 80% report being owned by a hospital or health system, and 67% report holding not-for-profit status (11).

> *The growing relationship between the fitness industry and the healthcare field is evidenced by the steady growth of medical fitness centers and the establishment of the Medical Fitness Association.*

A central mission of many MFCs is integration of services for both the "sick" and the "healthy." It is not uncommon for patients in cardiovascular rehabilitation or physical therapy programs to exercise next to healthy community members. Using the same space and equipment saves on overhead, space, and staffing needs. While there currently are not any specific guidelines for hiring Personal Trainers with specific degrees or certifications in these facilities, the focus on transitional programs may require a Personal Trainer to have higher qualifications than usual.

Corporate

> **Worksite health promotion** *can be defined as "a combination of educational, organizational, and environmental activities and programs designed to motivate and support healthy lifestyles among a company's employees and their families" (9).*

More than 50% of business profits are spent annually on employees' and dependents' healthcare (10). *Worksite health promotion* can be defined as "a combination of educational, organizational, and environmental activities and programs designed to motivate and support healthy lifestyles among a company's employees and their families" (9). The three chief goals of WHP programs are to:

➤ Assess health risks
➤ Reduce those health risk factors that can be reduced
➤ Promote socially and environmentally healthy lifestyles.

However, only about 55% of companies have a comprehensive WHP program. The National Employee Service and Recreation Association estimates that there are more than 50,000 organizations with on-site physical fitness programs in the United States and nearly 1,000 employing full-time program directors (9).

The kinds of fitness-specific offerings vary greatly in WHP programs, ranging from pedometer-based walking programs to group exercise classes to fully equipped health clubs. One of the primary determinants of facility and program size is the number of employees. Companies with more than 1,000 employees working in a central location (building or campus) are much more likely to offer traditional fitness facilities, because they have the financial means to do so and it makes economic sense. Smaller companies with a smaller employee base are much less likely to offer a WHP, especially one that includes fitness facilities.

Many corporate fitness programs are outsourced to companies that specialize in facility and program management. This makes it somewhat easier for the corporation because it can rely on someone else's expertise instead of having to develop it from within. Some choose to avoid development and management altogether by setting up a corporate account with an existing local fitness facility. A reduced membership fee is negotiated, and the company reimburses employees a portion or all of the fees. It is common, though, for the company to dictate that an employee must visit the facility a certain number of times per month to qualify for reimbursement.

Corporate fitness opportunities exist for Personal Trainers within both large and smaller companies. For larger companies, the typical route is to work as a traditional employee or independent contractor in the fitness center. For smaller companies, a more entrepreneurial approach is usually taken. Personal Trainers will typically need to approach the management about offering on-site services to the employees with the employer absorbing some of the cost. Because employers are often very cost-conscious and are typically unsure about investing in preventive programs, Personal Trainers will need to educate them about the benefits of their services to the health and well-being of their employees. Reporting client results, such as weight loss, reductions in blood pressure, and other health factors, also has a positive impact on their thinking and decision making. Because individual sessions are the most expensive option, small-group training sessions are potentially more appealing to the employer.

ACSM'S ROLE AND THE EDUCATIONAL CONTINUUM

The ACSM is a professional member association composed of a multidisciplinary mix of more than 20,000 exercise science researchers, educators, and medical practitioners. More specifically, member categories include physicians, nurses, athletic trainers, exercise physiologists, dietitians, and physical therapists, as well as many other allied healthcare professionals with an interest in sports medicine and the exercise sciences. The mission statement for ACSM is:

> *ACSM promotes and integrates scientific research, education and practical applications of sports medicine and exercise science to maintain and enhance physical performance, fitness, health, and quality of life.*

ACSM was founded in 1954, was the first professional organization to begin offering health and fitness certifications (in 1975), and continues to deliver the most respected, NCCA-accredited certifications within the health and fitness industry. Because of the multidisciplinary nature and diversity of its members, ACSM has evolved into the unique position of an industry leader for creating evidence-based best practices through the original research of its members, as well as disseminating this information through its periodicals, meetings and conferences, position stands and consensus statements, and certification workshops. ACSM's respect has earned them numerous health initiative partnerships and collaborative efforts with groups such as the AHA, American Medical Association, NSF International, American Cancer Society, Centers for Disease Control and Prevention, IHRSA, National Intramural-Recreational Sports Association, National Academy of Sports Medicine, the CAAHEP, the NCCA, the National Collegiate Athletic Association, the NCPAD, and many others.

> *ACSM was founded in 1954, was the first professional organization to begin offering health and fitness certifications (in 1975), and continues to deliver the most respected, NCCA-accredited certifications within the health and fitness industry.*

Identification of a Core Body of Knowledge

Shortly after ACSM began offering certifications, the first edition of *ACSM's Guidelines for Exercise Testing and Prescription* (1) was published along with its companion publication *ACSM's Resource Manual for Guidelines for Exercise Testing and Prescription* (2). These publications included, for the first time anywhere, the consensus of SMEs and so defined the core body of knowledge with respect to standards and guidelines for assessing fitness and prescribing exercise. Generally, all professions, regardless of the industry, have a core body of knowledge that provides guidance and clarity and also helps establish a specific profession's scope of practice. This initial publication proved so effective for practitioners that periodic review and revision of this book now takes place every 4 years. The year 2009 will mark the publication of the 8th edition of *ACSM's Guidelines for Exercise Testing and Prescription*. Also in 2009, the 6th edition of the *ACSM's Resource Manual for Guidelines for Exercise Testing and Prescription* as well as the 3rd edition of *ACSM's Certification Review Book* were published.

Development and Continuous Revision of Knowledge, Skills, and Abilities

Included in the appendices of every edition of *ACSM's Guidelines for Exercise Testing and Prescription* is a comprehensive list of knowledge, skills, and abilities (KSAs) relative to each ACSM certification. These KSAs represent the specific attributes necessary for success as a practitioner and usually are categorized across different content areas. The general process for the ongoing revision and/or addition to the KSAs follows industry-accepted best-practice models for ongoing quality assurance. First, a group of appropriate SMEs is convened to review the current set of KSAs. These SMEs include practitioners, academicians, researchers, and even potential employers. After their first round of review and revision, the first draft of updated KSAs is evaluated through a "job task analysis," in which a large number of randomly selected practitioners and employers further comment on the importance, frequency, and relevance of each specific KSA compared with the typical job demands and requirements in the real-world setting. Additionally, the participants in the job task analysis phase can comment and suggest other appropriate attributes as new KSAs, not appearing within the current KSA list.

Once the job task analysis results are compiled, the original group of SMEs further revises the KSAs as needed, based on the results and comments from the job task analysis. Finally, the KSAs are assigned to their appropriate content areas, and a certification examination blueprint is developed, which represents the combined work of the SMEs and the results of the job task analysis. This examination blueprint is the basis of the certification examination. The current examination test blueprint for the ACSM Certified Personal Trainer is found in Table 1.2. The examination has multiple-choice questions delivered in a computer-based testing format. Please check www.acsm.org for current pricing, testing locations, and dates.

ESTABLISHING YOUR KNOWLEDGE BASE

Everyone has strengths and weaknesses with respect to how much he or she knows or doesn't know about any given topic, including Personal Trainers. Even fitness professionals with college degrees have content areas that they are more knowledgeable in than others. Part of your commitment to the profession is to continuously evaluate your educational foundation or knowledge base. One way to focus on an action plan for your specific continuing education needs is to use the KSAs as your knowledge map.

TABLE 1.2	ACSM CERTIFIED PERSONAL TRAINER EXAMINATION BLUEPRINT[a]
The approximate percentage of questions from each content area is as follows:	
Percentage	**Content Areas**
28	Exercise prescription (training) and programming
24	Exercise physiology and related exercise science
13	Health appraisal and fitness exercise testing
10	Clinical and medical considerations (risk factor identification)
9	Nutrition and weight management
8	Safety, injury prevention, and emergency procedures
4	Program administration, quality assurance, and outcome assessment
4	Human behavior
Total 100	

NOTE: All certification examination candidates are encouraged to visit the American College of Sports Medicine Web site (www.acsm.org). Follow the links through certification to view the latest certification examination test blueprint.

[a]Percentages reflect approximate numbers of questions addressing each of the eight competencies.

Begin by performing a thorough review of the KSAs, rating your familiarity and competence against each specific KSA. Next, use this checklist to prioritize the KSA content areas from weakest to strongest. Over the course of a year, seek out and participate in continuing educational opportunities that focus on your weakest content areas. You should do this on a yearly basis, at a minimum, as content areas that were once weak may become stronger for you over time, especially as you devote additional study to these areas and, more importantly, develop a client base in which some content areas are relied upon more than others. If you can do this consistently one year to the next, recertifying becomes a pleasure as opposed to a chore. Some Personal Trainers procrastinate, waiting until the last minute to accumulate the required number of CEUs/CECs. Not only does this create a great deal of stress for you, but also it is not a very effective way to expand your knowledge base as a Personal Trainer.

The Exercise Sciences

The competent Personal Trainer should have a strong knowledge foundation in the exercise sciences. Exercise science is a broad term that includes multiple disciplines. These disciplines often include but are not limited to anatomy and physiology, exercise physiology, motor learning/motor control, nutrition (dietetics), biomechanics/applied kinesiology, and exercise (sports) psychology. Good-quality educational programs (workshops or online opportunities offered by certification organizations or curriculums offered by academic institutions) may offer a course of study that includes content or courses

The competent Personal Trainer should have a strong knowledge foundation in the exercise sciences.

dedicated to helping the Personal Trainer develop an understanding of these more specific disciplines.

ACSM has worked collaboratively with Fitness Resource Associates to offer both 1-day and 3-day workshops to help you prepare for the ACSM Certified Personal Trainer Certification examination. The workshops review the knowledge, skills, and abilities relevant to the content areas tested on the examination. Taking a workshop in no way guarantees passing an examination; however, many candidates find it helpful to review at the workshop what they have already learned. For current pricing, workshop locations, and dates, see www.acsm.org.

Developing Your Tool Kit

In addition to a strong knowledge foundation in the exercise sciences, effective Personal Trainers are constantly adding skills to their "tool kit." Additional tools include

- ➤ effective communication skills (in-person, phone, and written such as e-mail),
- ➤ ability to motivate appropriately,
- ➤ ability to influence behavior change,
- ➤ effective interviewing and screening,
- ➤ effective use of goals and objectives,
- ➤ effective and safe exercise program design,
- ➤ ability to instruct appropriate exercise movements, and
- ➤ using a sound business model.

These are the minimum tools you should not only include in your tool kit but also master using effectively, either individually or in combination with others. As you progress through your professional career, you should be continuously adding tools to make you more effective as a Personal Trainer.

COMMUNICATING SKILLS (MOTIVATING AND INFLUENCING BEHAVIORAL CHANGE)

Perhaps the most overlooked yet important skill for the Personal Trainer tool kit is that of communication. Communication is more than just verbal, as it includes nonverbal elements such as visual (what is observed) and kinesthetic (what is felt). Additionally, effective communication involves much more than information exchange. Communication also relies on the emotional state of both individuals. For example, is the client "ready" to accept information or is there temporary resistance to the new information being provided? Likewise, are you an effective motivator who can create an optimal emotional state for clients so they are ready not only to take in the information that you are providing but also to put it to good use? As a complex and important skill, communication is discussed throughout this book.

SCREENING, ASSESSMENT, AND REFERRALS

Another set of tools required for the Personal Trainer includes interviewing, screening, risk stratification, and the ability to recognize when to refer a client to a medical healthcare provider such as a physician or registered dietitian. When health screening forms are used appropriately, these tools help establish a foundation of trust that facilitates the development of the trainer–client relationship. Combined with effective communication skills, these tools further improve the possibility of achieving the client's goals.

Typically, a Personal Trainer conducts an initial interview with a potential client in which basic demographic information is obtained, along with the client's heath history. Two types of forms are used at a minimum: the health history form and the PAR-Q form. (Examples of these and other forms are available in this text, "Screening and the ACSM Risk Stratification Process.") In addition, it is appropriate during this initial interview to ask clients about their specific expectations for working with a Personal Trainer, what initial goals they may have, as well as any other lifestyle information they can share. Examples include

➤ recent and past history of physical activity (if any);
➤ history of previous injuries (if any);
➤ level of social support from family and friends; and
➤ potential stressors that may impose challenges on their exercise regimen, such as excessive work hours, physically demanding work, and multiple recurring commitments within the community or with family.

Finally, this initial consultation should be used to synchronize the Personal Trainer–client expectations, obtain or request any medical clearance forms (if required), as well as obtain signatures on required waivers, informed consent forms, and/or other contractual forms and agreements as required by your employer.

Risk stratification (ranking the client into a category of "low," "medium," or "high" risk, based on the presence or absence of various risk factors for cardiovascular disease) of your new client is the next step and should be based on the ACSM's risk stratification system (1), which is described in detail in this text. It is important to note that Personal Trainers do not diagnose or treat disease, disorders, injuries, or other medical conditions under any circumstance. The presence of specific and/or multiple risk factors requires that the Personal Trainer refer the client to the appropriate medical–healthcare provider for additional guidance and/or a medical release before designing and implementing an exercise program. Also, even if the client fails to initially disclose information that becomes known at a later time, the Personal Trainer still has a legal obligation to refer the client to his or her healthcare provider before additional training guidance can be provided. Personal Trainers who provide services outside their scope of practice place both themselves and their clients at risk.

> *The presence of specific and/or multiple risk factors requires that the Personal Trainer refer the client to the appropriate medical–healthcare provider for additional guidance and/or a medical release before designing and implementing an exercise program.*

Assessments are tests and measurements that Personal Trainers use with their clients to evaluate their current physical and functional status. Assessments may include:

➤ resting and exercise heart rate;
➤ resting and exercise blood pressure;
➤ body weight and height;
➤ body composition estimates using skinfold calipers, etc.;
➤ circumference measurements of limbs, hips, and waist;
➤ calculation of body mass index;
➤ calculation of waist-to-hip ratio;
➤ measurements of flexibility using a sit and reach, etc.;
➤ tests for muscular strength/muscular endurance; and
➤ tests for cardiorespiratory fitness via walking, biking, stepping, etc.

Assessments provide a current snapshot of the functional ability of your client. When combined with the data from the PAR-Q and other health-related questionnaires, the Personal Trainer can begin developing a draft of a customized exercise regimen for the client.

ETHICS AND PROFESSIONAL CONDUCT

Ethics can be described as standards of conduct that guide decisions and actions, based on duties derived from core values. Specifically, core values are principles that we use to define what is right, good, and/or just. When a professional demonstrates behavior that is consistent, or aligned, with widely accepted standards in their respective industry, that professional is said to behave "ethically." On the other hand, "unethical" behavior is behavior that is not consistent with industry-accepted standards. As a fitness professional, you have an obligation to stay within the bounds of the defined scope of practice for a Personal Trainer, as well as to abide by all industry-accepted standards of behavior at all times. Furthermore, as a certified or registered professional through ACSM, it is your responsibility to be familiar with all aspects of the ACSM's Code of Ethics for certified and registered professionals.

Code of Ethics for ACSM Certified and Registered Professionals

PURPOSE

This Code of Ethics is intended to aid all certified and registered American College of Sports Medicine Credentialed Professionals (ACSMCPs) to establish and maintain a high level of ethical conduct, as defined by standards by which ACSMCPs may determine the appropriateness of their conduct. Any existing professional, licensure, or certification affiliations that ACSMCPs have with governmental, local, state, or national agencies or organizations will take precedence relative to any disciplinary matters that pertain to practice or professional conduct.

This Code applies to all ACSMCPs, regardless of ACSM membership status (to include members and nonmembers). Any cases in violation of this Code will be referred to the ACSM Committee on Certification and Registry Boards (CCRB).

PRINCIPLES AND STANDARDS

Responsibility to the Public

➤ ACSMCPs shall be dedicated to providing competent and legally permissible services within the scope of the KSAs of their respective credential. These services shall be provided with integrity, competence, diligence, and compassion.
➤ ACSMCPs provide exercise information in a manner that is consistent with evidence-based science and medicine.

> ACSMCPs respect the rights of clients, colleagues, and healthcare professionals, and shall safeguard client confidences within the boundaries of the law.
> Information relating to the ACSMCP–client relationship is confidential and may not be communicated to a third party not involved in that client's care without the prior written consent of the client or as required by law.
> ACSMCPs are truthful about their qualifications and the limitations of their expertise and provide services consistent with their competencies.

Responsibility to the Profession

> ACSMCPs maintain high professional standards. As such, an ACSMCP should never represent himself or herself, either directly or indirectly, as anything other than an ACSMCP unless he or she holds other license/certification that allows him or her to do so.
> ACSMCPs practice within the scope of their KSAs. ACSMCPs will not provide services that are limited by state law to provision by another healthcare professional only.
> An ACSMCP must remain in good standing relative to governmental requirements as a condition of continued credentialing.
> ACSMCPs take credit, including authorship, only for work they have actually performed and give credit to the contributions of others as warranted.
> Consistent with the requirements of their certification or registration, ACSMCPs must complete approved, additional educational course work aimed at maintaining and advancing their KSAs.

Principles and Standards for Candidates of ACSM Certification Examinations

Candidates applying for a credentialing examination must comply with candidacy requirements and, to the best of their abilities, accurately complete the application process. In addition, the candidate must refrain from any and all behavior that would be interpreted as "irregular."

Public Disclosure of Affiliation

> Any ACSMCP may disclose his or her affiliation with ACSM credentialing in any context, oral or documented, provided it is currently accurate. In doing so, no ACSMCP may imply college endorsement of whatever is associated in context with the disclosure, unless expressly authorized by the college. Disclosure of affiliation in connection with a commercial venture may be made provided the disclosure is made in a professionally dignified manner; is not false, misleading, or deceptive; and does not imply licensure or the attainment of specialty or diploma status.
> ACSMCPs may disclose their credential status.
> ACSMCPs may list their affiliation with ACSM credentialing on their business cards without prior authorization.
> ACSMCPs and the institutions employing an ACSMCP may inform the public of an affiliation as a matter of public discourse or presentation.

Discipline

Any ACSMCP may be disciplined or lose his or her certification or registry for conduct that, in the opinion of the Executive Council of the ACSM Committee on CCRB, goes against the principles set forth in this Code. Such cases will be reviewed by the ACSM CCRB Ethics Subcommittee, which will include a liaison from the ACSM CCRB executive council, as appointed by the CCRB chair. The ACSM CCRB Ethics Subcommittee will make an action recommendation to the executive council of the ACSM CCRB for final review and approval.

SUMMARY

The rapidly expanding fitness industry offers Personal Trainers many potential work environments in which to gain experience and to develop a career, including commercial clubs, not-for-profit clubs, university recreation centers, corporate fitness centers, MFCs, and more. Although compensation varies greatly for trainers, they are overall very satisfied with their career choice and see opportunities for advancement and growth. With a nation on the verge of a healthcare crisis due primarily to the prevalence of lifestyle-related conditions, highly qualified and motivated Personal Trainers are needed now more than ever to lead individuals down the road to good health and well-being. As the fitness industry grows and the demographics/characteristics of the population continue to change, it is likely that the role of Personal Trainers will change too. This changing role will likely be an expansion of Personal Trainers' scope of practice so that Personal Trainers may soon be seen as allied healthcare professionals. In the future, Personal Trainers may be commonplace in areas where they are seldom seen now, such as medical clinics, with a role of helping low-risk individuals cleared by a doctor to become more active, as the medical profession turns to the prevention of disease and not just the treatment of it. As an emerging professional in this rapidly growing field, you can contribute to this expanding sphere of influence by being the utmost professional at all times for your clients and for the best interests of the profession.

REFERENCES

1. American College of Sports Medicine. *ACSM's Guidelines for Exercise Testing and Prescription.* 8th ed. Baltimore: Lippincott Williams & Wilkins; 2010.
2. American College of Sports Medicine. *ACSM's Resource Manual for Exercise Testing and Prescription.* 6th ed. Baltimore: Lippincott Williams & Wilkins; 2010.
3. American College of Sports Medicine and American Medical Association. ACSM & AMA Launch Exercise is Medicine program. [Internet]. [cited 2007 Nov 5]. Available from: http://www.acsm.org/AM/Template.cfm?Section=Home_Page&TEMPLATE=/CM/ContentDisplay.cfm&CONTENTID=859
4. American College of Sports Medicine. ACSM American Fitness Index: Actively moving U.S. cities to better health—May 2008 pilot phase pilot report. [Internet] [cited 2008 May 1]. Available from: http://www.americanfitnessindex.org
5. Bureau of Labor Statistics, U.S. Department of Labor. Occupational outlook handbook. 2008–09 ed. [Internet]. [cited 2008 Aug 21]. Available from: http://www.bls.gov/oco/ocos296.htm
6. Centers for Disease Control and Prevention. U.S. obesity trends 1985–2007 [Internet]. [cited 2008 Aug 21]. Available from: http://www.cdc.gov/nccdphp/dnpa/obesity/trend/maps/
7. Centers for Disease Control and Prevention. U.S. physical activity statistics, 2007 [Internet]. [cited 2008 Aug 21]. Available from: http://www.cdc.gov/nccdphp/dnpa/physical/stats/index.htm
8. Central Intelligence Agency. Life expectancy. In: *The CIA World Factbook 2008.* [Internet]. New York: Skyhorse Publishing; [cited 2007, Oct 1]. Available from: https://www.cia.gov/library/publications/the-world-factbook/geos/us.html
9. Chenowith D. *Worksite Health Promotion.* Champaign (IL): Human Kinetics; 1998.
10. Ethics Resource Center. [Internet] [cited 2008 Aug 21]. Available from: http://www.ethics.org
11. International Health, Racquet and Sportsclub Association. Fair competition annual report. [Internet] [cited 2003]. Available from: http://download.ihrsa.org/gr/faircomp.pdf
12. International Health, Racquet and Sportsclub Association. Industry Statistics. IHRSA 2008 Global Report: The state of the health club industry [Internet]. [cited 2008 June 3]. Available from: http://www.ihrsastore.com/fiintef.html
13. National Association for Sport and Physical Education. State physical education requirements, 2008 [Internet]. [cited 2008 Aug 21]. Available from: http://www.drwoolard.com/commentary/state_pe_requirements.htm
14. Pennington B. Baby boomers stay active, and so do their doctors. *The New York Times* [Internet]. [cited 2006 Apr 16]. Available from: http://www.nytimes.com/2006/04/16/sports/16boomers.html

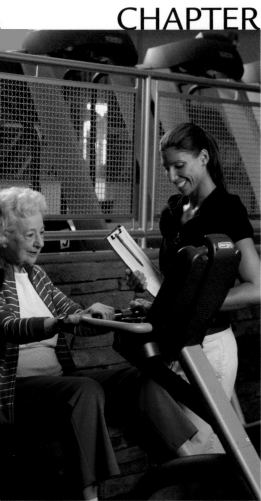

 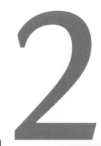

Career Track for Professional Personal Trainers

OBJECTIVES

- Describe a career as a professional Personal Trainer
- Identify areas of specialization
- Set a timeline for becoming a Personal Trainer
- Identify educational options
- Develop a successful professional foundation
- Dedicate yourself to excellence

A lthough fitness professionals have been providing exercise advice for decades, the reality is that the term "Personal Trainer" did not become popular until the late 1970s. In the early days, the only prerequisite for a Personal Trainer was an engaging personality, a drill sergeant mentality, and the physical appearance of a Marine recruit. Today, however, a career in personal training is positioned to evolve into a highly respectable profession and a rewarding career.

As the personal training industry grew, so did the number of untrained, uneducated, but well-intentioned people wanting to teach others how to get fit regardless of their academic training or experience. Even though the early Personal Trainers had a knowledge base that was minimal at best, the training business continued to grow, as it expands exponentially today.

> *As the personal training industry grew, so did the number of untrained, uneducated, but well-intentioned people wanting to teach others how to get fit regardless of their academic training or experience.*

The personal training field is expected to grow 27% by 2016 (1). Much of this growth will likely be due to aging baby boomers, large corporations seeking healthcare professionals to keep employees well, and more people becoming aware of the need for physical fitness. A career in personal training is positioned for an exciting growth trend.

This chapter covers many content areas that should be considered when choosing a career in personal training. The following questions may help determine your career interest.

Why do I want to become a Personal Trainer? As with any profession, it is important that you be clear about your reasons for wanting to dedicate your life to a particular career. Did you decide to become a Personal Trainer because you have had your own experience that drew you into the health and fitness business? Do you know someone who is involved in the industry? Are you at a place in your life where a career in personal training seems like a great fit? Do you want to help people? Do you enjoy seeing your clients achieve healthy results? Whatever your objectives, make sure that they resonate with your personal values. An exciting part about becoming a professional Personal Trainer is that your specialty options are numerous (7).

Do I possess the compassion and empathy that are required in a profession that deals with people's physical and mental strengths and weaknesses? Being a Personal Trainer requires that you have a well-developed ability to connect with people. This skill will enhance your success as well as that of your clients. You must also be able to understand where and when clients need support at various points in your relationship. You may have clients who are focused on and clear about their goals, whereas others struggle to commit to goals. Even clients who are committed to clearly stated goals sometimes struggle with making the lifestyle changes necessary to their achievement. Whatever the situation, you must be prepared to deal with clients' frustrations and disappointments to help them move forward with optimism rather than feeling defeated, frustrated, and isolated. You must be able to interview your clients in a way that empowers them to believe that they are ultimately in charge of the goals they achieve. You are their facilitating expert but the real reason for success is internally driven. Today's successful personal trainers are experts when needed and facilitators always.

What specialty option holds the greatest interest for me? There are several venues where you can practice personal training including: a client's home, a commercial health club or fitness center, a specialized personal training studio, a corporate fitness facility, a hospital-based wellness center, a medically based outpatient clinic that offers rehabilitation, a fitness center based in an educational institution, a senior living center, a professional sports team, or a residential complex that offers a fitness center exclusively for the residents. Each one has a unique financial model and a different set of prospective clients whom you must train successfully to have a viable personal training business. Begin by asking yourself what part of personal training most interests you. If you enjoy working with seniors, then concentrate your efforts there. You may like the idea of joining a large commercial health club that provides numerous training opportunities, or you may prefer working with children in an after-school program. Whatever your choice of specialization, you should take the time to explore the options and where and when you want to work with your client. Your must match the client's culture. Go where it seems the least like work or where the time always flies or where at the end of the day you have had the most fun and professional satisfaction. If you do, the economic rewards will follow.

Do I have superior time management skills? When you begin creating your own personal training business or managing your own schedule, time management is crucial. There is a direct correlation between time management and high performance. Time management skills are critical when it comes to scheduling clients. Clients generally seek times that are convenient for them, and they count on you to keep their appointments consistent (4). If you fail to keep consistent client schedules or don't keep appointments because you are unable to manage your time efficiently, you will soon find yourself with no clients. Being well-prepared at each training session (which takes time and organizational skills) is something your clients appreciate (and deserve), and this is one of the secrets to growing a successful personal training business. Create clear policies in writing regarding time-based training sessions so there is no confusion with your clients about late cancellations or no-shows by either party.

Do I pay close attention to details? Many people believe that being a Personal Trainer means creating an exercise program and counting the repetitions—nothing could be further from the truth. In the personal training field, to achieve desired results, retain clients, and obtain client referrals and recommendations for safety purposes as well as for legal purposes, you must pay attention to your client's every move during each session and make sure that he or she is committed to following your directions (5). Details must be carefully noted after each session so that you can track client results. Your notes should be relative to the training objectives and also specific enough for a colleague to follow if he or she has to cover for you in a subsequent training session. In addition to the training sessions and depending upon your field of specialization, there will be daily responsibilities such as maintaining records, phone calls, and billing. If you own your own facility, the list will include equipment upkeep, marketing, advertising, and payroll. No matter what your role is, each area of responsibility must be attended to in precise detail to meet the needs of your clients and grow a successful business. If any of these details are not your strong suit, then recruiting the right person to get these tasks done while you maximize your own individual strengths is a must. Hire people who can complement you, not ones who replicate you.

What traits do I possess that will contribute to my success as a Personal Trainer? As a Personal Trainer, you are required to teach. You are there to provide your client with all the necessary information that will enhance his or her overall health. If you are able to communicate efficiently the information your client needs to know, your success rate as well as that of your client will be impressive. Practice your ability to demonstrate specific skills, especially ones that you may not perform on a regular basis. Get the stance, grip, and breathing right too. Your picture of technique is worth a thousand words to your clients. Motivation is a key part of your communication skill set. You must ask yourself if you can adequately motivate your clients to do the work necessary to achieve their goals. To do so, you must know what motivates them. Watch their body language, listen to their verbal cues, and look at their faces for the excitement of accomplishment. When in doubt, ask the clients what motivates them effectively, listen to their answers, and use it liberally.

> *Practice your ability to demonstrate specific skills, especially ones that you may not perform on a regular basis.*

Whether it is a client wishing to lose weight or a runner intent on improving his or her speed, you will need to provide the necessary motivation to help him or her succeed. Another key trait is self-discipline. Being a Personal Trainer requires that you maintain a dedication not only to the health of your clients but also to your own health. Leading a healthy lifestyle is not possible without self-discipline. Clients learn as much from what you show them as what you tell them. Being a positive role model usually leads to being a positive mentor.

What strengths do I have that can contribute to the fitness industry? Regardless of your career path, it's helpful to know what strengths you bring to your chosen profession so that you can build on them and facilitate your growth personally as well as professionally. The more you know about your industry, the more you will be able to grow your business, given the insight you gain from your involvement. Very often people are so consumed by their day-to-day activities (a result of poor time management) that they find they have little time or energy to participate in extracurricular events that can have a positive impact on their professional success. There are many different ways that you can become involved in the fitness industry. For example, if you believe you have strong writing skills, why not share your expertise and experience with magazines and journals? Publications in the health and fitness field are always looking for writers who can provide timely and insightful articles. If writing is a strength of yours, explore the possibilities. Perhaps you have strong public speaking skills. Find an opportunity to speak or be a panel member at industry conferences. Becoming a speaker is a great way to enhance your credibility, as it shows your clients that you have the knowledge necessary to teach others. In addition, your public speaking skills may lead you to local organizations, which will raise your profile and allow the opportunity for business growth.

The industry also offers many opportunities for professional growth that do not require you to write or speak publicly. Serve on a committee for the regional chapter of your organization to help with fund-raising, events planning, strategic brainstorming, or member recruitment. Volunteer to work for the local charity events leading a preevent warm-up or a postevent cool-down routine. Teach a class pro bono at a senior center or teen recreational program. Get and stay involved in the industry outside of your comfort zone. This is where professional and personal growth lives.

Am I passionate about my chosen career? Publisher and philanthropist Malcolm Forbes once said, "Success follows doing what you want to do. There is no other way to be successful" (6). Nothing lays the foundation for success better than being passionate about your chosen profession. Because the personal training industry is relatively new and has grown so rapidly, there are many Personal Trainers who jumped aboard strictly because of the money-making potential or because of the perceived glamour that follows the profession. It doesn't matter how much money you make or how much of a power trip you get from personal training; if you

> *It doesn't matter how much money you make or how much of a power trip you get from personal training; if you are not passionate about your career choice, it will come across in your business interactions.*

are not passionate about your career choice, it will come across in your business interactions. Your clients will pick up on the fact that your focus is not on their success but on your own personal gain. This is one of the fastest ways to lose clients and your credibility. Passion is obvious to you internally but may not be so to those who observe you in action. In fact, unbridled passion can come out as sheer annoyance if not focused and controlled, and distributed with some objectives in mind. It starts with the look on your face. Direct eye contact and clear thoughtfully chosen words can say a lot about your ability to communicate. How's your posture: upright or uptight? There is a difference. Are you meticulous about your uniform? Do you wear a nametag? Do you address your clients by name and show them a smile in your voice over the phone? Are you in a position to spot correctly with hands held in position and eyes on their form and not on the TV, your black-berry or worse yet, on your self in the mirror? Passion does not have to be loud or hyperac-tive, but it does need to be yours.

Am I willing to take responsibility as a role model and mentor? This is a question that needs serious consideration. As a Personal Trainer, you are setting an example in the fitness industry. People will be looking to you as a model of what constitutes health and fitness. This does not necessarily mean that you need to qualify for the cover of *Muscle & Fitness*. Start with a positive attitude that radiates from within. Preparation for each and every client, whether it's your first or last, speaks volumes as a role model who is willing to take responsibility for your task at hand. Realistic goal setting especially in regards to any individual client's body weight or percent body fat objectives is essential. Most people have unrealistic expectations for their body weight and body fat percentage, the time it will take to achieve these goals and the self-discipline needed to maintain a healthy body weight. A good mentor will effectively manage these expectations from the beginning. A good role model will lead by example in his or her own representations and communications about these weight-related goals and objectives. A mentor by definition is someone deemed as wise and trusted. Are your motivations and actions with each and every client worthy of these adjectives? Are you researching the most effective and intelligent training regimen for your clients or recycling the same canned routines regardless of their current training status or personalized objectives? Are you really committed to the clients' long-term health, or just to renewing the next block of sessions?

Have I created my Mission and Values? The start of a personal training career is in essence a business of YOU. The clients are paying for you, and you are promising to work with them for a predetermined number of sessions to achieve a set of goals related to health, fitness, or sports performance. All credible businesses, big and small, have a Mission and Values. The mission is a written statement of what you want your business to stand for over time. A mis-sion does not change with the business environment, annual strategic goals, budgets, or op-erating principles. For example, the mission of the American College of Sports Medicine is to "promote and integrate scientific research, education, and practical applications of sports medicine and exercise science to maintain and enhance physical performance, fitness, health, and quality of life." The mission for your personal training business could be as simple as "training my clients to be fit without me." A mission describes your business ideals, whereas values articulate clear behaviors that demonstrate the mission in action. The delineation and description of values makes it possible for you to focus on the few (sometimes as little as two to six) essential actions that will make your career a success. For example, you may establish a simple value for each of your clients that you will be 100% sure of their primary goal for each and every training session. If you act accordingly and are very aware of what your clients want to get out of each hour spent with you, and you work toward achieving this end, your clients will return time and time again. Consistent execution of this value will ensure desired results, eliminate guesswork, and provide a positive experience for your clients and for you. The last word about both your Mission Statement and Values is to com-municate them clearly to yourself, your clients, and your team.

BECOMING A PERSONAL TRAINER

As you consider a career as a Personal Trainer, it is wise to learn as much as you can about the fit-ness industry. You can begin to do this by interviewing health and fitness professionals. Sitting down one-on-one with a qualified expert in the field is a great starting point, as it will provide insight that you typically cannot get through formal academic training or in a classroom setting. Attending in-dustry conferences, attending continuing education opportunities, and interacting with others will also help enhance your knowledge.

TABLE 2.1	ACSM EXAMINATION ELIGIBILITY REQUIREMENTS
ACSM Certification	**Examination Eligibility Requirements**
ACSM Certified Personal Trainer	High school diploma or equivalent Current adult CPR (with practical skills component) 18 years of age or older
ACSM Certified Health Fitness Specialist	Associate's degree (see www.acsm.org/certfication for a list of eligible degrees) in a health-related field Eligible to sit for examination if in last semester of degree program Current adult CPR (with practical skills component)
ACSM Certified Clinical Exercise Specialist	Bachelor's degree in an allied health field 600 hours of practical experience in a clinical exercise program Current basic life support or CPR for the Professional Rescuer certification
ACSM Registered Clinical Exercise Physiologist	Master's degree in exercise science, exercise physiology or kinesiology 600 hours of practical experience in a clinical exercise program Current basic life support or CPR for the Professional Rescuer certification

According to the U.S. Department of Labor, Bureau of Labor Statistics, more and more employers are requiring fitness employees to have a bachelor's degree in a health- or fitness-related field such as exercise science or physical education (2). Some employers accept certification in lieu of a college degree, whereas others may require both certification and a college degree. In 2006, the International Health, Racquet and Sportsclub Association (IHRSA), a global trade organization of more than 7,000 health club owners, recommended that personal trainers attain a certification from an accredited organization similar to the National Commission for Certifying Agencies of the National Organization for Competency Assurance (www.noca.org).

According to the U.S. Department of Labor, Bureau of Labor Statistics, more and more employers are requiring fitness employees to have a bachelor's degree in a health- or fitness-related field such as exercise science or physical education (2).

The Personal Trainer gains increased credibility by seeking out high-quality certification and formal education. ACSM's four certifications have increasing educational requirements as you move up from Personal Trainer to Health Fitness Specialist and to Clinical Exercise Specialist to Registered Clinical Exercise Physiologist. Table 2.1 contains the educational requirements for the four ACSM certifications. As the Personal Trainer profession matures, there will be a natural evolution for increased educational requirements specific to the field of exercise science. This serves the public, the profession, and the fitness field as a whole. Table 2.1 identifies the ACSM exam eligibility requirements for three certifications.

In addition, don't lose sight of the value of meeting and networking with other healthcare professionals. It is always recommended that you do so and that you look beyond health clubs and include hospitals and educational environments in your networking activities. The more insight you gain into the various areas of the business, the greater the chance you will discover the direction that is most appropriate for you. Remember that continuing education is required with or without a degree. Commit yourself to learning as much as you can about physiology, psychology, kinesiology, biomechanics, and anatomy along with current industry know-how, good interpersonal skills, and a desire to be your best.

ORGANIZING YOUR CAREER PATHWAY

As you begin to develop your career pathway, it is important to clarify your objectives and decide on your specific area of interest. You may want to complete your four-year degree at a university with an emphasis on exercise science. An internship with one or several businesses that work in your

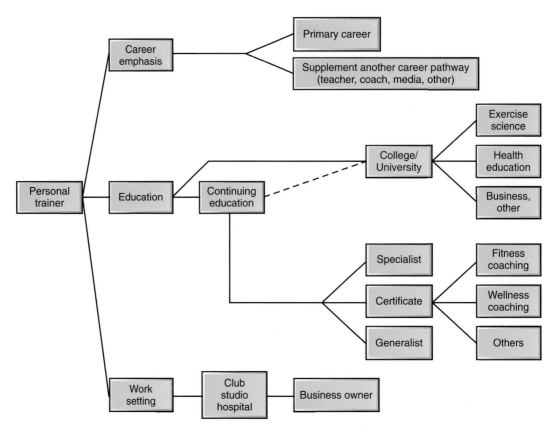

FIGURE 2.1. ACSM career path development.

interest areas is also recommended (usually it is part of a college curriculum, counts toward college credits, and is required or at least encouraged for both baccalaureate and graduate programs). Or, you may already hold a degree in another field and simply want to complete a credible certification in the industry. Either way, you should explore your options, consider continuing your education with a degree, and obtain a certification. Refer to the career path flowchart to determine your educational options (Fig. 2.1).

Consider looking to colleges and universities that provide specialized curriculum and education in personal training and the exercise sciences that meet your career needs (8). Note that some universities may have ACSM's university endorsement or accreditation, which can add significant value to your educational pursuit.

Focus on the aspect of the industry that interests you most and in which you can see yourself being involved. Your area of specialization should engage your passion and dedication to becoming the best in your chosen field. As mentioned above, don't dismiss the value of connecting with experts in the area you would like to pursue. Participation in professional organizations specific to your areas of interest is an effective way to connect with these professionals. A regional clinic or convention provides you with a venue to hear these individuals speak about their experiences and expertise. It also gives you a face-to-face opportunity to network with them so you can start to build your contact list of professionals in your field. And, do not forget to have a business card on hand and to get one of theirs. With the new contact management Internet applications like Plaxo (www.plaxo.com) and LinkedIN (www.linkedin.com), it makes it easy to build and manage your network of professional contacts and keep them abreast of your career developments. The more you learn from them, the better prepared you will be to lay out a realistic career path and timeline.

It is best to start by setting up a timeline outlining the steps you need to take to reach your desired goals. Keep in mind that your educational/career path should match your goals. For

TABLE 2.2 CAREER PATH CONTRAST	
Personal Trainer A	**Personal Trainer B**
BA degree–finance	Health Club Manager/Personal Trainer (2 years)
Master's degree in education	Associates degree in fitness management (2 years)
Specialization in biomechanics	Fitness Practitioner Certification (1 year)
Pursuing a PhD	AFAA Certification, ACE Certification
ACSM Health/Fitness Instructor Certification	Research and study of physiology, kinesiology, biomechanics, and anatomy (ongoing)
Started Personal Training and Fitness Consulting Business	Started In-home Personal Training Business
Medically-Based Affiliations	NASM Certification
Community/Professional Affiliations	Opened Personal Training Studio
Local/International Presenter and Writer	Contributing Writer for major industry magazines
Volunteer for IDEA Committee	Health and Fitness Columnist for suburban newspaper
Former Chair of the Senior Fitness Subcommittee Governor's Council on Physical Fitness and Sports	Family Fitness Columnist for major e-zine.
Recognitions: Personal Trainer of the Year Award, nationally and internationally	Author of health and fitness book published by large publishing firm
Program Coordinator for College of Extended Studies Certificate program for Personal Fitness Training	Presenter at numerous health and fitness conferences
Program Coordinator for 4-year college—undergraduate degree in personal fitness training	Numerous awards for excellence in business, management, and customer service
Committee member for numerous health and fitness organizations	Active member of numerous health and fitness organizations
American Alliance for Health, Physical Education, Recreation & Dance (AAHPERD) Exercise Science Committee	
Authoring books and instructional videos/DVDs	

example, if your goal is to work in a hospital environment, you should begin by speaking with individuals in that environment and discover what credentials will best support your goals. Once you gain a clear idea about what is involved by speaking to others, you can begin to develop a specific timeline.

By referring to the career pathways of Personal Trainer A and Personal Trainer B in Table 2.2, you will see two vastly different approaches for two persons involved in the same industry. This contrast may help illustrate the different options available to you as you organize your own career path. Note that although their paths are different, they both became certified, which is a vital part of the Personal Training profession.

EDUCATION

Among the many certification options available to you, you may choose to consider one from the ACSM. You can research which certification program is best for you by visiting the ACSM Web site. If you are reading this book, you are probably studying for ACSM's Certified Personal Trainer examination (considered by many in the fitness industry to be the most rigorous) or studying for some other ACSM certification. The ACSM programs are often viewed as the best measures of competence and require a high level of knowledge, skills, and abilities.

ACSM provides an internal recognition system of academic programs through its University Connection Endorsement program. As of this printing, there are more than 50 undergraduate and graduate programs nationwide with "ACSM-Endorsed" status. This program is currently being phased out, however, in favor of academic program accreditation. ACSM is a sponsoring organization of the Committee on Accreditation for the Exercise Sciences (CoAES) of the Commission on Accreditation of Allied Health Education Programs (CAAHEP) (3). The primary role of the CoAES is to establish standards and guidelines for academic programs that facilitate the preparation of students seeking employment in the health, fitness, and exercise industry. The CoAES also works to establish and implement a process of self-study, review, and recommendation for all programs seeking CAAHEP accreditation (3). Academic program accreditation through CAAHEP is specifically intended for exercise science or related departments (e.g., physical education, kinesiology) with a professional preparation track designed for students seeking employment opportunities in the health, fitness, and exercise industry. CAAHEP reviews and accredits more than 2,000 educational

> *The primary role of the CoAES is to establish standards and guidelines for academic programs that facilitate the preparation of students seeking employment in the health, fitness, and exercise industry.*

programs in 21 health science occupations across the United States and Canada. Accreditation in the health-related disciplines serves an important public interest. Along with certification and licensure, accreditation is a tool intended to help ensure a well-prepared and qualified workforce providing healthcare services. Search academic institutions that offer the appropriate programs to help you achieve your career goals. If you are looking for colleges and universities in which to pursue your career, the following courses are examples of some that help prepare you for a personal training career:

➤ applied anatomy and kinesiology,
➤ exercise physiology,
➤ biomechanics,
➤ motor skills and learning,
➤ exercise psychology,
➤ health and fitness in clinical and work site settings,
➤ health behavior and health promotion,
➤ health screening and fitness evaluation and prescription,
➤ health and fitness program management,
➤ exercise program development,
➤ professional development and internship in health and fitness, and
➤ clinical practices in personal training.

Whether you are seeking certification through ACSM, are currently ACSM certified, or hold an undergraduate degree in the exercise sciences, it does not mean that you are finished with your education. You should make a commitment to education and continued learning. One degree or one certification is not all that is required to succeed. You should keep up with the industry through continuing education classes, business relationships, your client base, community involvement, and medical affiliations.

CONTINUING EDUCATION

The reality is that you need to make continuing education a part of your commitment right from the start. You should read good-quality professional periodicals that offer continuing education units or continuing education credits that are designed to inform you of changes in the industry. Get involved in conferences that put you in touch with different aspects of the industry, and provide you with opportunities for meeting and networking with people in your field. Subscribe to newsletters that keep you abreast of the latest research and developments in the industry. Many of these are part of your membership in professional organizations (e.g., ACSM membership can include a monthly subscription to *Medicine & Science in Sports & Exercise, ACSM's Health & Fitness Journal*, among others), whereas others are available via the

Internet directly from very credible health and fitness resources. Some examples include the following:

- www.acsm.org
- www.corpfittoday.blogspot.com
- www.ideafit.com
- www.exrx.net
- www.fitnessworld.com
- www.ihrsa.org
- www.dswfitness.com
- http://www.cdc.gov/physicalactivity/everyone/guidelines/index.html

Your selection of professional organizations for certification should be influenced by the quality of their offerings for continuing education. Are they affordable and regional to minimize related expenses? Are their educational opportunities virtual and scheduled so you can access them at your convenience. Some employers are also offering in-house educational opportunities for their personal trainers. Even working part-time with such an employer can be a valuable resource to meet your educational goals. You should be sure to create an annual budget for your own continuing education needs and do not forget to factor in the lost revenue while away from your clients and the travel-related costs in addition to registration fees for the course. And, make sure to spend your money allocated for continuing education. Many Personal Trainers get caught up in the day-to-day activities of their careers and do not carve out enough time to stay abreast of the new information available every year.

> *Many personal trainers get caught up in the day-to-day activities of their careers and do not carve out enough time to stay abreast of the new information available every year.*

DEVELOPING BUSINESS RELATIONSHIPS

There is no better way to understand the nuances of a business than through the voice of experience. Talking with seasoned professionals can help you avoid the mistakes they made and teach you the secrets to building a successful career. It is important to meet new business contacts throughout your career, not just in the beginning. For example, if you are interested in writing for health and fitness journals and you read an article that focuses on sports-specific training and it piques your interest, why not contact the author? By contacting the author, you will have a chance to ask specific questions and have the author elaborate not only on the article but also on how he or she got into writing for health and fitness journals. Industry publications (e.g., IHRSA's Club Business International) feature successful entrepreneurs every month. Read and learn from their stories and reach out to them for additional information specific to your career path. Start to build a detailed contact list including the individual's special area of interest, how you met them, and a trail of communication that happens throughout your career. This list can become both your source of work and a resource of potential employees. Make contact at periodic intervals not just when you need something specific from any of your contact resources. Think about how you can send business to them when appropriate. On many occasions your clients will need a personal training resource while traveling or for a family member or friend. This is a perfect opportunity to reach out to colleagues in other cities or countries and send them some business opportunities.

ESTABLISHING A CLIENT BASE

To develop a client base, you need to determine the type of client you are seeking. This can be done only if you have contact with people of varying ages and personalities who have different needs, goals, and other physical challenges. Once you have established the clientele with whom you are interested in working, you need to find a venue that hosts that type of clientele. For example, if you like working with seniors, you will most likely find them at a community center, senior center, or health club. Once you have found a location with the clientele you are seeking, see if you can gain employment there on a full- or part-time basis. Create business cards, as mentioned above, offer to do public speaking as a way to introduce yourself to your community, and establish yourself as a health and fitness expert. Consider writing articles or a column for a local newspaper or a popular Web site or blog (e.g., www.about.com or www.ivillage.com) as another way to raise your profile and credibility within the community.

If you start working the floor at a health club, it is a great opportunity to meet members and to introduce yourself. When members see your enthusiasm for assisting them, they will remember when they are seeking a qualified Personal Trainer. Teaching large groups is also a great way to develop relationships and to establish yourself in a new facility. The more you are able to engage with your potential clients, the greater the likelihood of attracting and retaining a healthy clientele.

COMMUNITY INVOLVEMENT

It is unfortunate that many believe that community involvement is only for those who have a lot of time. It is not uncommon for people to get so caught up in their business that they lose sight of the industry and the community that supports their vocation. Overlooking the value of working within your community or industry might be the difference between a successful business and a marginal business. Look into donating your time at a senior center teaching group classes or after-school programs for kids. You will find literally hundreds of opportunities within your community that will enable you to get involved. A community that knows who you are and sees that you are involved will become one of your best business referral sources.

MEDICAL AFFILIATIONS

Another great way to help develop a client base is forming partnerships with professionals in the health field such as a registered dietician, a physician, a mental health specialist, and others, all of whom can have a profound effect on the development of your business. You can offer to train these professionals so that they are able to see your capabilities or you can offer to present a program on developing a sound fitness program for their patients and/or clients. Establishing relationships with allied professionals serves to elevate your credibility within the community and the fitness industry. Set aside time to sit and discuss your philosophies and find out how you can develop a reciprocal relationship in which mutual referral of clients occurs.

BUILDING A SOLID PROFESSIONAL FOUNDATION

Your reputation will be based upon the perception of how well you work with your clients and how you have positioned yourself within the community and within the fitness industry.

One of the best ways to establish yourself as a professional is to develop a reputation that is credible and respected. Your reputation will be based upon the perception of how well you work with your clients and how you have positioned yourself within the community and within the fitness industry.

PERSONAL TRAINER'S ROLE AS A TEACHER, COACH, AND EDUCATOR

Excellent communication skills are an absolute necessity to enhance your role as a Personal Trainer. Personal Trainers must be able to teach with a clear and succinct message. This book will show how you, as a Personal Trainer, can create and develop personal training sessions that have a sound educational, scientific, and practical approach. Unfortunately, there is a glut of bogus health and fitness information in the media. It is the responsibility of Personal Trainers to be able to disseminate correct and scientifically valid information and avoid fads and gimmicks that detract from professional and client success. Planning the client's training experience for the entire course of your regimen is also important to achieving the desired results. Creating a 12-week plan that is broken down into biweekly cycles and following the plan with appropriate levels of flexibility are signs of a good teacher. Motivating your client throughout the training cycle is the sign of a good coach. This process starts with effective interviewing skills that pinpoint the client's motivating factors that are driving him or her to proceed and succeed.

BEING WELL-ROUNDED—IT'S MORE THAN COUNTING REPETITIONS

A Personal Trainer who simply counts repetitions has no business in an industry that requires focus, listening, and leadership skills. From the time a personal training session starts to the time it is completed, the job of a Personal Trainer is to guide a client through a series of exercises that are designed to help that client achieve his or her stated goals. The job also requires that you inspire the client to a lifelong commitment to physical activity for health well after the personal training experience ends. To do this effectively, it is important to have interpersonal skills that will allow your client to feel comfortable and safe in the knowledge that you are committed to their success. One of the most valuable skills that a Personal Trainer can have is the ability to know when to talk and when to listen. Whether it is reviewing client goals and training him or her accordingly or laying out specific guidelines, being able to provide your client with personal attention will make you a successful Personal Trainer. The ability to ask questions that empower the client to formulate his or her own strategies for success is also a valuable skill to help the client realize that while you are creating the recipe he or she is in fact responsible for the action and discipline necessary to achieve success.

PRACTICES, STANDARDS, AND ETHICS

Part of what creates a successful and rewarding career is a clear understanding of ethical practice and standards. To run a business with integrity, you must follow clear guidelines of standards and ethics. They should be in writing and clearly understood and communicated to your clients and other members of your business team. An example of an ethical practice is a fair and honest policy for late cancellation or no-show fees by either party.

To run a business with integrity, you must follow clear guidelines of standards and ethics.

When working with a client if you are charging them for an hour of personal training, then that is what they should get: a full 60 minutes of your undivided attention. Another example is how you approach goal setting with your clients. If your client proposed an unrealistic, unhealthy, or unsafe set of goals, how do you disclose your philosophies about these goals and time frames for achievement? Another opportunity for setting good business practices comes with your policies for talking with clients about other clients and about disclosing personal health information (see Chapter 22). You should remember that although the client will want to hear about others, would they really want you talking about them in the same way? Social interactions with clients should be professional in every way. Close bonds are formed in the Personal Trainer–client relationships and should be treated like all other business relationships. It is your way to make a living and support your family. Treat your profession and business accordingly.

SUMMARY

It is an exciting time to be a part of the personal training industry. Make sure that you do your homework and assess all of the different options available to you before selecting an area of specialization. The field is vast, so take the time to explore it. Regardless of the career path you choose, it is important to take the necessary steps to position yourself for a long and successful career. The career is demanding physically and mentally. Take care of your own health by exercising regularly and eating right. Schedule breaks between clients and make time for vacations and family life. The job requires focus, personalized planning, research, continuing education, and attention to many details. At the same time it is fun and rewarding and helps give your clients a priceless reward: better health. The Personal Trainer makes a commitment to excellence in the areas of education, community–industry involvement, customer service, and time management, and embraces the highest ethical standards. If you pay close attention to each of these aspects of your career, you will find yourself in a business that is rewarding and satisfying and ultimately successful.

REFERENCES

1. Bureau of Labor Statistics, U.S. Department of Labor. Fitness workers (O*NET 39-9031.00) [Internet]. [cited 2008 Aug 21]. Available from: http://www.bls.gov/oco/pdf/ocos296.pdf

2. Bureau of Labor Statistics, U.S. Department of Labor. Occupational outlook handbook, 2008–09 ed, recreation and fitness workers. [Internet]. [cited 2008 Aug 21]. Available from: http://www.bls.gov/oco/ocos058.htm

3. Commission on Accreditation of Allied Health Education Programs. [Internet]. [cited 2008 Aug 21]. Available from: www.caahep.org

4. Cooper J, Fazio R. A new look at dissonance. *Adv Exp Psychol*. 1984;17:229–66.

5. Herbert DL, Herbert WG. Legal considerations. In: Roitman JL, Kelsey M, editors. *ACSM's Resource Manual for Guidelines for Exercise Testing and Prescription*. 3rd ed. Baltimore: Lippincott Williams & Wilkins; 1998. p. 614.

6. Klein A. *The Change-Your-Life Book*. New York: Gramercy Books; 2000. p. 116.

7. Kravitz L, Rochey C. Career growth tips for the 21st century: a resource guide to career opportunities. [Internet]. [cited 2008 Aug 21]. Available from: http://www.unm.edu/~lkravitz/Article%20folder/career.html

8. Prime Media Business Magazines and Media Inc. Club industry's fitness business pro. Purdue to offer 4-year degree in personal training. [Internet]. [cited 2008 Aug 21]. Available from: http://fitnessbusinesspro.com/news/purdue_personaltraining_092804/index.html

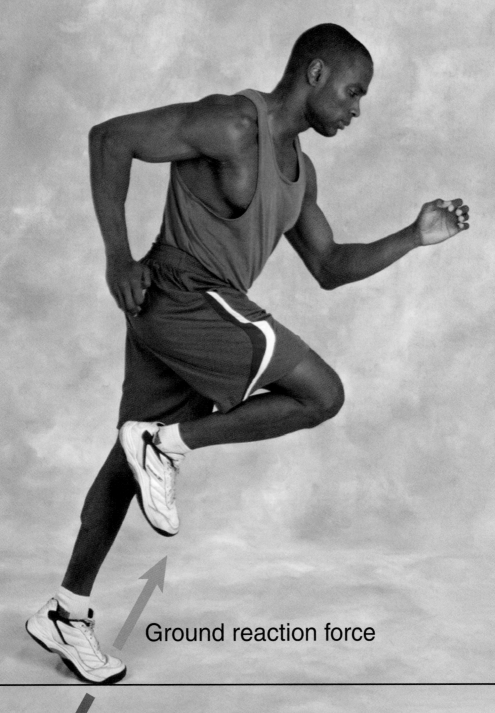

The Science of Personal Training

PART **II**

Ground reaction force

Driving action

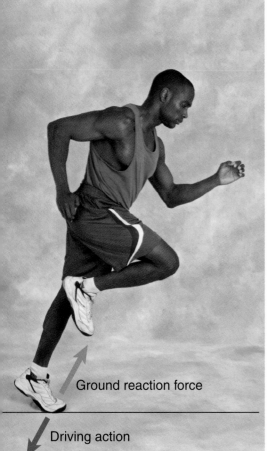

CHAPTER 3

Ground reaction force

Driving action

Anatomy and Kinesiology

OBJECTIVES

- Provide an overview of anatomical structures of the musculoskeletal system
- Explain the underlying biomechanical and kinesiological principles of musculoskeletal movement
- Identify the key terms used to describe body position and movement
- Describe the specific structures, movement patterns, range of motion, muscles, and common injuries for each major joint of the body

A major goal of exercise training is to improve cardiovascular and musculoskeletal fitness. The physiological adaptation of muscle to exercise training is evidenced by improvements in muscle strength, endurance, flexibility, and resistance to injury (12). The objective of this chapter is to gain an understanding of musculoskeletal functional anatomy of the major joint structures during exercise movements, with emphasis on body alignment and kinesiological principles. A thorough understanding of these principles is essential for the Personal Trainer to design safe, effective, and efficient exercise training programs to improve musculoskeletal fitness.

Personal Trainers teach clients how to perform exercise movements and how to use exercise or rehabilitation equipment. The disciplines primarily involved in describing and understanding human movement are biomechanics and kinesiology. Biomechanics is the study of the motion and causes of motion of living things, using a branch of physics known as mechanics (31). The study of biomechanics is essential for Personal Trainers because it forms the basis for documenting human motion (kinematics) and understanding the causes of that motion (kinetics). Chapter 4 covers this information in more detail. Kinesiology is the study of the mechanics of human movement and specifically evaluates muscles, joints, and skeletal structures and their involvement in movement (38). Kinesiology is primarily based on three fields of science—biomechanics, musculoskeletal anatomy, and neuromuscular physiology. Kinesiology includes the study of gait, posture and body alignment, ergonomics, sports and exercise movements, and activities of daily living and work. A variety of healthcare practitioners, including Personal Trainers, exercise physiologists, athletic trainers, physicians, physical educators, occupational therapists, physical therapists, chiropractors, and ergonomists, use biomechanical and kinesiological principles (4).

> *The disciplines primarily involved in describing and understanding human movement are biomechanics and kinesiology.*

DESCRIBING BODY POSITION AND JOINT MOVEMENT

Anatomical Position

Anatomical position is the universally accepted reference position used to describe regions and spatial relationships of the human body and to refer to body positions (e.g., joint motions) (18). In the anatomical position, the body is erect with feet together and the upper limbs positioned at the sides, palms of the hands facing forward, thumbs facing away from the body, and fingers extended (Fig. 3.1). Other common terms to describe anatomical spatial relationships and positions are shown in Table 3.1 (4).

Planes of Motion and Axes of Rotation

There are three basic imaginary planes that pass through the body (Fig. 3.2). The sagittal plane divides the body or structure into the right and left sides. The frontal plane (also called the coronal plane) divides the body or structure into anterior and posterior portions. The transverse plane (also called the cross-sectional, axial, or horizontal plane) divides the body or structure into superior and inferior portions (18). Activities of daily living, exercise, and sports usually involve movement in more than one plane at a given joint structure. If movement occurs in a plane, it must rotate about an axis that has a 90° relationship to that plane. Thus, movement in the sagittal plane rotates about an axis with a frontal arrangement, movement in the frontal plane rotates about an axis with a sagittal arrangement, and movement in the transverse plane rotates about an axis with a vertical arrangement (38).

Center of Gravity, Line of Gravity, and Postural Alignment

An object's center of gravity is a theoretical point where the weight force of the object can be considered to act. Center of gravity changes with movement and depends on body position. When a person is standing in a neutral position, the body's center of gravity is approximately at the second sacral

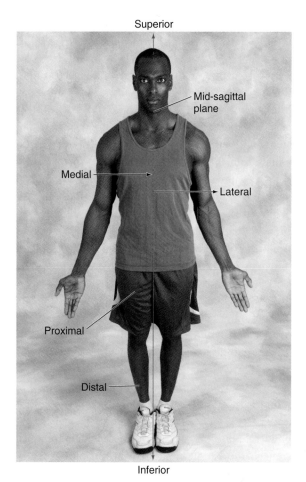

Superior

Mid-sagittal plane

Medial

Lateral

Proximal

Distal

Inferior

FIGURE 3.1. Anatomical position. Body is erect with the feet together, upper limbs hanging at the sides, palms of the hands facing anteriorly, thumbs facing laterally, and fingers extended. Typically, all anatomical references to the body are relative to this position.

TABLE 3.1	DEFINITIONS OF ANATOMICAL LOCATIONS AND POSITIONS

Term	Definition
Anterior	The front of the body; ventral
Posterior	The back of the body; dorsal
Superficial	Located close to or on the body surface
Deep	Below the surface
Proximal	Closer to any reference point
Distal	Farther from any reference point
Superior	Toward the head; higher (cephalic)
Inferior	Away from the head; lower (caudal)
Medial	Toward the midline of the body
Lateral	Away from the midline of the body; to the side
Ipsilateral	On the same side
Contralateral	On the opposite side
Unilateral	One side
Bilateral	Both sides
Prone	Lying face down
Supine	Lying face up
Valgus	Distal segment of a joint deviates laterally
Varus	Distal segment of a joint deviates medially
Arm	The region from the shoulder to elbow
Forearm	The region from the elbow to the wrist
Thigh	The region from the hip to the knee
Leg	The region from the knee to the ankle

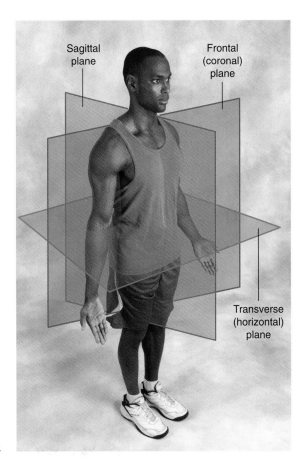

FIGURE 3.2. Anatomical planes of the body.

segment (31). The kinematics (variation in height and horizontal distance) of the center of gravity relative to the base of support (31) are often studied to examine balance exhibited by the performer. In a sit-to-stand movement, for example, the center of gravity is shifted over the base of support when there is a transition from primarily horizontal motion to a vertical or lifting motion (Fig. 3.3).

The line of gravity of the body is an imaginary vertical line passing through the center of gravity and is typically assessed while the subject is standing (18). The line of gravity helps define proper body alignment and posture, using various superficial landmarks from the head, upper extremity, trunk, and lower extremity regions as guides. From the lateral view, the line of gravity should be slightly posterior to the apex of the coronal suture, through the mastoid process, through the midcervical vertebral bodies, through the shoulder joint, through the midlumbar vertebral bodies, slightly posterior to the axis of the hip joint, slightly anterior to the axis of the knee joint, and slightly anterior to the lateral malleolus. From the posterior view, the line of gravity should pass through the midline of the body, and bilateral structures such as the mastoid, shoulder, iliac crest, knee, and ankles should be in the same horizontal plane (18) (Fig. 3.4). Personal Trainers should consider the ideal line of gravity when describing postural abnormalities.

> *The line of gravity helps define proper body alignment and posture, using various superficial landmarks from the head, upper extremity, trunk, and lower extremity regions as guides.*

Joint Movement

Joint movement is often described by its spatial movement pattern in relation to the body, typically in terms of anatomical position. Terms used to describe joint movement are listed below (18) and discussed in detail for the major joints in the next section:

➤ *Flexion:* Movement resulting in a decrease of the joint angle, usually moving anteriorly in the sagittal plane

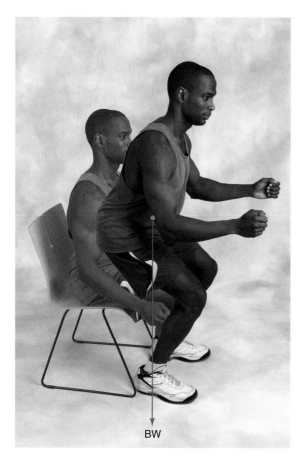

FIGURE 3.3. The initial phase of the sit-to-stand movement involves trunk lean and horizontal weight shift to position the center of gravity over the new base of support (feet). The movement of the center of gravity in several directions is often used to study balance. BW, body weight.

➤ *Extension:* Movement resulting in an increase of the joint angle, usually moving posteriorly in the sagittal plane

➤ *Abduction:* Movement away from the midline of the body, usually in the frontal plane

➤ *Adduction:* Movement toward the midline of the body, usually in the frontal plane

➤ *Horizontal abduction:* Movement away from the midline of the body in the transverse plane, usually used to describe horizontal humerus movement when the shoulder is flexed at 90°

➤ *Horizontal adduction:* Movement toward the midline of the body in the transverse plane, usually used to describe horizontal humerus movement when the shoulder is flexed at 90°

➤ *Internal (medial) rotation:* Rotation in the transverse plane toward the midline of the body

➤ *External (lateral) rotation:* Rotation in the transverse plane away from the midline of the body

➤ *Lateral flexion (right or left):* Movement away from the midline of the body in the frontal plane, usually used to describe neck and trunk movement

➤ *Rotation (right or left):* Right or left rotation in the transverse plane, usually used to describe neck and trunk movement

➤ *Elevation:* Movement of the scapula superiorly in the frontal plane

➤ *Depression:* Movement of the scapula inferiorly in the frontal plane

➤ *Retraction:* Movement of the scapula toward the spine in the transverse plane

➤ *Protraction:* Movement of the scapula away from the spine in the transverse plane

➤ *Upward rotation:* Superior and lateral movement of the inferior angle of the scapula in the frontal plane

➤ *Downward rotation:* Inferior and medial movement of the inferior angle of the scapula in the frontal plane

➤ *Circumduction:* A compound circular movement involving flexion, extension, abduction, and adduction, circumscribing a cone shape

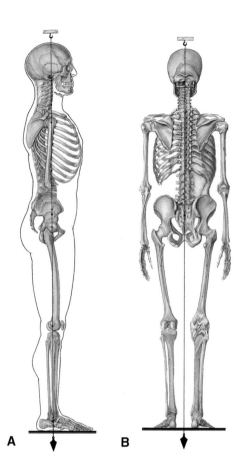

FIGURE 3.4. Line of gravity of the skeletal system. Panel A: Lateral view. Panel B: Posterior view. (Asset provided by Anatomical Chart Co.)

A   **B**

➤ *Radial deviation:* Abduction of the wrist in the frontal plane
➤ *Ulnar deviation:* Adduction of the wrist in the frontal plane
➤ *Opposition:* Diagonal movement of thumb across the palmar surface of the hand to make contact with the fifth digit
➤ *Eversion:* Abducting the ankle
➤ *Inversion:* Adducting the ankle
➤ *Dorsiflexion:* Flexing the ankle so that the foot moves anteriorly in the sagittal plane
➤ *Plantarflexion:* Extending the ankle so that the foot moves posteriorly in the sagittal plane
➤ *Pronation (foot/ankle):* Combined movements of abduction and eversion resulting in lowering of the medial margin of the foot
➤ *Supination (foot/ankle):* Combined movements of adduction and inversion resulting in raising of the medial margin of the foot

MUSCULOSKELETAL ANATOMY

The three primary anatomical structures of the musculoskeletal system that are of interest to the Personal Trainer are bones, joints, and muscles. Mechanically, the interaction of the bones, joints, and muscles determines the range of motion (ROM) of a joint, the specific movement allowed, and the force produced. This section provides an overview of these structures. For in-depth study, the reader is referred to a variety of excellent sources (1,16,28,29,33).

Mechanically, the interaction of the bones, joints, and muscles determines the range of motion of a joint, the specific movement allowed, and the force produced.

Skeletal System

The skeletal system consists of cartilage, periosteum, and bone (osseous) tissue. The bones of the skeletal system support soft tissue, protect internal organs, act as important sources of nutrients and blood constituents, and serve as rigid levers for movement. There are 206 bones in the human body, 177 of which engage in voluntary movement. The skull, vertebral column, sternum, and ribs are considered the axial skeleton; the remaining bones, in particular those of the upper and lower limbs and their respective girdles, are considered the appendicular skeleton (36). The major bones of the body are illustrated in Figure 3.5.

The structure of a bone can be explained using a typical long bone such as the humerus (the long bone of the upper arm). The main portion of a long bone or shaft is called the "diaphysis" (Fig. 3.6). The ends of the bone are called the "epiphyses" (singular is "epiphysis"). The epiphyses are covered by articular cartilage. Cartilage is a resilient, semirigid form of connective tissue that reduces the friction and absorbs some of the shock in synovial joints. The region of mature bone where the diaphysis joins each epiphysis is called the "metaphysis." In an immature bone, this region includes the epiphyseal plate, also called the "growth plate." The medullary cavity, or marrow cavity, is the space inside the diaphysis. Lining the marrow cavity is the endosteum, which contains cells necessary for bone development. The periosteum is a membrane covering the surface of bones, except at the articular surfaces. The periosteum is composed of two layers, an outer fibrous layer and an inner highly vascular layer that contains cells for the creation of new bone. The periosteum serves as a point of attachment for ligaments and tendons and is critical for bone growth, repair, and nutrition (31).

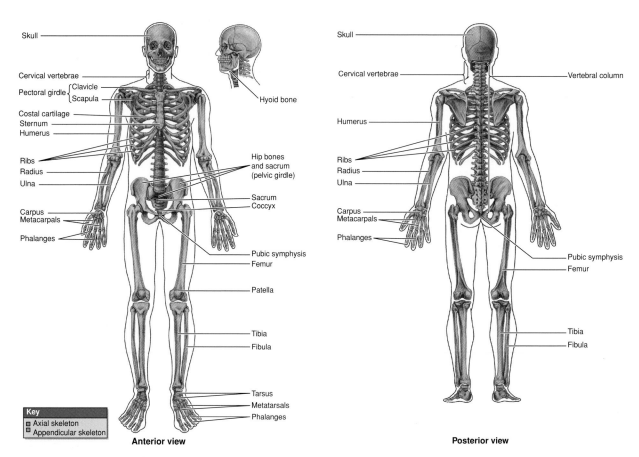

FIGURE 3.5. Divisions of the skeletal system (From Moore KL, Dalley AF II. *Clinical Oriented Anatomy*. 4th ed. Baltimore: Lippincott Williams & Wilkins; 1999.)

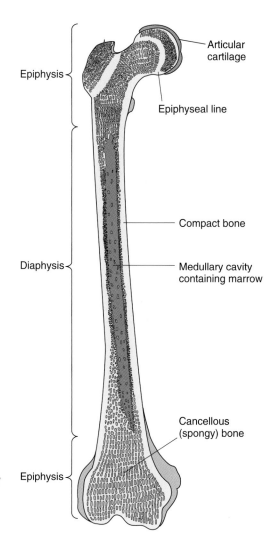

Articular
cartilage

Epiphyseal line

Compact bone

Medullary cavity
containing marrow

Cancellous
(spongy) bone

Epiphysis

Diaphysis

Epiphysis

FIGURE 3.6. Bone anatomy. (From Willis MC. *Medical Terminology: A Programmed Learning Approach to the Language of Health Care.* Baltimore: Lippincott Williams & Wilkins; 2002.)

There are two types of bones (2): compact and cancellous (spongy). The main differences between the two types are the architecture and amount of matter and space they contain. Compact bone is architecturally arranged in "osteons" that contain few spaces. It forms the external layer of all bones of the body and a large portion of the diaphysis of the long bones, where it provides support for bearing weight. In contrast, spongy bone is characterized as being much less dense. It consists of a three-dimensional lattice composed of beams or struts of bone called "trabeculae." Open spaces are present between the trabeculae, unlike in compact bone. The trabeculae are oriented to provide strength against the stresses normally encountered by the bone. In some bones, the space within these trabeculae is filled with red bone marrow, which produces blood (31).

Bones are also classified according to their shape. Long bones contain a diaphysis with a medullary canal (e.g., femur, tibia, humerus, ulna, and radius). Short bones are relatively small and thick (e.g., carpals and tarsals). Flat bones are plate-like (e.g., sternum, scapulae, ribs, and pelvis). Irregular bones are oddly shaped (e.g., vertebrae, sacrum, and coccyx). Finally, sesamoid bones are found within tendons and joint capsules and are shaped like sesame seeds (e.g., patella) (38).

Articular System

Joints are the articulations between bones, and along with bones and ligaments, they constitute the articular system. Ligaments are tough, fibrous connective tissues anchoring bone to bone. Joints are classified as synarthrodial, amphiarthrodial, or diarthrodial (synovial) (31). Synarthrodial joints (e.g., sutures of the skull) do not move appreciably. Amphiarthrodial joints move slightly and are held together by ligaments (syndesmosis; e.g., inferior tibiofibular joint) or fibrocartilage (synchondrosis; e.g., pubic symphysis). Synarthrodial and amphiarthrodial joints do not contain an articular cavity, synovial membrane, or synovial fluid (31).

SYNOVIAL JOINTS

The most common type of joint in the human body is the synovial joint. Synovial joints contain a fibrous articular capsule and an inner synovial membrane that encloses the joint cavity. Figure 3.7 illustrates a synovial joint's unique capsular arrangement. There are five distinct features of a synovial joint (31):

1. It is enclosed by a fibrous joint capsule.
2. The joint capsule encloses the joint cavity.
3. The joint cavity is lined with synovial membrane.
4. Synovial fluid occupies the joint cavity.
5. The articulating surfaces of the bones are covered with hyaline cartilage, which helps absorb shock and reduces friction.

The synovial membrane produces synovial fluid, which provides constant lubrication during movement to minimize the wearing effects of friction on the cartilaginous covering of the articulating bones (31). Ligaments sometimes reinforce synovial joints. These ligaments are either separate structures (extrinsic) or a thickening of the outer layer of the joint capsule (intrinsic). The collagen fibers of ligaments are typically arranged to counteract multidimensional stresses. Some synovial joints have other structures such as articular discs (e.g., meniscus of the knee), bursae, or fat pads. There are six major types of synovial joints classified by the shape of the articulating surfaces or types of movement allowed. Table 3.2 summarizes the joint classifications and examples in the human body. Table 3.3 summarizes the motions of the major joints and the planes in which they occur.

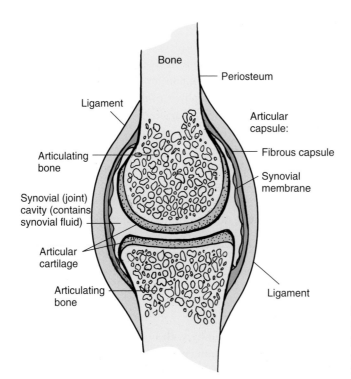

FIGURE 3.7. A synovial joint. (From Oatis CA. *Kinesiology. The Mechanics and Pathomechanics of Human Movement.* Baltimore: Lippincott Williams & Wilkins; 2003.)

TABLE 3.2   CLASSIFICATION OF JOINTS IN THE HUMAN BODY

Joint Classification	Features and Examples
Fibrous	
Suture	Tight union unique to the skull
Syndesmosis	Interosseous membrane between bone (e.g., the union along the shafts of the radius and ulna, tibia, and fibula)
Gomphosis	Unique joint at the tooth socket
Cartilaginous	
Primary (synchondroses; hyaline cartilaginous)	Usually temporary to permit bone growth and typically fuse (e.g., epiphyseal plates); some do not (e.g., at the sternum and rib [costal cartilage])
Secondary (symphyses; fibrocartilaginous)	Strong, slightly movable joints (e.g., intervertebral discs, pubic symphysis)
Synovial	
Plane (arthrodial)	Gliding and sliding movements (e.g., acromioclavicular joint)
Hinge (ginglymus)	Uniaxial movements (e.g., elbow, knee extension and flexion)
Ellipsoidal (condyloid)	Biaxial joint (e.g., radiocarpal extension, flexion at the wrist)
Saddle (sellar)	Unique joint that permits movements in all planes, including opposition (e.g., the carpometacarpal joint of the thumb)
Ball-and-socket (enarthrodial)	Multiaxial joints that permit movements in all directions (e.g., hip and shoulder joints)
Pivot (trochoidal)	Uniaxial joints that permit rotation (e.g., proximal humeroradial and atlantoaxial joints)

TABLE 3.3   MAJOR JOINT MOTIONS AND PLANES OF MOTION

Major Joints	Type of Joints	Joint Movements	Planes
Scapulothoracic	Not a true joint ("physiological" or "functional" joint)	Elevation–depression Upward–downward rotation Protraction–retraction	Frontal Frontal Transverse
Glenohumeral	Synovial: ball-and-socket	Flexion–extension Abduction–adduction Internal–external rotation Horizontal abduction–adduction Circumduction	Sagittal Frontal Transverse Transverse Multiple
Elbow	Synovial: hinge	Flexion–extension	Sagittal
Proximal radioulnar	Synovial: pivot	Pronation–supination	Transverse
Wrist	Synovial: ellipsoidal	Flexion–extension Abduction–adduction	Sagittal Frontal
Metacarpophalangeal	Synovial: ellipsoidal	Flexion–extension Abduction–adduction	Sagittal Frontal
Proximal and distal interphalangeal	Synovial: hinge	Flexion–extension	Sagittal
Intervertebral	Cartilaginous	Flexion–extension Lateral flexion Rotation	Sagittal Frontal Transverse
Hip	Synovial: ball-and-socket	Flexion–extension Abduction–adduction Internal–external rotation Circumduction	Sagittal Frontal Transverse Multiple
Knee	Synovial: hinge	Flexion–extension	Sagittal
Ankle: talocrural	Synovial: hinge	Dorsiflexion–plantarflexion	Sagittal
Ankle: subtalar	Synovial: gliding	Inversion–eversion	Frontal

Synovial joints are typically perfused by numerous arterial branches and are innervated by branches of the nerves supplying the adjacent muscle and overlying skin. Proprioceptive feedback is a significant joint sensation, as is pain, because of the high density of sensory fibers in the joint capsule. This feedback has obvious importance in regulating human movement and preventing injury (31).

JOINT MOVEMENTS AND RANGE OF MOTION

Joint movement is a combination of rolling, sliding, and spinning of the joint surfaces (4). "Open chain" movements occur when the distal segment of a joint moves in space. An example of an open chain movement for the knee joint is leg extension exercise on a machine. "Closed chain" movements occur when the distal segment of the joint is fixed in space. An example of a closed chain movement for the knee joint is standing barbell squats. A joint is in a "closed pack" position when there is both maximal congruency of the joint surfaces and maximal tautness of the joint capsule and ligaments (4). A joint is in an "open pack" (loose) position when there is the least joint congruency and the joint capsule and ligaments are most loose. Movement at one joint may influence the extent of movement at adjacent joints because a number of muscles and other soft tissue structures cross multiple joints. For example, finger flexion decreases in the presence of wrist flexion because muscles that flex both the wrist and fingers cross multiple joints (4).

> *"Open chain" movements occur when the distal segment of a joint moves in space.*
> *"Closed chain" movements occur when the distal segment of the joint is fixed in space.*

The degree of movement within a joint is called the ROM. It can be active (the range that can be reached by voluntary movement from contraction of skeletal muscle) or passive (the ROM that can be achieved by external means). Joints with excessive ROM are called "hypermobile," and joints with restricted ROM are called "hypomobile" (4). Joint ROM is quantified using goniometers or inclinometers, and each joint has normal ROM values for reference purposes (18). ROM measures at baseline help guide the exercise prescription, and ROM measures at follow-up help document progress.

JOINT STABILITY

The stability of a joint is its resistance to displacement. All joints do not have the same degree of stability, and in general, ROM is gained at the expense of stability. Five factors account for joint stability (4):

1. Ligaments check normal movement and resist excessive movement.
2. Muscles and tendons that span a joint also enhance stability, particularly when the bony structure alone contributes little stability (e.g., shoulder).
3. Fascia contributes to joint stability (e.g., iliotibial band of the tensor fasciae latae).
4. Atmospheric pressure creates greater force outside of the joint than internal pressure exerts within the joint cavity (the suction created by this pressure is an important factor in aiding joint stability).
5. The bony structure of a joint is an important contributor to joint stability (e.g., limitation of elbow extension by the olecranon process of the ulna) (4).

Muscular System

Bones provide support and leverage to the body, but without muscles, movement would not be possible. There are three types of muscle tissue: skeletal, cardiac, and smooth muscle. Skeletal muscle is primarily attached to bones and is under voluntary control. Skeletal muscle is responsible for moving the skeletal system and stabilizing the body (e.g., maintaining posture). There are more than 600 skeletal muscles in the human body (38), approximately 100 of which are primary movement muscles with which Personal Trainers should be familiar (4). The superficial muscles of the body are shown in Figures 3.8 and 3.9.

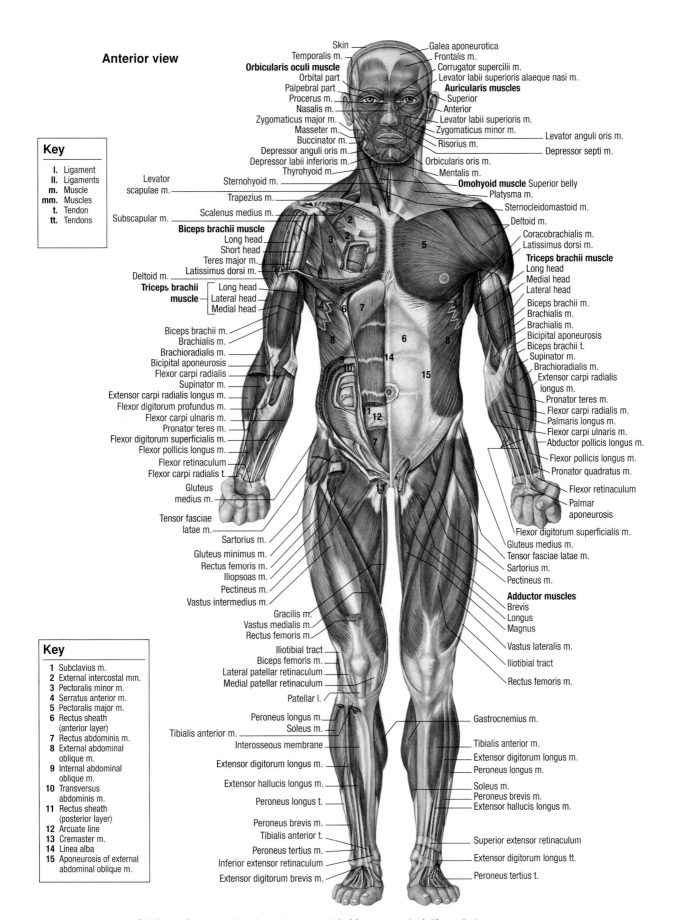

Anterior view

Skin
Temporalis m.
Orbicularis oculi muscle
Orbital part
Palpebral part
Procerus m.
Nasalis m.
Zygomaticus major m.
Masseter m.
Buccinator m.
Depressor anguli oris m.
Depressor labii inferioris m.
Thyrohyoid m.

Galea aponeurotica
Frontalis m.
Corrugator supercilii m.
Levator labii superioris alaeque nasi m.
Auricularis muscles
Superior
Anterior
Levator labii superioris m.
Zygomaticus minor m.
Risorius m.
Orbicularis oris m.
Mentalis m.

Levator anguli oris m.
Depressor septi m.

Levator scapulae m.
Sternohyoid m.
Trapezius m.
Scalenus medius m.
Subscapular m.

Omohyoid muscle Superior belly
Platysma m.
Sternocleidomastoid m.
Deltoid m.

Biceps brachii muscle
Long head
Short head
Teres major m.
Latissimus dorsi m.
Deltoid m.
Triceps brachii muscle
Long head
Lateral head
Medial head

Coracobrachialis m.
Latissimus dorsi m.
Triceps brachii muscle
Long head
Medial head
Lateral head
Biceps brachii m.
Brachialis m.
Brachialis m.
Bicipital aponeurosis
Biceps brachii t.
Supinator m.
Brachioradialis m.
Extensor carpi radialis longus m.
Pronator teres m.
Flexor carpi radialis m.
Palmaris longus m.
Flexor carpi ulnaris m.
Abductor pollicis longus m.
Flexor pollicis longus m.
Pronator quadratus m.
Flexor retinaculum
Palmar aponeurosis
Flexor digitorum superficialis m.
Gluteus medius m.
Tensor fasciae latae m.
Sartorius m.
Pectineus m.
Adductor muscles
Brevis
Longus
Magnus
Vastus lateralis m.
Iliotibial tract
Rectus femoris m.

Biceps brachii m.
Brachialis m.
Brachioradialis m.
Bicipital aponeurosis
Flexor carpi radialis
Supinator m.
Extensor carpi radialis longus m.
Flexor digitorum profundus m.
Flexor carpi ulnaris m.
Pronator teres m.
Flexor digitorum superficialis m.
Flexor pollicis longus m.
Flexor retinaculum
Flexor carpi radialis t.
Gluteus medius m.
Tensor fasciae latae m.
Sartorius m.
Gluteus minimus m.
Rectus femoris m.
Iliopsoas m.
Pectineus m.
Vastus intermedius m.

Gracilis m.
Vastus medialis m.
Rectus femoris m.
Iliotibial tract
Biceps femoris m.
Lateral patellar retinaculum
Medial patellar retinaculum
Patellar l.
Peroneus longus m.
Tibialis anterior m.
Interosseous membrane
Extensor digitorum longus m.
Extensor hallucis longus m.
Peroneus longus t.
Peroneus brevis m.
Tibialis anterior t.
Peroneus tertius m.
Inferior extensor retinaculum
Extensor digitorum brevis m.

Soleus m.
Gastrocnemius m.
Tibialis anterior m.
Extensor digitorum longus m.
Peroneus longus m.
Soleus m.
Peroneus brevis m.
Extensor hallucis longus m.
Superior extensor retinaculum
Extensor digitorum longus tt.
Peroneus tertius t.

Key

I.	Ligament
II.	Ligaments
m.	Muscle
mm.	Muscles
t.	Tendon
tt.	Tendons

Key

1 Subclavius m.
2 External intercostal mm.
3 Pectoralis minor m.
4 Serratus anterior m.
5 Pectoralis major m.
6 Rectus sheath (anterior layer)
7 Rectus abdominis m.
8 External abdominal oblique m.
9 Internal abdominal oblique m.
10 Transversus abdominis m.
11 Rectus sheath (posterior layer)
12 Arcuate line
13 Cremaster m.
14 Linea alba
15 Aponeurosis of external abdominal oblique m.

FIGURE 3.8. Superficial muscles—anterior view. (Asset provided by Anatomical Chart Co.)

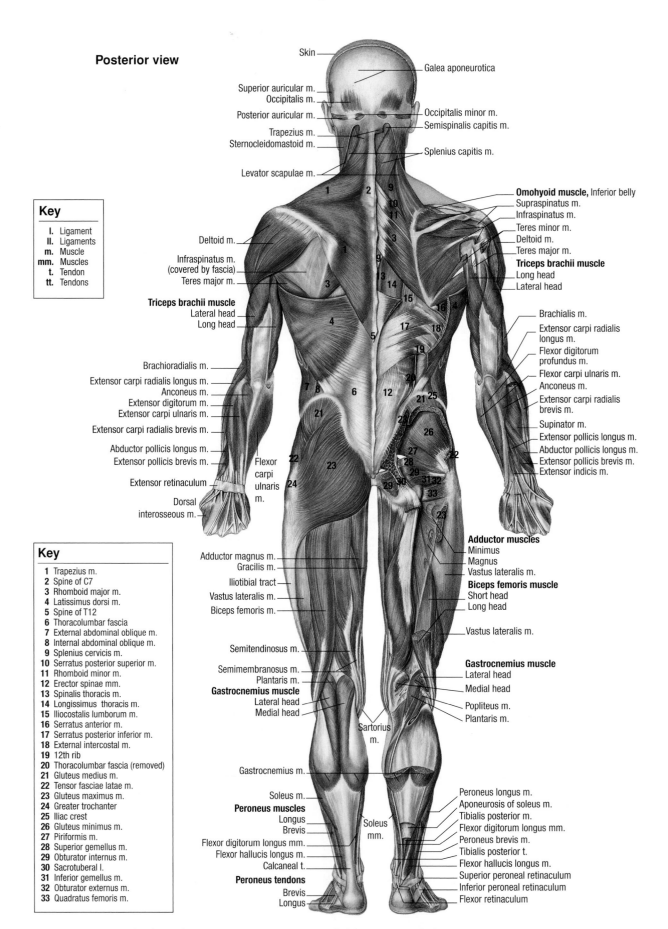

Posterior view

Skin

Galea aponeurotica

Superior auricular m.
Occipitalis m.
Posterior auricular m.
Trapezius m.
Sternocleidomastoid m.
Levator scapulae m.

Occipitalis minor m.
Semispinalis capitis m.
Splenius capitis m.

Omohyoid muscle, Inferior belly
Supraspinatus m.
Infraspinatus m.
Teres minor m.
Deltoid m.
Teres major m.
Triceps brachii muscle
Long head
Lateral head

Deltoid m.
Infraspinatus m.
(covered by fascia)
Teres major m.
Triceps brachii muscle
Lateral head
Long head

Brachialis m.
Extensor carpi radialis
longus m.
Flexor digitorum
profundus m.
Flexor carpi ulnaris m.
Anconeus m.
Extensor carpi radialis
brevis m.
Supinator m.
Extensor pollicis longus m.
Abductor pollicis longus m.
Extensor pollicis brevis m.
Extensor indicis m.

Brachioradialis m.
Extensor carpi radialis longus m.
Anconeus m.
Extensor digitorum m.
Extensor carpi ulnaris m.
Extensor carpi radialis brevis m.
Abductor pollicis longus m.
Extensor pollicis brevis m.
Extensor retinaculum
Dorsal
interosseous m.

Flexor
carpi
ulnaris
m.

Key

I. Ligament
II. Ligaments
m. Muscle
mm. Muscles
t. Tendon
tt. Tendons

Key

1 Trapezius m.
2 Spine of C7
3 Rhomboid major m.
4 Latissimus dorsi m.
5 Spine of T12
6 Thoracolumbar fascia
7 External abdominal oblique m.
8 Internal abdominal oblique m.
9 Splenius cervicis m.
10 Serratus posterior superior m.
11 Rhomboid minor m.
12 Erector spinae mm.
13 Spinalis thoracis m.
14 Longissimus thoracis m.
15 Iliocostalis lumborum m.
16 Serratus anterior m.
17 Serratus posterior inferior m.
18 External intercostal m.
19 12th rib
20 Thoracolumbar fascia (removed)
21 Gluteus medius m.
22 Tensor fasciae latae m.
23 Gluteus maximus m.
24 Greater trochanter
25 Iliac crest
26 Gluteus minimus m.
27 Piriformis m.
28 Superior gemellus m.
29 Obturator internus m.
30 Sacrotuberal l.
31 Inferior gemellus m.
32 Obturator externus m.
33 Quadratus femoris m.

Adductor muscles
Minimus
Magnus
Vastus lateralis m.
Biceps femoris muscle
Short head
Long head

Vastus lateralis m.

Adductor magnus m.
Gracilis m.
Iliotibial tract
Vastus lateralis m.
Biceps femoris m.

Semitendinosus m.
Semimembranosus m.
Plantaris m.
Gastrocnemius muscle
Lateral head
Medial head

Sartorius
m.

Gastrocnemius muscle
Lateral head
Medial head
Popliteus m.
Plantaris m.

Gastrocnemius m.

Soleus m.
Peroneus muscles
Longus
Brevis
Flexor digitorum longus mm.
Flexor hallucis longus m.
Calcaneal t.
Peroneus tendons
Brevis
Longus

Soleus
mm.

Peroneus longus m.
Aponeurosis of soleus m.
Tibialis posterior m.
Flexor digitorum longus mm.
Peroneus brevis m.
Tibialis posterior t.
Flexor hallucis longus m.
Superior peroneal retinaculum
Inferior peroneal retinaculum
Flexor retinaculum

FIGURE 3.9. Superficial muscles—posterior view. (Asset provided by Anatomical Chart Co.)

Skeletal muscles are generally anchored to the skeleton by tendons. Tendons are dense cords of connective tissue that attach a muscle to the periosteum of the bone. The collagen fibers of tendons are in parallel arrangement, which makes the tendon suitable for unidirectional stress. When the tendon is flat and broad, it is called an "aponeurosis." Tendons and aponeuroses provide the mechanical link between skeletal muscle and bone. Bursae are often positioned between tendons and bony prominences to allow the tendons to slide easily across the bones (31).

CLASSIFICATION OF SKELETAL MUSCLES

Skeletal muscles can be classified according to their muscle fiber architecture (i.e., the arrangement of muscle fiber relative to the line of pull of the muscle) (Fig. 3.10). Muscles typically have either a parallel arrangement or a pennate arrangement. In parallel muscle, the muscle fibers run in line with the pull of the muscle. Fusiform muscles have a parallel arrangement and are spindle shaped, tapering at each end (e.g., biceps brachii). Longitudinal muscles are strap-like, with parallel fibers (e.g., sartorius). Quadrate muscles are four-sided, are usually flat, and consist of parallel fibers (e.g., rhomboids). Fan-shaped or triangular muscles contain fibers that radiate from a narrow attachment at one end to a broad attachment at the other (e.g., pectoralis major) (38).

In pennate muscle, the fibers run obliquely or at an angle to the line of pull. Pennate muscles can be classified as unipennate (fibers only on one side of the tendon; e.g., flexor pollicis longus), bipennate (fibers on both sides of a centrally positioned tendon; e.g., rectus femoris), or multipennate (two or more fasciculi attaching obliquely and combined into one muscle; e.g., subscapularis) (38).

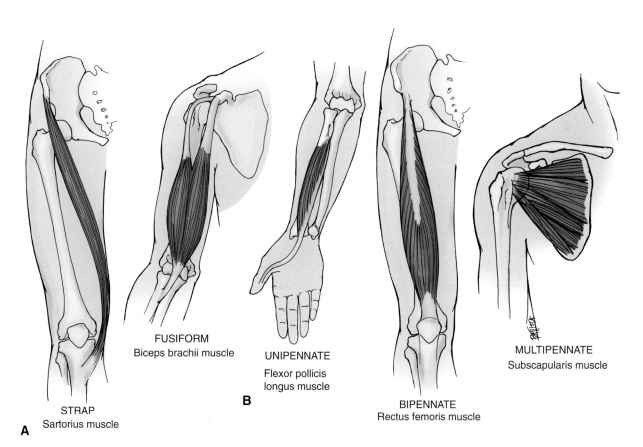

FUSIFORM
Biceps brachii muscle

UNIPENNATE
Flexor pollicis
longus muscle

B

MULTIPENNATE
Subscapularis muscle

BIPENNATE
Rectus femoris muscle

STRAP
Sartorius muscle

A

FIGURE 3.10. Skeletal muscle architecture **(A)** and shape **(B)**. (From Oatis CA. *Kinesiology. The Mechanics and Pathomechanics of Human Movement*. Baltimore: Lippincott Williams & Wilkins; 2003.)

Muscles can also be described on the basis of the number of joints upon which they act. For example, a muscle that causes movement at one joint is uniarticular (e.g., brachialis). Muscles that cross more than one joint are referred to as biarticular (having actions at two joints, e.g., hamstring muscles and biceps brachii) or multiarticular (e.g., erector spinae). The main advantage of bi- and multiarticular muscles is that only one muscle is needed to generate tension in two or more joints. This is more efficient and conserves energy. In many instances, the length of the muscle stays within 100%–130% of the resting length. As one side of the muscle shortens, the other side lengthens, maintaining a near constant overall length. This property of bi- and multiarticular muscles enhances tension production (4).

HOW MUSCLES PRODUCE MOVEMENT

Skeletal muscles produce force that is transferred to the tendons, which in turn pull on the bones and other structures, such as the skin. Most muscles cross a joint, so when a muscle contracts, it pulls one of the articulating bones toward the other. Usually, both articulating bones do not move equally; one of the articulating bones remains relatively stationary. The attachment that is usually more stationary and proximal (especially in the extremities) is called the "origin." The muscle attachment located on the bone that moves more and is usually located more distally is called the "insertion" (4).

> *Skeletal muscles produce force that is transferred to the tendons, which in turn pull on the bones and other structures, such as the skin.*

Muscle Roles

Movements of the human body generally require several muscles working together rather than a single muscle doing all the work. Keep in mind that muscles cannot push, they can only pull; therefore, most skeletal muscles are arranged in opposing pairs such as flexor–extensor, internal–external rotator, and abductor–adductor. Muscles can be classified according to their roles during movement (38). When a muscle or a group of muscles is responsible for the action or movement, it is called a "prime mover" or "agonist." For example, during a biceps curl, the prime movers are the elbow flexors, which include the biceps brachii, brachialis, and brachioradialis muscles. The opposing group of muscles is called the antagonist (e.g., the triceps brachii and anconeus muscles in biceps curl). Antagonists relax to permit the primary movement and contract to act as a brake at the completion of the movement. In addition, most movements also involve other muscles called "synergists." The role of synergists is to prevent unwanted movement, which helps the prime movers perform more efficiently. Synergists can also act as fixators or stabilizers. In this role, the muscles stabilize a portion of the body against a force (38). For example, the scapular muscles (e.g., rhomboids, serratus anterior, and trapezius) must provide a stable base of support for the upper extremity muscles during the throwing motion. Co-contraction is the simultaneous contraction of the agonist and antagonist. Co-contraction of the abdominal and lumbar muscles, for example, helps stabilize the lower trunk during trunk movements (25).

SPECIFIC JOINT STRUCTURES

Muscle actions produce force that causes joint movement during exercise. Personal Trainers need a solid working knowledge of the functional anatomy and kinesiology of major joint structures. Tables 3.4 and 3.5 summarize the major joint movements, muscles that produce those movements, normal ROM values, and example resistance exercises for the muscles. This knowledge is the basis for the development of exercise programs to be used in training (8). In this section, we describe the structure and function of each of the major joints of the body in four steps:

1. *Structure:* What are the initial considerations of the joint's structure (e.g., bones, muscles, tendons, ligaments, cartilage, bursae) and ability to move?

TABLE 3.4 — MAJOR UPPER EXTREMITY JOINTS: MOVEMENTS, RANGE OF MOTION, MUSCLES, AND EXAMPLE RESISTANCE EXERCISES

Joint	Movement	Range of Motion (°)	Major Agonist Muscles	Examples of Resistance Exercises
Scapulothoracic	Fixation		Serratus anterior, pectoralis minor, trapezius, levator scapulae, rhomboids	Push-up, parallel bar dip, upright row, shoulder shrug, seated row
	Upward rotation		Trapezius	
	Downward rotation		Rhomboids, pectoralis minor, levator scapulae	
	Elevation		Rhomboids, levator scapulae, trapezius	Shoulder shrug
	Depression		Pectoralis minor, trapezius	
	Protraction		Serratus anterior, pectoralis minor	Supine dumbbell serratus press, push-up
	Retraction		Rhomboids, trapezius	Seated row
Glenohumeral (shoulder)	Flexion	90–100	Anterior deltoid, pectoralis major (clavicular head), Biceps brachii (long head)	Dumbbell front raise, incline bench press
	Extension	40–60	Latissimus dorsi, teres major, pectoralis major (sternocostal head)	Dumbbell pullover, chin-up
	Abduction	90–95	Middle deltoid, supraspinatus	Dumbbell lateral raise, dumbbell press
	Adduction	0	Latissimus dorsi, teres major, pectoralis major	Lat pull-down, seated row, cable crossover, flat bench dumbbell fly
	Horizontal abduction	45	Posterior deltoid, teres major, latissimus dorsi	Prone reverse dumbbell fly, reverse cable fly
	Horizontal adduction	135	Pectoralis major, pectoralis minor, anterior deltoid	Flat bench chest fly, pec dec, cable crossover
	Internal rotation	70–90	Latissimus dorsi, teres major, subscapularis, pectoralis major, anterior deltoid	Lat pull-down, bent over row, dumbbell row, rotator cuff exercises, dumbbell press, parallel bar dip, front raises
	External rotation	70–90	Infraspinatus, teres minor, posterior deltoid	External rotator cuff exercises—dumbbell side-lying, cable in, rotator cuff exercises—dumbbell side-lying, cable
Elbow	Flexion	145–150	Biceps brachii, brachialis, brachioradialis	Dumbbell curl, preacher curl, hammer curl
	Extension	0	Triceps brachii, anconeus	Dip, pulley triceps extension, close grip bench press, push-downs, dumbbell kickback
Radioulnar	Supination	80–90	Biceps brachii, supinator	Dumbbell curl (with supination)
	Pronation	70–90	Pronator quadratus, pronator teres	Dumbbell pronation
Wrist	Flexion	70–90	Flexor carpi radialis and ulnaris, palmaris longus, flexor digitorum superficialis	Dumbbell wrist curl
	Extension	65–85	Extensor carpi radialis longus, brevis, and ulnaris, extensor digitorum longus	Dumbbell reverse wrist curl
	Adduction	25–40	Flexor and extensor carpi ulnaris	Wrist curl, reverse wrist curl
	Abduction	15–25	Extensor carpi radialis longus and brevis, flexor carpi radialis	Wrist curl, reverse wrist curl

TABLE 3.5 **MAJOR SPINE AND LOWER EXTREMITY JOINTS: MOVEMENTS, RANGE OF MOTION, MUSCLES, AND EXAMPLE RESISTANCE EXERCISES**

Joint	Movement	Range of Motion (°)	Major Agonist Muscles	Examples of Resistance Exercises
Cervical spine	Flexion	50	Sternocleidomastoid, anterior scalene, longus capitis/colli	Machine neck flexion
	Extension	60	Suboccipitals, splenius capitus/cervicus, erector spinae	Machine neck extension
	Lateral flexion	45	Unilateral contraction of flexor–extensor muscles above	Machine neck lateral flexion
	Rotation	80	Unilateral contraction of flexor–extensor muscles above	Machine neck rotation
Lumbar spine	Flexion	60	Rectus abdominis, internal/external oblique abdominus	Crunch, leg raise, machine crunch, high pulley crunch
	Extension	25	Erector spinae, multifidus	Roman chair, machine trunk extension, dead lift, squat, good morning
	Lateral flexion	25	Quadratus lumborum, internal/external oblique abdominals, unilateral erector spinae	Roman chair side bend, dumbbell side bend, hanging leg raise
	Rotation		Internal/external oblique abdominals, intrinsic spinal rotators, multifidus	Broomstick twist, machine trunk rotation
Hip	Flexion	130	Iliopsoas, rectus femoris, sartorius, pectineus, tensor fascia latae	Leg raise, sit-up, machine crunch
	Extension	30	Gluteus maximus, hamstrings	Squat, leg press, lunge, machine leg extension
	Abduction	35	Tensor fascia latae, sartorius, gluteus medius and minimus	Cable or machine hip abduction
	Adduction	30	Adductor longus, brevis, and magnus, gracilis, and pectineus	Power squats, cable or machine hip adduction, lunge
	Internal rotation	45	Semitendinosus, semimembranosus, gluteus medius and minimus, tensor fascia latae	
	External rotation	50	Biceps femoris, sartorius, gluteus maximus, deep rotators (piriformis, superior and inferior gemelli, internal and external obturators, quadrates femoris)	
Knee	Flexion	140	Hamstrings, gracilis, sartorius, popliteus, gastrocnemius	Leg curl (standing, seated, prone)
	Extension	0–10	Quadriceps femoris	Lunge, squats, machine leg extension
	Internal rotation	30	Gracilis, semimembranosus, semitendinosus	
	External rotation	45	Biceps femoris	
Ankle: talocrural	Dorsiflexion	15–20	Tibialis anterior, extensor digitorum longus, extensor hallucis longus	Ankle dorsiflexion resistance band
	Plantarflexion	50	Gastrocnemius, soleus, tibialis posterior, flexor digitorum longus, flexor hallucis longus	Standing/seated calf raise, donkey calf raise
Ankle: subtalar	Eversion	5–15	Peroneus longus and brevis	Elastic band eversion
	Inversion	20–30	Tibialis anterior and posterior	Elastic band inversion

2. *Movements:* What movements occur at the joint? What are the normal ROMs for each movement?

3. *Muscles:* What specific muscles are being used to create the movements? How are the muscles being used (e.g., agonist, synergist, stabilizer)?

4. *Injuries:* What common injuries occur to the joint structure?

Upper Extremity

SHOULDER

The shoulder complex is a multijoint structure that provides the link between the thoracic cage and upper extremity. The shoulder has a high degree of mobility; as a result, the shoulder region is very unstable. Because the bony structures of the shoulder provide relatively little support, much of the responsibility for stabilizing this region falls on the soft tissues—the muscles, ligaments, and joint capsules. The shoulder is more likely to be injured than the hip, a ball-and-socket joint (3).

> *The shoulder has a high degree of mobility; as a result, the shoulder region is very unstable.*

Bones. The bones of the shoulder region include the humerus, scapula, and clavicle (Fig. 3.10). The humerus is a long bone and is the major bone of the arm. The humeral head is rounded and articulates with the glenoid fossa of the scapula. The greater and lesser tubercles of the humerus are attachment sites for many of the muscles that act on the shoulder. The scapula is a large triangular bone that rests on the posterior thoracic cage between the second rib and the seventh rib in the normal position. The scapula lies in the scaption plane, that is, obliquely at 30° to the frontal plane. The glenoid fossa of the scapula faces anterolaterally. The acromion process is located at the superior aspect of the scapula and articulates with the clavicle. The clavicle runs obliquely at 60° to the scapula and provides the link between the upper extremity and the axial skeleton. The clavicle provides protection for the neural bundle called the "brachial plexus," the vascular system supporting the upper extremity; supports the weight of the humerus; and helps maintain the position of the scapula and the humerus (36).

Ligaments and Bursae. The ligaments and bursae of the shoulder region are shown in Figure 3.11, and some of these structures are discussed in this section. The coracohumeral ligament spans

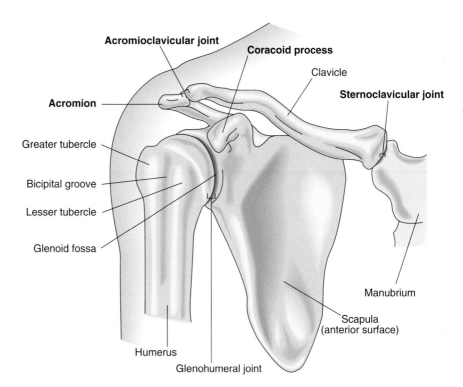

FIGURE 3.11. Ligaments and bursae of the shoulder region—anterior view. (From Hendrickson T. *Massage for Orthopaedic Conditions.* Baltimore: Lippincott Williams & Wilkins; 2002.)

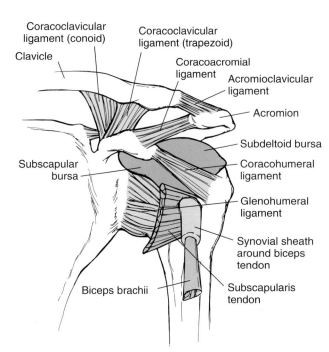

FIGURE 3.12. Bones and articulations of the shoulder region—anterior view. (From Bickley LS, Szilagyi P. *Bates' Guide to Physical Examination and History Taking.* 8th ed. Philadelphia: Lippincott Williams & Wilkins; 2003.)

the bicipital groove of the humerus and provides anteroinferior stability to the glenohumeral joint. The glenohumeral ligament (anterior, middle, and anteroinferior bands) reinforces the anterior capsule and provides stability to the shoulder joint in most planes of movement. The coracoacromial ligament, located superior to the glenohumeral joint, protects the muscles, tendons, nerves, and blood supply of the region and prevents superior dislocation of the humeral head. The acromioclavicular ligament is the major ligament that provides stability to the acromioclavicular joint. The coracoclavicular ligament (trapezoid and conoid bands) prevents superior dislocation of the acromioclavicular joint. The sternoclavicular ligaments (anterior and posterior) help strengthen the capsule of the sternoclavicular joint. The costoclavicular ligament connects the first rib and clavicle, and the interclavicular ligament connects the two clavicles and manubrium. The subacromial (subdeltoid) bursa, which lies between the supraspinatus and deltoid tendons and the acromion, allows gliding and cushioning of these structures, especially upon shoulder abduction (4).

Joints. The shoulder region is a complex of four joints: the glenohumeral (shoulder), acromioclavicular, sternoclavicular, and scapulothoracic joints (see Fig. 3.12). The glenohumeral joint is a ball-and-socket joint and is the most freely moveable joint in the body. It consists of the articulation of the spherical head of the humerus with the small, shallow, and somewhat pear-shaped glenoid fossa of the scapula. The glenoid labrum (which is composed of fibrocartilage) of the scapula deepens the fossa and cushions against impact of the humeral head in forceful movements (4) (Fig. 3.13).

The acromioclavicular joint is a plane synovial joint of the articulation of the acromion and the distal end of the clavicle. The acromioclavicular joint moves in three planes simultaneously with scapulothoracic motion. The sternoclavicular joint, the articulation of the proximal clavicle with the sternum and cartilage of the first rib, is a saddle synovial joint. The sternoclavicular joint moves in synchronization with the other three joints of the shoulder region and, importantly, provides the only bony connection between the humerus and the axial skeleton (38).

The scapulothoracic joint is not a true joint, but a physiological ("functional") joint. It is formed by the articulation of the scapula with the thoracic cage. In the kinematic chain, any movement of the scapulothoracic joint results in movement of the acromioclavicular, sternoclavicular, and glenohumeral joints. The scapulothoracic joint provides mobility and stability for the orientation of the glenoid fossa and the humeral head for arm movements in all planes (31).

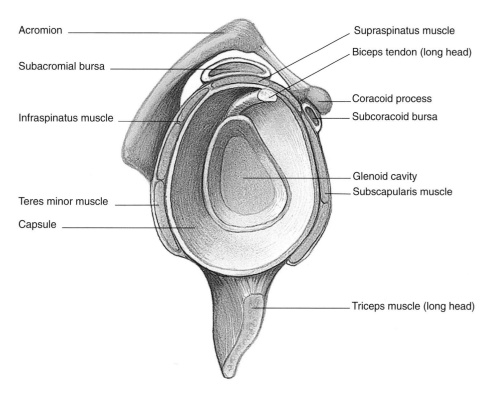

Acromion

Subacromial bursa

Infraspinatus muscle

Teres minor muscle

Capsule

Supraspinatus muscle

Biceps tendon (long head)

Coracoid process

Subcoracoid bursa

Glenoid cavity

Subscapularis muscle

Triceps muscle (long head)

FIGURE 3.13. Shoulder joint socket. (Asset provided by Anatomical Chart Co.)

Movements. Because the glenohumeral joint is a ball-and-socket joint, it is capable of motion in three planes: abduction–adduction in the frontal plane, flexion–extension in the sagittal plane, and internal–external rotation and horizontal abduction–adduction in the transverse plane. Furthermore, the multiplanar movement of circumduction is possible at the glenohumeral joint (38). Glenohumeral movements are demonstrated in Figure 3.14, and normal ROM values are listed in Table 3.4.

The center of rotation of the glenohumeral joint occurs at the humeral head within the glenoid fossa. At 0°–50° of abduction, the lower portion of the humeral head is in contact with the glenoid fossa, while at 50°–90° of abduction, the upper portion of the humeral head is in contact with the glenoid fossa. Because shear force creates friction across surfaces, the rolling of the humeral head within the glenoid reduces stress on the joint (4).

The scapulothoracic joint is also capable of motion in three planes. These motions include upward–downward rotation, retraction–protraction, elevation–depression, anterior–posterior tilting, and winging (4). Scapulothoracic joint movements are shown in Figure 3.15.

Scapulohumeral Rhythm. Full abduction of the arm requires simultaneous movement of the glenohumeral and scapulothoracic joints. This dual movement is called "scapulohumeral rhythm" (Fig. 3.16). Scapulohumeral rhythm allows a greater abduction ROM, maintains optimal length–tension relationships of the glenohumeral muscles, and prevents impingement between the greater tubercle of the humerus and the acromion. At about 120° of abduction, the greater tubercle of the humerus hits the lateral edge of the acromion. Lateral rotation of the scapula in the frontal plane causes the glenoid fossa of the scapula to face upward, making further elevation of the arm above the head possible (32). Overall, for every 3° of abduction of the arm, 2° of abduction occurs at the glenohumeral joint and 1° of rotation occurs at the scapula (37).

Muscles. The numerous muscles of the shoulder region are typically characterized as either shoulder joint muscles or shoulder girdle muscles. The shoulder joint and shoulder girdle muscles work together to perform upper extremity movements. The shoulder joint muscles directly move the arm,

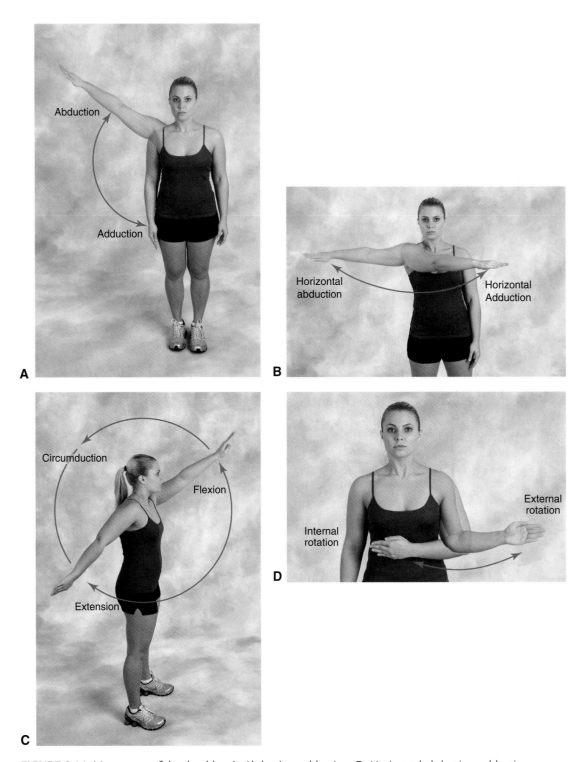

FIGURE 3.14. Movements of the shoulder. **A.** Abduction–adduction. **B.** Horizontal abduction–adduction. **C.** Flexion–extension and circumduction. **D.** Internal–external rotation.

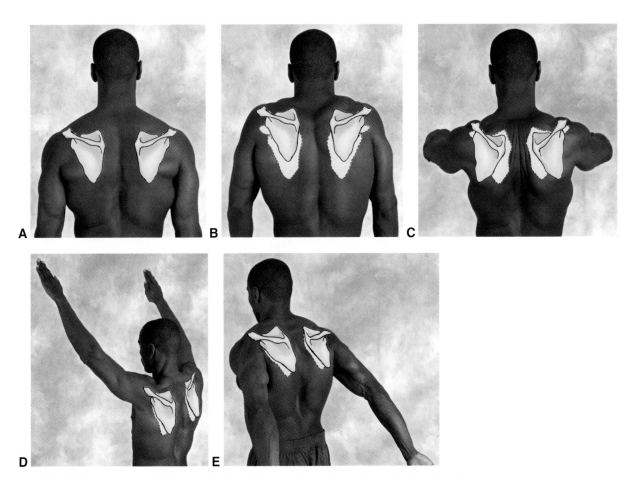

FIGURE 3.15. Movements of the scapulothoracic joint. **A.** Starting position. **B.** Elevation–depression. **C.** Protraction–retraction. **D.** Internal–external rotation. **E.** Anterior–posterior tilt.

whereas the shoulder girdle muscles mainly stabilize the scapula on the thoracic cage and are particularly important in maintaining proper posture (38). The muscles of the shoulder region are shown in Figures 3.17 and 3.18.

Shoulder Joint. The anterior muscles of the shoulder joint are the pectoralis major, subscapularis, coracobrachialis, and biceps brachii. The posterior muscles of the shoulder joint are the infraspinatus and teres minor. The superior muscles are the deltoid and supraspinatus, and the inferior muscles include the latissimus dorsi, teres major, and long head of the triceps brachii. The pectoralis major is a large and powerful muscle that is a prime mover in adduction, horizontal adduction, and internal rotation of the humerus. The pectoralis major is triangular, originating along the medial clavicle and sternum and attaching to the intertubercular groove of the humerus. The clavicular portion of the muscle primarily flexes the humerus, whereas the sternocostal portion extends the humerus from a flexed position (4). The coracobrachialis, a small muscle, assists with shoulder flexion and adduction. The biceps brachii is a two-joint, two-head muscle that crosses the shoulder and elbow. At the shoulder, the long head of the biceps brachii assists with horizontal adduction, flexion, and internal rotation (4). Its primary functions and anatomical considerations are discussed in the "Elbow" section of this chapter.

The deltoid muscle has three heads: anterior, middle, and posterior. All heads insert at the deltoid tuberosity on the lateral humerus. The anterior deltoid originates from the anterolateral aspect of the clavicle. It is chiefly responsible for shoulder flexion, horizontal adduction, and internal rotation of the glenohumeral joint. The middle deltoid originates from the lateral aspect of the acromion and

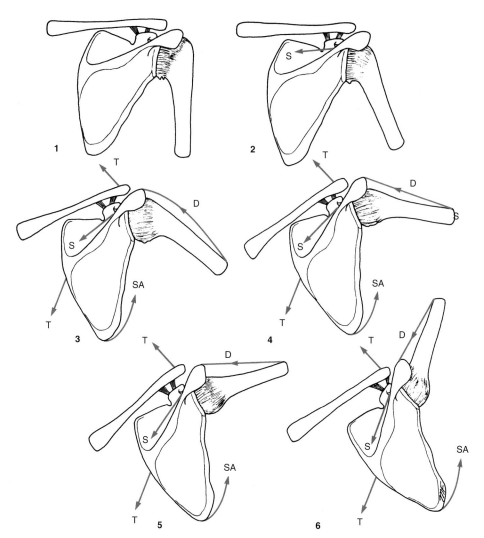

FIGURE 3.16. Scapulohumeral rhythm: Movements of shoulder abduction and scapular rotation, and the muscles that produce these movements at various stages of abduction. For every 3° of abduction of the arm, 2° of shoulder abduction and 1° of scapular rotation occur. *S, supraspinatus*; D, deltoid; *T, trapezius*; SA, serratus anterior. (From Snell RS. *Clinical Anatomy*. 7th ed. Baltimore: Lippincott Williams & Wilkins; 2003.)

is a powerful abductor of the glenohumeral joint. The posterior deltoid originates from the inferior aspect of the scapular spine, and its actions of glenohumeral extension, horizontal abduction, and external rotation oppose those of the anterior deltoid (18). The anterior and posterior deltoids should be approximately the same size. However, in most individuals, the anterior deltoid is much more developed than the posterior deltoid. This imbalance can cause postural abnormalities (shoulder forward and internally rotated) and may be related to shoulder problems such as impingement syndrome (4).

The rotator cuff muscles include the supraspinatus, infraspinatus, teres minor, and subscapularis, often remembered by the acronym "SITS," which describes their insertions on the greater and lesser tubercles of the humerus (Fig. 3.19). The rotator cuff muscles originate from the scapula and insert at the greater or lesser tubercle of the humerus (6). The supraspinatus primarily initiates abduction at the glenohumeral joint, the infraspinatus and teres minor externally rotate the glenohumeral joint, and the subscapularis internally rotates the glenohumeral joint.

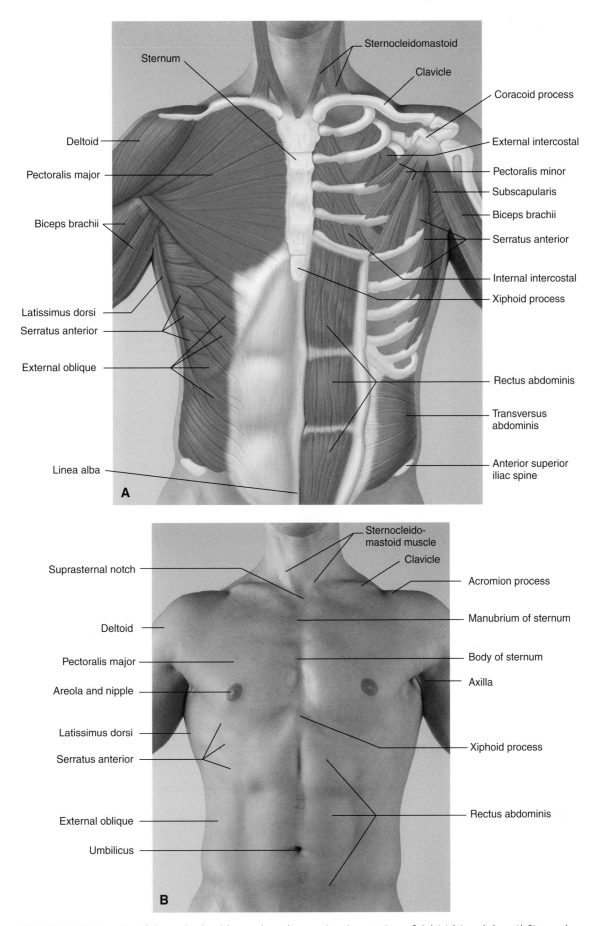

FIGURE 3.17. Muscles of the neck, shoulder, and trunk—anterior view. **A.** Superficial (*right*) and deep (*left*) muscles. **B.** Surface landmarks. (From Premkumar K. *The Massage Connection Anatomy and Physiology*. Baltimore: Lippincott Williams & Wilkins; 2004.)

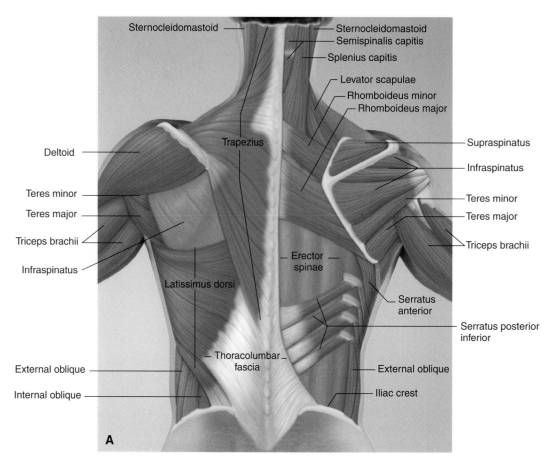

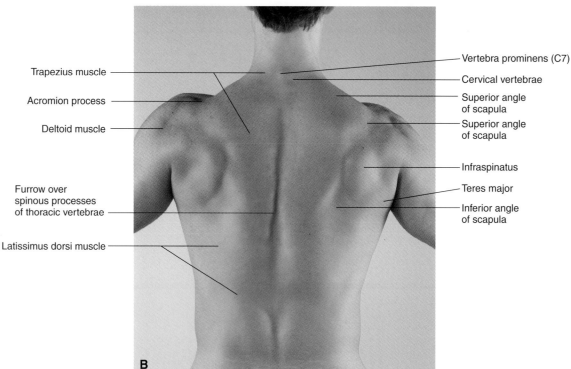

FIGURE 3.18. Muscles of the neck, shoulder, and trunk—posterior view. **A.** Superficial (*right*) and deep (*left*) muscles. **B.** Surface landmarks. (From Premkumar K. *The Massage Connection Anatomy and Physiology*. Baltimore: Lippincott Williams & Wilkins; 2004.)

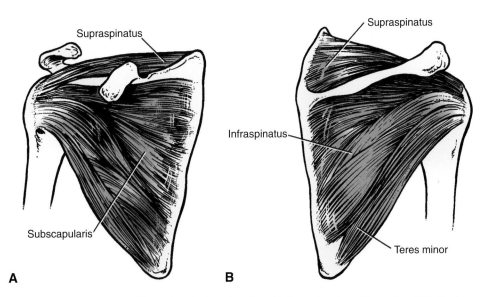

FIGURE 3.19. Rotator cuff muscles. **A.** Anterior view. **B.** Posterior view. (From Koval KJ, Zuckerman JD. *Atlas of Orthopaedic Surgery: A Multimedial Reference.* Philadelphia: Lippincott Williams & Wilkins; 2004.)

The rotator cuff muscles are important stabilizers of the glenohumeral joint and aid in glenohumeral positional control (6). These muscles act like a strong ligament, holding the humeral head tightly in the glenoid fossa during arm movements initiated by the larger shoulder muscles. The rotator cuff stabilizes the shoulder through four mechanisms: (a) passive muscle tension, (b) contraction of the muscles causing compression of the articular surface, (c) joint motion that results in secondary tightening of the ligamentous restraints, and (d) the barrier effect of contracted muscle (2).

The latissimus dorsi is a large fan-shaped muscle that originates from the iliac crest and the posterior sacrum (via thoracolumbar fascia), lower six thoracic vertebrae, and lower three ribs. It inserts at the intertubercular groove of the humerus. The latissimus dorsi is a strong extensor, internal rotator, and adductor of the glenohumeral joint. The angle of pull of the latissimus dorsi increases when the arm is abducted to 30°–90°. The teres major muscle has actions similar to those of the latissimus dorsi. The triceps brachii is typically known as an elbow muscle, but its long head acts to extend the shoulder as well (18).

Shoulder Girdle. The muscles of the anterior shoulder girdle include the pectoralis minor, serratus anterior, and subclavius. The pectoralis minor originates from the anterior aspects of the third to fifth ribs and inserts at the coracoid process of the scapula. Contraction of the pectoralis minor causes protraction, downward rotation, and depression of the scapula. The pectoralis minor has a lifting effect on the ribs during forceful inspiration and postural control. The serratus anterior contains several bands that originate from the upper nine ribs laterally and insert on the anterior aspect of the medial border of the scapula. The serratus anterior protracts the scapula and is active in reaching and pushing. Winging of the scapula results from serratus anterior dysfunction, possibly related to long thoracic nerve dysfunction. The subclavius is a small muscle that protects and stabilizes the sternoclavicular joint (18).

The posterior shoulder muscles are the levator scapulae, rhomboids (major and minor), and trapezius. The levator scapulae originate from the transverse processes of the upper four cervical vertebrae, run obliquely, and insert at the medial border of the scapular spine. The levator scapulae produce elevation and downward rotation of scapula and also act on the neck. The rhomboids originate from the spinous processes of the last cervical and upper five thoracic vertebrae and insert along the entire length of the medial border of the scapula. Rhomboid action results in scapular retraction, downward rotation, and slight elevation. Along with the trapezius, proper rhomboid activity is necessary for good posture (i.e., squeezing shoulder blades together) (4).

The trapezius muscle is a large triangular muscle and one of the largest muscles of the shoulder region. It contains three distinct regions: the upper, middle, and lower fibers. The origin of the trapezius covers a broad area from the base of the occiput to the spinous process of the 12th thoracic vertebra, and its insertion runs from the lateral clavicle, medial border of the acromion, and scapular spine. Contraction of the upper trapezius causes scapular elevation, of the middle trapezius causes scapular retraction, and of the lower trapezius causes scapular depression (18). Together, the upper and lower fibers cause upward rotation of the scapula.

Injuries. Impingement syndrome is probably the most common nontraumatic cause of shoulder pain (17). Impingement syndrome results from approximation of the acromion and greater tubercle of humerus, which causes entrapment of the rotator cuff tendons (6). Shoulder impingement may also be associated with subacromial bursitis, biceps tendonitis, and degenerative tears of the rotator cuff tendons (3). A primary factor of impingement syndrome is muscular imbalance at the shoulder exacerbated by external rotator cuff muscle weakness and highly trained internal rotator muscles (particularly the prime movers) (17). This imbalance can lead to postural abnormalities, such as anterior shoulder carriage with excessive internal rotation (shoulder rounded forward), adaptive shortening and fibrosis of the internal rotators, and inflamed rotator cuff tendons. The progressive loss of external rotation, due to fibrosis or adaptive shortening of the internal rotators, is the most common factor in chronic rotator cuff disorders. Some of the predisposing factors for impingement syndrome include biomechanically unsound exercises, sports activities (e.g., swimming), lifting weights with poor form, and training the same area of the body too often (overtraining anterior deltoids, pectoralis major, and latissimus dorsi) (17). Treatment of impingement syndrome is heavily focused on retraining proper exercise and posture. This includes strengthening and improving the function of the external rotators, stretching the internal rotators, and eliminating the training errors that started the dysfunction in the first place (17). All too often, however, a person who suffers from impingement syndrome is noncompliant with appropriate rehabilitation, and the condition becomes chronic, leading to permanent degenerative changes and dysfunction.

> *A primary factor of impingement syndrome is muscular imbalance at the shoulder exacerbated by external rotator cuff muscle weakness and highly trained internal rotator muscles (particularly the prime movers) (17).*

Thoracic outlet syndrome is another condition of the shoulder that can be related to faulty biomechanics, poor posture, and shoulder muscle imbalance (7). Thoracic outlet syndrome is compression of the neurovascular bundle (brachial plexus and axillary artery/vein) in the axillary region and results in symptoms of pain, numbness, and tingling in the upper extremity, usually ulnar distribution or C8 dermatome (fourth and fifth digits of the hand). The three sites of compression in thoracic outlet syndrome occur between the first rib and anterior scalene muscle, pectoralis minor muscle or clavicle (7). Treatment of thoracic outlet syndrome includes correcting faulty biomechanics, strengthening the rotator cuff, and stretching the shoulder internal rotators and scalenes. As with impingement syndrome, complete recovery may take several months or longer.

The shoulder is also susceptible to traumatic injuries such as joint separation or dislocation and tearing of tendons, ligaments, or joint capsules. Glenohumeral joint dislocation usually occurs anteriorly because of capsular tears (4). The mechanism of glenohumeral joint dislocation is typically excessive abduction, external rotation, and extension of the shoulder. Stabilizing the shoulder after suspected glenohumeral joint dislocation is important to prevent any further damage, particularly to the neurological structures. Acromioclavicular joint separation is classically due to a direct blow to the shoulder or fall on an outstretched arm (3). Signs and symptoms of acromioclavicular joint separation include elevation of the distal clavicle and sharp pain in the joint. Rotator cuff tendon tears (particularly of the supraspinatus muscle) can be caused by forceful throwing (e.g., baseball) and improper weight-lifting techniques (3).

ELBOW

The elbow is an important joint involved in lifting and carrying, throwing, swinging, and most upper extremity exercise movements. The elbow is commonly injured and is the second most injured joint from overuse or repetitive motion (15,23).

> **The elbow is commonly injured and is the second most injured joint from overuse or repetitive motion (15,23).**

Bones. The elbow consists of the humerus, radius, and ulna bones. The humeroulnar joint is the articulation of the distal humerus with the proximal ulna, the humeroradial joint is the articulation of the distal humerus with the proximal radius, and the proximal radioulnar joint is the articulation of the proximal radius with the proximal ulna (38) (Fig. 3.20).

With the arms held at the side of the body and the palms of the hand facing anteriorly, the forearm and hands are usually held slightly away from the body. This is due to the carrying angle of the elbow, which is normally 5°–15° in males and 20°–25° in females. Carrying angle allows the forearm to swing free of the side of the hips during walking and provides a mechanical advantage when carrying objects (4).

Ligaments. Three major ligaments stabilize the elbow: the ulnar (medial) collateral ligament, which connects the humerus with the ulna; the radial (lateral) collateral ligament, which connects the humerus with the radius; and the annular ligament, which connects the radius with the ulna. The collateral ligaments provide support for stresses in the frontal plane, the medial collateral for valgus forces, and the lateral collateral for varus forces. The annular ligament provides stability for the radius, securing it to the ulna (38) (Fig. 3.20).

Joints. The elbow joint complex is a compound synovial joint that consists of two articulations: humeroulnar and humeroradial. It is continuous with the proximal radioulnar joint, responsible for allowing the radial head to rotate during pronation and supination of the forearm. The distal humerus articulates with both the proximal ulna and proximal radius, and the two articulations are enclosed by one capsule and share a single synovial cavity. On the lateral side of the elbow, the capitulum of the humerus articulates with the head of the radius to form the humeroradial joint; medially, the trochlea of the humerus articulates with the trochlear notch of the ulna to form the humeroulnar joint. The proximal radioulnar joint, whose joint capsule is continuous with that of the humeroulnar and humeroradial joints, is the articulation of the radial head with the radial notch of the ulna (38) (Fig. 3.20).

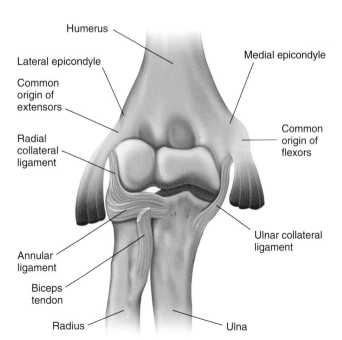

FIGURE 3.20. Bones and ligaments of the elbow joint—anterior view. (From Premkumar K. *The Massage Connection Anatomy and Physiology.* Baltimore: Lippincott Williams & Wilkins; 2004.)

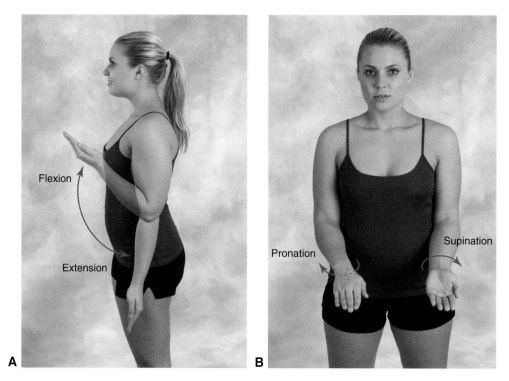

FIGURE 3.21. Movements of the elbow. **A.** Flexion-extension. **B.** Pronation-supination.

Movements. Both the humeroulnar and humeroradial are hinge joints that flex and extend the elbow in the sagittal plane (Fig. 3.21). The normal ROM for flexion–extension is 145°–150°, with the fully flexed position (elbow bent) represented by 145°–150° and the fully extended position (arm straight with forearm) represented by 0°. During sagittal movement of the elbow, the trochlear notch of the humerus slides into the trochlear groove of the ulna. Upon full flexion, the coronoid process of the ulna approximates the coronoid fossa of the humerus. At full extension, the olecranon process of the ulna hits the olecranon fossa of the humerus, which enhances stability of the elbow in full extension. The proximal radioulnar joint is a pivot joint, which permits axial rotation of the radial head during supination and pronation of the forearm. Normal ROM for supination (forearm rotated laterally—palms facing anteriorly) is 80°–90°; normal ROM for pronation (forearm rotated medially—palms facing posteriorly) is 80°–90° (38).

Muscles

Anterior. The anterior muscles of the arm mainly flex the elbow joint (5) and include the biceps brachii, brachialis, and brachioradialis (Fig. 3.22). The biceps brachii is a two-head, two-joint muscle that acts on both the shoulder and elbow. Its long head originates from the supraglenoid tubercle of the scapula, and the short head originates from the coracoid process of the scapula, with both heads inserting at the tuberosity of the radius. The biceps brachii is a strong supinator and flexes the elbow most effectively when the forearm is in supination. The long head of the biceps brachii also assists in shoulder flexion. To optimally train the biceps brachii, exercise movements should include both elbow flexion and forearm supination (e.g., dumbbell biceps curl). The brachialis is considered the elbow flexor workhorse (4). Hammer curls, with the forearms maintained in a neutral position, are ideal to develop the brachialis and brachioradialis. In the forearm, the pronator quadratus and pronator teres, as their names suggest, cause pronation. The pronator quadratus is the stronger of the two.

Posterior. The posterior muscles of the elbow primarily extend the elbow joint and include the triceps brachii and anconeus (Fig. 3.23). The triceps brachii is a three-head, two-joint (long head)

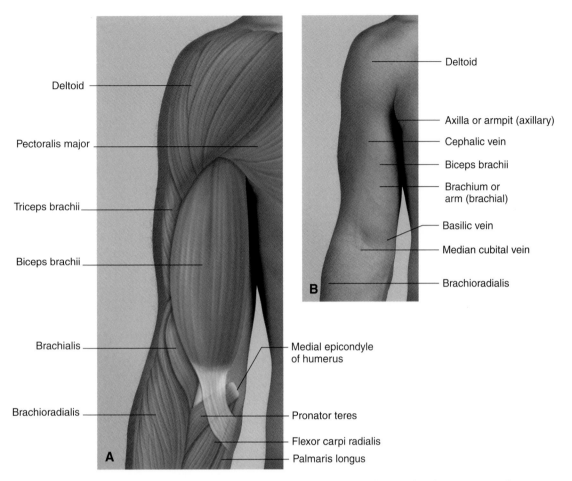

Deltoid

Pectoralis major

Triceps brachii

Biceps brachii

Brachialis

Brachioradialis

Medial epicondyle of humerus

Pronator teres

Flexor carpi radialis

Palmaris longus

A

Deltoid

Axilla or armpit (axillary)

Cephalic vein

Biceps brachii

Brachium or arm (brachial)

Basilic vein

Median cubital vein

Brachioradialis

B

FIGURE 3.22. Muscles of the upper arm—anterior view. **A.** Muscles. **B.** Surface landmarks. (From Premkumar K. *The Massage Connection Anatomy and Physiology*. Baltimore: Lippincott Williams & Wilkins; 2004.)

muscle that acts on the elbow and shoulder. Its long head originates from the infraglenoid tubercle of the scapula, whereas the medial and lateral heads originate from the upper humerus. All three heads insert on the olecranon of the ulna. The triceps brachii is the main elbow extensor, getting minor assistance from the anconeus. The anconeus, a small muscle, also adds stability to the posterior elbow joint (18).

Injuries. Because of its use in most upper extremity daily living activities, exercise, and sport activities, the elbow is frequently injured from chronic overuse or repetitive motion (3). Tendonitis is evident in a variety of muscular insertion points at the elbow. "Tennis elbow" (lateral epicondylitis), which creates lateral elbow pain, is the most widespread overuse injury of the adult elbow (15,23).

Because of its use in most upper extremity daily living activities, exercise, and sport activities, the elbow is frequently injured from chronic overuse or repetitive motion (3).

It is usually caused by eccentric overload of the forearm extensor muscles (e.g., gripping a racquet too tightly, wrong grip size, faulty backhand technique, excessive racquet weight) (11). "Golfer's elbow" (medial epicondylitis), which produces medial elbow pain, is often caused by repeated valgus stresses placed on the arm during swinging of racquets or clubs. Triceps tendonitis, which produces pain over the olecranon, is caused by repetitive posterior stresses during elbow extension. Resistance and flexibility exercises for elbow flexion, extension, pronation, and supination are often incorporated to prevent and treat these injuries. Medial collateral ligament sprain often results from repetitive microtrauma and excessive valgus force (3).

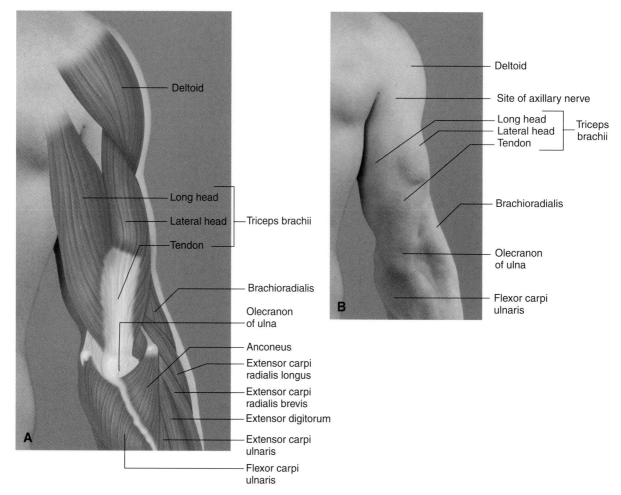

FIGURE 3.23. Muscles of the upper arm—posterior view. **A.** Muscles. **B.** Surface landmarks. (From Premkumar K. *The Massage Connection Anatomy and Physiology*. Baltimore: Lippincott Williams & Wilkins; 2004.)

The elbow is also the site for traumatic injuries. Olecranon bursitis, which typically produces a large red swelling over the posterior elbow, usually results from a fall directly on the elbow. Ulnar dislocation typically results from violent hyperextension or varus or valgus forces. Ulnar dislocation, which is most common in individuals younger than 20 years, results in obvious elbow deformity and may present with neurological symptoms into the hand (fifth digit) because of entrapment of the ulnar nerve at the elbow (3).

WRIST, HAND, AND FINGERS

The wrist, hand, and fingers are required for most daily living, work, and sports activities, including tasks such as gripping, lifting, writing, typing, eating, and throwing. Because adequate wrist and hand function is necessary for these activities, injuries to the wrist and hand are often disabling. This section focuses mainly on the functional anatomy of the wrist. The reader is referred to other sources (1,16,28,29,33) for the functional anatomy of the intrinsic hand and fingers.

> *The wrist, hand, and fingers are required for most daily living, work, and sports activities, including tasks such as gripping, lifting, writing, typing, eating, and throwing.*

Bones. The wrist, hand, and fingers consist of 29 bones: the distal ulna, distal radius, eight carpals, five metacarpals, and 14 phalanges (36) (Fig. 3.24). The carpals are small oddly shaped bones arranged in two rows. The proximal row from lateral to medial includes the scaphoid (navicular),

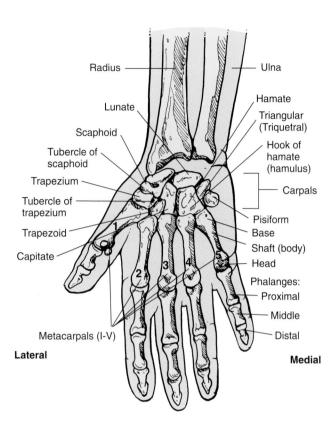

FIGURE 3.24. Bones of the wrist and hand—anterior view. (From Anderson M, Hall SJ. *Sports Injury Management.* 2nd ed. Baltimore: Lippincott Williams & Wilkins; 2000.)

lunate, triquetrum, and pisiform. The distal row from lateral to medial includes the trapezium, trapezoid, capitate, and hamate. There is one metacarpal per digit, which connects the carpals to the phalanges. Each digit has three phalanges, except the thumb, which has two (36).

Ligaments. The volar radiocarpal, dorsal radiocarpal, radial collateral, and ulnar collateral ligaments support the radioulnar joint. The radiocarpal ligaments provide stability in the sagittal plane, whereas the collateral ligaments provide stability in the frontal plane (36). There are numerous other ligaments that stabilize the wrist, hand, and fingers, many of which have clinical implications for healthcare professionals other than Personal Trainers.

Joints. The primary wrist joint (radiocarpal joint) is a condyloid (ellipsoidal) joint consisting of the articulation of the distal radius with three proximal carpal bones: scaphoid, lunate, and triquetrum. The joint surface of the radius is concave, allowing the convex carpals to approximate it. The proximal and distal rows of carpal bones form the complex midcarpal joint. The distal radioulnar joint, a pivot joint, is situated medial to the radiocarpal joint and allows forearm supination and pronation (36).

Movements. The wrist allows approximately 70°–90° of flexion and 65°–85° of extension in the sagittal plane and 15°–25° of abduction (radial deviation) and 25°–40° of adduction (ulnar deviation) in the frontal plane (Fig. 3.25). Flexion–extension and abduction–adduction movements occur mainly at the radiocarpal joint. However, gliding motions at the midcarpal joint, which are facilitated by ligaments, allow full ROM in both planes. Circumduction of the wrist is also possible through the compound action of the radioulnar and midcarpal joints. The closed pack position of the wrist joint is full extension, whereas the open pack position is 0° of extension with slight adduction (4).

Muscles

Anterior. The wrist flexor muscles, which are located on the anteromedial aspect of the wrist and generally originate from the medial epicondyle of the humerus, include the flexor carpi radialis, flexor carpi ulnaris, flexor digitorum superficialis, and palmaris longus (Fig. 3.26). In addition to the

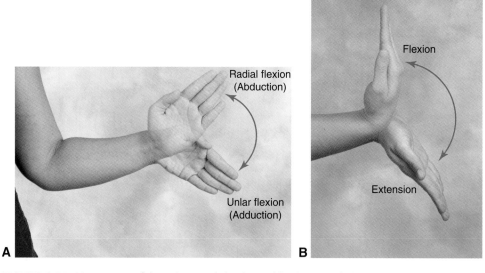

FIGURE 3.25. Movements of the wrist. **A.** Abduction–adduction. **B.** Flexion-extension.

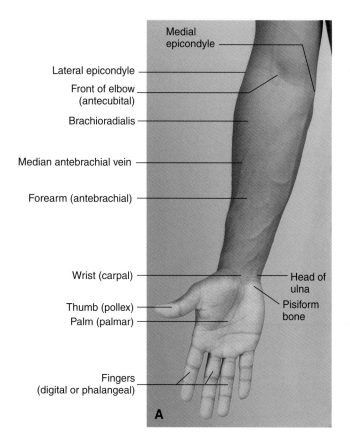

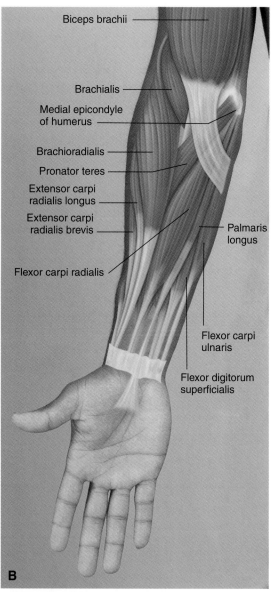

FIGURE 3.26. Muscles of the forearm—anterior view. **A.** Muscles. **B.** Surface landmarks. (From Premkumar K. *The Massage Connection Anatomy and Physiology*. Baltimore: Lippincott Williams & Wilkins; 2004.)

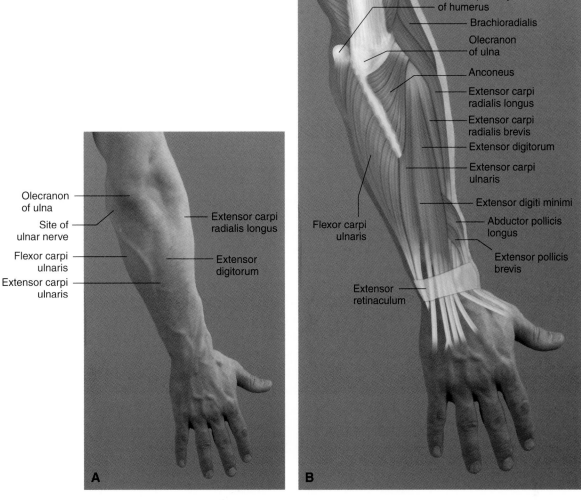

FIGURE 3.27. Muscles of the forearm—posterior view. **A.** Muscles. **B.** Surface landmarks. (From Premkumar K. *The Massage Connection Anatomy and Physiology*. Baltimore: Lippincott Williams & Wilkins; 2004.)

flexor activity, the flexor carpi radialis abducts the wrist, the flexor carpi ulnaris adducts the wrist, and the flexor digitorum superficialis flexes the phalanges as well (18).

Posterior. The wrist extensor muscles, which are located on the posterolateral aspect of the wrist and generally originate at or near the lateral epicondyle of the humerus, include the extensor carpi radialis longus and brevis, extensor digitorum, extensor digiti minimi, and the extensor carpi ulnaris (Fig. 3.27). In addition to their extensor activity, the extensor carpi radialis longus abducts the wrist and the extensor carpi ulnaris adducts the wrist, and extensor digitorum, extensor digiti minimi extend the phalanges as well (18).

Injuries. Dislocations, fractures, and sprains are common at the wrist following falls. Falling on an outstretched arm with the wrist extended may cause lunate bone dislocation (usually anteriorly) or scaphoid bone fracture. Colles and Smith fractures are serious fractures affecting both the distal ulna and radius, which many times require fixation with rigid screws and plates to restore function (14). Wrist ligament sprains are frequently caused by axial loading of the palm during a fall on an outstretched arm (3).

Carpal tunnel syndrome is a widespread cumulative trauma disorder that is caused by median nerve entrapment at the anterior wrist (7). It usually results from repeated microtrauma to the carpal tunnel and flexor retinaculum due to prolonged manual work with the wrist in a flexed position

Carpal tunnel syndrome usually results from repeated microtrauma to the carpal tunnel and flexor retinaculum due to prolonged manual work with the wrist in a flexed position (e.g., in individuals who work with computer keyboards, assembly line workers, cyclists).

(e.g., in individuals who work with computer keyboards, assembly line workers, cyclists). Its symptoms include pain, numbness, tingling, and weakness in thumb, index, and middle finger (median nerve distribution). Carpal tunnel syndrome usually requires physical rehabilitation, surgery, or ergonomic correction to restore function.

Lower Extremity

PELVIS AND HIP

The pelvic girdle is the link between the axial skeleton (trunk) and lower extremities. This region assists with motion, stability, and shock absorption and helps distribute body weight evenly to the lower extremities (4).

The pelvic girdle is the link between the axial skeleton (trunk) and lower extremities.

Bones. The bones of the pelvic girdle (pelvis) are the sacrum, innominate (os coxae), and two femurs. The innominate bone includes the fused ilium (largest pelvic bone), ischium, and pubis on each side (which typically fuse by the end of puberty). The two sides of the pelvis join anteriorly at the pubic symphysis and posteriorly at the sacroiliac joints. The pelvis of females is usually wider than that of males, which contributes to the increased "Q angle" of the knee in females (4). The anterior superior iliac spine (ASIS) of the ilium is a bony protuberance that provides an attachment point for several muscles of the anterior thigh. The sacrum articulates with the pelvis on each side, forming the sacroiliac joints, and the pelvis articulates with each femur at the acetabulum, forming the hip joints (36) (Fig. 3.28).

Anterior view

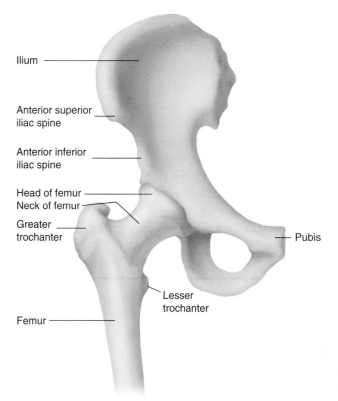

FIGURE 3.28. Bones of the pelvis and hip region—anterior view. (Asset provided by Anatomical Chart Co.)

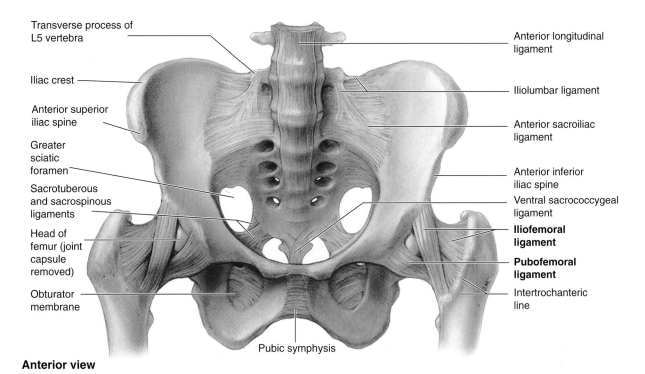

Transverse process of
L5 vertebra

Iliac crest

Anterior superior
iliac spine

Greater
sciatic
foramen

Sacrotuberous
and sacrospinous
ligaments

Head of
femur (joint
capsule
removed)

Obturator
membrane

Anterior longitudinal
ligament

Iliolumbar ligament

Anterior sacroiliac
ligament

Anterior inferior
iliac spine

Ventral sacrococcygeal
ligament

**Iliofemoral
ligament**

**Pubofemoral
ligament**

Intertrochanteric
line

Pubic symphysis

Anterior view

FIGURE 3.29. Ligaments of the pelvis and hip regions—anterior view. (From Moore KL, Dalley AF II. *Clinical Oriented Anatomy.* 4th ed. Baltimore: Lippincott Williams & Wilkins; 1999.)

Ligaments. The anterior, posterior, and interosseous ligaments bind the sacroiliac joint. The highly mobile hip joint is stabilized by several intrinsic ligaments, forming a strong, dense joint capsule (42). They include iliofemoral, pubofemoral, and ischiofemoral ligaments. The iliofemoral ligament ("Y" ligament) is an extraordinarily strong band that checks hip extension and rotation. The pubofemoral ligament prevents excessive abduction. The ischiofemoral ligament is triangular and limits hip rotation and adduction in the flexed position (38) (Fig. 3.29). The transverse acetabular ligament is a sturdy band that bridges the acetabular notch and completes the acetabular ring of the hip joint. The ligamentum teres (ligament of the femoral head) ligament ties the head of the femur to the acetabulum, providing reinforcement from within the joint (Fig. 3.30).

Joints. The pubic symphysis connects each side of the pelvic girdle anteriorly and is an amphiarthrodial joint. The sacroiliac joint connects the sacrum to the ilium on each side and is sometimes described as a gliding joint. These joints are capable of relatively little movement (38).

The hip joint is a ball-and-socket (enarthrodial) joint and is one of the most mobile joints in the body. The hip joint is formed by the articulation of the proximal femur (femoral head) with the acetabulum of the pelvis. The femoral head is covered with hyaline cartilage, except at the fovea capitis, and the acetabulum is lined with hyaline cartilage as well. The acetabular labrum is a fibrocartilaginous "lip" that adds depth to the acetabulum and serves as a cushion for the femoral head (4) (Fig. 3.30).

Movements. The pelvic girdle allows movement in three planes. These movements are shown in Figure 3.31. Movement at the pelvis during normal activities usually involves simultaneous motion of the hip and lumbar spine (38). In the sagittal plane, the pelvis is capable of anterior–posterior tilt. With anterior pelvic tilt, the pubic symphysis moves inferiorly, the lumbar spine extends, and the hips flex, resulting in an increased lumbosacral angle. With posterior pelvic tilt, the pubic symphysis moves superiorly, the lumbar spine flexes, and the hips extend, resulting in a decreased lumbosacral angle. Lateral tilt of the pelvis occurs in the frontal plane, and rotation of the pelvis occurs in the axial plane. Locomotion (walking or running) typically involves small oscillations of the pelvis in all three planes (38).

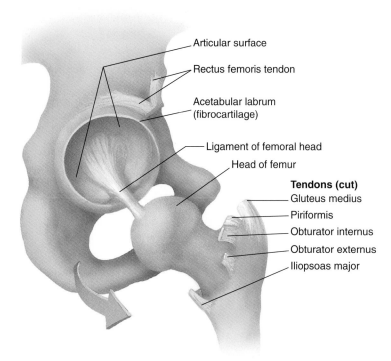

Articular surface

Rectus femoris tendon

Acetabular labrum
(fibrocartilage)

Ligament of femoral head

Head of femur

Tendons (cut)
Gluteus medius
Piriformis
Obturator internus
Obturator externus
Iliopsoas major

FIGURE 3.30. Acetabulum of the hip joint.
(Asset provided by Anatomical Chart Co.)

The highly mobile hip joint allows movement in three planes: flexion–extension in the sagittal plane, abduction–adduction in the frontal plane, internal–external rotation in the axial plane, and the combined plane movement of circumduction (38). Hip movements are shown in Figure 3.32.

Pelvic Muscles. The muscles of the pelvis include the muscles that act on the lumbar spine, lower trunk, and hip, which are discussed elsewhere in this chapter. In general, anterior pelvic tilt results from contraction of the hip flexors and lumbar extensors. Posterior pelvic tilt results from contraction of the hip extensors and lumbar flexors. Lateral tilt results from contraction of the lateral lumbar muscles (e.g., quadratus lumborum) and hip abductor–adductor muscles, and axial rotation occurs through the action of the hip and spinal rotator muscles (4).

Hip Muscles. The muscles that act on the hip are shown in Figures 3.33 through 3.36.

Anterior. The anterior muscles of the hip region include the iliopsoas, pectineus, rectus femoris, sartorius, and tensor fasciae latae. The iliopsoas muscle group, which consists of the psoas major and iliacus muscles, is a strong hip flexor. The pectineus is a small muscle that attaches the anterior pubis to the posteromedial side of the proximal femur. It assists in hip flexion, adduction, and internal rotation. The rectus femoris is a large two-joint muscle that flexes the hip and extends the knee. The rectus femoris originates from the anterior inferior iliac spine and inserts at the tibial tuberosity via the patellar ligament. The sartorius, a two-joint muscle, is the longest muscle in the body, originating from the anterior superior iliac spine (ASIS) and inserting at the medial tibial surface. The sartorius flexes, abducts, and externally rotates the hip (it also assists with knee flexion). The tensor fasciae latae, a two-joint muscle, originates from the anterior iliac crest of the ilium and inserts at the anterolateral tibial condyle via a long band of fascia—the iliotibial band. The tensor fasciae latae abducts and flexes the hip and stabilizes the hip against external rotation when the hip is flexed (18) and also assists with extension and stabilization of the knee.

Medial. The medial muscles of the hip include gracilis and the adductors longus, brevis, and magnus. These muscles primarily adduct the hip. Variably, they may participate in hip flexion (adductor

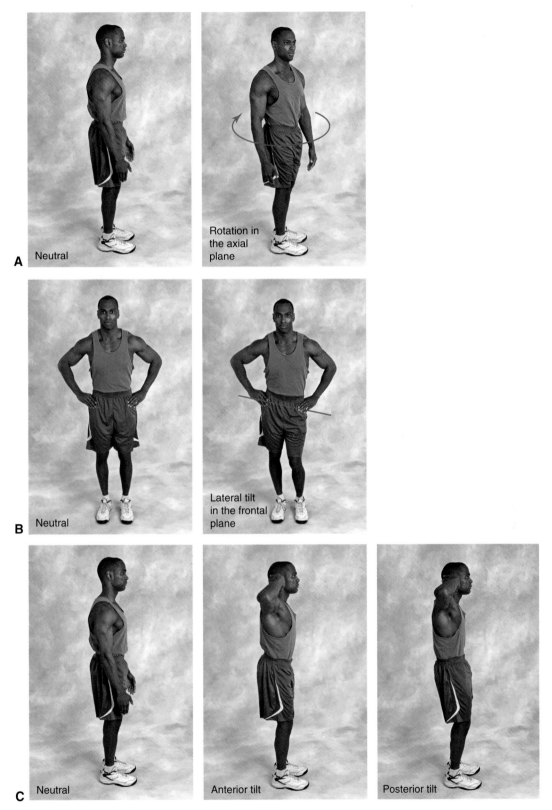

FIGURE 3.31. Movements of the pelvis. **A.** Rotation in the axial plane. **B.** Lateral tilt in the frontal plane. **C.** Anterior and posterior tilt in the sagittal plane.

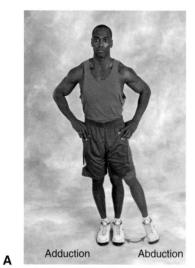

A   Adduction   Abduction

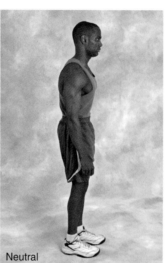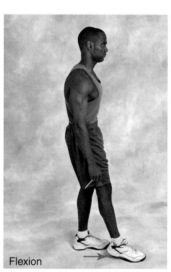

B   Extension   Neutral   Flexion

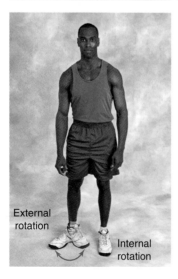

External rotation   Internal rotation

C

FIGURE 3.32. Movements of the hip joint. **A.** Abduction–adduction. **B.** Flexion–extension. **C.** Internal–external rotation.

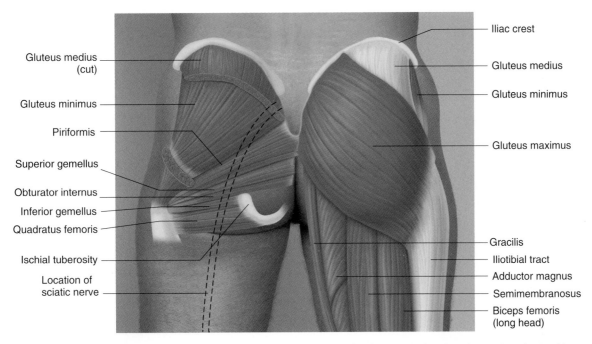

FIGURE 3.33. Superficial (*right*) and deep (*left*) muscles of the hip and pelvis—posterior view. (From Premkumar K. *The Massage Connection Anatomy and Physiology*. Baltimore: Lippincott Williams & Wilkins; 2004.)

longus and brevis, upper fibers of adductor magnus) or extension (lower fibers of adductor magnus) and medial rotation (adductors longus, brevis, and magnus). Pectineus, a muscle previously considered with the anterior hip muscles, also participates in hip adduction. These muscles originate generally from the pubis and insert on the linea aspera of the femur. Gracilis, which is a two-joint muscle inserting on tibia (pes anserine), may also assist with knee flexion.

Posterior. The posterior muscles of the hip include gluteus maximus, medius and minimus, the six deep lateral rotators (piriformis, gemellus superior and inferior, obturators internus and externus, and quadratus femoris), and hamstrings (biceps femoris, semimembranosus, and semitendinosus). Gluteus maximus, which forms the bulk of the buttock regions, has an extensive origin from ilium, sacrum, and coccyx and inserts on the gluteal tuberosity, located on the lateral aspect of femur. In addition to being a powerful extensor of the hip, it also participates in lateral rotation and adduction. Gluteus medius and minimus lie deep to gluteus maximus and are abductors and medial rotators of the hip. Additionally, these muscles are important postural muscles to keep the pelvis level during locomotion. They arise from the external surface of ilium and insert on the greater trochanter of femur with most of the deep lateral rotators. The hamstrings (semimembranosus, semitendinosus, and biceps femoris) are two-joint muscles, which extend the hip (except the short head of biceps femoris) and flex the knee. Biceps femoris originates from the ischial tuberosity (long head) and proximal femur (short head) and inserts on the lateral tibial condyle and fibular head. The long head extends the hip, flexes the knee, and causes lateral rotation at both joints, whereas the short head acts only on the knee. Semimembranosus and semitendinosus are also two-joint muscles that extend the hip, flex the knee, and internally rotate both joints. They originate on the ischial tuberosity and insert on the medial aspect of the tibia.

Injuries. The hip and pelvis have a strong structural anatomy, so traumatic sports injuries at these locations are relatively infrequent compared with injuries to other joints (3). However, the soft tissues of the thigh are often injured in sports (3), and the hip and pelvis are sites of several chronic overuse disorders.

Traumatic injuries of the pelvis and hip include dislocation, fracture, contusion, and muscle strain. Hip dislocation results from violent twisting of the hip or jamming the knee into the dashboard of

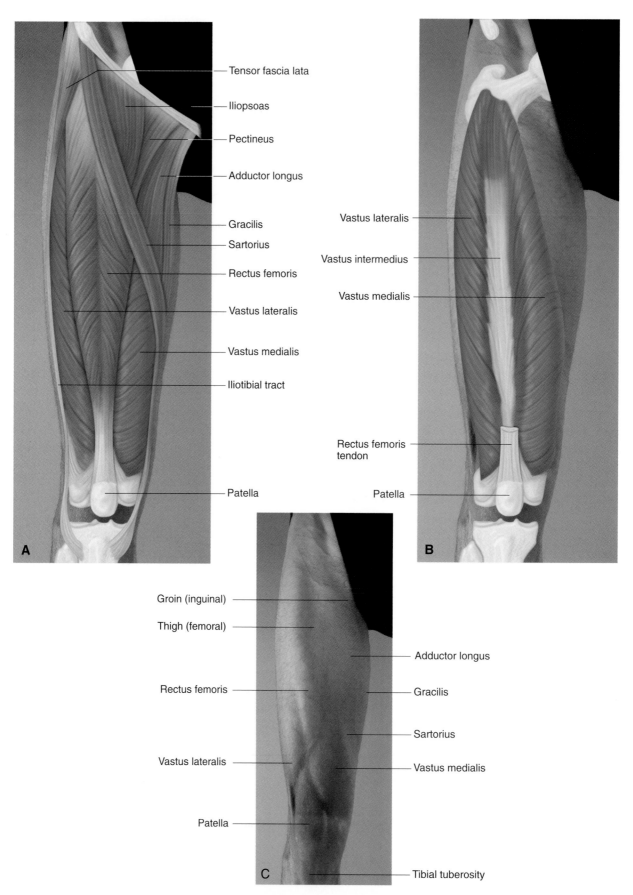

FIGURE 3.34. Muscles of the thigh—anterior view. **A.** Muscles. **B.** Quadriceps femoris. **C.** Surface landmarks. (From Premkumar K. *The Massage Connection Anatomy and Physiology*. Baltimore: Lippincott Williams & Wilkins; 2004.)

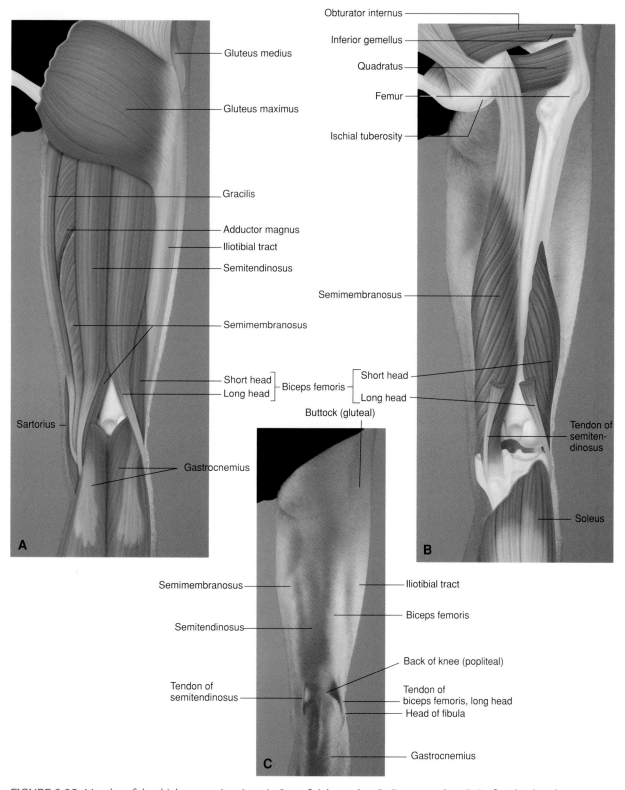

FIGURE 3.35. Muscles of the thigh—posterior view. **A.** Superficial muscles. **B.** Deep muscles. **C.** Surface landmarks. (From Premkumar K. *The Massage Connection Anatomy and Physiology*. Baltimore: Lippincott Williams & Wilkins; 2004.)

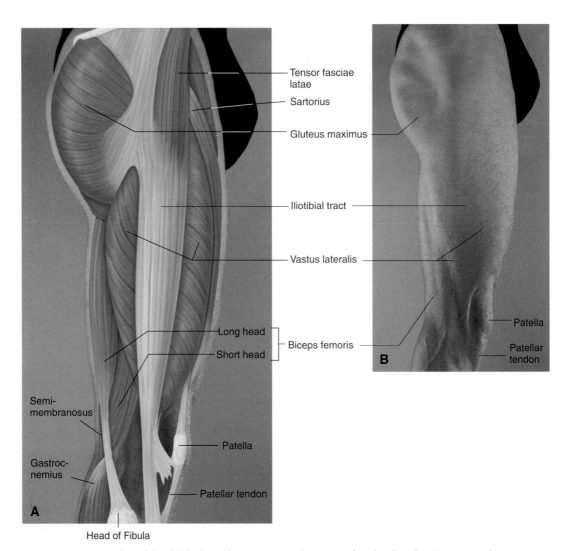

FIGURE 3.36. Muscles of the thigh—lateral view. **A.** Muscles. **B.** Surface landmarks. (From Premkumar K. *The Massage Connection Anatomy and Physiology.* Baltimore: Lippincott Williams & Wilkins; 2004.)

a car. Some 85% of hip dislocations are posterior. Hip fractures (fractures of the femoral neck) are common in older adults with osteoporosis and can cause permanent disability. Contusions (crush injuries of muscle against bone) are common in the region. Iliac crest contusion ("hip pointer") is caused by a direct blow to the pelvis region. Quadriceps contusion ("charley horse") and tearing can result in permanent muscle abnormality called "myositis ossificans," in which bone tissue is deposited within the muscle (3). Hamstring muscle strains and tears are often caused by sudden changes in direction and speed, with underlying factors of muscular imbalance, fatigue, and a deconditioned athlete (3). Hamstring injuries are frequent in preseason or early season activities.

Chronic and overuse injuries to the hip and pelvis include arthritis, bursitis, and tendonitis. Degenerative arthritis of the hip results from abnormal articular cartilage wear from either too much or too little resistance. Avascular necrosis of the hip is caused by the lack of proper blood flow to the femoral head and typically results in severe hip degeneration. Trochanteric bursitis involves irritation of the bursa between the iliotibial band and greater trochanter of the femur. Chronic bursitis in this region can lead to "snapping hip syndrome" (3). Iliotibial band friction syndrome is a chronic overuse injury that causes pain along the lateral aspect of the thigh. Piriformis syndrome is a myofascial

Traumatic injuries of the pelvis and hip include dislocation, fracture, contusion, and muscle strain.

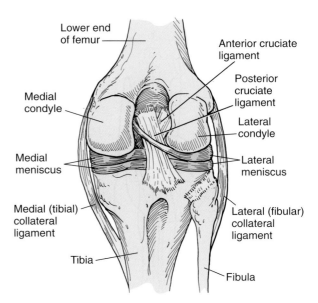

FIGURE 3.37. Bones, ligaments, and menisci of the knee region—posterior view—with the knee extended. (From Cipriano J. *Photographic Manual of Regional Orthopaedic and Neurological Tests*. 2nd ed. Baltimore: Lippincott Williams & Wilkins; 1991.)

disorder that can be caused by faulty lower extremity biomechanics. The hypertonic piriformis muscle may compress the sciatic nerve, because the nerve may course through the muscle. This results in pain and neurological symptoms of the posterior aspect of the lower extremity ("sciatica") (7).

KNEE

The knee joint is the largest joint in the body. Because the knee joint bears the load of the upper body and trunk and is crucial for locomotion, it is frequently subject to overuse and traumatic injuries (38).

> *Because the knee joint bears the load of the upper body and trunk and is crucial for locomotion, it is frequently subject to overuse and traumatic injuries (38).*

Bones. The knee joint consists of the distal femur, proximal tibia, and patella (Fig. 3.37). The tibia is the major weight-bearing bone of the leg. The fibula is not considered part of the knee joint (38). The patella (kneecap) is a triangular sesamoid bone that is located within the patellar tendon of the quadriceps muscle group. The patella protects the anterior knee (3) and creates an improved angle of pull for the quadriceps muscles, which results in a mechanical advantage during knee extension (38).

Ligaments. There are two major pairs of ligaments in the knee: the cruciate and collateral ligaments (Fig. 3.37). The cruciate ligaments cross within the joint cavity between the femur and tibia and are important in maintaining anterior–posterior and rotational stability at the knee. The anterior cruciate ligament is slightly longer and thinner than the posterior ligament (4).

The collateral ligaments connect the femur with the leg bones—the medial collateral with the tibia and the lateral collateral with the fibula. The collateral ligaments aid in stability of the knee, counteracting valgus and varus forces. The medial collateral ligament attaches to the medial meniscus of the knee, but the lateral collateral ligament does not attach to the lateral meniscus (4).

Menisci. The knee is equipped with fibrocartilage discs (menisci) that are attached to the tibial plateaus and knee joint capsule (4) (Fig. 3.37). The menisci improve congruency of the joint surfaces (allowing better distribution of joint pressure), add stability, aid in shock absorption, provide joint lubrication, aid in load bearing, add anterior–posterior stability, and protect articular cartilage. The medial meniscus is larger, thinner, and more "C"-shaped than the lateral meniscus (4).

Joints. The knee consists of the tibiofemoral and patellofemoral joints (Fig. 3.37). The proximal tibiofibular joint, although an important attachment site for knee structures, is typically not considered

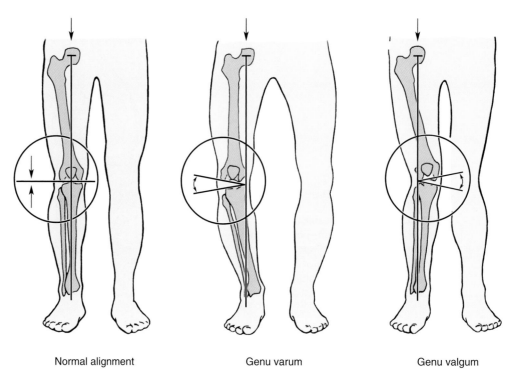

Normal alignment   Genu varum   Genu valgum

FIGURE 3.38. Q angle of the knee: Normal alignment, genu varum, and genu valgum. (From Moore KL, Dalley AF II. *Clinical Oriented Anatomy*. 4th ed. Baltimore: Lippincott Williams & Wilkins; 1999.)

a compartment of the knee joint (38). The tibiofemoral joint is the primary joint of the knee and primarily a hinge joint allowing flexion and extension; however, with its rotational components about the vertical axis, it is better considered bicondylar. The tibiofemoral joint is formed by the articulation of the medial and lateral femoral condyles with the medial and lateral tibial plateaus. The medial femoral condyle typically extends more distally than the lateral condyle, giving the knee a slight valgus arrangement (38).

The patellofemoral joint is an arthrodial joint formed by the posterior aspect of the patella and patellofemoral groove between the condyles of the femur. The "Q angle" is the angle formed from the line connecting ASIS to the center of the patella and the line connecting the center of the patella to the tibial tuberosity (4) (Fig. 3.38). The Q angle determines the line of pull of the patella at the patellofemoral joint. A normal Q angle is 18° in females and 13° in males. A Q angle that is below normal (negative) results in a genu varum position of the knee (bow-legged), whereas a Q angle that is above normal results in a genu valgum position (knock-kneed) (4).

Movements. The major movements at the tibiofemoral joint are flexion and extension in the sagittal plane (Fig. 3.39). The knee has a normal ROM in the sagittal plane of 140°, with 0° representing full extension (knee straight) and 140° representing full flexion (knee bent). When the knee is flexed, the tibiofemoral joint is also capable of internal and external rotation in the transverse plane. Approximately 30° of internal rotation and 45° of external rotation can be achieved at the knee (4). During the final few degrees of extension, the tibia externally rotates on the femur, which brings the knee into a closed packed, or locked, position. This phenomenon is known as the "screwing home" mechanism (3).

Muscles

Anterior. Large and powerful thigh muscles cross the knee joint, several of which are two-joint muscles acting on the hip joint as well. The quadriceps muscles (i.e., rectus femoris, vastus lateralis, vastus intermedius, and vastus medialis) are anterior knee muscles and act to extend the knee joint (Fig. 3.34). The quadriceps muscles insert into the superior aspect of the patella and ultimately to

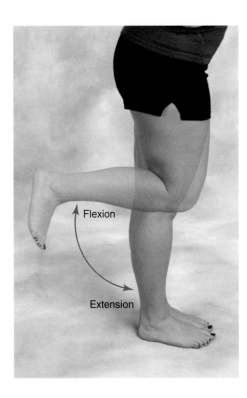

FIGURE 3.39. Movements of the knee joint (flexion–extension).

the tibial tuberosity by the patellar ligament. The rectus femoris is a large, two-joint muscle that originates from the anterior inferior iliac spine. The rectus femoris flexes the hip in addition to extending the knee. The three vasti muscles originate from the proximal femur. The vastus lateralis and vastus medialis are pennate muscles that pull on the patella at oblique angles (20).

Posterior. The muscles of the posterior knee joint are the hamstrings (biceps femoris, semitendinosus, and semimembranosus), sartorius, gracilis, popliteus, and gastrocnemius (Fig. 3.35). The biceps femoris (lateral hamstrings) muscle contains a long head (which originates from the ischial tuberosity and is a two-joint muscle) and a short head (which originates from the mid-femur). The biceps femoris inserts into the lateral condyle of the tibia and head of the fibula. It acts to flex and externally rotate the knee and extend and externally rotate the hip. The semimembranosus and semitendinosus (medial hamstrings) are two-joint muscles that act to flex and internally rotate the knee and extend and internally rotate the hip. The sartorius muscle, which originates from the ASIS, acts on both the knee and hip joints. The tendons of the sartorius, gracilis, and semimembranosus join together to form the pes anserinus, which inserts to the anteromedial aspect of the proximal tibia just inferior to the tibial tuberosity. The gastrocnemius muscle is a two-head and two-joint muscle that acts to flex the knee and plantarflex the ankle (18). The gastrocnemius is discussed in detail in the "Ankle and Foot" section of this chapter. The popliteus is a weak flexor of the knee but, more importantly, "unlocks" the extended knee by laterally rotating the femur on the fixed tibia.

Injuries. As mentioned above, the knee is a frequently injured joint, with its ligaments, menisci, and patellofemoral joint vulnerable to acute and repetitive use damage. Most knee injuries require exercise training for rehabilitation, and some require surgery as well. Predisposing factors to knee injury include the following (3,7,36):

➤ Lower extremity malalignment (e.g., Q angle abnormalities, flat feet)
➤ Limb length discrepancy
➤ Muscular imbalance and weakness
➤ Inflexibility
➤ Previous injury
➤ Inadequate proprioception

➤ Joint instability
➤ Playing surface and equipment problems
➤ Slight predominance in females (particularly for patellofemoral problems)

Ligamentous sprains and tears are common in the knee, particularly in athletes. Because of its structure and insertion points, the anterior cruciate ligament is more frequently injured than the posterior cruciate ligament. Classically, the anterior cruciate ligament is injured when external rotation of the tibia is coupled with a valgus force on the knee (e.g., direct force from the lateral side of the knee, planting the foot and twisting the knee) (3).

> *Ligamentous sprains and tears are common in the knee, particularly in athletes.*

The menisci are also frequently injured, particularly in athletes. The medial meniscus is more frequently torn than the lateral meniscus, due in part to its attachment to the medial collateral ligament. The menisci are poorly innervated and relatively avascular; thus, they are not very pain sensitive and are slow to heal following injury. The "terrible triad" is a traumatic sports injury in which the anterior cruciate ligament, medial collateral ligament, and medial meniscus are damaged simultaneously (4).

Patellofemoral pain syndrome is a common disorder in young athletes (particularly females) that produces anterior knee pain. Often, patellofemoral pain syndrome is caused by an off-center line of pull of the patella, which irritates the joint surfaces and retinaculum of the knee (40). An off-center pull of the patella can result from insufficiency muscular imbalance during knee extension (24) and from excessive varus and valgus stresses from Q angles outside of the normal range of 13°–18°.

ANKLE AND FOOT

Ankles and feet are responsible for weight bearing and ambulation. Proper function and mechanics of ankles and feet are essential for most sports activities and performance of activities of daily living. Slight abnormalities in the feet and ankles (e.g., muscular imbalance, proprioceptive dysfunction, and structural changes) are transmitted via the kinetic chain to most joints superior to them in the body (4). Thus, knee, hip, low back, neck, shoulder, and body alignment and postural problems can at times be traced to dysfunctional ankles and feet. This section focuses on ankle functional anatomy. For the functional anatomy of the intrinsic foot, the reader is referred to other sources (1,16,28,29,31).

> *Proper function and mechanics of ankles and feet are essential for most sports activities and performance of activities of daily living.*

Bones. The foot has 26 articulating bones contained in three functional units: the anterior (forefoot), middle (midfoot), and posterior (hindfoot) (Fig. 3.40). The forefoot contains the five metatarsals (one for each digit) and 14 phalanges (toes), three each for digits 2–5 and two for the great toe. The midfoot contains the five tarsal bones: the navicular, cuboid, and three cuneiforms. The hindfoot contains the talus and calcaneus bones. The dome of the talus articulates with the distal tibia and fibula and provides the link between the leg and foot at the talocrural joint. The ankle is formed by the fibrous union of the distal tibia, the medial malleolus of the tibia, and the lateral malleolus of the fibula (7). The location of the talus is superior to the calcaneus, between the malleoli of the tibia and fibula. Most of the calcaneus represents the posterior projection of the heel. The calcaneus provides important attachment sites for the ankle plantarflexor muscles.

Ligaments. There are approximately 100 ligaments in the ankle and foot region (Fig. 3.41). On the lateral side of the ankle, the major ligaments include the anterior and posterior talofibular and the calcaneofibular ligaments. The deltoid ligament complex is on the medial ankle and includes the tibiocalcaneal, anterior and posterior tibiotalar, and tibionavicular ligaments. The plantar calcaneonavicular ligament (spring ligament) of the foot helps support the talus and maintains the longitudinal arch (36).

There are two arches on the plantar aspect of the foot that give the foot its shape and distribute body weight from the talus to the foot during various load-bearing conditions (3). The various

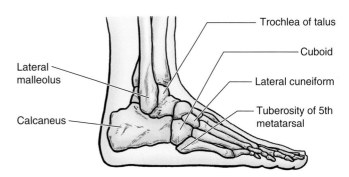

A Lateral foot

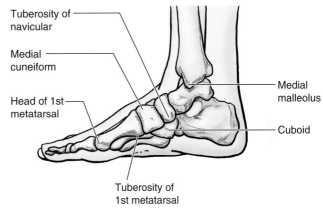

B Medial foot

FIGURE 3.40. Bones of the ankle and foot regions. **A.** Lateral view. **B.** Medial view. (From Moore KL, Dalley AF II. *Clinical Oriented Anatomy.* 4th ed. Baltimore: Lippincott Williams & Wilkins; 1999.)

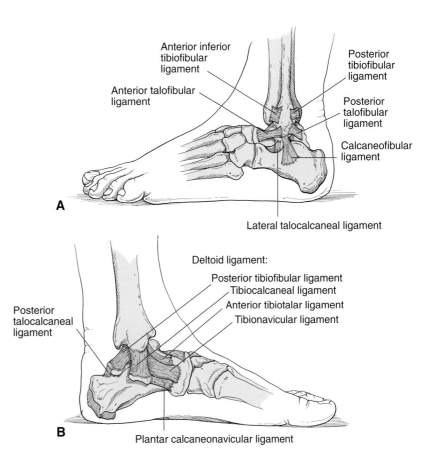

FIGURE 3.41. Ligaments of the ankle and foot regions. **A.** Lateral view. **B.** Medial view. (From Cipriano J. *Photographic Manual of Regional Orthopaedic and Neurological Tests.* 2nd ed. Baltimore: Lippincott Williams & Wilkins; 1991.)

ligaments and bones primarily support the arches, with muscles providing secondary support. The longitudinal arch extends from the calcaneal tuberosity to the five metatarsals, whereas the transverse arch extends crosswise from medial to lateral in the midtarsal region. The plantar fascia, or plantar aponeurosis, is a strong fibrous connective tissue that provides support for the longitudinal arch. The plantar fascia acts as an extension of the calcaneal (Achilles) tendon of the plantarflexor muscles. During weight-bearing phase of gait, the plantar fascia acts like a spring to store mechanical energy that is then released during foot push-off (38).

Joints. The ankle joint is a synovial, hinge-type joint between the distal tibia and fibula and the dome of talus. A tight fibrous syndesmosis between tibia and fibula unites the distal ends of the bones and forms a "malleolar mortise" into which the trochlea or "dome" of talus fits. The subtalar joint is a plane synovial joint between talus and calcaneus. There are many other joints between the other tarsal bones that allow varying degrees and types of movements. Additionally there are tarsometatarsal, intermetatarsal, metatarsophalangeal, and interphalangeal joints (36).

Movements. The talocrural joint allows approximately 15°–20° of dorsiflexion and 50° of plantarflexion in the sagittal plane. The subtalar joint allows approximately 20°–30° of inversion and 5°–15° of eversion in the frontal plane. The midtarsal and tarsometatarsal joints permit gliding motion. The metatarsophalangeal and interphalangeal joints primarily allow flexion and extension of the digits in the sagittal plane. Pronation and supination are combination movements at the ankle and foot that allow the foot to maintain contact with the ground in a variety of stances or on uneven ground. Pronation is a combination of talocrural dorsiflexion, subtalar eversion, and forefoot abduction. Supination is a combination of talocrural plantarflexion, subtalar inversion, and forefoot adduction (38) (Fig. 3.42).

Muscles. The major muscles that act on the ankle and foot are located in the leg, and these muscles are typically grouped by their compartmental location—anterior, lateral, superficial posterior, and deep posterior (38).

Anterior and Lateral. The anterior muscles, tibialis anterior, peroneus tertius, extensor digitorum longus, and extensor hallucis longus, are ankle dorsiflexors (Fig. 3.43). The tibialis anterior also inverts the foot and extends the second through fifth digits, whereas the peroneus tertius everts the foot. The extensor hallucis longus acts to extend the big toe. The lateral muscles, peroneus longus and brevis, evert the foot and assist with plantarflexion as well (18) (Fig. 3.44).

Superficial and Deep Posterior. The superficial posterior muscles, gastrocnemius, soleus, and plantaris, are ankle plantarflexors (Fig. 3.45). The gastrocnemius is a two-head and two-joint muscle, which is a powerful plantarflexor of the ankle as well as a flexor of the knee. The gastrocnemius has relatively more fast twitch fibers than the soleus. Thus, the gastrocnemius is used more during dynamic, higher-force activities, and the soleus is more active during postural and static contractions (4). Because the gastrocnemius crosses the knee and ankle, the position of the knee during

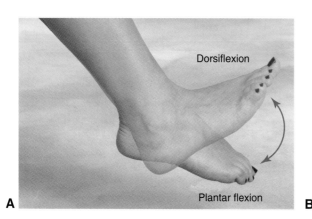
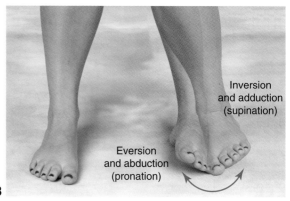

FIGURE 3.42. Movements of the ankle and foot. **A.** Dorsiflexion–plantarflexion. **B.** normal, inversion, and eversion.

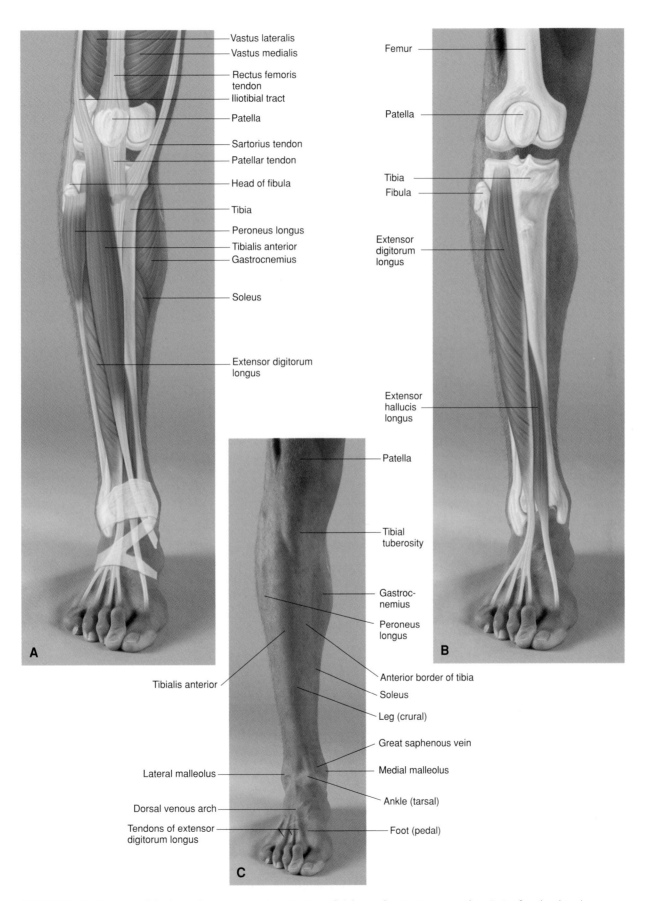

FIGURE 3.43. Muscles of the lower leg—anterior view. **A.** Superficial muscles. **B.** Deep muscles. **C.** Surface landmarks. (From Premkumar K. *The Massage Connection Anatomy and Physiology*. Baltimore: Lippincott Williams & Wilkins; 2004.)

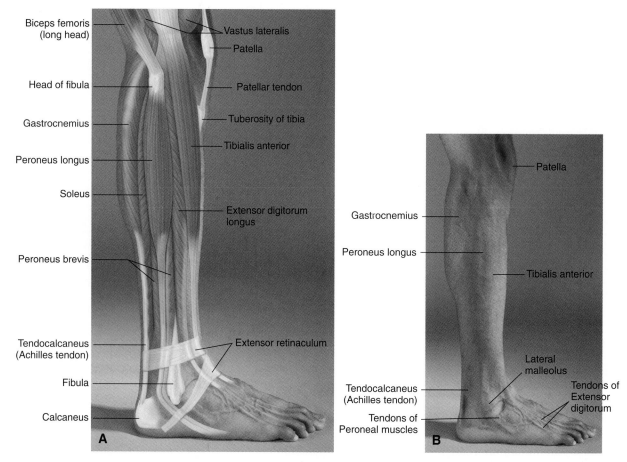

FIGURE 3.44. Muscles of the lower leg—lateral view. **A.** Muscles. **B.** Surface landmarks. (From Premkumar K. *The Massage Connection Anatomy and Physiology*. Baltimore: Lippincott Williams & Wilkins; 2004.)

plantarflexion resistance exercise affects the activity of the gastrocnemius. At 90° of knee flexion, the gastrocnemius experiences passive insufficiency and thus is less active than when the knee is straight (0° of flexion). In other words, during calf raise exercise, keep the knees straight to emphasize the gastrocnemius and bend the knees to emphasize the soleus. The deep posterior muscles—flexor digitorum longus, flexor hallucis longus, tibialis posterior, and popliteus—are ankle plantarflexors (except for the popliteus) and inverters (42). Additionally, the tibialis posterior inverts the foot. The flexor digitorum and hallucis longus flex their respective digits.

Injuries. Because of the burden placed on the ankle and foot during activities such as walking, running, jumping, and lifting, traumatic and overuse injuries frequently occur to these structures (3). Numerous acute muscular strains and cramps occur in the lower leg and foot, and many ligament sprains occur in this region as well. Ankle sprains are more common on the lateral side than on the medial side because there is less bony stability and ligamentous strength on the lateral side. The mechanism of injury for lateral ankle sprains is excessive inversion (rolling out of the ankle), as occurs when landing on someone's foot after jumping in basketball. The anterior talofibular ligament is the most frequently sprained ligament in inversion injuries (3).

> *Numerous acute muscular strains and cramps occur in the lower leg and foot, and many ligament sprains occur in this region as well.*

Achilles tendon rupture is possibly the most serious acute injury of the leg (3). Nearly 75% of Achilles tendon ruptures are seen in male athletes between 30 and 40 years of age. The typical mechanism is forceful plantarflexion while the knee is extended. These injuries almost always require surgical repair and extensive, long-term rehabilitation. Achilles tendon rupture is often a career-ending injury for athletes, especially if it occurs in the later stages of their careers (3).

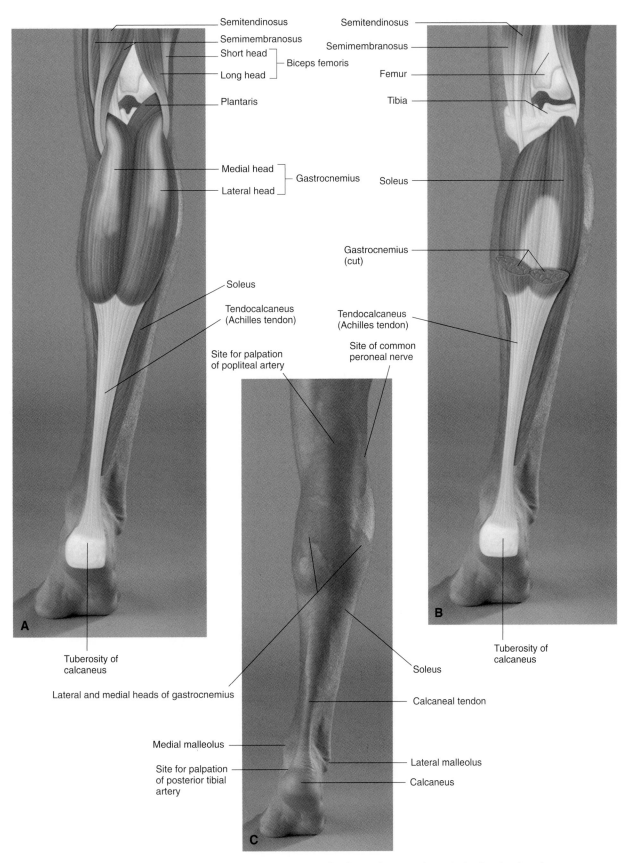

FIGURE 3.45. Muscles of the lower leg—Posterior view. **A.** Superficial muscles. **B.** Soleus. **C.** Surface landmarks. (From Premkumar K. *The Massage Connection Anatomy and Physiology*. Baltimore: Lippincott Williams & Wilkins; 2004.)

Plantar fasciitis is a chronic inflammatory condition that typically results in pain at the calcaneal insertion of the plantar fascia (3). Plantar fasciitis is usually caused by chronic pulling on the plantar fascia, tight Achilles tendon, hyperpronation (flat feet or pes planus), or other factors that overload the fascia (e.g., obesity). Treatment of plantar fasciitis includes stretching and strengthening exercises for the posterior calf muscles, orthoses to correct hyperpronation, and physiotherapy modalities and medication to reduce inflammation. Sometimes surgery is required to release the plantar fascia. Plantar fasciitis is often associated with calcaneal heel spurs (3).

Other chronic conditions of the foot and ankle include bunions, neuromas, Achilles tendonitis, and calcaneal bursitis. These conditions are frequently related to structural problems of the foot and ankle, such as hyperpronation or hypersupination (high arch or pes cavus). Unilateral hyperpronation or hypersupination may cause instability and proprioceptive difficulties at the ankle and postural imbalances and mechanical problems to proximal joint structures in the kinetic chain.

SPINE

The spine is an intricate multijoint structure that plays a crucial role in functional mechanics. The spine provides the link between the upper and lower extremities, protects the spinal cord, and enables trunk motion in three planes (3). Moreover, the rib cage of the thoracic spinal region protects the internal organs of the chest. Because of its intricacies, the spine is susceptible to injuries that may severely impair physical function.

> *The spine provides the link between the upper and lower extremities, protects the spinal cord, and enables trunk motion in three planes (3).*

Bones. The spinal column contains a complex of irregular bones called "vertebrae" that are stacked upon one another (Fig. 3.46). There are 24 individual vertebrae: 7 cervical (neck), 12 thoracic (mid back), and 5 lumbar (low back) (36). The most superior cervical vertebra (C1) articulates with the

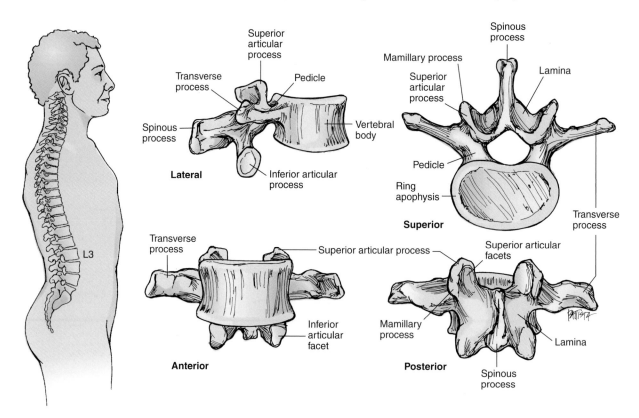

FIGURE 3.46. A typical lumbar vertebra (L3) in four views identifying the relevant landmarks. (From Oatis CA. *Kinesiology. The Mechanics and Pathomechanics of Human Movement.* Baltimore: Lippincott Williams & Wilkins; 2004.)

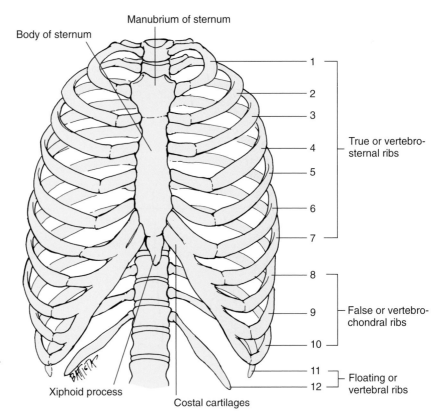

FIGURE 3.47. The thoracic cage—anterior view. (From Oatis CA. *Kinesiology. The Mechanics and Pathomechanics of Human Movement.* Baltimore: Lippincott Williams & Wilkins; 2003.)

occipital bone of the skull, whereas the most inferior lumbar vertebra (L5) articulates with the sacrum. The size of the vertebrae increases from the cervical to the lumbar region because of an increase in load-bearing responsibilities. Each vertebra contains anterior and posterior elements. The anterior element, called the "vertebral body," is oval with flat superior and inferior surfaces for articulation with the adjacent vertebral bodies. The posterior element, or posterior arch, consists of pedicles and laminae, which join anteriorly at the body and posteriorly at the spinous process to form the vertebral foramen (canal). The vertebral foramen provides a space through which the spinal cord passes. The posterior arch also contains facets on each side and top and bottom for articulation with adjacent vertebrae. The spinous and transverse processes are bony protuberances that provide attachment points for the spinal musculature (36).

Ribs attach to each of the 12 thoracic vertebrae bilaterally and form the thoracic cage (Fig. 3.47). The seven most superior pairs of ribs are considered true ribs and attach directly to the sternum. The five lower pairs of ribs are considered false ribs. Three pairs of false ribs attach indirectly to the sternum by the costal cartilages. Two most inferior pairs of false ribs do not attach to the sternum and are considered floating ribs (38).

The spinal column also contains a sacrum and coccyx, which are situated at the lower spine, immediately inferior to the fifth lumbar vertebra. The sacrum is a large triangular bone that acts as the transition point between the spine and pelvis. The coccyx is a bone formed of three to five fused vertebrae located at the distal sacrum (36).

In the sagittal plane, the spinal column normally demonstrates four curves instead of a straight line (Fig. 3.48). These curves give the spine mechanical advantage and improved load-bearing capabilities. When the convexity of the curve is posterior, the curve is known as kyphosis, and when the convexity of the curve is anterior, the curve is known as lordosis. The cervical and lumbar regions have lordosis, and the thoracic and sacral regions have kyphosis. Deviations in the sagittal plane are referred to as "hyperlordosis" or "hyperkyphosis." In the frontal plane, the spinal column should normally be positioned in the midline. Lateral deviation is referred to as "scoliosis" (Fig. 3.49) (4).

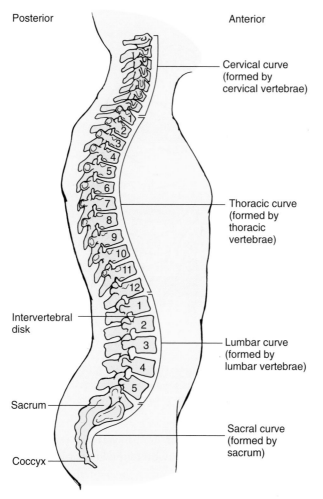

Posterior

Anterior

Cervical curve
(formed by
cervical vertebrae)

Thoracic curve
(formed by
thoracic
vertebrae)

Intervertebral
disk

Lumbar curve
(formed by
lumbar vertebrae)

Sacrum

Sacral curve
(formed by
sacrum)

Coccyx

FIGURE 3.48. Vertebral column—lateral view showing the four normal curves and regions. (From Oatis CA. *Kinesiology. The Mechanics and Pathomechanics of Human Movement.* Baltimore: Lippincott Williams & Wilkins; 2003.)

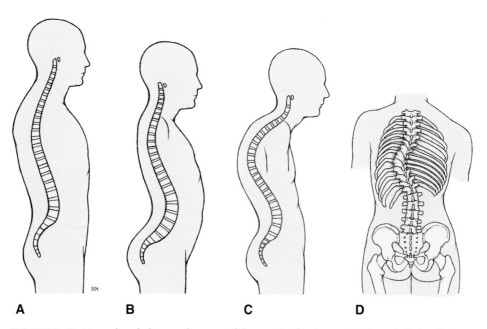

A   B   C   D

FIGURE 3.49. Normal and abnormal curves of the vertebral column. **A.** Normal. **B.** Lordosis. **C.** Kyphosis. **D.** Scoliosis (Courtesy of Neil O. Hardy, Westpoint, CT).

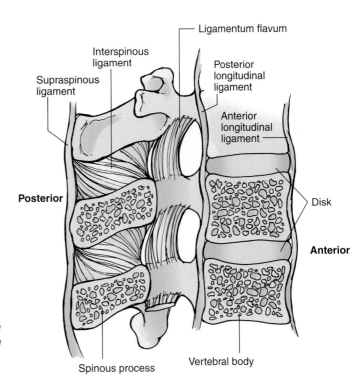

FIGURE 3.50. Ligaments and discs of the lumbar spine—mid-sagittal view. (From Oatis CA. *Kinesiology. The Mechanics and Pathomechanics of Human Movement.* Baltimore: Lippincott Williams & Wilkins; 2003.)

Ligaments. The main supporting ligaments of the spinal column are the anterior and posterior longitudinal ligaments and the ligamentum flavum, which span from the upper cervical to lower lumbar region (Fig. 3.50). The anterior and posterior longitudinal ligaments attach to the vertebral bodies, and the ligamentum flavum connects the posterior arches and forms the posterior border of the vertebral canal. The interspinous and supraspinous ligaments attach to adjacent posterior arch structures (4).

Intervertebral Discs. The intervertebral discs are important structures that provide load bearing, shock absorption, and stability to the vertebral column. The discs are located between the vertebral bodies and compose about 20%–33% of the height of the vertebral column (31) (Fig. 3.50). Each intervertebral motion segment contains a disc, except for the articulation between the first and second cervical vertebrae (the atlas and axis, respectively). The intervertebral disc consists of the nucleus pulposus, annulus fibrosis, and endplates. These structures are composed of various concentrations of water, collagen, and proteoglycans. The nucleus pulposus, located in the center of the disc, is gel-like and more liquid than the annulus fibrosis. The nucleus pulposus dehydrates with age, which is one of the reasons why overall body height reduces with age (31). The annulus fibrosis, located at the periphery of the disc, is a more rigid structure and contains more collagen fibers than the nucleus. The oblique arrangement of the collagen fibers of the annulus helps the annulus resist tensile and compressive forces in various planes. However, the annulus is most susceptible to tearing with movements involving rotation and flexion under load. The vertebral endplates are thin layers of fibrocartilage that cover the inferior and superior aspects of the vertebral body and help anchor the disc to the vertebrae (25).

Joints. The spinal column consists of numerous motion segments (two adjacent vertebrae). Each motion segment of spine contains five articulations: one intervertebral joint and four zygapophysial ("facet") joints. The intervertebral joint connects adjacent bodies, whereas the zygapophysial joints connect adjacent facets (superior and inferior on each side). The lumbar zygapophysial joints are angled to allow flexion and extension and restrict axial rotation. The cervical and thoracic zygapophysial joints, on the other hand, are angled to accommodate axial rotation (4).

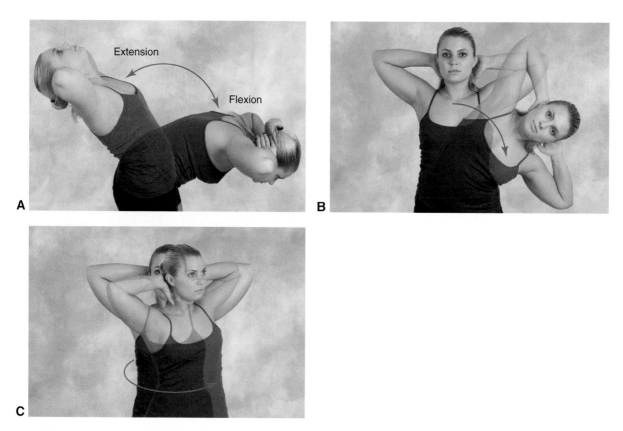

FIGURE 3.51. Movements of the lower trunk. **A.** Flexion–extension. **B.** Lateral flexion. **C.** Rotation.

Movements. The spine is capable of motion in all planes, and the extent of motion varies with region. In the cervical spine, the atlantooccipital joint allows flexion and extension and slight lateral flexion. The atlantoaxial joint allows primarily rotation. The remaining cervical joints allow flexion and extension, lateral flexion, and rotation. The thoracic joints allow moderate flexion, slight extension, moderate lateral flexion, and rotation. The lumbar joints allow flexion and extension, lateral flexion, and slight rotation (4) (Fig. 3.51). Refer to Table 3.5 for normal cervical and lumbar ROM values.

Compound Trunk Extension. Trunk motion in the sagittal plane during normal activities, such as lifting and bending, requires the compound movement of the lumbar spine, pelvis, and hip joints (22). This action is called "compound trunk extension" or "lumbopelvic rhythm." From a position of full trunk flexion, the lumbar extensors (erector spinae and multifidus) and hip extensors (gluteals and hamstrings) work together to actively rotate the trunk through approximately 180° in the sagittal plane (7) (Fig. 3.52). Lumbar movement accounts for approximately 72° of this motion, whereas hip and pelvis movement accounts for the remaining 108° (34). The relative contribution of individual muscle groups to force production during compound trunk extension is unknown, but it is assumed that the larger hip extensors generate most of the force (7). Because the pelvis remains free to move during activities of daily living such as lifting and bending, it is assumed that the small lumbar muscles play only a minor role in trunk extension torque production. Thus, they are considered to be the weak link in trunk extension movements (13). The rationale behind isolating the lumbar spine through pelvic stabilization mechanisms during exercise training is to force the lumbar muscles to be the primary trunk extensors, thereby providing the overload stimulus for strength gains (13). Dynamic progressive resistance exercise protocols on devices that stabilize the pelvis have produced unusually large gains (greater than 100%) in lumbar extension strength, even with training frequencies as low as one time per week (13). Clinically, patients with low back pain have displayed

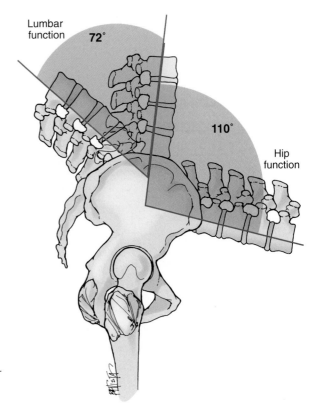

FIGURE 3.52. Compound trunk extension (lumbopelvic rhythm). Compound trunk extension involves the simultaneous movement of the lumbar spine (72°) and pelvis/hips (110°).

significant improvements in symptoms, disability, and psychosocial function following intensive exercise training with pelvic stabilization (19,26).

Muscles. The spine and trunk muscles exist in pairs, one on each side of the body. In general, bilateral contraction results in movement in the sagittal plane. The anterior muscles flex the spine, whereas the posterior muscles extend the spine. Unilateral contraction results in lateral bend or axial rotation.

Cervical

Anterior. The major anterior muscles of the cervical region include the sternocleidomastoid, scalenes (anterior, middle, and posterior), longus capitis, and longus colli muscles. On unilateral contraction, these muscles laterally flex and rotate the neck and head. On bilateral contraction, the anterior scalene, longus capitis and colli, and sternocleidomastoid muscles flex the neck and head. The scalenes attach proximally to the upper cervical transverse processes and distally to the upper two ribs. The sternocleidomastoid attaches proximally to the mastoid process of the occiput and distally to the sternum (medial head) and clavicle (lateral head) (Fig. 3.17). The longus muscles run from the transverse processes of the upper cervical vertebrae to the anterior aspect of the superior cervical vertebrae (longus colli) or the base of the occiput (longus capitis) (18).

Posterior. The suboccipital muscles, which attach the upper cervical vertebrae to the occiput, extend the head when they contract bilaterally and laterally bend and rotate the neck when they contract unilaterally. Similarly, the splenius (capitis and cervicis) and erector spinae (spinalis, longissimus, and iliocostalis) muscles extend the neck when they contract bilaterally and laterally bend and rotate the neck when they contract unilaterally (18) (Fig. 3.18).

Lateral. The lateral muscles of the neck and head include the levator scapulae and upper trapezius muscles, both of which laterally bend and rotate the neck on unilateral contraction. The upper trapezius extends the neck as well on bilateral contraction. The levator scapulae attaches proximally to the transverse processes of the upper four cervical vertebrae and distally to the vertebral border

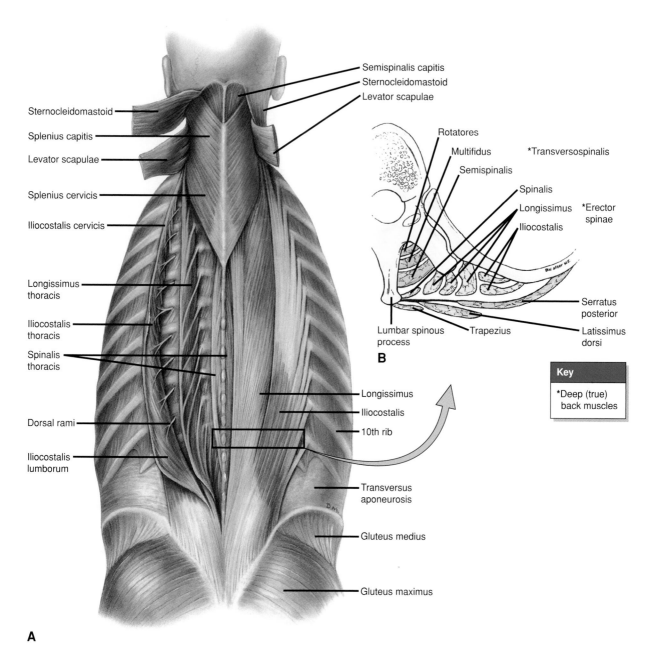

A

FIGURE 3.53. Deep muscles of the back. **A.** *Right,* the three columns of the erector spinae. *Left,* the spinalis is displayed by reflecting the longissimus and iliocostalis. **B.** Transverse section of the back showing arrangement of the erector spinae, multifidus, and rotator muscles. (From Moore KL, Dalley AF II. *Clinical Oriented Anatomy.* 4th ed. Baltimore: Lippincott Williams & Wilkins; 1999.)

of the scapula. The upper trapezius attaches proximally to the occiput and spinous processes of the cervical vertebrae and distally to the clavicle and acromion of the scapula (18). The levator scapulae and upper trapezius muscles also cause movement of the scapulothoracic joint, as discussed in the "Shoulder" section of this chapter.

Lumbar

Posterior. The posterior musculature of the lumbar spine consists of three muscle groups, namely, the erector spinae, multifidus muscles, and intrinsic rotators (Fig. 3.53). Additionally, the latissimus dorsi, which is usually considered a muscle that acts on the shoulder, extends and stabilizes the lumbar spine through its attachment to the thoracolumbar fascia (25). The erector spinae group, which lies lateral and superficial to the multifidus, is divided into the iliocostalis lumborum and longissimus thoracis muscles (5). These muscles are separated from each other by the lumbar intramuscular aponeurosis, with the longissimus lying medially. The longissimus and iliocostalis are composed of several multisegmental fascicles, which allow for extension and posterior translation when the muscles are contracted bilaterally. The fascicular arrangement of the multifidus muscle suggests that the multifidus acts primarily as a sagittal rotator (extension without posterior translation) (21). Lateral flexion and axial rotation are possible for both the multifidus and erector spinae musculature during unilateral contraction. The iliocostalis may be better suited to exert axial rotation on the lumbar vertebral motion segment than either the longissimus or multifidus muscles (5). Because of their anatomical and biomechanical properties, the posterior lumbar muscles are particularly adapted to maintain posture and stabilize the spine and trunk (5). The intrinsic rotators, rotatores and intertransversarii muscles, are primarily length transducers and position sensors for the vertebral segment (30).

Lateral. The lateral muscles of the lumbar spine include the quadratus lumborum and psoas (major and minor). The quadratus lumborum originates from the iliac crest and inserts at the 12th rib and transverse process of the lower four lumbar vertebrae. The quadratus lumborum produces lateral bending of the lumbar spine with unilateral contraction and stabilizes the trunk with bilateral contraction. The psoas major muscle originates from the anterior surfaces of the transverse processes of all the lumbar vertebrae and inserts at the lesser trochanter of the femur. The psoas major flexes the trunk and the hip (18).

Anterior. The anterior muscles of the lumbar region consist of the abdominal group: the rectus abdominis, internal and external abdominal oblique and transversus abdominis (see Fig. 3.17). The rectus abdominus originates from the pubic bone and inserts at the fifth through seventh ribs and xiphoid process. The rectus abdominis exists as two vertical muscles separated by a connective tissue band, the linea alba. Horizontally, the rectus abdominis appears to be separated by three distinct lines. These lines represent areas of connective tissue that support the muscle in place of attachment to bones (38). The rectus abdominis is the primary trunk flexor, and through its attachment to the pubic bone, it also tilts the pelvis posteriorly. The internal and external obliquus abdominis muscles rotate the trunk on unilateral contraction and flex the trunk on bilateral contraction. The transversus abdominis runs horizontally, attaching medially to the linea alba via the abdominal aponeurosis and laterally to the thoracolumbar fascia, inguinal ligament, iliac crest, and the lower six ribs. Contraction of the transversus abdominis stabilizes the lumbar spine and increases intra-abdominal pressure, and aberrant firing patterns of the transversus abdominis appear to be related to low back pain (35).

To isolate the abdominal muscles during trunk flexion exercise, it is advisable to shorten the psoas and other hip flexor muscles (active insufficiency) by flexing the hips and knees (38). Thus, crunches with the hips and knees flexed may be more effective in conditioning the abdominals than straight knee sit-ups (18).

Injuries

Cervical. The cervical region is the most mobile region of the spine, and relatively small cervical muscles are responsible for supporting the head. These factors make the cervical region vulnerable to instability and injury (3). The most dangerous injuries to the cervical region are traumatic fractures and dislocations that result in instability of the column. The combination of axial compression and hyperflexion is a common mechanism for severe cervical injuries such as these (39). Examples of activities with these mechanisms include diving into a

The most dangerous injuries to the cervical region are traumatic fractures and dislocations that result in instability of the column.

shallow pool or a football player making a head-on tackle. The most dire consequence of upper cervical dislocation or fracture is neural damage to the upper spinal cord, which may result in paralysis or death (3). Thus, any traumatic neck injury should be treated as a medical emergency (41).

Sprains and strains of the neck muscles and ligaments are frequently the result of violent hyper-extension–hyperflexion from sudden acceleration–deceleration, such as a head-on car collision. This condition, commonly called "whiplash," can cause tears of the anterior and posterior structures of the cervical region, including the muscles (e.g., sternocleidomastoid, upper trapezius, and cervical paraspinals) and ligaments (7). After ruling out fracture, dislocation, instability, and disc herniation, treatment of whiplash usually includes passive modalities, stretches, and strengthening exercises for the neck.

Lumbar. Low back pain is one of the leading causes of disability and consistently ranks as one of the top reasons for visits to physicians. Low back pain affects 60%–80% of the general population at some point during their lifetime, and 20%–30% suffer from this disorder at any given time (9,10). Attaching a specific diagnosis to low back pain is difficult and elusive, because there often is no identifiable source of the pain or injury (27).

> **Low back pain is one of the leading causes of disability and consistently ranks as one of the top reasons for visits to physicians.**

Some of the causes of low back pain include intervertebral disc herniation, facet joint inflammation, muscular strains, and ligamentous sprains. Injury to these structures can be traumatic, caused by events such as inappropriately lifting or falling, or degenerative, caused by a deconditioned lumbar spine, poor posture, prolonged mechanical loading, or poor body mechanics during work, home, or sports activities (3,7). A common cause of lumbar disc herniation is forceful flexion and rotation of the lumbar spine. A protruded lumbar disc that encroaches on the lumbar nerve roots may result in lower extremity sensory and motor problems such as pain, numbness, and muscular weakness and atrophy. Bowel and bladder dysfunction are serious conditions that can result from herniated lumbar discs and require immediate medical treatment (3).

Restorative exercise designed to improve the structural integrity of the lower trunk is commonly used for the treatment of low back pain, and generally, the efficacy of this approach has been supported (20). Many types of exercises, including aerobic, flexibility, muscular strength and endurance, and core stability, are used. The Personal Trainer should be particularly well versed in low back exercise techniques, incorporating those needed when appropriate.

SUMMARY

This chapter provides an overview of musculoskeletal functional anatomy of the major joint structures of the human body. These principles play a major role in nearly all aspects of the Personal Trainer's practice, including exercise testing, exercise prescription, and analysis of exercise movements. Thus, the Personal Trainer is urged to master these principles so that safe, effective, and efficient exercise training programs can be designed to improve musculoskeletal fitness.

REFERENCES

1. Agur A, Lee M, Anderson J. *Grant's Atlas of Anatomy*. 9th ed. Baltimore: Williams & Wilkins; 1991.
2. An K, Morrey B. Biomechanics of the shoulder. In: Matsen F, editor. *The Shoulder*. Philadelphia: WB Saunders; 1990. p. 213–265.
3. Anderson M, Hall S. *Fundamentals of Sports Injury Management*. Baltimore: Williams & Wilkins; 1997.
4. Baldwin K. *Kinesiology for Personal Fitness Trainers*. New York: McGraw-Hill; 2003.
5. Bogduk N, Twomey LT. *Clinical Anatomy of the Lumbar Spine*. New York: Churchill Livingstone; 1990.
6. Burkhead W. *Rotator Cuff Disorders*. Baltimore: Williams & Wilkins; 1996.
7. Cailliet R. *Soft Tissue Pain and Disability*. 3rd ed. Philadelphia: FA Davis; 1996.
8. DeLavier F. *Strength Training Anatomy*. Champaign (IL): Human Kinetics; 2001.
9. Deyo R, Tsui-Wu Y. Descriptive epidemiology of low back pain and its related medical care in the United States. *Spine*. 1987;12:264–8.
10. Frymoyer J. An overview of the incidences and cost of low back pain. *Orthop Clin North Am*. 1991;22:263–71.
11. Garrick J, Webb D. *Sports Injuries: Diagnosis and Management*. Philadelphia: WB Saunders; 1990.

12. Graves J, Franklin B. Introduction. In: Graves J, Franklin B, editors. *Resistance Training for Health and Rehabilitation*. Champaign (IL): Human Kinetics; 2001. p. 1–20.

13. Graves JE, Webb DC, Pollock ML, et al. Pelvic stabilization during resistance training: its effect on the development of lumbar extension strength. *Arch Phys Med Rehabil*. 1994;75(2):210–15.

14. Griggs S, Weiss A. Bony injuries of the wrist, forearm, and elbow. In: Plancher KD, editor. *Clinics in Sports Medicine*. Philadelphia: WB Saunders; 1996.

15. Halikis M, Taleisnik J. Soft-tissue injuries of the wrist. In: Plancher KD, editor. *Clinics in Sports Medicine*. Philadelphia: WB Saunders; 1996.

16. Hall-Craggs E. *Anatomy As the Basis for Clinical Medicine*. 3rd ed. Baltimore: Williams & Wilkins; 1995.

17. Horrigan J, Robinson J. *The 3-Minute Rotator Cuff Solution*. Los Angeles: Health for Life; 1990.

18. Kendall F, McCreary E. *Muscles: Testing and Function*. 4th ed. Philadelphia: Lippincott Williams & Wilkins; 1993.

19. Leggett S, Mooney V, Matheson L, et al. Restorative exercise for clinical low back pain: a prospective two-center study with 1-year follow-up. *Spine*. 1999;24(9):889–98.

20. Liemohn W, editor. *Exercise Prescription and the Back*. New York: McGraw-Hill; 2001.

21. MacIntosh J, Bogduk N. The attachments of the lumbar erector spinae. *Spine*. 1991;16(7):783–92.

22. Mayer L, Greenberg B. Measurement of the strength of trunk muscles. *J Bone Joint Surg*. 1942;4:842–56.

23. McCue F, Hussamy O. Hand and wrist injuries. In: Magee D, Quillen W, editors. *Athletic Injuries and Rehabilitation*. Philadelphia: WB Saunders; 1996.

24. McGee D. *Orthopedic Physical Assessment*. Philadelphia: WB Saunders; 1987.

25. McGill S. *Low Back Disorders: Evidence-Based Prevention and Rehabilitation*. Champaign (IL): Human Kinetics; 2002.

26. Mooney V, Kron M, Rummerfield P, Holmes B. The effect of workplace based strengthening on low back injury rates: a case study in the strip mining industry. *J Occup Rehabil*. 1995;5:157–67.

27. Mooney V. Functional evaluation of the spine. *Curr Opin Orthop*. 1994;5(11):54–7.

28. Moore K, Agur A. *Essentials of Clinical Anatomy*. 2nd ed. Baltimore: Williams & Wilkins; 2002.

29. Moore K. *Clinically Oriented Anatomy*. 4th ed. Baltimore: Williams & Wilkins; 2004.

30. Nitz A, Peck D. Comparison of muscle spindle concentrations in large and small human epaxial muscles acting in parallel combinations. *Am Surg*. 1986;52:273–7.

31. Norkin C, Levangie P. *Joint Structure & Function*. Philadelphia: FA Davis; 1992.

32. Oatis C. *Kinesiology—The Mechanics and Pathomechanics of Human Movement*. Baltimore: Lippincott Williams & Wilkins; 2004.

33. Olson T, Pawlina W. *A.D.A.M. Student Atlas of Anatomy*. Baltimore: Williams & Wilkins; 1996.

34. Pollock ML, Leggett SH, Graves JE, et al. Effect of resistance training on lumbar extension strength. *Am J Sports Med*. 1989;17(5):624–9.

35. Richardson C, Jull G, Hodges P, Hides J. *Therapeutic Exercise for Spinal Segmental Stabilization in Low Back Pain*. Edinburgh, Scotland: Churchill Livingstone; 1999.

36. Rosse C, Clawson D. *The Musculoskeletal System in Health and Disease*. Hagerstown (MD): Harper & Row; 1980.

37. Snell R. Clinical *Anatomy*. 7th ed. Baltimore: Lippincott Williams & Wilkins; 2003.

38. Thompson C, Floyd R, editors. *Manual of Structural Kinesiology*. 14th ed. New York: McGraw-Hill; 2001.

39. Torg J, Vegso J, O'Neill MJ, Sennett B. The epidemiologic, pathologic, biomechanical and cinematographic analysis of football-induced cervical spine trauma. *Am J Sports Med*. 1990;18(1):50–7.

40. Westfall D, Worrell T. Anterior knee pain syndrome: role of the vastus medialis oblique. *J Sports Rehabil*. 1992;1(4):317–25.

41. Wiesenfarth J, Briner W. Neck injuries: urgent decisions and actions. *Phys Sports Med*. 1996;24(1):35–41.

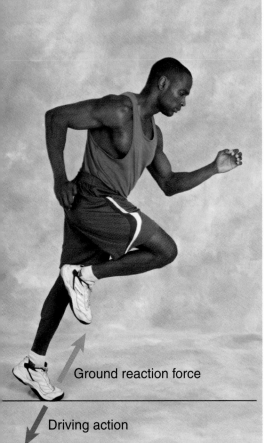

Ground reaction force

Driving action

CHAPTER 4

Applied Biomechanics

OBJECTIVES

- Introduce the concept of levers so that there is a distinction between a 1st-class lever, a 2nd-class lever, and a 3rd-class lever
- Describe the mechanical concepts of linear work, linear power, and power
- Describe the effect of gravity acting on a weight of a lever to the left of the axis causing the muscle to lengthen
- Identify the differences between angular work and angular power
- Illustrate rotary motion at the elbow
- Explain translation and rotation that occurs at the knee
- Illustrate the concept of force–time
- Describe the relationship between external torque, the moment of inertia, and angular acceleration
- Describe the concept of ground reaction forces

Biomechanics is a field of science that involves application of mechanical principles to the study of living organisms. The prefix "bio" denotes life. The term "mechanics" indicates analysis of forces. The term is used in a broad sense to define how biological and material properties of the skeletal, neuromuscular, and articular systems are governed by the laws and principles of physics. Biomechanics is however not simply a field that has application in the sports or physical activity or physical training setting; rather, it is broad and includes human factor design, ergonomics, improvement of physical function and activities of daily activity, and numerous medical applications including stress and strain and load deformation of various biological materials. Numerous professional fields use an understanding of biomechanics for pragmatic application including engineers, surgeons, dentists, teachers, coaches, and personal trainers (8,16,18).

Terms commonly used in association with the field of biomechanics include anthropometrics, dynamics, fulcrum, kinematics, kinesiology, kinetics, levers (1st, 2nd, and 3rd classes), moments, moment arm, torque, and units of measurement. See Box 4.1 for a complete list.

NEWTON'S LAWS AND THE APPLICATION TO MOVEMENT

Human movement is based on Newton's Laws of Motion. Table 4.1 outlines the three laws and the application from a linear and angular perspective.

LEVERS

There are three types of levers mechanically as shown in Figure 4.2. Most of the muscles in the human body act as 3rd-class levers because the muscles act through a much shorter moment arm than the segment and any resistance that the person might be attempting to overcome.

A 1st-class lever has the fulcrum or axis between the force and the resistance.

A 2nd-class lever has the axis or fulcrum at the distal end with the resistance between the axis and the force arm.

A 3rd-class lever has the resistance toward the end of the lever and the muscle moment arm between the external resistance or load and the axis.

A 1st-class lever has the fulcrum or axis between the force and the resistance. The simplest method for thinking about this is a seesaw. There are few examples of this in the human body. Extending the elbow against resistance is an example of a 1st-class lever. Extension of the neck (between the first two cervical vertebrae) is another example of a 1st-class lever in the body.

A 2nd-class lever has the axis or fulcrum at the distal end with the resistance between the axis and the force arm. A good example of this is a wheelbarrow. In the body, an example of a 2nd-class lever is plantarflexion at the ankle as during the push-off phase in the gait cycle.

TABLE 4.1	**NEWTON'S LINEAR AND ANGULAR LAWS**	
Law	**Linear Component**	**Angular Component**
1st Law of Inertia	A body at rest will remain at rest or uniform velocity unless changed by an external force	A body will remain at constant angular velocity unless changed by an external torque
2nd Law of Acceleration	Linear acceleration is proportional to force and inversely proportional to mass	Angular acceleration is proportional to torque causing acceleration and inversely proportional to moment of inertia
3rd Law of Action–Reaction	Every force has an equal and opposite directed force	Every torque has an equal and opposite torque

Adapted from Nawoczenski DA, Neumann DA. Biomechanical principles. In: Neumann DA, editor. *Kinesiology of the Musculoskeletal System—Foundations for Physical Rehabilitation*. St. Louis (MO): Mosby; 2002. p. 56–87.

| BOX **4.1** | **Definitions of Common Biomechanical Terms** |

Anthropometrics is a term associated with the field of anthropology and is concerned with comparative measurements of the human body. Typically in the field of personal training, the application would be to the width, length, girth, and/or circumference of body segments (e.g., upper arm circumference).

Dynamics is the field of a science, like biomechanics that deals with the science of motion due to application of forces and typically describes bodies that are accelerating.

Fulcrum is sometimes used interchangeably with the term **axis.** This is the point about which a lever rotates. In the human body, because most articulations are unconstrained, the fulcrum changes, depending on where a person is in the range of motion (ROM).

Ground reaction force (GRF) is a contact force, typically displayed in three cardinal planes (*xy*, ml, and vertical). The *xy* plane is typically the horizontal plane, which is forward and backward. The ml plane is the mediolateral plane and commonly refers to movement from side to side, sometimes also called medial and lateral movement, depending on the starting position. The vertical plane is the plane that defines movement up and down and of all the GRFs is typically the greatest in magnitude. Figure 4.1 provides a pragmatic example of how GRF would be displayed.

Joint reaction force is the net force acting across a joint in the body. For example, in single-leg stance the upper body and thigh on the stance side is exerting a compressive force downwardly across the knee and foot/ankle complex. The JRF exerts a force equal and opposite upward against the femoral condyles in stance. In most instances this is unknown and is an estimated value (8).

Kinematics is the geometry of motion or a description of motion without regard to the forces that cause that motion. The linear and curvilinear and angular variables included under this term include position, distance, displacement, speed, velocity, and acceleration.

Kinesiology is the science or study of movement and is an umbrella term that can encompasses anatomy, physiology, and psychology of movement.

Kinetics is the study of the action of forces.

Levers (1st, 2nd, and 3rd classes) are rigid or semirigid segments that rotate about an axis. In the human body, typically our limbs (arms and legs) or some component of our limbs rotate about a point on the body. For example, when knee extension occurs, the leg (defined from the knee distal to the foot and ankle) rotates about some point at the knee. In this case, the leg is a lever and the knee extensor muscle group creates the force that allows this movement to occur.

Moment, used interchangeably with the term **torque,** is the product of force and perpendicular distance. To remain in a static position (equilibrium), the body's levers and muscles acting through a perpendicular distance create an internal moment to offset the external moment generated by body weight and any other external load that may be applied.

Moment arm also referred to as the lever arm, force arm, or torque arm is the perpendicular distance that the force acts through to create a moment or torque.

Torque is also known as moment, which is defined previously.

Units of measurement are the values used to report results from a biomechanical perspective. The metric system is used in most countries (base units include mass [kg], length [m], and time [s]); however, in the United States the English system is still in use (base units include weight [lb], length [ft], and time [s]).

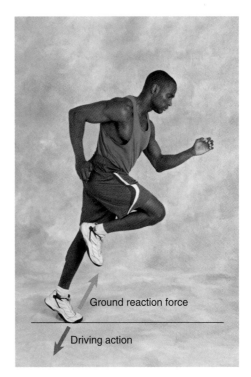

FIGURE 4.1. Ground reaction force (GRF) has practical application in a simple activity such as running. In this case the GRF, based on Newton's 3rd Law, exerts an equal and opposite GRF. This force is provided by the surface upon which one is moving. The ground pushes back against the person who is bearing weight based on Newton's 3rd Law— every action has an equal and opposite reaction.

A 3rd-class lever has the resistance toward the end of the lever and the muscle moment arm between the external resistance or load and the axis. Most muscles in the human body act as 3rd-class levers.

MECHANICAL CONCEPTS CRITICAL FOR THE PERSONAL TRAINER

Resistance activities are a key component for the Personal Trainer. Resistance can be in many forms. The body itself is a primary source for resistance. This is seen in commonly used activities such as sit-ups, push-ups, and pull-ups. The resistance for participants is their body weight. Body weight in the United States is mostly quantified in pounds, which is mass × acceleration or slugs (the term used in the English system to quantify mass) × 32.2 ft/s^2. In the metric system, the unit for body weight is newton, which is kg × 9.81 m/s^2.

If we assume that the person being trained has either less or more upper body strength, which is defined as the ability to exert force, simple geometry can be used to increase or decrease resistance (23). An incline push-up creates less resistance for the person performing a push-up for example (Fig. 4.3). The reason for this is that the body's resistance or body weight acts through a shorter distance, depending on the angle of incline. On the other hand, a decline push-up increases the resistance that is felt by the exercising person because the exerciser has to move his body weight through a greater distance (Fig. 4.4). Both of these are examples of 2nd-class levers in action.

Linear Work

The term "work" has numerous meanings, but essentially work requires mental and physical efforts on the part of the person working. For example, mowing the grass requires work, especially if the mower is not self-propelled. In the mechanical sense, work has a different meaning. "Linear mechanical work" is defined as the product of force and the parallel distance through which the force acts.

$$\text{Linear work} = \text{Force} \times \text{Distance}$$

For example, when weight training as the exerciser moves a 20-pound dumbbell (~90 N) vertically through a distance of 4 feet (~1.22 m), they have generated 80 pound · feet (~110 N · m) of linear work (8).

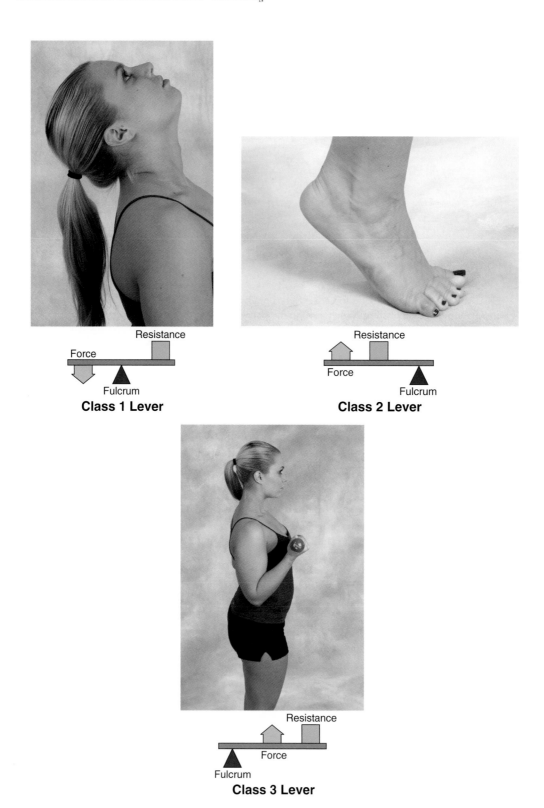

FIGURE 4.2. Display of three lever types within the human body for resistance, force, and the fulcrum (axis).

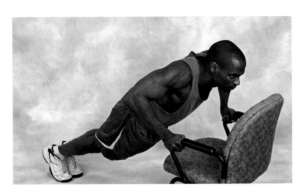

FIGURE 4.3. An incline push-up.

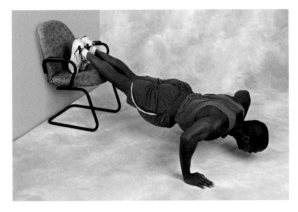

FIGURE 4.4. A decline push-up.

The rate of work production is termed linear power. Power is quantified as work/time.

$$\text{Linear Power} = \text{Work/Time}$$

When work is quantified, the amount of time needed to lift the object is not considered. However, when power is calculated, time is considered. As the time over which work is accomplished decreases, the power increases. In the example above, if the time needed to perform the work was 0.75 seconds, the power would be quantified as 106.7 pound · feet/s or (80 pound · feet/0.75 s) or in the metric system work would be quantified as 110 N · m/0.75 s (see Box 4.2 for the specific calculations). If the time was decreased to 0.5 seconds, the power would be increased to 160 pound · feet/s and 220 N · m/s or J/s. This simple mathematical example demonstrates how when time for work is decreased the power exerted is greater.

Power can also be quantified by an alternate method by rearranging the power equation and substituting mechanical work into the equation below

$$\text{Power} = \text{Force} \times \text{Displacement/Time}$$

Therefore, because velocity (V) is equal to displacement/time, power can be summarized as in the equation below.

$$P = F \times V$$

In this case, power is the product of force and velocity. Power is an important component in many sports and athletic movements from power lifting to jumping, throwing, and most ballistic movements including striking as in tennis, baseball, and badminton.

BOX **4.2**   **Power Calculations**

Linear power (LP) = Work/Time
English system calculations
LP = 80 pound · feet/0.75 s
LP = 106.7 pound · feet/s
Metric calculations
LP = 110 N · m/0.75 s
N · m also is known as a joule
LP = 146.7 N · m/s or J/s
J/s = watts
The power would be quantified as N · m /s or joules (a.k.a. N · m).

BOX **4.3**	**How Radians Are Calculated**

Remember from geometry that there are 360° in a circle. One revolution is also 360°. 360° is also equal to 2π radians ($\pi = 3.14$). Therefore, one radian is equal to 57.3°. Therefore, if the degree measurement is 51, the radian equivalent is 0.89 radians. If the measurement is given in revolutions, to convert to radians, multiply by 2. In the case given above, 51° is 0.14 revolutions. To convert to radians, multiply 0.14 by 2π. When torque magnitude and angular measurement magnitude are multiplied, the radian unit disappears (radians is unitless). Therefore, if 50 N · m is multiplied by 0.89 radians. the value is 44.5 N · m.

Work in Angular Movements

Work and power also must be considered when rotational movement in the body occurs. Angular work is the product of torque and the angular distance that the torque acts through.

$$\text{Angular work} = \text{Torque} \times \Delta\theta$$

$\Delta\theta$ is a change in angular distance or position. Torque units are in N · m. Angular distance units can be measured as degrees, revolutions, or radians, but in this case the units need to be in radians because radians are unitless. If the value seen is in degrees or revolutions, these units must be converted to radians. See Box 4.3 for an explanation of how radians are calculated.

When skeletal muscles contract, they can produce either positive work or negative work. This occurs through the action of muscles creating tension and pulling on a lever, or a segment of the body. Rotation of the segment occurs about an axis so the body segment moves through an angular displacement. The skeletal muscles do the mechanical work to cause the movement to occur. Positive work is associated with muscle shortening under a load (concentric action). For example, when a weight lifter flexes at the elbow, the forearm and dumbbell move through some angular displacement as the elbow flexors shorten. This is an example of positive angular work. Negative work in this example occurs when the elbow flexors lengthen under a load (eccentric action). Eccentric action occurs when the dumbbell and the weight of the forearm are lowered under a load so the arm returns to a position with the elbow extended. The metabolic costs of positive and negative muscle work are beyond the scope of this chapter. More muscle force can be exerted eccentrically than concentrically. This concept is demonstrated frequently in the weight training setting by doing "negatives." Negatives in this case refer to negative muscle work.

To expand on the previous example, assume that you work out the elbow flexors until the muscles are fatigued to the point that you cannot shorten the elbow flexors one more time. If a partner places a dumbbell in your hand with the elbow flexed, most people will be able to lower the weight under control so the elbow is in an extended position. This is an example of negative work. Caution must be adhered to in this case because of the risk of cellular muscle damage with excessive eccentric muscle work, although when used judiciously this weight training technique can provide useful benefits to the participant (8,19).

The effect of gravity acting on the weight of the lever to the left of the axis causes the muscle to lengthen, not the action of the muscle pushing the lever into that position.

It is important to remember that muscles can only pull, not push. As demonstrated in Figure 4.5, when the muscle pulls, the lever is moved to a more vertical upward position. The muscle, however, cannot push the lever into an angled downward position. The effect of gravity acting on the weight of the lever to the left of the axis causes the muscle to lengthen, not the action of the muscle pushing the lever into that position.

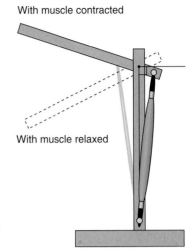

With muscle contracted

With muscle relaxed

FIGURE 4.5. The position of the lever changes more vertically oriented position when the muscle shortens or pulls (© Shadow Robot Company; www.shadowrobot.com).

Power in Angular Movements

The linear definition of power is work/time or the product of force and velocity. Angular power can be quantified in a similar method, but the units used are different from those with linear power, just as angular work and linear work use different units for measurement.

$$\text{Angular power} = \text{Angular Work/Time}$$

or

$$\text{Angular power} = T \times \omega$$

In the equation above, T is torque and ω (omega) is the Greek symbol for angular velocity, which is expressed in radians/s. Angular velocity may be expressed as degrees/s and revolutions/s, both of which are correct, however, by convention radians/s needs to be used because radian is a unitless value. The unit for angular power is N · m/s or J/s, which is equivalent to a watt.

Muscle power is frequently expressed in the literature as the product of net muscle moment and angular velocity. The net muscle moment is not for a single muscle, but rather for specific groups of muscles that serve a specific function (i.e., flexors/extensors) across a joint. Net muscle activity is described as either extension or flexion. Biarticular muscles complicate the understanding of this concept. For example, the hamstring muscles (biceps femoris, semitendinosus, semimembranosus) extend the hip and flex the knee. When muscle moment is combined with joint angular velocity, concentric and eccentric muscle activity can be determined. Muscle power is the rate of change in work based on time (the work of muscles is seldom constant) or expressed another way, the product of net muscle moment and angular velocity. Muscle power can be either positive or negative with positive muscle power representing positive muscle work (concentric muscle action) and negative muscle power representing negative muscle work (eccentric muscle action). If the muscle moment and angular velocity are both positive or both negative, the power will be positive. If one is negative, the muscle power will be negative (8).

Power output can be quantified in a number of ways including in the action of cycling. In an article published almost 10 years ago, to break the world record for cycling for 1 hour, the cyclist would have had to deliver greater than 440 W at sea level (1). Commonly, in the field of exercise science we see watts expressed as a result of ergometric work either as a leg or arm ergometer (Fig. 4.6).

Free Body Diagram

A free body diagram (FBD) is a simplified sketch that represents the interaction among forces and the distances through which they act. The system may be simple as seen in the sprinter sketch

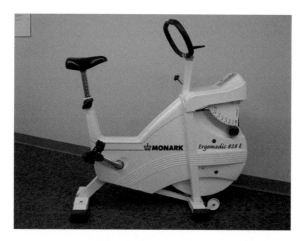

FIGURE 4.6. A cycle ergometer.

(Fig. 4.7). The only forces seen are the ground reaction forces in two directions (*x* and *y*), the sprinter's body weight and air resistance that will be negligible in most cases (19). Box 4.4 outlines important points to consider when establishing an FBD.

Figure 4.8 illustrates an FBD of the right arm with the weight of the arm and the resistance weight illustrated being offset by the static force of the flexor muscles. In this case, the weight of the arm and the weight (resistance) in the hand would tend to rotate the arm portion of the FBD in a clockwise direction about the axis of rotation. The force of the arm flexors would act in a counterclockwise direction to keep the system static or quasistatic.

The joint reaction force (JRF) in this figure implies that as the proximal humerus pushes against the glenoid fossa of the scapula, the glenoid fossa pushes against the humerus. JRF is the summative effect of force from one segment to another (5). Reducing JRF is a common focus in the healthcare field and can be accomplished noninvasively through weight reduction and reduction of walking or running velocity. In Figure 4.9 JRF is affected at the ankle by muscle force through the Achilles tendon, vertical ground reaction force (GRF), and weight of the foot.

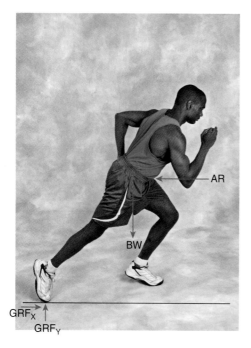

FIGURE 4.7. A simple free body diagram (FBD) demonstrating the horizontal and vertical forces on the push-off foot in running. (Adapted from Nawoczenski DA, Neumann DA. Biomechanical principles. In: Neumann DA, editor. *Kinesiology of the Musculoskeletal System—Foundations for Physical Rehabilitation*. St. Louis (MO): Mosby; 2002. p. 56–87.)

> BOX **4.4**   **Free Body Diagram Setup**

The steps in setting up the FBD are outlined below.
- Isolate the system to be considered
- Establish a reference frame (for most simple mechanics this will be an *x* axis with *x* being horizontal and a *y* axis with *y* representing vertical)
- Identify the internal and external forces. The internal forces will be muscle forces and frequently is defined as a single force vector. External forces or masses must be properly identified
- Indicate the distances that the forces act from the axis of rotation

---

Reference Frames

To accurately describe motion, a frame of reference must be established. This allows for the position and direction of a point, segment, or whole-body movement to be described with respect to a known point or axis of rotation. Reference frames are either relative or global (a.k.a. as a local coordinate system). The relative reference frame typically describes the movement of one body segment with respect to another. For example, it might be the position of the thigh with respect to the trunk. The relative reference system is used with goniometric measurements. The global system is based on a horizontal *x* axis and a vertical *y* axis and is used to analyze motion with respect to the ground. Figure 4.10 illustrates the differences in the two reference systems (19).

Joint Angle

Most body movement occurs about a joint. The joint angle in turn affects the moment that the muscles that cross that joint can exert. Joint angle can affect

1. muscle length,
2. moment arm distance,
3. resistance arm distance,
4. exercise type (i.e., eccentric, concentric, isometric, isotonic, isokinetic),

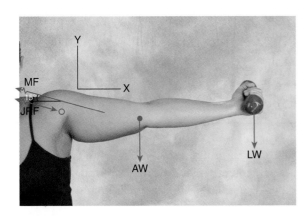

FIGURE 4.8. Free body diagram (FBD) of the right arm demonstrating muscle force (MF), arm weight (AW), load weight (LW), and joint reaction force (JRF). (Adapted from Nawoczenski DA, Neumann DA. Biomechanical principles. In: Neumann DA, editor. *Kinesiology of the Musculoskeletal System—Foundations for Physical Rehabilitation*. St. Louis (MO): Mosby; 2002. p. 56–87.)

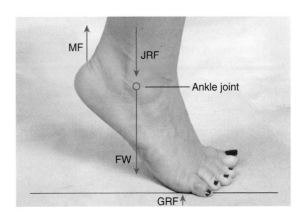

FIGURE 4.9. Free body diagram (FBD) demonstrating muscle force (MF), foot weight (FW), ground reaction force (GRF), and joint reaction force (JRF).

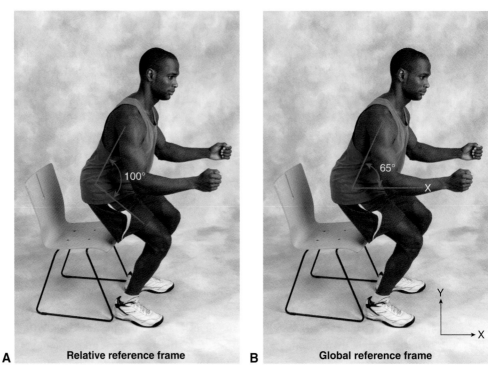

A   Relative reference frame   **B**   Global reference frame

FIGURE 4.10. Demonstration of relative reference system **(A)** and the global reference system **(B)**. (Adapted from Nawoczenski DA, Neumann DA. Biomechanical principles. In: Neumann DA, editor. *Kinesiology of the Musculoskeletal System—Foundations for Physical Rehabilitation*. St. Louis (MO): Mosby; 2002. p. 56-87).

5. movement direction (flexion/extension; abduction/adduction, internal rotation/external rotation), and

6. speed of movement.

Muscle torque is affected by the muscle moment arm length, which is affected by the range of motion. It is also important to note that the distance changes based on the articulation being considered. For example, the elbow is a constrained joint, primarily because of the bony architecture; therefore, the change in the axis of rotation and the subsequent change in the moment arm for the muscles, whether flexing or extending the joint, does not change as much as would be seen at the knee. Because the knee joint is not as constrained as the elbow, there will be greater changes in the axis of rotation and therefore the moment arm for the muscles that cause flexion and extension. Motion at the elbow involves primarily rotary motion, whereas even in a normal knee with no pathology there is a considerable amount of translation and rotation that occurs which affects the muscle moment arm. As the moment arm for the muscle shortens, the muscle force that is required increases because the muscle moment is the multiplication of these two components.

> *Motion at the elbow involves primarily rotary motion, whereas even in a normal knee with no pathology there is a considerable amount of translation and rotation that occurs which affects the muscle moment arm.*

When the pull of the muscle is at a 90° angle, the muscle force that is causing rotation is 100%. At angles greater than or less than 90°, some percentage of the force of muscle action is causing either a dislocation force or a stabilizing force but is not causing rotation to occur. So the optimal angular position for rotation at a joint is 90°. The problem here is that at 90° the muscle has shortened, which lessens the force that the muscle can potentially exert because skeletal muscle is able to exert the greatest force at approximately resting length or slightly greater than resting length if

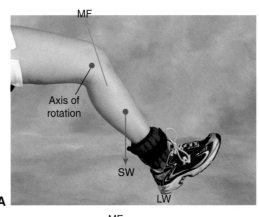

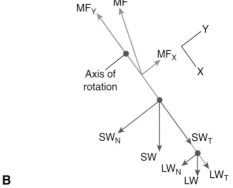

FIGURE 4.12. An example of how muscle force (MF), segment weight (SW), and load weight (LW) are resolved into X and Y components in static loading. (Adapted from Nawoczenski DA, Neumann DA. Biomechanical principles. In: Neumann DA, editor. *Kinesiology of the Musculoskeletal System—Foundations for Physical Rehabilitation*. St. Louis (MO): Mosby; 2002. p. 56-87).

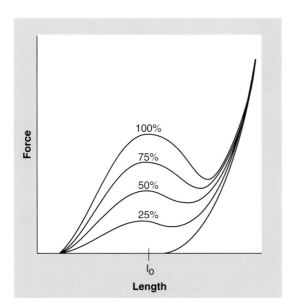

FIGURE 4.11. Elbow flexion alters the amount of force the muscle can exert. Extremes of extension and flexion lessen the force generated. (Adapted from Winter D. *Biomechanics and Motor Control of Human Movement*. New York: John Wiley & Sons; 1990, 174 p.)

the muscle takes advantage of the parallel and series elastic elements. Figure 4.11 is a practical example of this concept. In this example, the biceps has shortened to overcome the weight of the can in the hand. Although the muscle is shortening to cause flexion at the elbow, not all the muscle force is being used to cause rotation because the muscle has shortened and is not pulling at a 90° angle. Therefore, it is not possible to have optimal mechanical advantage and optimal anatomic advantage in the muscle concurrently. Of course, all of this is dependent on the muscle moment arm, the type of contraction, the velocity of contraction, and the physiological cross-sectional area of the muscle (9).

Resolution of Forces

Resolution of forces for human movement can be through graphical methods or analytical methods. In both methods, when considering two-dimensional motion, there will be a normal and a tangential component. The normal component represents the component of muscle force that acts perpendicularly to the long axis of the body segment; therefore, this component of the muscle force is what causes rotation. The tangential component of the muscle force represents the force that is directed parallel to the long axis of the body segment and provides for stabilization of the joint as in Figure 4.12 (19).

A change in the knee joint angle affects the magnitude of the two components of muscle force. The graphic method has the drawback of a high degree of precision to accurately represent the

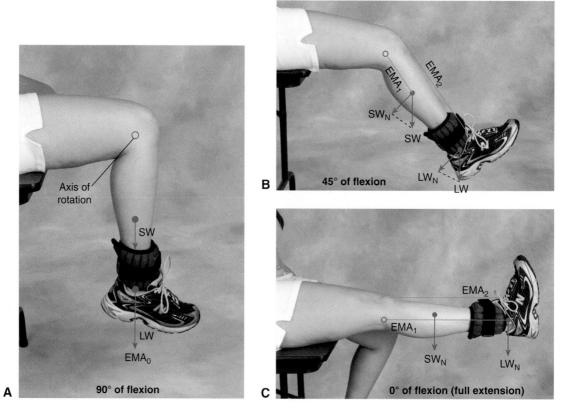

FIGURE 4.13. Changes in the moment arm distance based on the knee position between 90° and 0°.

forces. The analytic method requires some basic trigonometry to accurately represent forces when angles are known. Of course, the external angle that the relative joint angle represents is one part of the analytic method for resolution of forces.

The other component that is equally important is the angle that the muscle is pulling internally and the distance that the muscle is pulling to create the internal moment. As shown in Figure 4.13, the normal force represented by the lower leg (knee joint distal to the foot and ankle) and the load weight creates no moment when the knee is flexed at 90° because there is no distance for the normal force to act through; therefore, the moment is zero. However, when the knee is extended (or flexed depending on your perspective), the normal force changes both at 45° and at 90°, when the knee is fully extended. Although not shown, the tangential force would also change as the knee moves into an extended position (19).

As shown in Figure 4.14, body weight and the depth of flexion at the knee also affect the magnitude of the external moment that is created. Clearly, the difference in moments is a function of a longer moment arm in part A of the figure compared with part B. In part A, knee flexion is greater; therefore, the external moment arm is longer. The message this figure conveys is that the greater the flexion of the knees the larger the external moment arm becomes. To stabilize the body in this position, the internal moment, especially the muscle force, must correspondingly increase to keep the body in a quasi-static position.

Application of External Loads to Alter the External Moment (Torque)

External loads are frequently applied in fitness and training environments. The distance that loads are applied from the axis of rotation and the magnitude of loads both affect the internal moment that is applied to either stabilize the limb or move the limb through a prescribed range of motion.

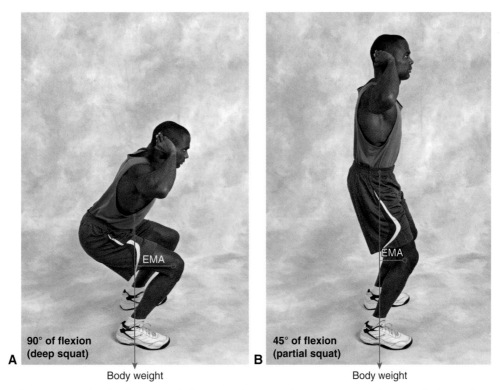

FIGURE 4.14. The depth of knee flexion alters the external moment arm and in turn the internal moment required to stabilize the knee.

In terms of strengthening the muscle, the further the load application is from the axis the greater the moment generated. As demonstrated in Figure 4.15, the same external torque or moment can be generated by two different load magnitudes based on the distance that the load is applied from the axis of rotation. As seen in A, the load is 100 N and the distance from the axis is 15 cm. In part B, the load magnitude is half of that seen in A, but the distance that the load is applied is twice that seen in A (30 cm). These cases show the importance of load and distance and the effect these two components have on torque (19).

Friction

Friction is the product of the coefficient of friction and the normal force. Coefficient of friction is symbolized by lowercase Latin mu (μ); the value of μ ranges from 0 to 1.0 and as a general rule the

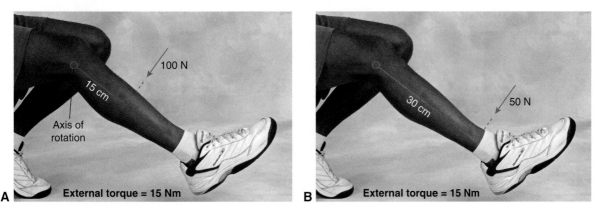

FIGURE 4.15. Distance from the knee axis and load magnitude affect the external moment.

closer μ is to 1.0 the higher the magnitude. The normal force is commonly symbolized by the uppercase letter N. The coefficient of static friction is higher than kinetic friction. This mechanical concept has several applications in the field of strength and conditioning. The chalk that is frequently used in strength and conditioning is to increase the coefficient of friction between the lifter's hands and the bar. In the sliding boards used in the field of personal training, the coefficient of friction is typically reduced to enhance sliding. This can occur by using a sock of some type. There are other devices on the market that are designed to enhance the throwing motion through the use of friction. These devices typically work through the use of a cable that runs over a braking device of some type. The braking typically can be adjusted to increase or decrease the frictional force experienced by the thrower. The limitation is that the thrower, for example, in javelin, is exposed to concentric work, but not eccentric work (9).

MECHANICAL APPLICATIONS IN WEIGHT TRAINING

Any external load whether dumbbells, barbells, or other forms of resistance acts downward and the moment arm for this load is horizontal from the center of the resistance. The resistance does not change during movement of levers about articulations; however, the distance that the resistance is acting from the axis of rotation changes, which in turn affects the external torque or moment. To maintain either equilibrium or a controlled change in joint position requires a change in the internal moment. If the resistance acts through the axis of rotation, there is not a moment created because the moment arm is equal to zero; therefore, no moment is generated. See Figure 4.16 for this concept.

The position of the weight with respect to the body also affects muscle activation. During the squat exercise, the further the lifter leans forward from the trunk the further the weight (resistance) acts from the axis of rotation at the hip, increasing the external moment that is produced. This in turn affects how the muscles that cross the hip act to keep the body in a quasi-equilibrium position. As the external resistance moves further forward horizontally, the resistance from the hip extensors (gluteus maximus and hamstrings) is greater and the knee extensor force is less. Conversely, if the bar is held higher on the upper shoulders or the bar is held in front of the shoulders and the trunk leans forward less, the knee

> *During the squat exercise, the further the lifter leans forward from the trunk the further the weight (resistance) acts from the axis of rotation at the hip, increasing the external moment that is produced.*

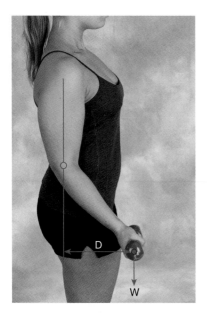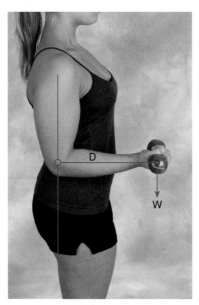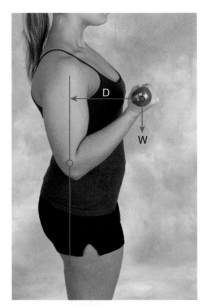

FIGURE 4.16. Distance from the elbow affects the external moment arm distance.

extensors will act more than the hip extensors (9). The application of this concept is that the training routine can be altered to suit individual needs and specific requirements.

FACTORS THAT AFFECT SKELETAL MUSCLE FORCE

Three factors that affect the mechanical action of muscle action include force–time, force–length, and force–velocity. As discussed earlier, the angle of muscle pull and the moment arm affect muscle force generation; however, there are three factors in the muscle itself that affect generation of force.

Force–Time

Force–time is related to the angle of muscle pull. When the muscle receives a stimulus to contract, the muscle develops tension by lengthening nonlinearly over time because of the passive elastic components in muscle and tendon (parallel and series elastic elements). After the elastic components are lengthened, muscle force progresses linearly until maximum muscle force is achieved. The time to maximum force is dependent on the joint position. If the tendon is in a lax position with the muscle shortened, the time to maximum muscle force will be greater than if the muscle is partially tensed (lengthened) (8). The pragmatic point is, however, that the time component is in milliseconds; therefore, practically there may be no noticeable effect. As shown in Figure 4.17 the time to achieve maximum force is approximately 1,500 milliseconds (1.5 seconds), further supporting the position that we cannot generate muscle force instantaneously.

Force–Length

Force–length is a concept that dictates the magnitude of muscle force generation is related to the length of the muscle (5). Maximum tension in the muscle can be generated when the muscle is between 80% and 120% of resting length (8,20). The tension or force that the muscle can generate is reduced when the muscle is in both short and elongated positions. In the shortened position (near the end of the flexion range of motion), the contractile components have become redundant, creating incomplete cross-bridge activation, thereby reducing the force that the muscle can generate (12,22). In the elongated position, slippage of cross-bridge results is less force generation capability.

The contractile components in muscle force generation are not the only factors that contribute to maximum muscle force. The parallel and series elastic elements in muscle also play a role. When the muscle is lengthened, tension is developed in the passive structures and this tension, when combined with force from the contractile proteins, adds to the total tension that the muscle can generate. Therefore, the optimal muscle length for muscle tension is slightly greater than resting length due to the contribution from active (muscle contraction) and passive structures (elastic components).

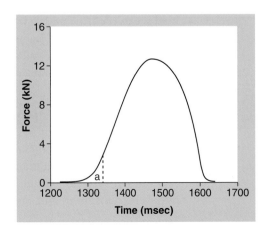

FIGURE 4.17. Force–time curve for skeletal muscle. (From *AAPS Pharm Sci Tech.* 2007;8(4):Article 89. Available from: http://www.aapspharmscitech.org/ articles/pt0804/pt0804089/pt0804089.pdf)

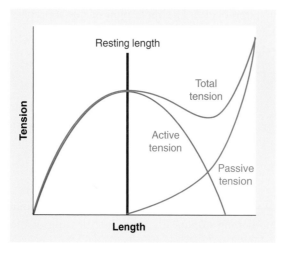

FIGURE 4.18. Force–length curve for skeletal muscle showing how active and passive components combine to optimize total muscle force. (From www.mfi.ku.dk/PPaulev/chapter2/images/n2-7.jpg)

The practical value of this is seen when pitchers and kickers wind up when throwing or kicking and when jumpers in sports create a countermovement by flexing the joints of the lower extremities before they take off when jumping (8). As shown in Figure 4.18, when active and passive components are summed, the total force that the muscle can generate is increased.

Force–Velocity

Force–velocity is a mechanical concept that dictates that the maximal force a muscle can develop is governed by both the velocity of muscle contraction and whether the muscle is shortening or lengthening. This concept was first described by Hill in 1938 (13). Because this concept is true only for maximally activated muscle, the relationship has limited application in daily activity. The concept does not imply that it is impossible to move a heavy object fast or a light object slowly. For example, a soccer ball can be kicked with a small amount of muscle force or with a large muscle force if the objective is to strike the ball forcefully. Most activities of daily living require skeletal muscle control; therefore, volitional control affects how the muscle responds (7).

> *The optimal muscle length for muscle tension is slightly greater than resting length due to the contribution from active (muscle contraction) and passive structures (elastic components).*

In concentric muscle movement when the muscle is shortening, force and velocity are inversely related. If velocity increases, the cycling rate of cross-bridge attachment increases, leaving fewer cross-bridges to act, thereby lessening muscle force production (8,14). Maximal force can be generated at zero velocity (isometrically). The force–velocity relationship, when the muscle is lengthening under a load, is opposite that seen in concentric muscle action. When a load that a muscle can isometrically hold is exceeded, the muscle lengthens under the load. If the load is as much as 50% greater than the force that can be handled isometrically, tension increases rapidly in the muscle as the speed of lengthening increases. The force–velocity curve ends abruptly when the muscle can no longer control the weight (8). Figure 4.19 provides a graphic representation of the force–velocity relationship.

WEIGHT TRAINING THROUGH THE USE OF WEIGHT MACHINES

The use of weight machines affects the multiplanar movement that is present with free weights. With free weights, the resistance can move in three orthogonal planes (anterior/posterior, mediolateral, and vertical), but with weight machines the direction the resistance moves is controlled by levers, cams, gear, and pulleys (Fig. 4.20). Because the leverage varies on the basis of the

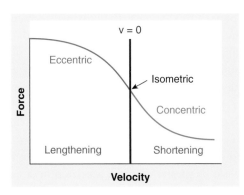

FIGURE 4.19. Force–velocity curve for skeletal muscle showing the relationships between force and velocity when the muscle is shortening and lengthening. (From www.bgs.qld. edu.au/.../news_2_clip_image007.jpg)

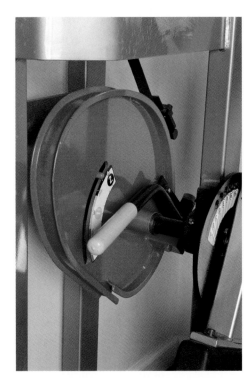

FIGURE 4.20. A machine with a cam-like device.

> *With free weights, the resistance can move in three orthogonal planes (anterior/posterior, mediolateral, and vertical), but with weight machines the direction the resistance moves is controlled by levers, cams, gear, and pulleys.*

machine, the exact resistance moved by the person who is weight training is different from that stamped on the weight plates. Because human movement at most skeletal articulations is mostly multiplanar, how strength is gained will be affected when weight training occurs with resistance other than free weights. Weight plates that are cabled over a single circular pulley are equal to the weight lifted. Cams that are "kidney" or oval shaped affect the resistance moved. The number of pulleys the cable encircles affects the resistance moved. The objective in some forms of accommodating weight training equipment is to resist the motion most when a person is strongest in the range of motion and least when they are at the weakest point.

Although this is an intriguing idea, the challenge with this is that there are a number of factors that affect when a person is strongest or weakest in the range of motion. Studies have demonstrated that the effectiveness of this type of training has deficits (9,10,15). Some of these devices have been shown to have limited correlation when machine resistive torque patterns were compared with human torque capacity (10). Generally, some weight training relative segment angles and positions will be more advantageous than others. When the muscle length changes, there is a corresponding change in the angle of pull for that particular muscle group. Both of these affect the stimulus that the muscle needs to overcome to achieve overload, which is the basis of all training. Because of these factors and human size and strength differences, constructing a weight machine that accommodates everyone is challenging.

INERTIA

Inertia is the resistance of a body to movement whether the body is moving or static.

Inertia is the resistance of a body to movement whether the body is moving or static. Inertia has no units of measurement but is directly proportional to the mass of the object, or in the case of the human body either the entire body or a segment of the body (7).

In the body, inertial force is generated as movement and transfer of momentum occurs from a proximal segment to a more distal segment. For example, in throwing a baseball the proximal segment of the arm (defined from the shoulder distal to the elbow) exerts an inertial force on the forearm as the ball is propelled. The same can be seen in kicking as the proximal segment creates an inertial force on the lower leg (8). The magnitude of inertial resistance is equal to the product of the mass of the object and acceleration. When lifting an object off the ground, the person's muscle torque generated must exceed the inertia of the object and the inertia of the body segments used to move the object. Once the object is in motion, the resistance is not as great because the initial inertia has been overcome.

In athletic movements when jumping to get the body off the ground or floor (e.g., in basketball, volleyball, football, and soccer), the performer must accelerate the body mass upward. Standing still is equal to the performer's body weight based on Newton's 3rd Law. This means that to get the body mass into the air the acceleration upward must be greater than the acceleration downward. Because of this, the vertical GRF seen in jumping can be two to three times body weight (11). In activities such as dance aerobics and step aerobics, the movement of body parts involves acceleration and deceleration, therefore requiring high levels of muscle force to accelerate and decelerate body segments.

MOMENT OF INERTIA

Moment of inertia (MOI) is the rotational equivalent of mass and is the quantity that indicates the resistance to a change in angular velocity. MOI is different from mass, which is a scalar value, meaning that mass has no direction. MOI is a more complex concept and indicates the resistance of an object to change in angular motion. MOI is dependent not only on the mass of an object but also on how the mass of the object is distributed with respect to the axis of rotation (19).

MOI will have different values, depending on the axis that is considered and the planes of motion about which the body is rotating. For example, when a gymnast rotates about the vertical or longitudinal axis through the center of the body, the distribution of the body's mass is much different from rotating about a transverse axis through the center of the body. What this means is that there is a greater MOI about the transverse axis than about the vertical axis because the distribution of the masses is further from the axis of rotation. Another example of this can be seen during the swing phase of walking. The swing limb functionally shortens as the hip and knee flex and the foot dorsiflexes. The masses of the leg in this example do not change, but the masses of the leg and where they act with respect to the axis of rotation at

When a gymnast rotates about the vertical or longitudinal axis through the center of the body, the distribution of the body's mass is much different from rotating about a transverse axis through the center of the body.

the hip shorten because of the joint movements. The mass is the same, but the distribution of the masses is different. This means that the muscle force required from the hip flexors is reduced (19).

In Figure 4.21, the gymnast changes the MOI from the top position to the bottom position. In the top position the gymnast has a larger MOI because the masses are distributed further from the axis of rotation at the hip. The larger MOI means that angular velocity is slowed. Conversely, when the MOI is smaller, as is shown in the bottom figure, angular velocity is increased. MOI plays a major role in the distribution of masses in a golf club, drivers, irons, and putters.

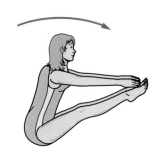

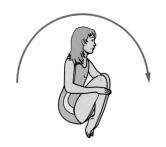

FIGURE 4.21. A change in body position affects the moment of inertia of the whole body in a rotational movement. (Adapted from Nawoczenski DA, Neumann DA. Biomechanical principles. In: Neumann DA, editor. *Kinesiology of the Musculoskeletal System—Foundations for Physical Rehabilitation*. St. Louis (MO): Mosby; 2002. p. 56–87).

MOI also plays a role in running. During the swing phase of gait, the limb is brought forward through the force of the hip flexors. After a toe-off, the swing limb is flexed at the hip, knee, foot, and ankle. The flexion of the limb effectively reduces the MOI of the swing limb by reducing the distance that the masses of the leg are acting from the axis of rotation at the hip joint. This allows the limb to move forward more effectively (8).

ANGULAR MOMENTUM

Angular momentum is the equivalent of Newton's 2nd Law and is expressed algebraically as follows:

$$T = I\alpha$$

T is the external torque and I is the MOI. Alpha (α) is angular acceleration and can be expressed as degrees/s^2, revolutions/s^2, or radians/s^2. Rearranging the equation produces:

$$H \text{ (angular momentum)} = I \text{ (MOI) } \omega \text{ (angular velocity)}$$

In this case, angular momentum is the product of MOI and angular velocity that will be expressed in radians per second. The application for this mechanical concept can be appreciated in several circumstances. For example, when divers leave the end of the diving board, they can alter the MOI of their body, which will either speed up the rotation or slow down the rotation. If the divers have their body in a tucked position, the body will tend to rotate faster about the center of gravity for the body. If the body is extended, the MOI increases, which tends to slow the rotation of the body. Other examples are seen in gymnastics and figure skating and track and field including the high jump and pole vaulting. As shown by Dapena et al. in the Fosbury flop, body momentum is conserved once the feet leave the ground (2). That is, the body, or the center of mass of the body, acts like a projectile. Figure 4.22 demonstrates how the Fosbury technique is executed. Notice as the jumper goes over the bar backward the change in the position of the body segments (arms and legs) with respect to the trunk. This change in body position changes the MOI for the body, optimizing the technique.

> *When divers leave the end of the diving board, they can alter the MOI of their body, which will either speed up the rotation or slow down the rotation.*

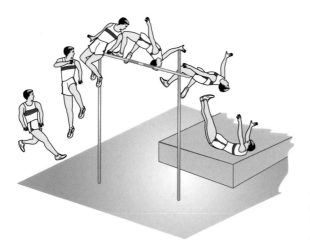

FIGURE 4.22. The change in body position after the jumper leaves the ground, which alters the body moment of inertia. (From motivate. maths.org/conferences/conf23/john5.gif)

IMPULSE–MOMENTUM

The mechanical concept of impulse–momentum is derived from Newton's 2nd Law, which is $F = ma$

$$F = m \times \Delta v / t$$

$$F \times t = m \times v$$

In the equation above, the left-hand side of the equation ($F \times t$) is impulse and the right-hand side is momentum ($m \times v$). Either side of the equation can be manipulated. When a moving mass is slowed or decelerated, a force must be exerted to slow the movement. This occurs in running, landing from a jump, or catching an object such as a ball that is thrown. We may not consider the impact of forces that we overcome daily. For example, when we walk on a level surface and when we walk up and down steps, we decelerate and accelerate the body. Other examples of impulse–momentum include catching a thrown ball. In catching as a person brings the ball to a stop, the elbows flex and absorb some of the force with the shoulders. If flexion did not occur, the force that the person catching the object would feel would be high because the time would be short; however, by "giving" with the arms and shoulders the time over which the force is felt is increased lessening the force felt by the body (16).

The same concept can be demonstrated when landing from a jump. If a person landed with "stiff legs" and failed to flex at the hips, knees, and ankles, the force that the body would experience would be elevated greater than normal because the time over which the force from landing would be short. One study found that a "soft" landing reduced the overall force that the muscular system was exposed to by approximately 20% when compared with a stiff landing (3). Basketball rebounders and volleyball players have demonstrated peak GRF of 3–6 times body weight (4). Clearly, this force needs to be lessened to reduce the potential risk of injury, both repetitive and acute.

An example of the impulse–momentum relationship from Hamill and Knutzen illustrates this concept (8). For a person with a body mass of 60 kg who jumps from a squat position, initial velocity is 0 and the velocity at take-off is found to be 4 m/s. Using impulse–momentum, we can estimate the force that the person exerts against the ground based on Newton's 3rd Law.

$$F \times t = m \times v_{\text{final}} - m \times v_{\text{initial}}$$

$$F \times t = (60 \text{ kg} \times 4 \text{ m/s}) - (60 \text{ kg} \times 0 \text{ m/s})$$

$$F \times t = 240 \text{ kg} \times \text{m/s}$$

If we assume the time of force exertion against the ground is 0.3 seconds, the average force can be estimated.

$$F \times 0.03 = 240 \text{ kg} \times \text{m/s}$$

$$F = 240 \text{ kg} \times \text{m/s/0.3}$$

$$F = 800 \text{ N}$$

In this example, the force exerted is approximately 1.3 × body weight (7).

Athletic shoes help reduce force through cushioning that serves to ameliorate the forces that the body experiences. Low-impact aerobics generates less force than high-impact aerobics. With high-impact aerobics, one or both feet are off the floor at any one time. The effect of impulse can be altered to increase the force and reduce the time component. Examples of this include changing directions quickly and accelerating an object or a projectile. For example, when striking a baseball for power, the objective is to increase the time component of the impulse side of the equation. The time component for the collision between the objects is short, typically in milliseconds and ranges in golf, baseball, and tennis between 1 and 5 milliseconds (16).

GAIT

Gait is classified as walking and running gait. In running, both feet are off the ground at any one time. In walking gait, there are two primary components, support or stance phase of gait, which is approximately 60% of the normal gait cycle and the swing phase that makes up the other 40%. All phases of gait are broken into specific components.

Generally, in stance there is initial contact, which is frequently heel contact in most people, although abnormal gait may involve forefoot contact first, or in pathologic conditions, other parts of the foot. Initial contact is also the initiation of the "braking" subphase of the gait cycle. This is the period of time when the body is slowed. Initial contact is preceded by the eccentric action of the hamstrings to slow extension of the knee on the support side so appropriate foot placement can occur. Braking is halted around the time of midsupport. Following initial contact, there is a loading response when lower extremity muscle activation is high to provide support for stabilization of the pelvis. At initial contact, based on GRF data, the foot generally rolls to the medial side followed by some magnitude of supination. The loading response is followed by midstance, terminal stance, and toe-off. Midstance is the time when the body begins to become propelled forward. Midstance ends at toe-off. On the swing side, there is initial swing, midswing, and then a slowing of the foot prior to initial contact before initiating the stance phase again.

In running, the GRFs will be greater than those seen in walking because in running there is a flight phase, which means that the body will be accelerated into the ground, whereas in walking there is not a flight phase and one foot stays in contact with the ground throughout the gait cycle. The biggest GRF vector will be the vertical component followed by the anterior posterior force and the mediolateral force will be least, although this may be the most important when examining pathology. Figure 4.23 demonstrates GRF for vertical, anterior–posterior, and mediolateral movement. Vertical force is bimodal. The two peaks and the partial unweighing are due to flexion of the lower extremity joints approximately midway through the time that the stance foot is on the force platform.

In running, the GRFs will be greater than those seen in walking because in running there is a flight phase, which means that the body will be accelerated into the ground, whereas in walking there is not a flight phase and one foot stays in contact with the ground throughout the gait cycle.

The periods of time when stumbling is most likely to occur is during initial contact and in midswing. At initial contact, the foot actually slides to a stop, which in some may cause a stumble. Midswing is when the toe of the swing foot is less than 2 cm from the ground and if either not enough dorsiflexion, knee flexion, or hip flexion occurs or there is an irregular surface, the chance

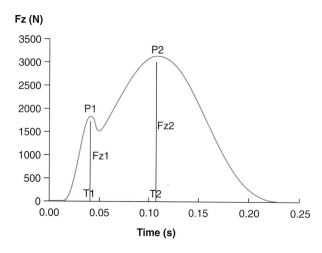

FIGURE 4.23. Typical GRF graph displaying vertical, medial, and anterior–posterior forces (modified from The Kistler Group, Multicomponent Force Platform [Internet]. 2008 [cited 2008 Nov 30]. Available from: http://www.kistler.com/mediaaccess/en-us/000-157e-10.08.pdf. The Kistler Group, Eulachstrasse 22, 8408 Winterthur, Switzerland.)

of stumbling is increased (8,9). See Box 4.5 for a list of mechanical errors often found in running and jogging.

Muscle Moments and Power in Gait

When estimating the muscle moment that occurs at the lower extremity articulations, the net muscle moment at the hip is lower than that at the knee and ankle. Intuitively, this would not seem to be plausible because the muscles that cross the hip are as a general rule larger and typically more powerful than those that cross the other two lower extremity joints. The difference at the hip is due to a leverage advantage compared with the other two joints. The vertical GRF vector at the hip passes close to the hip joint axis of rotation, thereby reducing the moment arm through which the force passes (24).

The mechanical power required in each step for steady pace running at the hip is also close to zero due to the lack of net change in the runner's potential and kinetic energy. Running uphill, however, changes the mechanical work due primarily to the increase in the moment arm distance through which the muscles have to work. During inclined running, the moment arm for the hip flexors moves forward, thereby increasing the joint moment and work as shown in Figure 4.24 (21).

CYCLING

Cycling is a form of exercise, which can be semistatic, in that the cycle does not move from one point to another or it may in fact involve movement from one place to another. In the field of exercise science, most of what we know today regarding cycling comes from cycle ergometry, which involves increasing

---

BOX **4.5**   **Mechanical Errors in Running and Jogging**

Common mechanical errors in the initial stages of running and jogging include the following.
- Running with a "stiff gait." Mechanically, a stiff gait decreases the time over which the force from running is dissipated, thereby increasing the impulse that the body is exposed to
- Asymmetrical upper and lower extremity motion, which compromises the desired linear movement of the body in a straight line
- In running, propelling yourself off the ground too far increases the energy costs, therefore making the motion of running less economical
- Overstriding, which decreases running speed and increases the "braking" motion during the gait cycle (17).

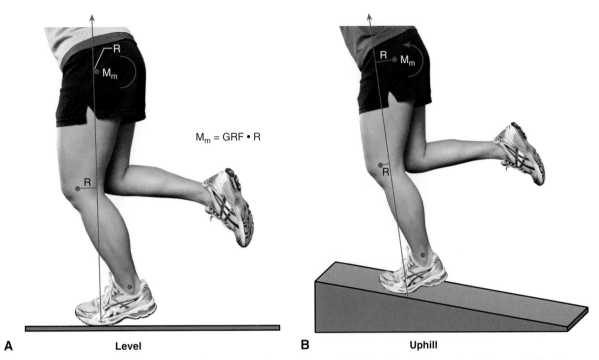

$$M_m = GRF \cdot R$$

A **Level** **B** **Uphill**

FIGURE 4.24. The change in the vertical GRF vector forward through the hip, thereby increasing the internal muscle moment at the hip.

> *Most of what we know today regarding cycling comes from cycle ergometry, which involves increasing the resistance of the wheel, thereby increasing the resistance or friction against which the rider pushes.*

the resistance of the wheel, thereby increasing the resistance or friction against which the rider pushes.

Cycling is an important event in many countries with some believing that the Tour de France is the toughest of all endurance events. Cycling power is typically quantified in watts and there is much sport-related research in this area that relates to power output and how this is affected by crank angles and pedaling rates and where during the movement the most power is generated by the cyclist (1).

LIFTING AND CARRYING

Proper technique in lifting is important to reduce the risk of injury, especially to the low back. The role that the knee extensors play is a function of posture. In Figure 4.25, the correct method to use when lifting an object is illustrated. Lifting with the knee in a semiextended position places the low back at increased risk of injury. In the right panel of Figure 4.25, the hamstrings assist in the lift from this position, but the low back is also at a disadvantage because of the increased moment arm for the weight of the upper body and the object being lifted. In the preferred lifting position, the quadriceps are primarily active, the object being lifted is closer to the center of gravity of the body, and the risk for injury is reduced because the internal moment required to lift the object is lessened, especially the muscle force component portion of the moment (8).

INJURY RISKS ASSOCIATED WITH BIOMECHANICS

As is true in a number of circumstances, the injury potential in an activity or sports setting is not necessarily based on speed. The speed is not what increases the risk for injury, but rather the time over which the force is dissipated as discussed above in the impulse–momentum section. If

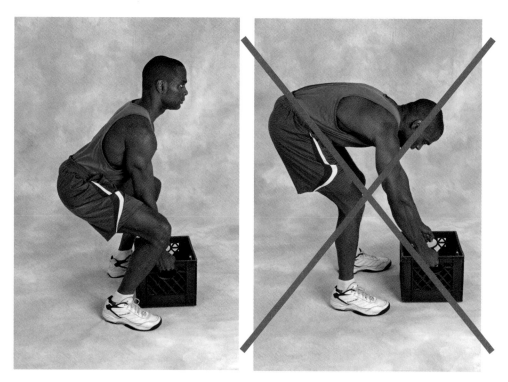

FIGURE 4.25. Correct (left-hand side of the figure) and incorrect (right-hand side of the figure) lifting techniques.

> *There is the risk of injury from improper mechanics associated with lifting and the strain this places on joints and muscles.*

the time can be increased, the risk of injury will likely be reduced. This occurs by reducing the force, especially that the muscles must overcome. There is the risk of injury from improper mechanics associated with lifting and the strain this places on joints and muscles.

SUMMARY

The field of biomechanics is an important component in the arsenal of personal trainers. Understanding the basics of movement, how to establish the proper training stimulus, how selected exercises bring about the proper training effect, how to most effectively train clients, and appropriate methods to reduce injury potential are key to having a successful practice.

REFERENCES

1. Bassett DR, Kyle CR, Passfield L, Broker JP, Burke ER. Comparing cycling world hour records, 1967–1996: modeling with empirical data. *Med Sci Sports Exer.* 1999;31(11):1665–76.
2. Dapena J. The rotation over the bar in the Fosbury-flop high jump. *Track Coach* 1995;132:4201–10.
3. Devita P Skelly WA. Effect of landing stiffness on joint kinetics and energetics in the lower extremity. *Med Sci Sports Exer.* 1992;24(1):108–15.
4. Dufek JS. Jump high … Then What? Making landings safe. *Strategies* 1992;5:92.
5. Edman KAP. Contractile performance of skeletal muscle fibers. In: Komi P, editor. *Strength and Power in Sport.* Boston: Blackwell Scientific; 1992. p.114–133.

6. Enoka RM. *Neuromechanical Basis of Kinesiology.* 2nd edition. Champaign (IL): Human Kinetics; 1994.

7. Hall SJ. *Basic Biomechanics.* 5th edition. Boston: McGraw-Hill; 2006.

8. Hamill J, Knutzen KM. *Biomechanical Basis of Human Movement.* 2nd edition. Philadelphia: Lippincott Williams & Wilkins; 2003.

9. Harman E. Biomechanics. In: Earle RW, Baechle TR, editors. *NSCA's Essentials of Personal Training.* Champaign (IL): Human Kinetics; 2004. p. 53–80.

10. Harman E. Resistance torque analysis of 5 Nautilus exercise machines. *Med Sci Sports Exer.* 1983;15(2):113.

11. Harman EA, Rosenstein MT, Frykman PN, Rosenstein RM. The effects of arms and countermovement of vertical jumping. *Med Sci Sports Exer.* 1990;22(6):825–33.

12. Herzog W, Leonard TR. The role of passive structures in force enhancement of skeletal muscles following active stretch. *J Biomech.* 2005;38:409–15.

13. Hill AV. *First and Last Experiments in Muscle Mechanics.* Cambridge: Cambridge University Press; 1970.

14. Huijing PA. Elastic potential of muscle. In: Komi P, editor. *Strength and Power in Sport.* Boston: Blackwell Scientific; 1992. p. 151–168.

15. Johnson JH, Colodny S, Jackson D. Human torque capability versus machine resistive torque for four Eagle resistance machines. *J Appl Sport Sc.* 1990;4(3):83–7.

16. Kreighbaum E, Barthels KM. *Biomechanics: A Qualitative Approach to Studying Human Movement.* 4th edition. Boston: Allyn and Bacon; 1996.

17. Lewis J. Functional anatomy and biomechanics. In: Howley E, Franks D, editors. *Health Fitness Instructor's Handbook.* 4th edition. Champaign (IL): Human Kinetics; 2003. p. 443–474.

18. McGinnis P. *Biomechanics of Sport and Exercise.* Champaign (IL): Human Kinetics; 1999.

19. Nawoczenski DA, Neumann DA. Biomechanical principles. In: Neumann DA, editor. *Kinesiology of the Musculoskeletal System—Foundations for Physical Rehabilitation.* St. Louis (MO): Mosby; 2002. p. 56–87.

20. Rassier DE, Herzog W, Wakeling J, Syme DA. Stretch-induced, steady-state force enhancement in single skeletal muscle fibers exceeds the isometric force at optimum fiber lengths. *J Biomech.* 2003;36:1309–16.

21. Roberts TJ, Belliveau RA. Sources of mechanical power for uphill running in humans. *J Exper Biol.* 2005;208:1963–70.

22. Sachachar R, Herzog W, Leonard TR. The effects of muscle stretching and shortening on isometric forces on the descending limb of the force–length relationship. *J Biomech.* 2004;37:917–26.

23. Siff M. Biomechanical foundations of strength and power training. In: Zatsiorsky VM, editor. *Biomechanics in Sport: Performance Enhancement and Injury Prevention.* London: Blackwell Science; 2000. p. 184–231.

24. Winter DA. Moments of force and mechanical power in jogging. *J Biomech.* 1983;16:91–7.

CHAPTER 5

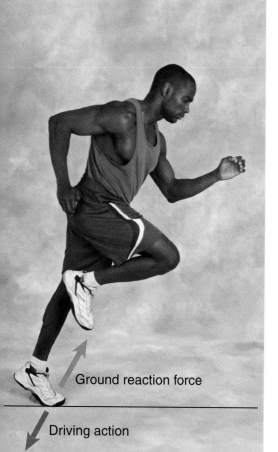

Ground reaction force

Driving action

Exercise Physiology

OBJECTIVES

- Provide fundamental background about the biological structure of the human body
- Introduce the physiological mechanism of various systems of the body and how they relate to exercise training
- Identify key elements that the body reacts and adapts to exercise stimulus so that effective exercise training can be prescribed

A thorough understanding of exercise physiology is essential to the success of a Personal Trainer. A solid foundation in exercise physiology principles is important for the Personal Trainer to prescribe appropriate exercise training programs to clients and to explain the rationale, process, and effects of the program for improving fitness. The Personal Trainer needs to provide brief and precise explanations about the physiological mechanisms involved in the activities and do so in a professional manner. During physical training, the exercise stimulation acts on a human body, creating significant physiological changes. Understanding these physiological changes and mechanisms allows a Personal Trainer to better understand the exercise and movement that has been prescribed to a client so that effective training that is safe and appropriate can be achieved. In this chapter, we attempt to introduce some basic but essential concepts of exercise physiology. Specifically, various biological systems such as the cardiovascular system, respiratory system, energy system, muscular and skeletal systems, and neurological system and their roles during exercise performance are presented.

OVERVIEW OF EXERCISE PHYSIOLOGY

Among the various disciplines in exercise science, exercise physiology perhaps is one of the most important for fitness professionals. Because exercise physiology is the study of the mechanism and effects of exercise on the body, it is important to enable a Personal Trainer to prescribe safe and effective exercise for improving physical function and fitness. Exercise physiology takes into account the effects of exercise on various systems of the body such as the cardiovascular or circulatory systems, respiration, muscles and bones, and the nervous system. These systems work together interactively to respond to an exercise stimulus so that an efficient and effective exercise outcome is produced. The Personal Trainer needs to understand all aspects of the body and the interaction of these systems as well as the nature of the exercise stimulus given to the body. For example, when a Personal Trainer needs to prescribe an exercise to improve the quadriceps muscles, knowledge of muscular structure will allow the Personal Trainer to identify the correct location and action associated with that muscle group. Then, the understanding of muscular contraction will allow the Personal Trainer to determine the appropriate types of exercise for the quadriceps. Knowledge of energy metabolism and adaptation of the muscle will allow the Personal Trainer to determine the suitable frequency, duration, and intensity of the exercise training.

> *Exercise physiology takes into account the effects of exercise on various systems of the body such as the cardiovascular or circulatory systems, respiration, muscles and bones, and the nervous system.*

Another example is the exercise prescription for a weight loss program. The important concept of energy metabolism allows a Personal Trainer to determine the appropriate type of exercise that is oxidative in nature and uses fat as the major energy source. The efficiency of such fat-burning mechanisms relies on the effectiveness of the cardiovascular system in maintaining blood circulation and the respiratory system in maximizing blood oxygenation. Understanding factors that limit or enhance these systems will allow a Personal Trainer to adjust the exercise training program as needed. Today, because of the rapid advances in technology and research, the depth and breadth of knowledge in exercise physiology is growing rapidly. Many of the more traditional beliefs of physiological concepts are being challenged, and new ideas and concepts are being generated every year. A Personal Trainer not only needs to master the foundations in all aspects of exercise physiology but also needs to pay attention to the development of current concepts of exercise physiology, to be a capable fitness professional of the 21st century.

DEFINITION OF EXERCISE PHYSIOLOGY

Exercise physiology is the study of the body's responses and its adaptation to the stress of exercise. Exercise physiology involves the scientific study of how exercise alters human systemic and cellular

> *Both the immediate (acute) and long-term (chronic) effects of exercise on all aspects of body function are fundamental concerns in exercise physiology.*

physiology both during and immediately after exercise, as well as in response to exercise training (49). Both the immediate (acute) and long-term (chronic) effects of exercise on all aspects of body function are fundamental concerns in exercise physiology. Many systems (muscular, skeletal, energy, cardiovascular) do not work independently but interactively to create the most efficient and effective responses to exercise demands.

CARDIOVASCULAR SYSTEM

The study of cardiovascular exercise physiology is one of the more prominent subdisciplines of exercise physiology. It examines how oxygen and other important nutrients are transported by the car-

> *The primary purpose of the cardiovascular system is to deliver nutrients to and remove metabolic waste products from the tissues.*

diovascular system and used by the muscles during exercise. The cardiovascular system consists of the heart and the blood vessels. There are more than 60,000 miles (96,000 km) of blood vessels in the body, which originate from and terminate at the heart and are structured in a continuous closed circuit (41). The primary purpose of the cardiovascular system is to deliver nutrients to and remove metabolic waste products from the tissues. The cardiovascular system assists with maintenance of normal function at rest and during exercise. The cardiovascular system performs the following specific functions (40):

1. Transports deoxygenated blood from heart to lungs and oxygenated blood from the lungs to the heart
2. Transports oxygenated blood from the heart to tissues and deoxygenated blood from the tissues to the heart
3. Distributes nutrients (e.g., glucose, free fatty acids, amino acids) to cells
4. Removes metabolic wastes (e.g., carbon dioxide, urea, lactate) from the periphery for elimination or reuse
5. Regulates pH to control acidosis and alkalosis
6. Transports hormones and enzymes to regulate physiological function
7. Maintains fluid balance to prevent dehydration
8. Maintains body temperature by absorbing and redistributing heat

The Heart

Figure 5.1 shows the anatomy of the heart. The heart is positioned at an angle within the chest cavity with the larger left ventricle (LV) pointed toward the left foot. It is anterior to (in front of) the thoracic vertebral column and posterior to (behind) the sternum. The lungs flank the heart on both sides and slightly overlap it. The heart has four chambers. The two upper chambers are the atria and the two lower chambers are the ventricles. The external deep grooves of the heart (called sulci) define the boundaries of the four chambers of the heart (55). The coronary sulcus separates the atria from the ventricles; the interventricular sulcus separates the LV and the right ventricle (RV). The sulci also contain the major arteries and veins that provide circulation to the heart.

The heart has a base and an apex. The base consists mainly of the left atrium (LA), the right atrium (RA), and parts of the proximal portion of the large veins that enter the heart from behind. It is located above and close to the right sternal border at the level of the second and third ribs. The apex of the heart is located below the base at the level of the fifth intercostal space.

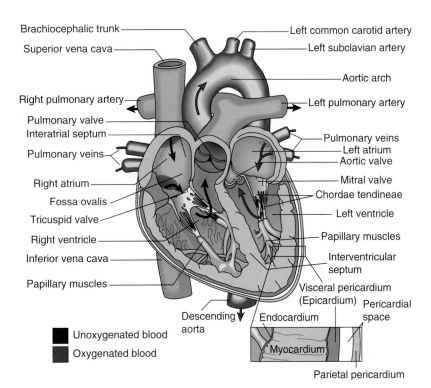

FIGURE 5.1. Anatomy of the heart and direction of blood flow. (From Smeltzer SCO, Bare BG. *Brunner and Suddarth's Textbook of Medical–Surgical Nursing.* 9th ed. Philadelphia: Lippincott Williams & Wilkins; 2002.)

Tissue Coverings and Layers of the Heart

The heart is covered by a double-walled, loose-fitting membranous sac called the pericardium. The outer wall of the pericardium has both a fibrous (tough) layer and a serous (smooth) layer. The interior lining of the heart is the epicardium. The thickest layer of tissue in the heart is the myocardium. The myocardium is the cardiac muscle. Within the myocardium is a network of crisscrossing connective tissue fibers, called the fibrous skeleton, separating the atria from the ventricles. This skeleton provides support for the myocardium and the valves of the heart.

Chambers, Valves, and Blood Flow

The heart has two pumps in a single unit with four chambers or cavities. The right-sided heart (RA and RV) and the left-sided heart (LA and LV) make up the two pumps. The right side of the heart collects deoxygenated blood from the periphery and pumps it through the lungs (pulmonary circuit). The left side of the heart collects blood from the lungs and pumps it throughout the body (systemic circuit) (42).

The heart has four valves, whose function is to maintain blood flow in one direction. The atrioventricular (AV) valves separate the atria from the ventricles. The semilunar valves separate the ventricles from the aorta and pulmonary artery. The right AV valve has three cusps and is called the tricuspid valve, whereas the left AV valve has only two cusps and is called the mitral (or bicuspid) valve. The tricuspid valve controls the flow of blood from the RA to the RV, whereas the mitral valve controls blood flow between the LA and LV. The chordae tendineae and papillary muscles help the AV valves stay closed, preventing them from swinging back into the atria, which would result in reversed blood flow (33).

There are two semilunar valves in the heart. The pulmonic valve lies between the RV and the pulmonary artery. The aortic valve is between the LV and the aorta. The cusps of the semilunar valves prevent the backflow of blood to the ventricles. Blood flow through the heart is accomplished by the following sequence of events, beginning with the return of systemic blood from the body to the RA:

1. Deoxygenated blood flows into the RA through the superior and inferior vena cavae, the coronary sinus, and anterior cardiac veins.
2. The RA contracts and blood moves through the tricuspid valve into the RV.
3. The RV contracts, the tricuspid valve closes, and blood flows through the pulmonic valve into the pulmonary arteries and the branches of the respiratory system.
4. Blood enters the alveolar capillaries from the pulmonary arteries, where gas exchange occurs. Oxygen is absorbed and carbon dioxide is removed.
5. Blood flows back to the LA through the pulmonary veins.
6. The LA contracts and blood flows through the mitral valve and into the LV.
7. The LV contracts, the mitral valve closes, and blood flows through the aortic valve into the aorta and its branches, where it is distributed to the coronary circulation and the systemic circulation (33).

Cardiac muscle has unique properties that allow it to contract without an external nervous system impulse. The components of the heart's conduction system include the sinoatrial (SA) node, AV node, AV bundle (bundle of His), right and left bundle branches, and the Purkinje fibers. The electrical impulse, which initiates cardiac contraction, begins at the SA node (the intrinsic pacemaker) of the heart. The electrical impulse is delayed at the AV node for approximately 0.12 seconds to allow the atria to contract and fill the ventricles with blood. The impulse then moves rapidly through the bundle of His, through the right and left bundle branches, and through the network of Purkinje fibers in the myocardium of both ventricles. This rapid conduction allows the two ventricles to contract at approximately the same time.

The Blood Vessels

After blood flows from the heart, it enters the vascular system, which is composed of numerous blood vessels. The blood vessels form a closed system to deliver blood to the tissues; help promote the exchange of nutrients, metabolic wastes, hormones, and other substances with cells; and return blood to the heart. Arteries carry blood away from the heart. Large arteries branch into smaller arteries and eventually to smaller arterioles. Arterioles branch into capillaries, which allow the exchange of blood and other nutrients with various tissues (e.g., digestive system, liver, kidneys, muscles). On the venous side of the circulation, capillaries converge into small venules, which converge to form larger vessels called veins. The largest veins return blood to the heart.

Arterioles play a major role in regulating blood flow to the capillaries because of their ability to vasoconstrict (narrow the opening of the blood vessel) or vasodilate (widen the opening of the blood vessel). Capillaries form dense networks that branch throughout all tissues. The average capillary is 1 mm in length and 0.01 mm in diameter. This is just large enough for a single red blood cell to pass through (4). Capillaries have extremely thin walls and are the site of exchange of nutrients between blood and the interstitial fluid. Veins receive blood from the venules. In general, the veins are thinner and more compliant than arteries and act as blood reservoirs. The walls of some veins, such as those in the legs, contain one-way valves that help maintain venous return to the heart by preventing backward blood flow even under relatively low pressures.

Cardiac Function

HEART RATE

Heart rate (HR) is the number of heart beats per minute (bpm). The average normal resting HR is approximately 60–80 bpm. The resting HR in women is typically 10 bpm higher than that in men.

Children have higher HRs than adults, whereas elderly people have lower HRs. In the same age group and gender, fit individuals have a lower resting HR than do unfit individuals because of a larger stroke volume (SV) of the heart as a result of exercise training so that the heart does not have to pump as many times as before to maintain the same cardiac output (36). HR can be measured by counting the number of pulses over a given time period.

BLOOD PRESSURE

The heart is an autonomic organ that contracts and relaxes alternatively throughout life. When the LV of the heart muscle contracts, a surge of blood is propelled into the aorta and arteries. The pressure being exerted on the arterial wall during contraction is the systolic blood pressure (SBP), whereas the pressure during the relaxation phase of the ventricles is termed diastolic blood pressure (DBP). An average resting blood pressure is 120 mm Hg for SBP and 80 mm Hg for DBP. When the SBP persistently exceeds 140 mm Hg and/or the DBP exceeds 90 mm Hg at rest, a medical condition known as hypertension may be present.

STROKE VOLUME

The amount of blood ejected from the LV in a single contraction is called SV. SV is equal to the difference between the end-diastolic volume (EDV) and end-systolic volume (ESV). EDV and ESV are the total volume of blood in the ventricles at the end of diastole and systole, respectively. In an upright posture, SV is lower in untrained individuals than in trained individuals. The SV of men is usually greater than that of women because of their larger heart size. SV is also sensitive to body position. In the supine or prone postures, SV increases.

CARDIAC OUTPUT

Cardiac output ($\dot{Q}$) is the volume of blood pumped by the heart per minute and is calculated by multiplying the HR by the SV. The resting $\dot{Q}$ for adults, both trained and untrained, is approximately 4 to 5 liters per minute. However, the maximal $\dot{Q}$ is higher in trained individuals than in untrained individuals.

ACUTE RESPONSE TO CARDIOVASCULAR EXERCISE

Many mechanisms function collectively to support the increased aerobic requirements of physical activity. The overall effect of changes in HR, SV, $\dot{Q}$, blood flow, blood pressure, arteriovenous oxygen difference, and pulmonary ventilation is to supply oxygenated blood that is delivered to the active tissues. As exercise intensity increases, oxygen consumption and carbon dioxide production by working muscles increase. The cardiorespiratory system is required to deliver oxygen to, and transport carbon dioxide from, these tissues in an attempt to maintain cellular homeostasis. The central nervous system (CNS) responds by increasing neural ventilatory and cardiac drive, resulting in increased activity of cardiac and respiratory muscles.

> *The cardiorespiratory system is required to deliver oxygen to, and transport carbon dioxide from, these tissues in an attempt to maintain cellular homeostasis.*

The lungs are largely passive, and the increased ventilatory and cardiac drives result in increasing blood and air flow and increased rate of transfer of oxygen and carbon dioxide across the gas-exchanging surfaces of the alveoli. However, limits to the degree to which increased air flow and blood flow can be supported can lead to pulmonary limitations to exercise either from mechanical ventilatory constraints or from compromised gas exchange. These limitations are generally not manifested in healthy individuals except in elite or older athletes.

Heart Rate

HR increases in a linear fashion with the work rate and oxygen uptake during dynamic exercise. The magnitude of the HR response is related to age, body position, fitness, type of activity, presence of heart disease, medications, blood volume, and environmental factors such as temperature and humidity. In contrast to SBP, which usually increases with age, maximum attainable HR decreases with age. The equation "max HR = 220 − age" provides an approximation of the maximum HR in healthy men and women, but the variance for any fixed age is considerable (standard deviation ∼ ±10 bpm) (19).

Stroke Volume

During exercise, SV increases curvilinearly with the work rate until it reaches a near-maximal level equivalent to approximately 40%–50% of aerobic capacity, increasing only slightly thereafter (43). When SV reaches maximum, the increase in oxygen demand is met by increasing the HR. At a higher HR, SV may actually decrease because of the disproportionate shortening of diastolic filling time in the heart (19).

Cardiac Output

$\dot{Q}$ in healthy adults increases linearly with increased work rate. However, maximum values of $\dot{Q}$ depend on many factors including age, posture, body size, presence of cardiovascular disease, and the level of physical conditioning. At exercise intensities up to 50% of maximum, the increase in $\dot{Q}$ is facilitated by increases in HR and SV (43). Thereafter, the increase results almost solely from the continued rise in HR.

Arteriovenous Oxygen Difference (a-v̄ O$_2$ Difference)

Oxygen extraction by tissues reflects the difference between oxygen content of arterial blood and the oxygen content of venous blood, yielding a typical a-v̄ O_2 difference at rest of 5 mL $O_2 \cdot dL^{-1}$ of blood. This approximates a use coefficient of approximately 25%. During exercise to exhaustion, the mixed venous oxygen content typically decreases to 5 mL $O_2 \cdot dL^{-1}$ of blood or less, thus widening the a-v̄ O_2 difference from 5 to 15 mL $O_2 \cdot dL^{-1}$ of blood, corresponding to a use coefficient of 75% (43).

Blood Flow

At rest, 15%–20% of the $\dot{Q}$ is distributed to the skeletal muscles; the remainder goes to visceral organs, the heart, and the brain (50). However, during exercise, as much as 85%–90% of the $\dot{Q}$ is selectively delivered to working muscles and shunted away from the skin and the splanchnic, hepatic, and renal vascular beds. Myocardial blood flow may increase four to five times with exercise, whereas blood supply to the brain is maintained at resting levels (56).

Blood Pressure

There is a linear increase in SBP with increasing levels of exercise. Maximal values typically reach 190–220 mm Hg (44); nevertheless, maximal SBP should not exceed 250 mm Hg (2). A SBP that fails to rise or falls with increasing workloads may signal a plateau or decrease in $\dot{Q}$ (16). Exercise testing should be terminated in persons demonstrating exertional hypotension (a decreasing SBP). DBP may decrease slightly or remain unchanged. This is due to the decrease in peripheral resistance caused by the vasodilation of arterioles in the active muscles during exercise (25).

Maximal Oxygen Consumption

The most widely recognized measure of cardiopulmonary fitness is the aerobic capacity or $\dot{V}O_{2max}$. This variable is defined physiologically as the highest rate of oxygen transport and use that can be achieved at maximal physical exertion. Oxygen consumption ($\dot{V}O_2$) may be expressed mathematically by a rearrangement of the Fick equation (42):

$$\dot{V}O_2 \, (\text{mL} \cdot \text{kg}^{-1} \cdot \text{min}^{-1}) = \text{HR (bpm)} \times \text{SV (mL} \cdot \text{beat}^{-1}) \times (\text{a-}\bar{\text{v}} \, O_2 \text{ difference})$$

Thus, it is apparent that both central (i.e., $\dot{Q}$) and peripheral (i.e., a-$\bar{\text{v}}$ O_2 difference) regulatory mechanisms affect the magnitude of $\dot{V}O_2$. $\dot{V}O_{2max}$ may be expressed on an absolute or relative basis. Absolute $\dot{V}O_{2max}$ usually uses the units of "liters per minute," reflecting total body energy output and caloric expenditure (i.e., 1 L $\approx$ 5 kcal), and does not account for differences in body weight. Relative $\dot{V}O_{2max}$ divides the absolute $\dot{V}O_{2max}$ value by body weight in kilograms (and is typically reported in mL $\cdot$ kg^{-1} $\cdot$ min^{-1} or METs). Because large persons usually have larger absolute $\dot{V}O_2$ by virtue of a larger muscle mass, the latter expression allows a more equitable comparison between individuals of different body masses. This measure is widely considered the single best index of physical work capacity or cardiorespiratory fitness (12). In terms of cardiovascular fitness, the higher the $\dot{V}O_{2max}$, the better.

RESPIRATORY SYSTEM

The respiratory system consists of the nose, nasal cavity, pharynx, larynx, trachea, bronchial tree, and the lungs. The primary function of the respiratory system is to filter air that enters the body and allow for gas exchange within microscopic air sacs in the lungs called alveoli. The structure of the respiratory system is illustrated in Figure 5.2. The lungs are situated inside the chest cavity above the diaphragm and protected by the ribs and pectoral muscles. The lungs are enclosed by a set of membranes called pleura. The breathing mechanism of the lungs is passively controlled by the involuntary movements of the respiratory muscles and diaphragm. The pressure inside the pleura cavity (intrapleural pressure) is less than atmospheric pressure and becomes even lower during inspiration, causing air to inflate the lungs, and prevents the collapse of the fragile air sacs within the lung. These pressure differences reverse during exhalation.

> *The primary function of the respiratory system is to filter air that enters the body and allow for gas exchange within microscopic air sacs in the lungs called alveoli.*

Control of Breathing

Respiratory muscles lack the ability to regulate their own contractions; therefore, the control of breathing in an awake person results from the interplay of brainstem and other respiratory pathways (7). Autonomic control structures are located in the brainstem, and voluntary control structures are located in the cerebral cortex of the brain.

Distribution of Ventilation

Ventilation of the pulmonary system is accomplished in two major divisions, the upper and lower respiratory tracts, illustrated in Figure 5.2.

UPPER RESPIRATORY TRACT

The upper respiratory tract, which includes the nose, sinuses, pharynx, and larynx, acts as a conduction pathway for the movement of air into the lower respiratory tract. The function of these structures is to purify, warm, and humidify air before it reaches the gas exchange units. During normal

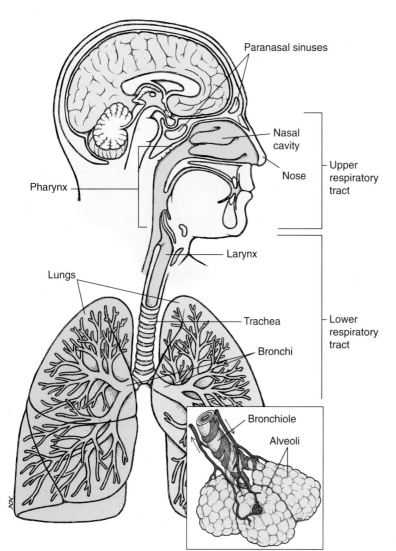

FIGURE 5.2. The structures of the respiratory system (anterior view). (From *Stedman's Medical Dictionary*. 27th ed. Baltimore: Lippincott Williams & Wilkins; 2000.)

quiet breathing, inspired air is heated to body temperature, and the relative humidity is increased to more than 90% during passage through the nose.

The pharynx is divided by the soft palate into the nasopharynx and the oropharynx. The epiglottis, located at the base of the tongue, protects the laryngeal opening during swallowing. The larynx contains the vocal cords, which contribute to speech and participate in coughing. Receptors throughout the upper respiratory tract may initiate a cough response. Coughing is produced by closure of the vocal cords along with contraction of the expiratory muscles to create increased intrathoracic (within the chest cavity) pressures. With sudden opening of the vocal cords, the positive airway pressure forces into the atmosphere air carrying any mucus or particles from the tracheobronchial tree. A cough can move gas from the lung at rates up to $10 \text{ L} \cdot \text{s}^{-1}$ during the expulsion phase.

LOWER RESPIRATORY TRACT

The lower respiratory tract begins in the trachea just below the larynx and includes the bronchi, bronchioles, and alveoli (Fig. 5.2). There are approximately 23 generations (divisions) of airways; the first 16 are conducting airways, and the last seven are respiratory airways ending blindly in approximately 300 million alveoli, which form the gas exchange surface. The structural components of the airways coincide with their functional properties. For example, the volume of the conducting zone is approximately 1 mL of air per pound of body weight and does not contribute to gas exchange, whereas gas exchange areas occupy a proportionately greater volume in the lungs. The trachea begins at the base of the neck and extends approximately 4–4.5 inches (10–12 cm) before it divides into the right and left main bronchi. It is anterior to the esophagus. The trachea consists of a series of anterior horseshoe-shaped cartilaginous rings and a posterior longitudinal muscle bundle.

The major bronchi contain cartilage that keeps the airway open as well as large numbers of mucous glands that produce secretions in response to irritation, infection, and/or inflammation. In the large airway, irritant receptors initiate the cough reflex when stimulated. The right main bronchus divides into three lobar bronchi: upper, middle, and lower. The left main bronchus divides into two lobar bronchi, upper and lower. Fissures separate the two lobes with two layers of visceral pleura. The lobar bronchi divide into segmental bronchi and segments, 10 on the right and 10 on the left.

Columnar cells lining the epithelium (inner lining) of the bronchi consist predominantly of ciliated cells that contain motile cilia, which move or beat in a coordinated manner to move the mucous layer toward the mouth ("mucociliary escalator"). The columnar epithelium is an important barrier for lung defense. Goblet cells interspersed among the ciliated cells secrete mucus. Segmental bronchi divide further into the terminal bronchioles, which have a diameter of about 1 mm. Beyond the terminal bronchioles are respiratory bronchioles, alveolar ducts, and the alveoli. Air flows through the conducting airways and at the level of the alveolar ducts and alveoli. Movement of air or gas is by diffusion.

Ventilatory Pump

The ventilatory pump consists of the chest wall, the respiratory muscles, and the pleural space.

CHEST WALL

The chest wall includes muscles of respiration (primarily intercostal muscles) and bones (spine, ribs, sternum). The ribs are hinged on the spine by ligaments and cartilage so that the ribs move upward and outward during inspiration and downward and inward during expiration. The hinging movement results in a change in thoracic volume and pressures. At rest and at the end of a normal expiration, the elastic properties of the chest wall exert an outward (expansion) force whereas the elastic properties of the lung structures exert an inward (recoil) force. Inspiration (airflow into the lungs) occurs by activation of the respiratory muscles, particularly the diaphragm, which creates a more negative pressure in the pleural space and the lungs than that in the atmosphere. Air enters the lungs until the intrapulmonary gas pressure equals atmospheric pressure. During expiration, when the respiratory muscles relax, air flows from the lungs into the atmosphere because of the positive pressure generated by the elastic recoil of the lungs.

RESPIRATORY MUSCLES

The muscles of respiration are the only skeletal muscles essential to life. The diaphragm, the major muscle of inspiration, is innervated by the phrenic nerve, which originates from the third to fifth cervical spinal segments. Spinal cord transection as a result of injury at or above this level compromises respiratory muscle function and consequently ventilation. An illustration of the role of the diaphragm in breathing is displayed in Figure 5.3. The diaphragm consists of a flattened centralized portion and vertical muscles called the costal portion. The diaphragm functions as a piston, with contraction and relaxation of the vertical muscle fibers. With contraction, the crural portion, or dome, moves downward and displaces the abdominal contents so that the abdomen moves outward, as does the chest wall. Expiration is normally passive under quiet breathing because of elastic recoil of the lung; it requires no work and is therefore passive. However, during active breathing, when ventilatory requirements are increased (e.g., during exercise), the muscles of expiration

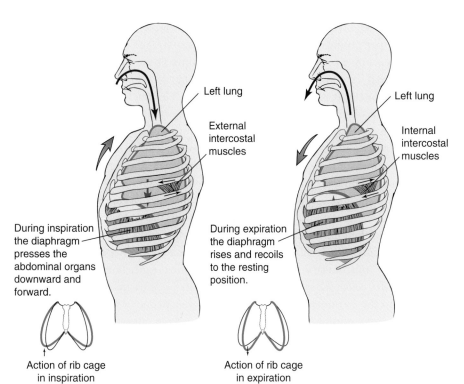

Left lung

External intercostal muscles

During inspiration the diaphragm presses the abdominal organs downward and forward.

Action of rib cage in inspiration

Left lung

Internal intercostal muscles

During expiration the diaphragm rises and recoils to the resting position.

Action of rib cage in expiration

FIGURE 5.3. Mechanics of normal—not deep, not shallow— inspiration (left) and expiration (right). (From Weber J, Kelley J. *Health Assessment in Nursing.* 2nd ed. Philadelphia: Lippincott Williams & Wilkins; 2003.)

are recruited. The major muscles of expiration are the internal intercostals and the abdominal muscles (rectus abdominis, external and internal oblique, and transverse abdominis). In clients with airflow obstruction (e.g., acute bronchoconstriction in asthma or emphysema), hyperinflation of the lungs stretches the lung tissue and leads to additional elastic recoil, forcing the crural portion of the diaphragm downward and shortening the vertical muscle fibers. This impairs the diaphragm's ability to contract.

PLEURA

The visceral (inner layer) and parietal (outer layer) pleura are thin membranes between the lung and the chest wall (39). The pleural space, which lies between the visceral and parietal pleura, contains a small amount of fluid. Because the pleural space is airtight and the chest wall and lung tissue pull against each other across the pleural space, negative pressure is produced at rest. During inspiration, both the visceral and parietal pleura expand outward and more negative pressure develops in the pleural space. Air can enter the pleural space (i.e., pneumothorax) by trauma to the chest wall (e.g., a fractured rib with penetration of the parietal pleura). With a pneumothorax, the lungs collapse whereas the chest wall expands because of its intrinsic elastic properties. The parietal pleura contains abundant pain fibers, and irritation of this membrane by a pneumothorax or an inflammation produces local chest pain exacerbated by motion of the pleura (e.g., deep inspiration).

DISTRIBUTION OF BLOOD FLOW

The lungs receive blood from the pulmonary arteries, which contain systemic venous blood from the RV and bronchial arteries. The pulmonary artery emerges from the RV and divides into the right and left main pulmonary arteries. The pulmonary arteries divide into branches corresponding to the divisions of the bronchial tree and supply the pulmonary arterioles. The pulmonary circulation is a low-pressure system with a normal mean pressure of approximately 15 mm Hg at rest. Most blood flow to the alveoli is derived from the pulmonary circulation, whereas the bronchial arteries supply the walls of the bronchi and bronchioles to the level of the alveoli. Pulmonary arterioles divide into pulmonary capillaries that form networks in the walls of the alveoli, where gas exchange occurs. The pulmonary veins carry oxygenated blood from the pulmonary capillaries. These veins converge to form the main pulmonary veins, which empty into the LA.

PULMONARY VENTILATION

Pulmonary ventilation ($\dot{V}_E$), the volume of air exchanged per minute, is approximately $6 \text{ L} \cdot \text{min}^{-1}$ at rest in the average sedentary adult male. At maximal exercise, however, $\dot{V}_E$ often increases 15- to 25-fold over resting values. Pulmonary ventilation is perhaps regulated more by the requirement for carbon dioxide removal than by oxygen consumption, and ventilation is not normally a limiting factor to aerobic capacity (18).

RESPIRATORY CHANGES

Several respiratory adaptations result from physical conditioning regimens. Although ventilation generally does not limit exercise in apparently healthy individuals, the limits of ventilation may be reached at $\dot{V}O_{2max}$ in elite athletes (6). Ventilation increases linearly with $\dot{V}O_{2max}$ up to about 50% $\dot{V}O_{2max}$, after which the increase is proportionately greater than the increase in work rate (6). Physically trained persons demonstrate larger lung volumes and diffusion capacity at rest and during exercise than their sedentary counterparts. Ventilation is either unaffected or only modestly affected by cardiorespiratory training. Maximal ventilatory capacity may be increased by exercise training, but it is unclear that this provides any advantage other than increased buffering capacity for lactate. Submaximal ventilation is probably not affected, but it may be decreased in some circumstances because a decrease in the production of lactate coincides with a decrease in the need to buffer lactate, which results in decreased ventilation.

ENERGY SYSTEMS

Energy is essential to produce mechanical work, maintain body temperature, and fulfill all biological and chemical activities inside the body. To release energy, foodstuff, particularly protein, carbohydrate, and fat, that is consumed must be metabolized to yield a high-energy compound called adenosine triphosphate (ATP). In the human body, all mechanical work that involves physical activity relies on the continuous supply of ATP. The manufactured ATP is stored inside muscles so that this immediate source of energy can be used for producing movement when a stimulus is given to the muscles.

> *To release energy, foodstuff, particularly protein, carbohydrate, and fat, that is consumed must be metabolized to yield a high-energy compound called adenosine triphosphate (ATP).*

The storage of ATP in the muscles, however, is limited. If ATP were the only form of energy available, mechanical movement would last for only a few seconds because of this limited storage capacity. Therefore, for movement that lasts longer than a few seconds, ATP must be further manufactured through the immediate breakdown of carbohydrate (in forms of glycogen and glucose inside muscle tissues).

This process of immediately breaking down muscle carbohydrate does not require the presence of oxygen and would provide an additional few minutes of ATP supply. This process is termed "anaerobic metabolism" or "anaerobic glycolysis." However, the metabolic end-product of lactate and resulting localized intramuscular acidosis limits muscular performance. Hence, anaerobic glycolysis is also called the "lactic acid system." With continuous movement lasting longer than a few minutes, the increased demand for ATP must be fulfilled by a greater capacity for energy production. Carbohydrate and fat can be broken down in the presence of oxygen, resulting in an abundant supply of ATP. This process is known as aerobic metabolism or oxidative phosphorylation. Only two molecules of ATP can be generated from breaking down a glucose molecule in anaerobic metabolism,

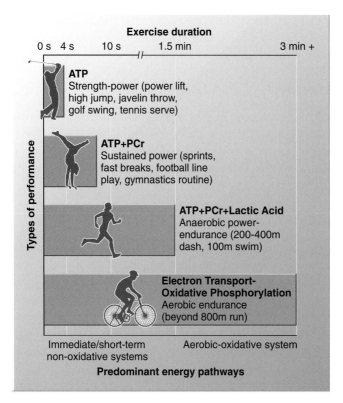

FIGURE 5.4. Comparison of activity with the energy pathways used (ATP = adenosine triphosphate, PCr = creatine phosphate, ATP + PCr + lactic acid = anaerobic glycolysis, electron transport-oxidative phosphorylation = aerobic oxidation). (From Premkumar K. *The Massage Connection, Anatomy and Physiology.* 2nd ed. Baltimore: Lippincott Williams & Wilkins; 2004.)

whereas the aerobic metabolism of a glucose molecule yields 36 ATP molecules (38 ATPs when starting with glycogen). The process of generating ATP aerobically, however, is a much slower process. The relationship between exercise duration and energy sources is illustrated in Figure 5.4.

Aerobic and Anaerobic Metabolism

The energy requirements of exercising human muscle increase substantially in the transition from rest to maximal physical exertion. Because the available stores of ATP are limited and capable of providing energy to maintain vigorous activity for only several seconds, ATP must be constantly resynthesized to provide continuous energy production. Therefore, exercising muscle must possess a large capacity of energy to produce sufficient ATP so that increased activity can continue. Energy production relies heavily on the respiratory and cardiovascular systems for the delivery of oxygen and nutrients and for the removal of waste products to maintain the internal equilibrium of cells.

Adenosine Triphosphate

ATP serves as the ideal energy-transfer agent that powers all of the cell's energy needs (42). The energy released through hydrolysis of the high-energy compound ATP to form adenosine diphosphate (ADP) and inorganic phosphate (Pi) powers skeletal muscle contractions. This reaction is catalyzed by the enzyme ATPase:

$$ATP \xrightarrow{(ATPase)} ADP + Pi + energy$$

The amount of ATP directly available in muscle at any time is small, so it must be resynthesized continuously if exercise lasts for more than a few seconds. Muscle fibers contain the metabolic machinery to produce ATP by three pathways: creatine phosphate (CP), anaerobic glycolysis, and aerobic oxidation of nutrients to carbon dioxide and water.

Creatine Phosphate

The CP system transfers high-energy phosphate from CP to rephosphorylate ATP from ADP (using the enzyme creatine kinase) as follows:

$$ADP + CP \xrightarrow{\text{(creatine kinase)}} ATP + C$$

This system is rapid because it involves only one enzymatic step (i.e., one chemical reaction). However, CP exists in finite quantities in cells as well, so the total amount of ATP that can be produced is limited. Oxygen is not involved in the rephosphorylation of ADP to ATP in this reaction, so the CP system is considered anaerobic (without oxygen).

Anaerobic Glycolysis

When glycolysis is rapid, it is capable of producing ATP without the involvement of oxygen. Glycolysis, the degradation of carbohydrate (glycogen or glucose) to pyruvate or lactate, involves a series of enzymatically catalyzed steps. Although glycolysis does not use oxygen and is considered anaerobic, pyruvate can readily participate in aerobic production of ATP when oxygen is available in the cell. Therefore, in addition to being an anaerobic pathway capable of producing ATP without oxygen, glycolysis can also be considered the first step in the aerobic degradation of carbohydrate (32) (Fig. 5.5).

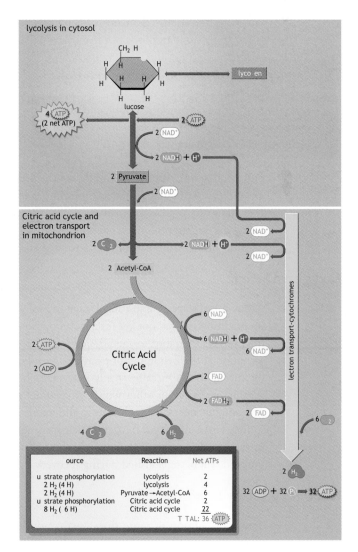

FIGURE 5.5. A net yield of 36 ATPs from energy transfer during the complete oxidation of one glucose molecule in glycolysis, the citric acid cycle, and electronic transport. (From McArdle WD, Katch FI, Katch VL. *Exercise Physiology: Energy Nutrition, and Human Performance.* 6th ed. Baltimore: Lippincott Williams & Wilkins; 2007.)

Aerobic Oxidation

The final metabolic pathway for ATP production combines two complex metabolic processes, the Krebs cycle and electron transport chain residing inside the mitochondria as illustrated in Figure 5.5. Oxidative phosphorylation uses oxygen as the final hydrogen acceptor to form water and ATP. Unlike glycolysis, aerobic metabolism can use fat, protein, and carbohydrate as substrates to produce ATP. Conceptually, the Krebs cycle can be considered a primer for oxidative phosphorylation. The primary function of the Krebs cycle is to remove hydrogens from four of the reactants involved in the cycle. The electrons from these hydrogens follow a chain of cytochromes (electron transport chain) in the mitochondria, and the energy released from this process is used to rephosphorylate ADP to form ATP. Oxygen is the final acceptor of hydrogen to form water, and this reaction is catalyzed by cytochrome oxidase (51). Although not all ATP is formed aerobically, the amount of ATP yielded by anaerobic glycolysis is extremely small (42). Nevertheless, anaerobic mechanisms provide a rapid source of ATP, which is particularly important at the beginning of any exercise bout and during high-intensity activity that can be sustained only for a brief period. As the duration of exercise increases, the relative contribution of anaerobic energy sources decreases (32).

The aerobic system requires adequate delivery and use of oxygen and uses glycogen, fats, and proteins as energy substrates, sustaining high rates of ATP production for muscular energy over long periods of time. The relative contributions of anaerobic and aerobic metabolism depend on oxygen exchange (respiration), delivery (cardiovascular), and use (muscular extraction) at rates commensurate with the energy demands of activity. The energy to perform most types of exercise does not come from a single source but from a combination of anaerobic and aerobic sources. The contribution of anaerobic sources (CP system and anaerobic glycolysis) to exercise energy metabolism is inversely related to the duration and intensity of the activity. The shorter and more intense the activity, the greater the contribution of anaerobic energy production. The longer the activity, however, and the lower the intensity, the greater the contribution of aerobic energy production. Although proteins can be used as a fuel for aerobic exercise, carbohydrates and fats are the primary energy substrates during exercise in a healthy, well-fed individual. In general, carbohydrates are used as the primary fuel at the onset of exercise and during high-intensity work (23). However, during prolonged exercise of low to moderate intensity (longer than 30 minutes), a gradual shift occurs from carbohydrate toward an increasing reliance on fat as a substrate.

> *The relative contributions of anaerobic and aerobic metabolism depend on oxygen exchange (respiration), delivery (cardiovascular), and use (muscular extraction) at rates commensurate with the energy demands of activity.*

Oxygen Deficit

At the initial stage or transitional stage of prolonged submaximal exercise, oxygen consumption builds up gradually and has not yet reached an optimal level of steady state for supporting energy demand of the exercise; therefore, oxygen deficit is incurred. Oxygen deficit is referred to the lag in oxygen consumption at the beginning of exercise. During this stage, part of the ATP supply relies on the anaerobic metabolism. Once the steady state is reached, all the ATP supply is sufficiently provided through aerobic oxidation. In other words, oxygen deficit describes the difference between the required oxygen amount necessary for meeting the energy demand of the exercise and the actual oxygen consumption. An additional oxygen deficit accumulates whenever energy demand is abruptly increased, as in sudden increase in exercise pace or intensity. After the exercise is ceased, the oxygen deficit accumulated will be replenished during recovery by consuming more than usual amounts of oxygen.

Recovery from Exercise

The consumption of more than usual amounts of oxygen after exercise is termed excess postexercise oxygen consumption (EPOC) (30). Oxygen uptake remains elevated above resting levels for

> *Oxygen uptake remains elevated above resting levels for several minutes during recovery from exercise.*

several minutes during recovery from exercise. In general, postexercise metabolism is higher following high-intensity exercise than after light or moderate work. Furthermore, EPOC remains elevated longer after prolonged exercise than after shorter-term exertion. The effect of EPOC is to restore PC in muscles and oxygen in blood and tissues.

MUSCULAR SYSTEM

All human movements require muscular action. Muscular action is illustrated through continuous alternations of muscular contraction and relaxation. There are three major types of muscles in the body: skeletal, smooth, and cardiac. Skeletal muscle is the muscle that attaches to the skeleton so as to produce physical movements. It is also called "striated muscle" because its fibers are composed of alternating light and dark stripes. Smooth muscle is the muscle that forms the internal organs. Cardiac muscle is the muscle of the heart. Skeletal muscle is voluntary muscle because it can be controlled, for the most part, by the individual. Smooth muscle and cardiac muscle are involuntary muscles because they are controlled by the autonomic nervous system (ANS), the involuntary division of the nervous system. All three kinds of muscles possess characteristics of extendibility, elasticity, excitability, and contractility. In this chapter, the focus is placed on skeletal muscle because it is strongly related to human movement during exercise.

Skeletal Muscles

Figure 5.6 shows the structure of skeletal muscle. Individual skeletal muscles are composed of a varying number of muscle bundles referred to as "fasciculi" (an individual bundle is a fasciculus). Fasciculi are likewise covered and thus separated by the perimysium. Individual muscle fibers are enveloped by the endomysium. Immediately beneath the endomysium is the thin, membranous sarcolemma, the cell membrane that encloses the cellular contents of the muscle fiber, nuclei, local stores of fat, glucose (in the form of glycogen), enzymes, contractile proteins, and other specialized structures such as the mitochondria.

Muscle Contraction

The smallest contractile unit of a muscle cell is the sarcomere. A sarcomere is composed of two types of muscle protein called "actin" (the thin filament) and "myosin" (the thick filament). Actin contains two other components called "troponin" and "tropomyosin." Myosin contains many cross bridges. Figure 5.7 illustrates the relationship between muscle contraction and microscopic action within the sarcomere. Two major principles describe the mechanism of muscle contraction: the "sliding-filament theory" and the "all-or-none principle."

> *The sliding-filament theory describes the events that occur between the actin and myosin filaments during muscle contraction and relaxation.*

The sliding-filament theory describes the events that occur between the actin and myosin filaments during muscle contraction and relaxation. When a nerve impulse is received, the cross bridges of the myosin will pull the actin filaments toward the center of the sarcomere and tension is created. The sliding motion between the actin and myosin causes the shortening of a sarcomere and subsequently the entire muscle fiber. Moreover, the nerve impulse that applies to the muscle cell, regardless of its "strength," causes the sarcomere to contract maximally or not all. This is called the all-or-none principle. The length of a muscle fiber during a contraction is determined by the number of muscle fibers (cells) being recruited for the contraction. The more sarcomeres recruited for contraction, the shorter the muscle length. The amount of force that is produced from a muscle contraction is determined by the number of motor units (one

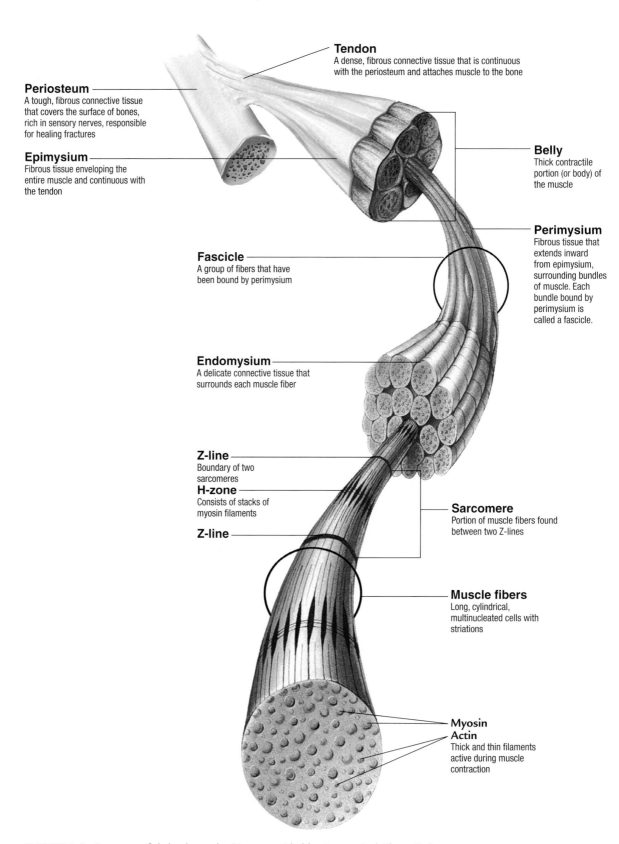

Tendon
A dense, fibrous connective tissue that is continuous with the periosteum and attaches muscle to the bone

Periosteum
A tough, fibrous connective tissue that covers the surface of bones, rich in sensory nerves, responsible for healing fractures

Epimysium
Fibrous tissue enveloping the entire muscle and continuous with the tendon

Belly
Thick contractile portion (or body) of the muscle

Perimysium
Fibrous tissue that extends inward from epimysium, surrounding bundles of muscle. Each bundle bound by perimysium is called a fascicle.

Fascicle
A group of fibers that have been bound by perimysium

Endomysium
A delicate connective tissue that surrounds each muscle fiber

Z-line
Boundary of two sarcomeres

H-zone
Consists of stacks of myosin filaments

Z-line

Sarcomere
Portion of muscle fibers found between two Z-lines

Muscle fibers
Long, cylindrical, multinucleated cells with striations

Myosin
Actin
Thick and thin filaments active during muscle contraction

FIGURE 5.6. Structure of skeletal muscle. (Asset provided by Anatomical Chart Co.)

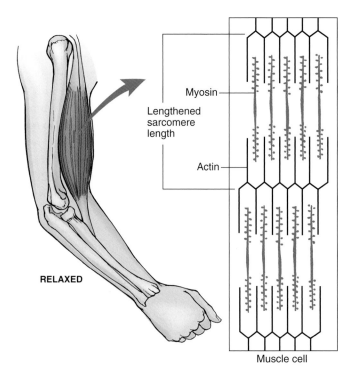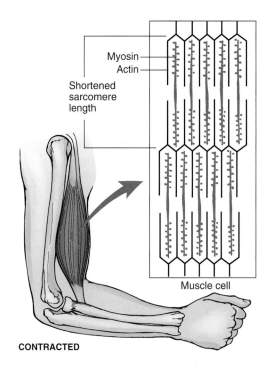

FIGURE 5.7. The sliding-filament model (contraction of skeletal muscle results from the sliding of the actin chains on the myosin chains). (From Oatis, Carol A. *Kinesiology—The Mechanics and Pathomechanics of Human Movement.* Baltimore: Lippincott Williams & Wilkins; 2004.)

motor nerve together with all the muscle fibers that it innervated) that are recruited and the number of fibers contained in each motor unit (46).

Muscle Contraction and Training

During static (isometric) contractions, the muscle or muscle group maintains a constant length as resistance is applied, and no change in joint position occurs. Research has demonstrated that static training produces significant improvements in muscular strength. The strength gains, however, are limited to the specific joint angles at which the static contractions are performed (23,31,37). As a result, static training may have limited value in enhancing functional strength. "Functional strength" is defined as performing work against a resistance specifically in such a way that the strength gained directly benefits the execution of activities of daily life and movements associated with sports. Static training has also been associated with short-term elevations in blood pressure, perhaps because of increased intrathoracic pressure during static contractions. Despite the limitations, static training appears to play a positive role in physical rehabilitation. For example, it is effective in maintaining muscular strength and preventing atrophy associated with the immobilization of a limb (e.g., application of a cast, splint, or brace) (21,23,31,37).

> *Functional strength is defined as performing work against a resistance specifically in such a way that the strength gained directly benefits the execution of activities of daily life and movements associated with sports.*

Dynamic (isotonic) resistance training is another common method. If movement of the joint occurs during contraction, it is dynamic. If force is sufficient to overcome resistance and the muscle shortens (e.g., the lifting phase of a biceps curl), the contraction is concentric. When resistance is greater than force and the muscle lengthens during contraction, it is eccentric (e.g., the lowering phase of the biceps curl). Most dynamic resistance training includes both concentric and eccentric actions. Significantly heavier loads can be moved eccentrically; in fact, in unfatigued muscle, the ratio of eccentric to concentric strength can be as high as 1.4:1 (21,23). For example, maximal eccentric weight is 1.4 times the maximal concentric weight in the same muscle group/movement. Furthermore, at the onset of fatigue, the relative level of eccentric strength and eccentric–concentric ratio increases even more. Greater force production during eccentric contraction than with the concentric contraction probably results from more motor units being recruited and a slow movement velocity. Individuals who are eccentrically trained are often subjected to delayed-onset muscular soreness (13). Eccentric training can, however, play an important role in preventing or rehabilitating certain musculoskeletal injuries. For example, eccentric training has been demonstrated to be effective for treating hamstring strains, tennis elbow, and patellofemoral pain syndrome (52).

The other major type of resistance training, isokinetic exercise, entails constant-speed muscular contraction against accommodating resistance. The speed of movement is controlled, and the amount of resistance is proportional to the amount of force produced throughout the full range of motion (ROM). The theoretical advantage of isokinetic exercise is the development of maximal muscle tension throughout the ROM. Research documents the effectiveness of isokinetic training (23,37). Strength gains achieved during high-speed training (i.e., contraction velocities of $180° \cdot s^{-1}$ or faster) appear to carry over to all speeds below that specific speed (17). Improvement in strength at slow speeds of movement, however, has not been shown to carry over to faster speeds.

Muscle Fiber Types

The human body has the ability to perform a wide range of physical tasks, combining varying composites of speed, power, and endurance. No single type of muscle fiber possesses the characteristics that would allow optimal performance across this continuum of physical challenges. Rather, muscle fibers possess certain characteristics that result in relative specialization. For example, certain muscle fibers are selectively recruited by the body for speed and power tasks of short duration, whereas others are recruited for endurance tasks of long duration and relatively low intensity. When the challenge requires elements of speed or power but also has an endurance component, yet another type of muscle fiber is recruited. These different fiber types should not be thought of as mutually exclusive. In fact, intricate recruitment and switching occurs in muscle over the performance of many tasks, and fibers designed to be optimal for one type of task can contribute to the performance of another. The net result is a functioning muscle that can respond to a wide variety of tasks, and although the composition of the muscle may lend itself to performing best in endurance activities, it still can accomplish speed and power tasks to a lesser degree (15).

Over the years, there has been a fair amount of controversy about the classification of muscle fiber types (4). In addition, there are questions about whether these types can change in response to an intervention such as endurance training (35). In either case, there is general agreement that relative to exercise performance, two distinct fiber types (type I or slow twitch and type II or fast twitch, with their proposed subdivisions) have been identified and classified by contractile and metabolic characteristics such as the chemical breakdown of carbohydrate, fat, and protein for energy within the muscle cell (10).

Type I Muscle Fibers

The characteristics of type I muscle fibers are consistent with those of muscle fibers that resist fatigue. Thus, type I fibers are selected for activities of low intensity and long duration. Within whole muscle, type I motor units contract, but the units do not all contract at the same time. In addition to their inherent fatigue resistance, endurance is prolonged by the constant switching that occurs to ensure freshly charged muscle as the exercise stimulus continues. Sedentary persons have approximately

Type I fibers are selected for activities of low intensity and long duration.

50% type I fibers, and this distribution is generally equal throughout the major muscle groups of the body (26). In endurance athletes, the percentage of type I fibers is greater, but this is thought to be largely a genetic predisposition, despite some evidence suggesting that prolonged exercise training can alter fiber type (11). Essentially, those most successful at endurance activities generally have a high proportion of type I fibers, and this is most likely due to genetic factors supplemented through appropriate exercise training. From a metabolic perspective, type I fibers are those frequently called "aerobic," because the generation of energy for continued muscle contraction is met through the ongoing oxidation (chemical breakdown using oxygen) of available energy substrates. Thus, with minimal accumulation of anaerobically (chemical breakdown without oxygen) produced metabolites, continued submaximal muscle contraction is favored in type I fibers.

TYPE II MUSCLE FIBERS

At the opposite end of the continuum, those who achieve the greatest success in power and high-intensity speed tasks usually have a greater proportion of type II muscle fibers distributed through the major muscle groups. Because force generation is so important, type II fibers shorten and develop tension considerably faster than type I fibers (54). These fibers are typically thought of as type IIB fibers, the "classic" fast-twitch fiber. Metabolically, these fibers are the classic anaerobic fibers, because they rely on energy sources from within the muscle, not the fuels used by type I fibers. When an endurance component is introduced, such as in events lasting upward of several minutes (800- to 1500-m races, for example), a second type of fast-twitch fiber, type IIA, is recruited. The type IIA fibers represent a transition of sorts between the needs met by the type I and type IIB fibers. Metabolically, while type IIA fibers have the ability to generate a moderately large amount of force, they also have some aerobic capacity, although not as much as that of type I fibers. This is a logical and necessary bridge between the types of muscle fibers and the ability to meet the variety of physical tasks imposed. Reference to the existence of the type IIC fiber is necessary in a complete description of human muscle fiber types. The type IIC fiber has been described as a rare and undifferentiated muscle fiber type that is probably involved in reinnervation of damaged skeletal muscle (38).

> *Those who achieve the greatest success in power and high-intensity speed tasks usually have a greater proportion of type II muscle fibers distributed through the major muscle groups.*

Neuromuscular Activation

Physical activity involves purposeful, voluntary movement. The stimulus for voluntary muscle activation comes from the brain. The signal is relayed through the brainstem and spinal cord and transformed into a specific motor unit activation pattern. To perform a specific task, the required motor units meet specific demands for force production by activating associated muscle fibers (22).

MOTOR UNIT ACTIVATION

The functional unit of the neuromuscular system is the motor unit (46). It consists of the motor neuron and the muscle fibers it innervates. Motor units range in size from a few to several hundred muscle fibers. Muscle fibers from different motor units can be anatomically adjacent to each other, and therefore a muscle fiber may be actively generating force whereas the adjacent fiber moves passively with no direct neural stimulation. Several nomenclatures have been used to classify skeletal muscle fibers, including color (red or white), action speed (fast or slow twitch), oxidative or glycolytic enzyme content (fast glycolytic, fast oxidative glycolytic, or oxidative), combination schemes (fast glycolytic), and myosin adenosine triphosphatase (ATPase) content. When maximal force is required, all available motor units are activated. Another adaptive mechanism affected by heavy resistance training is the muscle force effected by different motor unit firing rates and/or frequencies.

SKELETAL SYSTEM

Beyond supporting soft tissue, protecting internal organs, and acting as an important source of nutrients and blood constituents, the bones are the rigid levers for locomotion. The skull, vertebral column, sternum, and ribs are considered the axial skeleton; the bones of the upper and lower limbs make up the appendicular skeleton. An outer fibrous layer of connective tissue attaches the bone to muscles, deep fascia, and joint capsules. Just beneath the outer layer is a highly vascular inner layer that contains cells for the creation of new bone. The outer and inner layers that cover the bones constitute the periosteum. The periosteum, continuous with tendons and adjacent articulated structures, anchors muscle to bone. Tendons are likewise continuous with the epimysium, the outer layer of connective tissue covering muscle.

Structure and Function of Joints in Movement

The effective interaction of bone and muscle to produce movement depends somewhat on joint function. Joints are the articulations between bones, and along with bones and ligaments, they constitute the articular system. Ligaments are tough, fibrous connective tissues that connect bone to bone, whereas tendons connect muscle to bone. Joints are typically classified as fibrous, in which bones are united by fibrous tissue, cartilaginous (with cartilage or a fibrocartilaginous anchor), or synovial, in which a fibrous articular capsule and an inner synovial membrane lining enclose the joint cavity. The cavity is filled with synovial fluid, which provides constant lubrication during human movement to minimize the wearing effects of friction on the cartilaginous covering of the articulating bones. Joints are typically well perfused by numerous arterial branches and are innervated by branches of the nerves supplying the adjacent muscle and overlying skin.

Proprioception is defined as the receipt of information from muscles and tendons that enables the brain to determine movements and position of the body and its parts. Proprioceptive feedback is an important joint sensation, as is pain, owing to the high density of sensory fibers in the joint capsule. This feedback has obvious importance in regulating human movement and in preventing injury. The degree of movement within a joint is typically called the range of motion (ROM). ROM can be active (AROM), the range that can be reached by voluntary movement, or passive (PROM), the range that can be achieved by external means (e.g., an examiner or a device). Joints are typically limited in range by the articulations of bones (as in the limitation of elbow extension by the olecranon process of the ulna), ligamentous arrangement, and soft tissue limitations, as occurs in elbow or knee flexion. Movement at one joint may influence the extent of movement at adjacent joints, as a number of muscles and other soft tissue structures cross multiple joints. For example, finger flexion decreases in the presence of wrist flexion, because muscles that flex both the wrist and fingers cross multiple joints. More in-depth information about skeletal system is provided in Chapter 3.

> *Proprioception is defined as the receipt of information from muscles and tendons that enables the brain to determine movements and position of the body and its parts.*

NEUROLOGICAL SYSTEM

In the earlier discussion of a muscle contraction, we described the contraction as triggered by a nervous impulse of a motor unit. The nervous impulse is released from a motor neuron, which originates from the spinal cord. The spinal cord is a part of the CNS, which helps control all of the peripheral and internal organs. All muscular movements are controlled by the nervous system. To understand the complex control of human movement, understanding neural control is essential.

The nervous system consists of the brain, spinal cord, and peripheral nerves, and is divided into the CNS and the peripheral nervous system (PNS). The CNS consists of the brain and spinal cord, whereas the PNS consists of all other peripheral nerves of the voluntary system (Fig. 5.8) (40).

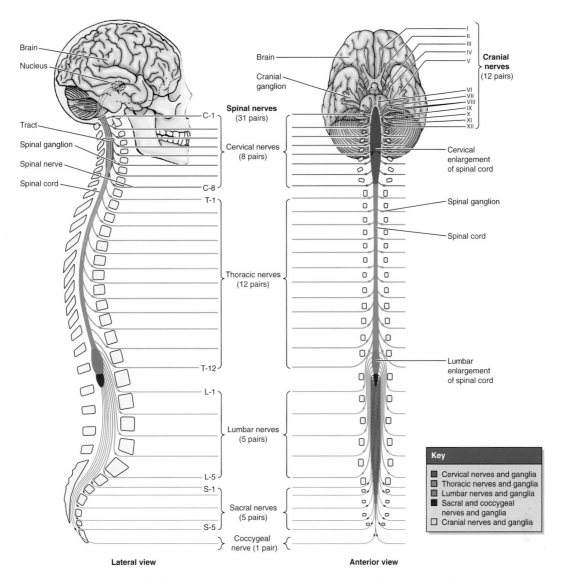

Lateral view   **Anterior view**

FIGURE 5.8. Basic organization of the nervous system. The brain and spinal cord constitute the CNS. A collection of nerve cell bodies in the CNS is a nucleus, and a bundle of nerve fibers connecting neighboring or distant nuclei in the CNS is a tract. The PNS consists of nerve fibers and cell bodies outside the CNS. Peripheral nerves are either cranial or spinal nerves. A collection of nerve cell bodies outside the CNS is a ganglion (e.g., a cranial or spinal ganglion). (From Moore KL, Dalley AF II. *Clinical Oriented Anatomy*. 4th ed. Baltimore: Lippincott Williams & Wilkins; 1999.)

CENTRAL NERVOUS SYSTEM

The CNS is the body's central control center where sensory stimuli are received, integrated, analyzed, and interpreted, and finally relayed as nerve impulses to muscles and glands for taking action.

The brain is the most important part of the CNS and is surrounded and protected by the bony skull. The spinal cord is the extension of the brain, which runs along and is surrounded and protected by the vertebral column. The CNS is the body's central control center where sensory stimuli are received, integrated, analyzed, and interpreted, and finally relayed as nerve impulses to muscles and glands for taking action.

Peripheral Nervous System

The PNS is composed of the cranial nerves associated with the brain and the spinal nerves associated with the spinal cord, as well as groups of nerve cell bodies called "ganglia." In other words, the PNS is made up of the nerve cells and their fibers that lie outside the brain and spinal cord (14). The PNS allows the brain and spinal cord to communicate with the rest of the body. There are two types of nerve fibers in the PNS, the afferent, or sensory, fiber and the efferent, or motor, fiber. The sensory nerve fiber is responsible for carrying nerve impulses from sensory receptors in the body to the CNS. Once the received signal is processed and analyzed in the CNS and an action is determined, then the motor nerve fiber is called to convey the nerve signal from the CNS to the effectors, either the muscles or other organs. The PNS can be subdivided into two functional branches, the somatic nervous system and the visceral nervous system. Both systems are composed of an afferent division and an efferent division. The somatic nervous system primarily regulates the voluntary contraction of the skeletal muscles, whereas the visceral system involves the motor activities that control internal organs such as the smooth (involuntary) muscles, cardiac muscle, and glands of the skin and viscera. The latter is also termed the "autonomic nervous system."

Autonomic Nervous System

The ANS regulates visceral activities such as HR, digestion, breathing, and the secretion of hormones. These activities normally are operated subconsciously and continue to function throughout life. However, they can also be altered to a certain limit consciously. These activities can be carried out even if the organs are deprived of innervation by the ANS. The ANS includes two pathways, the sympathetic pathway and the parasympathetic pathway, which complement each other. The sympathetic pathway stimulates visceral activities under stressful (or alarming) conditions, which results in acceleration of metabolism, HR, and breathing and adrenal hormone release. Exercise can be treated as a stressful stimulus to the body that triggers the sympathetic pathway for generating more energy and muscular force. When the stressful stimulus subsides, the parasympathetic pathway brings the visceral activities back to normal, for example, decreasing HR and breathing, relaxing the muscles, and increasing gastrointestinal activities. The parasympathetic pathway helps conserve and restore body resources.

Neuromuscular Control

The information transmitted and relayed by the sensory and motor nerves is in a form of electrical energy referred to as the "nerve impulse." The sensory stimulation received through vision or touching is transmitted to the CNS. A motor command is then released after the integration and decision making of the motor cortex of the brain. A nerve pulse is then transmitted to the targeted muscles through an efferent neuron for activating muscle contraction. The functional unit of the neuromuscular system is the motor unit (46). It consists of the motor neuron and the muscle fibers it innervates. When maximal force is required, all available motor units are activated. Another adaptive mechanism affected by heavy resistance training is the muscle force affected by different motor unit firing rates and frequencies (3).

Motor unit activation is also influenced by the size principle. This principle is based on the observed relationship between motor unit twitch force and recruitment threshold. Specifically, motor units are recruited in order according to recruitment thresholds and firing rates, resulting in a continuum of voluntary force. Whereas type I motor units are the smallest and possess the lowest recruitment thresholds, type IIa and IIb motor units are larger in size and have higher activation thresholds. Therefore, as force requirements of an activity increase, the recruitment order progresses from type I to IIa to IIb motor units. Thus, most muscles contain

> *Motor units are recruited in order according to recruitment thresholds and firing rates, resulting in a continuum of voluntary force.*

a range of motor units (type I and II fibers), and force production can span wide levels. Maximal force production requires not only the recruitment of all motor units, including high-threshold motor units, but also recruitment at a sufficiently high firing rate. It has been hypothesized that untrained individuals cannot voluntarily recruit the highest-threshold motor units or maximally activate muscles. Furthermore, electrical stimulation has been shown to be more effective in eliciting gains in untrained muscle or injury rehabilitation scenarios, suggesting further inability to activate all available motor units. Thus, training adaptation develops the ability to recruit a greater percentage of motor units when required.

Muscle Spindle and Golgi Tendon Organs

Other than the motor unit, muscular contraction is also affected by specialized sensory receptors in the muscles and tendons that are sensitive to stretch, tension, and pressure. These receptors are termed "proprioceptors." A sensory receptor called a "muscle spindle" is sensitive to the stretch of a muscle and is embedded within the muscle fiber. Anytime the muscle is stretched or shortened, the spindle is also stretched or shortened. The muscle spindles provide sensory information regarding the changes and rate of change in the length and tension of muscle fibers. Their main function is to respond to stretch of a muscle and, through reflex action, to initiate a stronger muscle action to reduce this stretch (42). This is known as the "stretch reflex." In contrast to the muscle spindles, the Golgi tendon organs are another type of specialized proprioceptor that attaches to the tendons near the junction of the muscle (Fig. 5.9). These receptors detect differences in the tension generated by active muscle rather than muscle length. When excessive tension is detected by the Golgi tendon organs, a continuous reflex inhibition signal is fired to prevent the muscle from contracting. Hence,

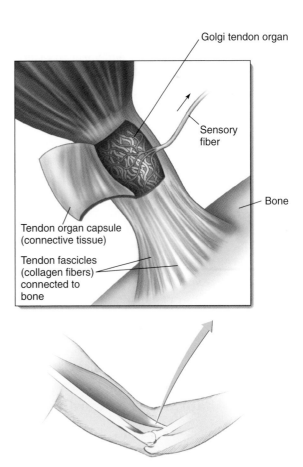

FIGURE 5.9. Structure of the Golgi tendon organ. (From Premkumar K. *The Massage Connection, Anatomy and Physiology*. 2nd ed. Baltimore: Lippincott Williams & Wilkins; 2004.)

the Golgi tendon organs serve as a protective sensory system to prevent muscle injury resulting from overcontraction.

EXERCISE SYSTEM ADAPTATIONS—STRENGTH, CARDIOVASCULAR, FLEXIBILITY

Long-term exercise training is important to overall health and physical fitness. A sound exercise training program leads to long-term physiological changes (adaptation), particularly improvement in muscular strength and endurance, cardiovascular function, and musculoskeletal flexibility. These improvements allow one to enhance athletic performance, engage in physically active leisure-time pursuits more efficiently, perform daily activities more easily, and maintain functional independence later in life.

Resistance Training

Resistance training is an effective exercise mode to improve muscular strength and endurance. Strength improves when sufficient tension is applied to the muscle fiber and its contractile proteins. The tension required for strength gain is about 60%–80% of the muscle's maximum force (23). Fleck and Kraemer (23) recommended a range of 75%–90% of one repetition maximum contraction (1 RM) for optimizing strength gain. For improvement to take place, the resistance work against a muscle must be large

Overload is accomplished when a greater than normal physical demand is placed on the muscles.

enough to impose a demand on the body system. This is the so-called overload principle. Overload is accomplished when a greater than normal physical demand is placed on the muscles. The amount of overload required depends on the current level of muscular fitness. To enhance muscular fitness, the muscular system must be progressively overloaded (e.g., increased resistance, repetitions, sets). The adaptation to strength training includes increase in muscular size, a condition called "hypertrophy." Hypertrophy is one of the most prominent adaptations among all other physiological changes. Increased muscle size is generally attributed to hypertrophy of existing muscle fibers. It is thought to occur through remodeling of protein within the cell and an increase in the number of myofibrils.

Strength training also improves aerobic enzyme systems. Increases in aerobic enzyme activity are reported with isokinetic and isometric training in humans and with isometric training in rats (53). Moreover, increases in oxidative enzymes have been demonstrated to be higher in type IIA fibers than in type IIB fibers. The increase in oxidative metabolism of muscles after long-term strength training is also associated with increases in capillary supply and the concentration of cellular mitochondria. Capillaries per unit area and per fiber are significantly increased in response to varying types of heavy resistance training (such as a combination of concentric and eccentric resistance exercise). Increased capillary density may facilitate performance of low-intensity weight training by increasing blood supply to active muscle. It also increases the ability to remove lactate and thereby improves the ability to tolerate training under highly acidic condition. All of these changes promote oxygen delivery and use within the muscle fiber, thereby improving muscular endurance (34).

Part of the strength gain resulting from strength training is attributed to changes in the nervous system. This is especially true during the early stages of strength training. Training tends to reduce the neuromuscular inhibition in both the CNS and proprioceptors (Golgi tendon organs). Other neural factors include the increased neural drive to muscle, increased synchronization of motor units, and increased activation of the contractile apparatus.

Chronic Adaptations to Cardiovascular Exercise

Physical inactivity is now classified as a major contributing risk factor for heart disease, with an overall weight for preventive value similar to that of elevated blood cholesterol level, cigarette smoking,

> *Longitudinal studies have shown that higher levels of aerobic fitness are associated with lower mortality from heart disease even after statistical adjustments for age, coronary risk factors, and family history of heart disease (9).*

and hypertension (24). Moreover, longitudinal studies have shown that higher levels of aerobic fitness are associated with lower mortality from heart disease even after statistical adjustments for age, coronary risk factors, and family history of heart disease (9). These findings and other recent reports in persons with and without heart disease have confirmed an inverse association between aerobic capacity and cardiovascular mortality (8).

Endurance exercise training increases functional capacity and provides relief of symptoms in many clients with coronary artery disease (CAD). This is particularly important because most clients with clinically manifest CAD have a subnormal functional capacity (50%–70% age, gender-predicted), and some may be limited by symptoms at relatively low levels of exertion. Improvement in function appears to be mediated by increased central and/or peripheral oxygen transport and supply, whereas relief of angina pectoris may result from increased myocardial oxygen supply, decreased oxygen demand, or both.

Most exercise studies on healthy subjects demonstrate 20% ($\pm10\%$) increases in aerobic capacity ($\dot{V}O_{2max}$), with the greatest relative improvements among the most unfit (47). Because a fixed submaximal work rate has a relatively constant aerobic requirement, the physically trained individual works at a lower percentage of $\dot{V}O_{2max}$, with greater reserve after exercise training. Enhanced oxygen transport, particularly increased maximal SV and cardiac output, have traditionally been regarded as the primary mechanism underlying the increase in $\dot{V}O_{2max}$ with training.

The effects of long-term exercise training on the ANS act to reduce myocardial demands at rest and during exercise. Exercise bradycardia may be attributed to an intracardiac mechanism (an effect directly on the myocardium, for example, increased SV during submaximal work) or an extracardiac mechanism (e.g., alterations in trained skeletal muscle) or both. The result is a reduced HR and SBP at rest and at any fixed oxygen uptake or submaximal work rate.

The increased oxidative capacity of trained skeletal muscle appears to offer a distinct hemodynamic advantage. Lactic acid production and muscle blood flow are decreased at a fixed external workload, whereas submaximal $\dot{Q}$ and oxygen uptake are unchanged or slightly reduced. As a result, there are compensatory increases in a-$\bar{v}$ O_2 difference at submaximal and maximal exercise.

Cardiovascular Adaptations

OVERALL CHANGES

The HR response plays a critical role in the delivery of oxygen to working skeletal muscle. The resting HR decreases by approximately 10–15 bpm as a result of cardiovascular training (29). Stroke volume will increase both at rest and during exercise up to a point, as a result of long-term cardiovascular training. $\dot{Q}$ will increase during exercise but will not change significantly at rest in cardiovascularly trained individuals. The a-$\bar{v}$ O_2 difference increases with long-term cardiovascular training, particularly near-maximal exertion. Both resting SBP and DBP may decrease (if elevated consistently before starting regular cardiovascular training) with long-term cardiovascular training. Resting lactate levels remain relatively unchanged with long-term cardiovascular training (5). As a result of proper cardiovascular training, less lactic acid will be produced at submaximal workloads during exercise (48). For responses to aerobic conditioning in untrained individuals, see Table 5.1.

GENDER-SPECIFIC IMPROVEMENT

The salutary effects of chronic endurance training in men are well documented (Table 5.2). Numerous studies now provide ample data on $\dot{V}O_{2max}$, cardiovascular hemodynamics, body composition, and blood lipids as well as changes with physical conditioning of middle-aged and older women. The results demonstrate that women with and without CAD respond to aerobic training

TABLE 5.1	**PHYSIOLOGICAL RESPONSES TO AEROBIC CONDITIONING IN UNTRAINED INDIVIDUALS**	
Variable[a]	**Unit of Measure**	**Response**
$\dot{V}O_{2max}$	mL/kg/min	↑
Resting heart rate	beats/min	↓
Exercise heart rate (submax)	beats/min	↓
Maximum heart rate	beats/min	↔ (or slight ↓)
a-$\bar{v}$ O_2 difference	mL O_2/100 mL blood	↑
Maximum minute ventilation	L/min	↑
Stroke volume	mL/beat	↑
Cardiac output	L/min	↑
Blood volume (resting)	L	↑
Systolic blood pressure	mm Hg	↔ (or slight ↑)
Blood lactate	mL/100 mL blood	↑
Oxidative capacity of skeletal muscle	Multiple variables[b]	↑

[a]At maximum exercise unless otherwise specified.

[b]Represents increase in skeletal muscle mitochondrial number and size, capillary density, and/or oxidative enzymes.

↑, increase; ↓, decrease; ↔, no change.

TABLE 5.2	**BENEFITS OF INCREASING CARDIORESPIRATORY ACTIVITIES AND/OR IMPROVING CARDIORESPIRATORY FITNESS[a]**

Decreased fatigue in daily activities

Improved work, recreational, and sports performance

Improved cardiorespiratory function
  Increased maximal oxygen uptake
  Increased maximal cardiac output and stroke volume
  Increased capillary density in skeletal muscle
  Increased mitochondrial density
  Increased lactate threshold
  Lower heart rate and blood pressure at a fixed submaximal work rate
  Lower myocardial oxygen demand at a fixed submaximal work rate
  Lower minute ventilation at a fixed submaximal work rate

Decreased risk of the following:
  Mortality from all causes
  Coronary artery disease
  Cancer (colon, perhaps breast and prostate)
  Hypertension
  Non–insulin-dependent diabetes mellitus
  Osteoporosis
  Anxiety
  Depression

Improved blood lipid profile
  Decreased triglycerides
  Increased high-density lipoprotein cholesterol
  Decreased postprandial lipemia

Improved immune function

Improved glucose tolerance and insulin sensitivity

Improved body composition

Enhanced sense of well-being

[a]Many of the health benefits accrue from physical activities that may have relatively little effect on increasing cardiorespiratory fitness (2,8–10).

in much the same way as men when subjected to comparable programs in terms of frequency, intensity, and duration (1). Improvement is negatively correlated with age, habitual physical activity, and initial $\dot{V}O_{2max}$ (which is generally lower in women than in men) and positively correlated with conditioning frequency, intensity, and duration (27). There are, however, large differences between individuals in the effects of physical conditioning independent of age, initial capacity, or conditioning program. These individual variations in response to aerobic exercise training may result from childhood patterns of activity, state of conditioning at the initiation of the program, or degree of physiological aging. Body compositional differences in trainability may also play an important role with respect to the results of physical conditioning. Obese women demonstrate lower aerobic capacity (per kilogram body weight), altered cardiovascular hemodynamics, and elevated serum lipids than leaner women (28). This initial varied profile may serve to modify the outcome of an aerobic conditioning program with respect to the magnitude of quantitative change.

Flexibility

Flexibility is another important, yet often neglected, component of health-related physical fitness. The level of flexibility is greatly reduced with age and physical inactivity. Lower back problems have been associated with poor flexibility of the lower back and hamstring muscles and weak abdominal muscles. Flexibility training should be promoted to improve ROM and joint mobility. Enhanced flexibility may also improve performance in some sports, especially those requiring obvious flexibility components such as gymnastics and wrestling.

Lower back problems have been associated with poor flexibility of the lower back and hamstring muscles and weak abdominal muscles.

Following a flexibility enhancement program, both long- and short-term adaptations exist. Immediately following the completion of a stretching program, the muscle's core temperature is increased. There is an increase in the blood flow to the working muscles, which positively alters the body's blood distribution to cope with the increasing demands placed on the musculature. Consequently, the body's ability to deliver hemoglobin (hence oxygen) to the working muscle is enhanced. There is also an increase in the interactions of the muscle's actin and myosin filaments, which increases the speed and force of each muscular contraction, thereby improving performance. Relaxation of the antagonist muscles is promoted. This reduces the resistance to movement and decreases the risk of muscle and tendon injuries, such as in strains and sprains. As muscle tension is reduced, the body becomes more relaxed and coordinated. This in turn promotes increased joint movement and enhances ROM (20).

For long-term adaptation, the ROM of the joint is increased, resulting in a decrease in muscle soreness. Furthermore, an inverse relationship has been demonstrated between neuromuscular tension and musculotendon extendibility. Improving flexibility reduces the likelihood of strains, tears, and tightness that may result in muscular pain, spasm, and cramping. Flexibility training also lengthens the fascia, which supports and stabilizes the muscles, organs, and most body tissues. From the physiological standpoint, this flexibility-enhancing effect may be traced to an inhibition of the spinal cord neurons by the Golgi tendon organs following an overly aggressive short-term application of a given flexibility-enhancing modality.

SUMMARY

This chapter was designed to introduce the Personal Trainer to the discipline of exercise physiology. Many concepts are not discussed in this chapter for reasons of length, not because they are unimportant. Emphasis is placed on cardiovascular physiology, pulmonary physiology, and muscle function because that is what the Personal Trainer works with every day. However, endocrine function and other body functions are also important so it is suggested that as you come across new issues with your clients, you seek out additional references that can assist you in understanding the function of the human being under conditions of physical stress.

REFERENCES

1. Ades PA, Waldmann ML, Polk DM, et al. Referral patterns and exercise response in the rehabilitation of female coronary patients aged ≥62 years. *Am J Cardiol.* 1992;69:1422–5.

2. American College of Sports Medicine. *ACSM's Guidelines for Exercise Testing and Prescription.* 6th ed. Baltimore (MD): Lippincott Williams & Wilkins; 2000. p. 104.

3. American College of Sports Medicine. *ACSM's Resources Manual for Guidelines for Exercise Testing and Prescription.* 4th ed. Baltimore (MD): Williams and Wilkins; 2001.

4. Armstrong RB. Muscle fiber recruitment patterns and their metabolic correlates. In: Horton ES, Terjunk RL, editors. *Exercise, Nutrition and Energy Metabolism.* New York: Macmillan; 1988. p. 9–26.

5. Astrand PO, Rodahl K. *Textbook of Work Physiology: Physiological Bases of Exercise.* 4th ed. New York: McGraw-Hill; 1985.

6. Beck KC, Johnson BD. Pulmonary adaptations to dynamic exercise. In: Durstine JL, editor. *Resource Manual for Guidelines for Exercise Testing and Prescription.* 2nd ed. Baltimore (MD): Williams & Wilkins; 1993.

7. Berger AJ. Control of breathing. In: Murray JF, Nadel JA, editors. *Textbook of Respiratory Medicine.* Vol 1. 2nd ed. Philadelphia: WB Saunders; 1994. p. 199–218.

8. Blair SN, Kampert JB, Kohl HW III, et al. Influences of cardiorespiratory fitness and other precursors on cardiovascular disease and all-cause mortality in men and women. *JAMA.* 1996;276:205–10.

9. Blair SN, Kohl HW III, Paffenbarger RS, et al. Physical fitness and all-cause mortality: a prospective study of healthy men and women. *JAMA.* 1989;262:2395–401.

10. Brooke MH, Kaiser KK. Muscle fiber types: how many and what kind? *Arch Neurol.* 1970;23:369–79.

11. Burke F, Cerny F, Costill D, Fink W. Characteristics of skeletal muscle in competitive cyclists. *Med Sci Sports Exerc.* 1977;9:109–12.

12. Buskirk E, Taylor HL. Maximal oxygen intake and its relation to body composition, with special reference to chronic physical activity and obesity. *J Appl Physiol.* 1957;2:72–8.

13. Byrnes W. Muscle soreness following resistance exercise with and without eccentric contractions. *Res Q.* 1985;56:283.

14. Carola R, Harley JP, Noback CR. *Human Anatomy and Physiology.* New York: McGraw-Hill; 1990.

15. Coggan AR, Spina RJ, King DS, et al. Skeletal muscle adaptations to endurance training in 60- to 70-yr-old men and women. *J Appl Physiol.* 1992;72:1780–5.

16. Comess KA, Fenster PE. Clinical implications of the blood pressure response to exercise. *Cardiology.* 198168:233–44.

17. Coyle E, Feiring DC, Rotkis, TC. Specificity of power improvements through slow and fast isokinetic training. *J Appl Physiol.* 1981;51:1437.

18. Davis JA, Vodak P, Wilmore JH, et al. Anaerobic threshold and maximal aerobic power for three modes of exercise. *J Appl Physiol.* 1975;41:544–50.

19. Dehn MM, Mullins CB. Physiologic effects and importance of exercise in patients with coronary artery disease. *J Cardiovasc Med.* 1977;2:365–87.

20. de Swardt A. Flexibility for cross country. *Track Field Coaches Rev.* 1995;95(2):28–9.

21. DiNubile NA. Strength training. *Clin Sports Med.* 1991;10:33.

22. Faulkner J, Claflin D, McCully K. Power output of fast and slow fibers from human skeletal muscles. In: Jones N, McCartney N, McComas A, editors. *Human Muscle Power.* Champaign (IL): Human Kinetics; 1986. p. 81–90.

23. Fleck SJ, Kraemer WJ. *Designing Resistance Training Programs.* 2nd ed. Champaign (IL): Human Kinetics; 1997.

24. Fletcher GF, Balady G, Blair SN, et al. Statement on exercise: benefits and recommendations for physical activity programs for all Americans. *Circulation.* 1996;94:857–62.

25. Foss ML, Keteyian SJ. *Fox's Physiological Basis for Exercise and Sport.* 6th ed. Boston: WCB McGraw-Hill; 1998. p. 238.

26. Fox EL, Bowers RW, Foss ML. *The Physiological Basis of Physical Education and Athletics.* 4th ed. Dubuque (IA): WC Brown; 1989. p. 106–7.

27. Franklin BA, Bonzheim K, Berg T. Gender differences in rehabilitation. In: Julian DG, Wenger NK, editors. *Women and Heart Disease.* London: Martin Dunitz; 1997. p. 151–71.

28. Franklin B, Buskirk E, Hodgson J, et al. Effects of physical conditioning on cardiorespiratory function, body composition and serum lipids in relatively normal-weight and obese middle-aged women. *Int J Obes.* 1979;3:97–109.

29. Frick M, Elovainio R, Somer T. The mechanism of bradycardia evoked by physical training. *Cardiologia.* 1967;51:46–54.

30. Gaesser G, Brooks C. Metabolic bases of excess post-exercise oxygen consumption: a review. *Med Sci Sports Exerc.* 1984;16:29.

31. Gardner G. Specificity of strength changes of the exercised and nonexercised limb following isometric training. *Res Q.* 1963;34:98.

32. Graham T. Mechanisms of blood lactate increase during exercise. *Physiologist.* 1984;27:299.

33. Hall-Craggs ECB. *Anatomy as a Basis for Clinical Medicine.* Baltimore (MD): Williams & Wilkins, 1995.

34. Jackson C, Dickinson A. Adaptations of skeletal muscle to strength or endurance training. In: Grana W, Lombardo J, Sharkey B, Stone J, editors. *Advances in Sports Medicine and Fitness.* Chicago: Year Book Medical; 1988. p. 45–9.

35. Jacobs I, Esbjornsson M, Slyvan C, et al. Sprint training effects on muscle myoglobin, enzymes, fiber types, and blood lactate. *Med Sci Sports Exerc.* 1987;19:368–74.

36. Karvonen MJ, Kentala E, Mustala O. The effects of training on heart rate: a longitudinal study. *Ann Med Exp Biol Fenn.* 1957;35:307.

37. Knapik JJ, Mawdsley RH, Ramos NU. Angular specificity and test mode specificity of isometric and isokinetic strength training. *J Orthop Sports Phys Ther.* 1983;5:58.

38. Komi PV, Karlsson J. Skeletal muscle fiber types, enzyme activities and physical performance in young males and females. *Acta Physiol Scand.* 1978;103:210.

39. Light RW. *Pleural Diseases*. 2nd ed. Philadelphia: Lea & Febiger; 1990. p. 1–7.

40. Marieb EN. *Human Anatomy and Physiology*. 3rd ed. Redwood City (CA): Benjamin/Cummings; 1998.

41. McArdle WD, Katch FI, Katch VL. *Essentials of Exercise Physiology*. 2nd ed. Baltimore (MD): Lippincott Williams & Wilkins; 1999.

42. McArdle WD, Katch FI, Katch VL. *Exercise Physiology, Energy, Nutrition, and Human Performance*. 4th ed. Baltimore (MD): Williams & Wilkins; 1995.

43. Mitchell JH, Blomqvist G. Maximal oxygen uptake. *N Engl J Med*. 1971;284:1018–22.

44. Naughton J, Haider R. Methods of exercise testing. In: Naughton JP, Hellerstein HK, Mohler IC, editors. *Exercise Testing and Exercise Training in Coronary Heart Disease*. New York: Academic Press; 1973. p. 79.

45. Newsholme E. The control of fuel utilization by muscle during exercise and starvation. *Diabetes*. 1979;28(Suppl 1):1.

46. Noth J. Motor units. In: Komi PV, editor. *Strength and Power in Sport*. Oxford (UK): Blackwell Scientific; 1992. p. 21–8.

47. Pate RR, Pratt M, Blair SN, et al. Physical activity and public health: a recommendation from the Centers for Disease Control and Prevention and the American College of Sports Medicine. *JAMA*. 1995;273:402–7.

48. Rerych SK, Sholz PM, Sabiston DC, et al. Effects of exercise training on left ventricular function in normal subjects: a longitudinal study by radionuclide angiography. *Am J Cardiol*. 1980;45:244–52.

49. Robergs RA, Roberts SO. *Exercise Physiology: Exercise, Performance and Clinical Applications*. St. Louis (MO): Mosby-Yearbook; 1997.

50. Rowell IB. Circulation. *Med Sci Sports*. 1969;1:15–22.

51. Senior A. ATP synthesis by oxidative phosphorylation. *Physiol Rev*. 1988;68:177.

52. Stanish WD, Rubinovich RM, Curwin S. Eccentric exercise in chronic tendinitis. *Clin Orthop*. 1986;208:65.

53. Tesch PA. Short- and long-term histochemical and biochemical adaptations in muscle. In: Komi P, editor. *Strength and Power in Sports: The Encyclopaedia of Sports Medicine*. Oxford: Blackwell Scientific; 1992. p. 239–48.

54. Vrbova G. Influence of activity on some characteristic properties of slow and fast mammalian muscles. *Exerc Sport Sci Rev*. 1979;7:181–213.

55. Williams PL, Warwick R, Dyson M, Bannister LH, eds. *Gray's Anatomy*. 38th ed. London: Churchill Livingstone; 1995.

56. Zobi EG, Talmers FN, Christensen RC, et al. Effect of exercise on the cerebral circulation and metabolism. *J Appl Physiol*. 1965;20:1289–93.

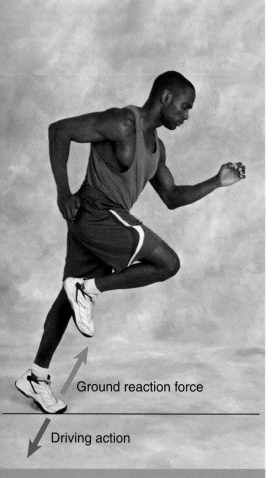

Ground reaction force

Driving action

CHAPTER 6

Nutrition and Human Performance

OBJECTIVES

- Understand the functions of the three energy substrates (carbohydrate, protein, and fat) in health and performance
- Know the interrelationships between vitamins and minerals in health and performance
- Understand the importance of hydration in maintaining health and achieving optimal performance
- Know the essential elements of energy balance as it relates to weight control, body composition, and performance
- Understand issues related to nutrient supplementation and strategies for discerning the circumstances under which specific supplements may be warranted
- Understand practical issues related to eating for performance, including eating on the road, the precompetition meal, during-competition nourishment, and postcompetition replenishment

Nutrition and athletic performance are closely linked, making it unlikely to experience success with a physical training program that has no parallel nutrition strategy. Personal Trainers who recommend the use of nutrition strategies for achieving an ideal weight or body composition without bearing in mind the impact this strategy could have on physical performance may be counterproductive and predispose clients to disease and injury.

An improvement in client conditioning cannot be realized by focusing only on time in the gym to improve flexibility, endurance, and/or power. The adjunct nutritional strategies clients should follow before arriving at the pool or gym, the foods and drinks they consume immediately following exercise and after they go home, and what they do to ensure an optimal flow of fluid and energy into their muscles are critical to improving power, sustaining concentration, and optimizing performance. Failure to consider nutrition as an integral component of the skills training and/or conditioning program will increase health risks and result in poor improvement rates. Well-nourished clients do better, recover more quickly from soreness and injuries, and derive more performance-improving benefits from long and strenuous training sessions. Unfortunately, Personal Trainers often fail to help clients match the dynamics of exercise with a supportive nutrition strategy.

Failure to consider nutrition as an integral component of the skills training and/or conditioning program will increase health risks and result in poor improvement rates.

A great deal of scientific information exists on the relationship between good nutrition and exercise performance, but the massive quantities of misinformation on nutrition makes it difficult for Personal Trainers to know when and what to eat before practice and competition; the foods that will best sustain energy levels; the best drinks and foods to consume before, during, and after exercise; how to balance an optimal energy intake with an ideal body composition; and how to make certain nutrient intake meets nutrient needs. These and other issues are covered in this chapter with the aim of helping the Personal Trainer to assist their clients in understanding the key nutritional strategies that are related to improving exercise performance.

SCOPE OF PRACTICE

Personal Trainers should be aware that, in most states, the profession of dietetics is regulated by law. The practice of dietetics is typically performed by a registered dietitian who has the academic degree and proper certifications or licenses to provide individual-specific meal plans or diet plans and to provide medical nutrition therapy for individuals suffering from specific diseases. The Personal Trainer must respect these professionals by always seeking out their assistance when governed by laws. Typically, Personal Trainers do not develop or provide meal/diet plans for clients, because this activity falls within the scope of practice for registered dietitians. However, Personal Trainers can, and should, recognize when it is appropriate to refer clients to a registered dietitian.

Typically, Personal Trainers do not develop or provide meal/diet plans for clients, because this activity falls within the scope of practice for registered dietitians.

Although laws typically have been written to protect the scope of practice for dietitians, the specific scope of practice for Personal Trainers regarding nutrition is not as clear. However, it appears that Personal Trainers can teach fundamentals of nutrition to clients (as outlined in this chapter) and also assist with a weight loss program that would include both diet and exercise (Fig. 6.1). Personal Trainers should also be aware of, and be able to recognize, patterns of disordered eating and make the appropriate referral to a healthcare practitioner who has the experience necessary to treat these conditions. Personal Trainers are urged to investigate any and all laws pertaining to the practice of dietetics in their local area.

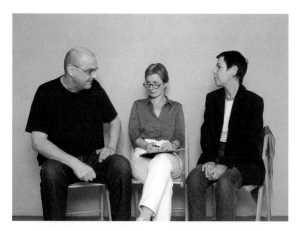

FIGURE 6.1. Scope of practice: professional trainer sitting at table with a client going over diet plan.

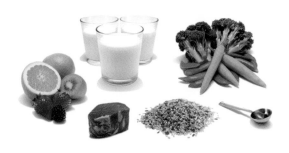

FIGURE 6.2. Nutrients that provide energy: oil, grains, legumes, meats, fruits, fruit juices, and vegetables.

ESSENTIAL NUTRITION CONCEPTS

Nutrients give metabolically active tissues, which include muscles, organs, and bones, the energy needed for work, tissue repair, and tissue development. Well-nourished clients are more likely to have better disease resistance and enhanced cardiovascular function, are more likely to grow normally and build needed muscle tissue, and will heal well if they are injured. For clients to be healthy and successful, they must consider nutritional needs as important as the skills training they may want to acquire.

Nutrients

There are six classes of nutrients: carbohydrates, proteins, fats, vitamins, minerals, and water. Clients should not think of any individual nutrient as more important than any other nutrient; rather, the focus should be on nutrient balance, which is critical to good health and performance. With your help, clients should try to find the appropriate balance between all the nutrients, because too much or too little of any single nutrient increases the risk of health and/or performance problems. For example, too little iron intake could lead to poor endurance and a lower ability to burn fat, whereas too much protein might increase urine production and increase the risk of dehydration. The best strategy for maintaining a nutrient balance is to eat a wide variety of foods, regularly consume fresh fruits and vegetables, and avoid a monotonous intake of the same few foods day after day (Fig. 6.2). Consumption

> *There are six classes of nutrients: carbohydrates, proteins, fats, vitamins, minerals, and water.*

of a wide variety of foods will ensure optimal nutrient exposure. No single food has all the nutrients a person needs to stay healthy, so eating a wide variety of foods helps people know that all the needed nutrients are available to them. An added benefit of eating a wide variety of foods is avoidance of potential nutrient toxicities that may result from an excess consumption of vitamins and/or minerals. Easily available and inexpensive nutrient supplements dramatically increase the possibility of nutrient toxicities. The common belief that "if a little bit of a nutrient is good, then more must be better" is wrong. Providing more nutrients than the body can use does not provide a benefit, and it forces cells into using valuable energy resources to excrete the surplus, with the additional risk of developing toxicity reactions.

There is a great deal of nutritional misinformation on television and in popular magazines, making it difficult for people to make the right nutritional decisions. Many of us often believe people (particularly celebrities) who sell nutritional supplements despite the lack of credible scientific evidence for what they're selling. Part of the problem is that the "placebo effect" is at play with nutrition (i.e., if you believe that something will work, it will actually work, even though there may be no biological reason for the result). Personal Trainers should ask for scientific evidence about whether nutritional products actually work, and when a claim is made, there should be immediate follow-up: "Show me the evidence." Scientific (peer-reviewed) journals are the best source of information. It should be clearly understood that one person's positive experience from taking a substance does not translate into a universal benefit. Claims that sound too good to be true probably are *not* true.

NUTRIENTS THAT PROVIDE ENERGY

Energy nutrients provide fuel for cellular work. Carbohydrates, proteins, and fats (Table 6.1) are considered energy nutrients because they all provide carbon (fuel) that can be "burned" for energy production. Energy nutrients allow us to do muscular work, transfer electrical energy between nerve cells, and help us maintain body temperature at 98.6°F (37°C). Energy is measured in calories, which in nutrition are often referred to as kilocalories (kcal) because they represent 1,000 times the calorie unit used in physics. In this chapter, the word "calories" is used synonymously with kilocalories (20).

Exercise causes an increase in the *rate* at which energy is burned. This process is not 100% efficient, so 40% or less of the burned energy is converted to mechanical energy whereas more than 60% of the energy is lost as heat. This extra heat causes body temperature to rise, which makes the body increase its sweat rate as a means of cooling down body temperature. Therefore, the two essential components of sports nutrition that Personal Trainers should focus on are:

1. Finding ways to provide enough extra energy at the right time to satisfy the needs of physical activity
2. Finding ways to provide enough fluid at the right time to maintain body water and replace the fluid that was lost as sweat

Meeting Energy Needs for Optimal Weight and Body Composition

The relationship between weight and caloric intake is relatively simple: If you eat more calories than you burn (expend), you will store the excess calories, and body weight will increase (Fig. 6.3). If you eat fewer calories than you burn, you will use some of your existing body tissues for needed energy, and body weight will drop. Consistently consuming too little energy will burn enough of your lean mass (muscles) that the *rate* at which you burn calories (called the "metabolic rate") will decrease. The end result of a lower metabolic rate is usually higher body weight (from more body fat) because you lose your ability to burn the calories you eat. Therefore, staying in an energy-balanced state or deviating from it only slightly is an important strategy for both body weight and body composition maintenance. Clients wishing to increase muscle mass should perform the exercises needed to enlarge muscle mass and

> *Consistently consuming too little energy will burn enough of your lean mass (muscles) that the **rate at which you burn calories (called the "metabolic rate")** will decrease.*

TABLE 6.1	IDEAL ENERGY (CALORIE) DISTRIBUTION FOR ATHLETES AND PHYSICALLY ACTIVE ADULTS
65% of total calories from carbohydrate or 6–10 gm carbohydrate/kg body weight	
15% of total calories from protein or 1.2–1.7 gm protein/kg body weight	
20%–35% of total calories	

Adapted from American College of Sports Medicine. Position statement: nutrition and athletic performance. *Med Sci Sports Exer.* 2000;32(12):2130–45 and American College of Sports Medicine. Position statement: nutrition and athletic performance. Med Sci Sports Exer. 2009;41(3):709–31.

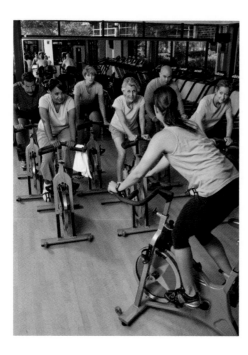

FIGURE 6.3. Meeting energy needs for optimal weight and body composition; fitness exercise class.

slightly increase (by 300–500 calories) daily caloric intake. Clients wishing to decrease body fat should make only subtle decreases (no more than 300–400 calories, depending on body size) in daily caloric intake while maintaining a vigorous conditioning schedule to maintain muscle mass.

For your athletic competitors, lower weight results in lower resistance, and all sports have resistance associated with them. Skaters must overcome the resistance of a skate blade going over the ice, cyclists must cope with air resistance, power lifters have the resistance from weights, and divers and gymnasts experience resistance as they tumble through the air. Sports performance is related to the ability of the athlete to overcome resistance (or drag) and the ability to sustain power output by overcoming this resistance on repeated bouts or long distances (16). Although these two factors (overcoming resistance and sustaining power output) are clearly related to performance, they are perceived by many athletes to be in conflict—a fact that causes many athletes problems with meeting energy needs. Athletes often view their ability to overcome resistance or drag with their ability to carry lots of muscle and relatively little fat. As fat mass does little to contribute to sports performance and may contribute to drag, this makes lots of sense. However, the *strategy* that athletes often use to reduce fat mass and maximize muscle mass is to diet by dramatically lowering total energy intake. This dieting strategy is counterproductive because it restricts the intake of energy that is needed to sustain power output.

Herein lies the dilemma: How can your clients maximize their ability to sustain power output while, at the same time, reducing body fat percentage? A number of studies suggest that the answer may lie in consuming small but frequent meals to stay in better energy balance throughout the day. Energy balance has typically been assessed in 24-hour units. That is, if you consume 3,000 calories during the day and you burn 3,000 calories during the day, you are in "energy balance." However, what happens *during* the day to achieve a state of energy balance makes a difference. If you spend most of the day in an energy-deficit state (i.e., you burned far more calories than you consumed) but then eat a huge meal at the end of the day to satisfy your energy needs, you might still be in energy balance at the end of the day. However, it appears that people who do this have different outcomes than those who maintain an energy-balanced state throughout the day. Eating small but frequent meals has the following benefits (10,12,14,15,17,18,21,27):

➤ Maintenance of metabolic rate
➤ Lower body fat and lower weight on higher caloric intakes

➤ Better glucose tolerance and lower insulin response (making it less likely that fats will be produced from the foods you eat)
➤ Lower stress hormone production
➤ Better maintenance of muscle mass
➤ Improved physical performance

Surveys have suggested that people (particularly athletes) tend to delay eating until the end of the day, and many experience severe energy deficits earlier in the day (particularly on days when they train hard and need the energy the most!). Problems with energy deficits include (6):

➤ Difficulty maintaining carbohydrate stores (this would impede endurance in high-intensity activities)
➤ Problems maintaining lean (muscle) mass
➤ Lower metabolic rate
➤ Difficulty meeting nutrient needs (foods carry both energy *and* other nutrients)
➤ Increased risk of injury (undernourished athletes may develop mental and muscular fatigue that, in some sports, would predispose them to injury)
➤ Missed opportunities to aid muscle recovery

Maintaining energy balance throughout the day by consuming small but frequent meals during the day is an excellent strategy for reducing these problems.

Maintaining energy balance throughout the day by consuming small but frequent meals *during* the day is an excellent strategy for reducing these problems.

Carbohydrate

The word **carbohydrate** is often referred to as if it is a single compound. In fact, carbohydrate comes in many different forms that have different nutritional outcomes. Some carbohydrates are digestible whereas others are not, some are considered "complex" whereas others are "simple," and some carbohydrates contain soluble fiber whereas others contain insoluble fiber (Fig. 6.4). The basic form of carbohydrate energy for human nutrition is the simple sugar glucose, and our bodies make a complex carbohydrate called glycogen, which is the storage form of glucose (Tables 6.2–6.4).

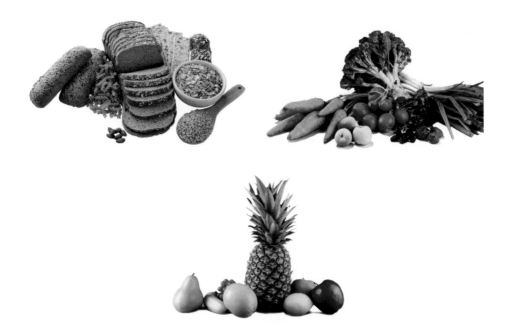

FIGURE 6.4. Carbohydrate foods—fruits, vegetables, grains (cereals, pasta, etc.), and potatoes.

TABLE 6.2	QUICK FACTS ABOUT CARBOHYDRATE
Minimum intake	50–100 g/day (200–400 calories) needed to avoid ketosis
Average U.S. intake	200–300 g/day (800–1200 calories)
Recommended fiber intake	20–30 g/day or more
Average U.S. fiber intake	10–15 g/day
Recommended intake of carbohydrate as percentage of total caloric intake	55% of total calories; up to 65% of total calories for athletes
Good sources of carbohydrate	Grains, legumes, seeds, pasta, fruits, vegetables

Carbohydrate Functions

➤ *Provide energy* (4 calories per gram). Carbohydrate is the preferred fuel for the body, and it is a quick energy source.

➤ *Protein sparing.* This is an often-overlooked, yet very important, function of carbohydrates. Because carbohydrate (glucose) is a preferred fuel, providing enough carbohydrate to meet most energy needs preserves (i.e., "spares") protein from being broken down and used as a source of energy.

➤ *Oxidation of fat.* It has been said that "fats burn in a carbohydrate flame." That is, to burn fats efficiently and completely, some carbohydrate is needed.

➤ *Part of other compounds.* Carbohydrates are essential components of other compounds essential in human nutrition.

➤ *Stored energy.* Carbohydrates have two storage forms: glycogen and fat. The ideal storage form for carbohydrate is glycogen because it can be easily converted back to glucose and used for energy.

TYPES OF CARBOHYDRATE

➤ *Simple carbohydrates (sugars).* These are sugars that include glucose, fructose (typically found in fruits and vegetables), galactose (one of the sugars in milk), sucrose (table sugar), lactose (milk sugar), and maltose (grain sugar).

➤ *Polysaccharides.* These are carbohydrates that contain many molecules of connected sugars. Polysaccharides can be digestible (starch, dextrins, and glycogen) or indigestible (cellulose, hemicellulose, pectin, gums, and mucilages). Dietary fiber is a carbohydrate that cannot be digested but is useful in the diet because it may lower fat and cholesterol absorption, improves blood sugar control, and may reduce the risk of colon cancer and heart disease.

Should the focus of your client's diet be carbohydrate, protein, or fat? Many studies show that *carbohydrates are the limiting energy substrate.* That is, when carbohydrates run out, people typically reach a point of exhaustion. For this reason, people should consume 55%–65% of total calories from

TABLE 6.3	SAMPLES OF GOOD HIGH-CARBOHYDRATE SNACKS	
Apple	Fruit cup	Orange juice
Bagel	Fruit smoothie	Popcorn
Baked corn chips	Energy bar	Rice
Baked potato	Grapes	Saltine crackers
Banana	Mashed potatoes	Spaghetti
Beans	Mixed berries	Whole-wheat toast
English muffin	Oatmeal	

TABLE 6.4	COMMON SOURCES OF FOODS HIGH IN CARBOHYDRATE	
Food	**Calories from Carbohydrate (%)**	**Total Calories**
Sugar (1 tbsp)	100	48
Pretzel sticks (10 small)	100	8
Maple syrup (1 tbsp)	100	64
Cranberry juice (1 cup)	100	152
Cola, regular (12 oz)	100	164
Apples (1 med)	100	84
Apricot juice (1 cup)	97	148
Sugar frosted flakes cereal (1 oz)	96	108
Raisins (1 cup)	94	489
Orange (1 raw)	94	64
Rice, white (1 cup)	93	216
Orange juice (1 cup)	93	112
Sweet potatoes (1 med)	93	120
Corn flakes cereal (1 oz)	92	104
Potato, baked (1 med)	91	224
Banana (1 raw)	89	121
Carrots (1 raw)	88	32
Potato, mashed with milk (1 cup)	86	173
Tomato sauce (1 cup)	86	84
Cantaloupe (1/2 melon)	84	105
Tomato (1 raw)	83	24
Green beans (1 cup)	83	48
Spaghetti (1 cup cooked)	82	157
Yogurt, low-fat fruit flavored (8 oz)	75	230
Bread, wheat (1 slice)	74	65
Bread, oatmeal (1 slice)	74	65
Beans (1 cup)	70	217
Broccoli (1 spear)	58	69

Adapted from USDA Nutrient Data Laboratory, Agricultural Research Service. *USDA National Nutrient Database for Standard Reference Release 17.* Washington, DC: Government Printing Office; 2004(13)

carbohydrates (1). However, because the body's storage capacity for carbohydrates is limited, carbohydrates should be provided throughout the day in small, frequent meals. A key reason for this is to sustain blood sugar, which is the primary fuel for the central nervous system (brain). If the brain receives insufficient glucose, mental fatigue will result, and mental fatigue leads to muscle fatigue. Blood sugar level reaches its peak approximately 1 hour after a meal and is back to premeal levels about 2 hours after that (2). This strongly suggests that meal frequency should be approximately every 3 hours to avoid the mental and muscle fatigue that could result from low blood sugar level. A person consuming a 3,000-calorie diet should consume between 1,650 and 1,950 calories from carbohydrates. Expressed another way, athletes should consume between 6 and 10 g of carbohydrate per kilogram of body weight. For a 75-kg (165-lb) person, that amounts to between 450 g (1,800 calories) to 750 g (3,000 calories) per day from carbohydrate alone.

Different activities have different carbohydrate requirements per unit of time. For instance, when walking at a brisk pace, 17% of the fuel comes from carbohydrate; when jogging at a medium pace, approximately 50% of the fuel comes from carbohydrate; and when running at a very fast pace, approximately 72% of the fuel comes from carbohydrate (23). However, because the length of time spent in these activities is usually much different (you can walk at a brisk pace much longer than you can run flat out), the **total** carbohydrate requirement may be similar when calculated over the total time invested in the activity.

> *By consuming a high-carbohydrate diet and carbohydrate-containing sports beverages, you can improve energy reserves and enhance performance of repeated bouts of high-intensity activity.*

A single 30-second bout of high-intensity activity could reduce muscle carbohydrate (glycogen) storage by more than 25%. By consuming a high-carbohydrate diet and carbohydrate-containing sports beverages, you can improve energy reserves and enhance performance of repeated bouts of high-intensity activity.

The Glycemic Index

The **Glycemic Index** is a measure of how different consumed carbohydrate foods affect the blood sugar level. Foods are compared with the ingestion of glucose, which has an index value of 100. It

> *It is generally believed that focusing on foods with a lower glycemic index helps maintain blood sugar, avoids an excessive insulin response that can encourage the production of fat, and keeps people feeling better longer.*

is generally believed that focusing on foods with a lower glycemic index helps maintain blood sugar, avoids an excessive insulin response that can encourage the production of fat, and keeps people feeling better longer. Although the glycemic index (Table 6.5) is a useful guide, you should be aware that different people have different responses to food. For instance,

TABLE 6.5 **GLYCEMIC INDEX OF SOME COMMON FOODS**		
High Glycemic Index (>85)	**Medium Glycemic Index (60–85)**	**Low Glycemic Index (<60)**
Glucose	All-bran cereal	Fructose
Sucrose	Banana	Apple
Maple syrup	Grapes	Applesauce
Corn syrup	Oatmeal	Cherries
Honey	Orange juice	Kidney beans
Bagel	Pasta	Navy beans
Candy	Rice	Chick-peas
Corn flakes	Whole grain rye bread	Lentils
Carrots	Yams	Dates
Crackers	Corn	Figs
Molasses	Baked beans	Peaches
Potatoes	Potato chips	Plums
Raisins		Ice cream
White bread		Milk
Whole wheat bread		Yogurt
Sodas (nondiet)		Tomato soup
Sports drinks		

Adapted from Rankin JW. *Glycemic Index and Exercise Metabolism.* Barrington (IL): Gatorade Sports Science Institute, Sports Science Exchange, Publication no. 64; 1997:10(1).

TABLE 6.6	QUICK FACTS FOR PROTEIN
Recommended intakes	Infants: 2.2 g/kg of body weight Children: 1.0–1.6 g/kg of body weight Adults: 0.8 g/kg of body weight Adult athletes: 1.2–1.7 g/kg of body weight (endurance athletes have a slightly higher requirement than strength athletes) (16)
Recommended intake of protein	12%–15% of total calories
Good sources of protein	Meat, poultry, fish, yogurt, eggs, milk; combinations of legumes (beans and dried peas) with cereal grains

people who exercise regularly are much more tolerant of foods with a high glycemic index than are people who rarely exercise (22). Young people must meet the combined energy needs of growth, exercise, and tissue maintenance and so will have a higher requirement for calories per unit of body weight (and therefore carbohydrate) than will adult athletes. Athletes interested in lowering either weight or body fat levels should consider focusing on foods with a medium to low glycemic index.

Protein

Proteins are complex compounds that are made of different connected amino acids, which uniquely contain nitrogen. Body proteins are constantly changing, with new proteins being made and old ones broken down. Growth hormone, androgen, insulin, and thyroid hormone are **anabolic** hormones (i.e., they cause new protein to be produced). Cortisone, hydrocortisone, and thyroxin are **catabolic** hormones (i.e., they cause the breakdown of proteins).

Despite the fact that the protein requirement for physically active people is about double that for nonathletes (Table 6.6), most athletes consume far more protein than they need. The nonathlete (average) adult requirement for protein is 0.8 g/kg of body weight, whereas the adult athlete requirement for protein ranges between 1.2 and 2.0 g/kg of body weight. An athlete who weighs 180 lb (about 82 kg) would require between 123 and 164 g of protein per day (19). At 4 calories per gram, this is between 492 and 656 calories from protein per day (Fig. 6.5). Most athletes far exceed this amount of protein just from the foods they consume. Consider that the protein in a hamburger, a chicken fillet sandwich, and one cup of milk combined provides more than half the total daily protein requirement for a 180-lb (82-kg) athlete (Table 6.7).

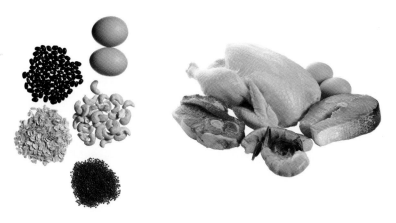

FIGURE 6.5. Protein foods—meats, poultry, dairy (cheese, milk, yogurt), and legumes.

TABLE 6.7	SAMPLE OF GOOD HIGH-PROTEIN SNACKS
Cheese	Tuna sandwich
Chicken	Hamburger
Cooked beef, lamb, or pork strips	Soy burger
Milk	Cottage cheese
Yogurt	Turkey sandwich

PROTEIN FUNCTIONS

➤ *Enzyme and protein synthesis.* There are hundreds of unique tissues and enzymes that are proteins.
➤ *Transports nutrients to the right places.* Proteins make "smart" carriers, enabling nutrients to go to the right tissues.
➤ *A source of energy.* The carbon in protein provides the same amount of energy per unit of weight as carbohydrates (4 calories per gram).
➤ *Hormone production.* Hormones control many chemical activities in the body, and these are made of unique proteins. For instance, testosterone (male hormone) is an important tissue-building hormone.
➤ *Fluid balance.* Protein helps control the fluid balance between the blood and surrounding tissues. This helps people maintain blood volume and sweat rates during physical activity.
➤ *Acid–base balance.* Proteins can make an acidic environment less acidic and an alkaline environment less alkaline. High-intensity activity can increase cellular acidity (through lactate buildup), which protein can help buffer.
➤ *Growth and tissue maintenance.* Protein is needed to build and maintain tissue. This is one reason why the protein requirement for growing children can be double that of adults and slightly higher for athletes (26).
➤ *Synthesis of nonprotein, nitrogen-containing compounds.* Phosphocreatine is a high-energy, nitrogen-containing compound that can quickly release energy over a short duration for quick-burst activities (Box 6.1).

PROTEIN QUALITY

Protein quality is determined by the presence (or absence) of essential amino acids. It is "essential" that we receive these amino acids from food because we are not capable of manufacturing them. Examples of foods containing protein with all the essential amino acids include meats, eggs, milk, cheese, and fish. Nonessential amino acids can be manufactured (synthesized), so it is not "essential" that we consume foods that contain them. Most foods contain both nonessential and essential amino acids, but it is the presence of a comprehensive set of essential amino acids that makes a high-quality protein.

> *Most foods contain both nonessential and essential amino acids, but it is the presence of a comprehensive set of essential amino acids that makes a high-quality protein.*

BOX 6.1	**Supplementation with Creatine Monohydrate**

Research has shown that creatine monohydrate supplementation may improve performance in repeated high-intensity activities, particularly in athletes with marginal caloric intakes. **However, creatine monohydrate supplementation has never been tested for safety. Until those tests are done, it should not be recommended to your clients.** A safer strategy would be to ensure that people have adequate caloric and protein intakes.

TABLE 6.8	COMMON SOURCES OF FOODS HIGH IN PROTEIN	
Food	Calories from Protein (%)	Total Calories
Tuna, canned in water (3 oz)	93	129
Shrimp, canned (3 oz)	87	97
Chicken, roasted, breast (3 oz)	80	185
Turkey, roasted light meat (3 oz)	79	127
Crab meat, canned (1 cup)	75	123
Chicken, roasted, drumstick (1.6 oz)	73	66
Clams, raw (3 oz)	72	61
Salmon, baked (3 oz)	65	129
Turkey, roasted dark meat (3 oz)	64	150
Beef steak, broiled (5 oz)	62	284
Halibut, broiled, with butter (3 oz)	60	134
Lamb, leg, roasted, lean (2.6 oz)	60	134
Salmon, canned (3 oz)	60	113
Pork, roasted (5 oz)	53	304
Cheese, cheddar (1 oz)	26	109
Peanut butter (1 tbsp)	19	104

People frequently take protein supplements, but these often contain proteins with an incomplete set of essential amino acids, making the supplements low in quality. The best protein supplement would be a few pieces of steak or fish or an egg. Vegetarians can ensure optimal protein quality by combining cereal grains (rice, wheat, oats) with legumes (dried beans or peas). Vegetarians are clearly more at risk for inadequate protein intake because the best source of high-quality protein is foods of animal origin (i.e., meat and fish). However, with some good dietary planning, vegetarians can consume enough high-quality protein.

Protein is the focus of many diets (Table 6.8), but there is a tendency to consume too much of it. Studies have found that people do best with protein intakes that supply approximately 15% of total calories or between 1.2 and 2.0 g of protein per kilogram of body weight. For a 75-kg (165-lb) person, that amounts to no more than 150 g (600 calories) of protein per day (26). Studies have shown that athletes often have protein intakes of 3 or more grams of protein per kilogram of body weight per day (19). It is possible that the perceived benefit from this much protein is actually a caloric rather than a protein benefit. That is, we must supply sufficient fuel to perform adequately, and the extra consumed protein may be helping people meet their *fuel* needs rather than their *protein* needs.

Although protein isn't the best fuel for physical activity, it is a fuel that can help satisfy energy needs if other fuels (i.e., carbohydrate and fat) are inadequate. There is no question that energy needs must be satisfied before you can consider the best way to distribute carbohydrate, protein, and fat.

Fat

Many people hold the mistaken belief that higher fat intakes can enhance athletic performance. The generally accepted healthy limit for fat intake is no more than 35% of total daily calories (Fig. 6.6). For someone consuming 2,500 calories per day, this amounts to 750 calories per day as fat (about 83 g of fat). Although this is considered the accepted healthy limit, people typically will do better with fat intakes that are no higher than 25% of daily calories. This level of intake will provide more room in the diet for needed carbohydrates (Tables 6.9 and 6.10).

The generally accepted healthy limit for fat intake is no more than 30% of total daily calories.

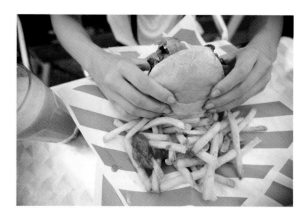

FIGURE 6.6. Fat foods—oil, butter, margarine, bacon, and fried foods.

FAT FUNCTIONS

➤ *Fat is a source of energy.* Fat provides 9 calories per gram (compared with 4 calories per gram from both carbohydrates and proteins).

➤ *Fat provides insulation from extreme temperatures.*

➤ *Cushion against concussive forces.* Fat protects organs against sudden concussive forces, such as a fall or a solid "hit" in football.

➤ *Satiety control.* Fat, because it stays in the stomach longer than other energy nutrients, makes us feel fuller longer.

➤ *Fat gives our food flavor.*

➤ *Fat carries essential nutrients.* Make sure that your clients get the necessary fat-soluble vitamins (A, D, E, and K) and essential fatty acids, which are found in vegetable and cereal oils.

FAT CLASSIFICATIONS AND DEFINITIONS

➤ *Fats and oils.* Fats are solid at room temperature and usually contain a high proportion of saturated fatty acids; oils are liquid at room temperature and typically (there are notable exceptions) contain a high proportion of unsaturated fatty acids.

➤ *Triglycerides, diglycerides, and monoglycerides.* Triglycerides are the most common form of dietary fats and oils, whereas diglycerides and monoglycerides are less prevalent but still commonly present in the food supply.

➤ *Short-chain, medium-chain, and long-chain fatty acids.* The most common dietary fatty acids are long-chain, containing 14 or more carbon atoms. Medium–chain triglycerides (MCT oil) have received some attention recently as an effective supplement for increasing caloric intake in athletes. Although MCT oil may hold some promise in this area, it has not been adequately tested.

TABLE 6.9	QUICK FACTS FOR FATS
Recommended intakes	Fat intake should provide between 20% and 35% of total calories
Essential fatty acid	Linoleic acid (and α-linoleic acid) is the essential fatty acid and must be provided in consumed foods; this fatty acid is found in corn, sunflower, peanut, and soy oils
Carrier of vitamins	Fat is the carrier of the fat-soluble vitamins: vitamins A, D, E, and K
Calorie-dense nutrient	Fats provide more than twice the calories, per equal weight, of carbohydrate and protein (9 calories vs. 4 calories per gram)
Cholesterol–fat relationship	High fat intakes (not just high cholesterol intakes) result in higher circulating blood cholesterol levels
Food sources	Oil, butter, margarine, fatty meats, fried foods, prepared meats (sausage, bacon, salami), and "whole-milk" dairy products

TABLE 6.10	FAT AND CALORIE CONTENT OF COMMON FOODS	
Food	Calories from Fat (%)	Total Calories
Butter (1 tbsp)	100	99
Margarine (1 tbsp)	100	99
Mayonnaise (1 tbsp)	100	99
Corn oil (1 tbsp)	100	126
Vegetable shortening (1 tbsp)	100	117
Olive oil (1 tbsp)	100	126
Blue cheese salad dressing (1 tbsp)	90	80
Cream cheese (1 oz)	88	102
1000 island salad dressing (1 tbsp)	87	62
Sour cream (1 tbsp)	87	31
Sausage, brown & serve (1 link)	85	53
Brazil nuts (1 oz)	84	203
Hazelnuts (1 cup)	83	780
Hotdog (1)	83	141
Cream, half & half (1 tbsp)	82	22
Bologna (2 slices)	80	180
Coconut, raw, shredded (1 cup)	80	303
Almonds, whole (1 oz)	74	183
Cheddar cheese (1 oz)	74	109
Feta cheese (1 oz)	73	74
Blue cheese (1 oz)	72	100
Avocado (1 whole)	65	371
Donuts, plain (1)	50	216
Milk, whole (1 cup)	49	148
Chicken, fried breast (1 breast)	46	354
Milk, 2% (1 cup)	36	125
Milk, 1% (1 cup)	25	107

➤ *Polyunsaturated fatty acids.* These fatty acids have a tendency to lower blood cholesterol level. The good thing about these fats is that they are typically associated with lots of vitamin E (found in vegetable and cereal oil, such as corn oil), which many people need.

➤ *Monounsaturated fatty acids.* These fatty acids tend to lower blood cholesterol level, while maintaining high-density lipoprotein (good) cholesterol (found in olive oil and canola oil).

➤ *Saturated fatty acids.* These fatty acids tend to increase serum cholesterol (found in meats and dairy products).

➤ *Low-density lipoproteins.* This is the major carrier of cholesterol and other lipids in the blood.

➤ *High-density lipoproteins.* These lipoproteins carry lipids away from storage and to the liver for metabolism and/or excretion. Because they are associated with removal of cholesterol, they are considered "good cholesterol."

For a 75-kg (165-lb) person consuming a 3,000-calorie diet, approximately 600–750 calories would come from fat if fat contributed about 25% of total calories. Because fats provide 9 calories per gram, this amounts to between approximately 65 and 85 g of fat per day. There has been a great deal of attention given to high-fat, high-protein, low-carbohydrate diets recently, but there is no evidence that these diets are useful for enhancing athletic performance. Cheuvront (8) described **The Zone** as a low-carbohydrate diet (in both relative and absolute terms). For instance, a male marathoner weighing 64 kg with 7.5% body fat would, following The Zone, have a 1,734-calorie intake, whereas his predicted caloric requirement is more than 3,200 calories. This is a calorically deficient diet by any standard. It is, therefore, quite true that people on The Zone would lose weight because it is an energy-deficient intake. However, your clients must meet energy requirements to sustain power output, so any severely energy-deficient diet, such as The Zone (whether it is high fat, high protein, or high carbohydrate), is not recommended for optimizing athletic performance.

Vitamins and Minerals

Vitamins are substances that help essential body reactions take place. The best strategy to make certain that an adequate amount of all the vitamins is consumed is to eat a wide variety of foods and consume plenty of fresh fruits and vegetables daily. Some vitamins are water soluble, whereas others are fat soluble. See Tables 6.11 through 6.13 for a summary of major vitamins and minerals. Remember that nutrient balance is a key to optimal nutrition, so

> *The best strategy to make certain that an adequate amount of all the vitamins is consumed is to eat a wide variety of foods and consume plenty of fresh fruits and vegetables daily.*

TABLE 6.11   WATER-SOLUBLE VITAMINS

Vitamin and Adult Requirement	Functions	Deficiency/Toxicity	Food Sources
Vitamin C (also called L-ascorbate) 75–90 mg/day	• Antioxidant • Collagen formation • Iron absorption • Carnitine synthesis • Norepinephrine synthesis **Athletic performance: conflicting study results; as antioxidant, may be useful in alleviating muscle soreness and in aiding muscle recovery**	Deficiency: scurvy, bleeding gums, fatigue, muscle pain, easy bruising, depression, sudden death	Fresh fruits and vegetables, particularly high in citrus fruits and cherries
Thiamin (also called vitamin B_1) 1.1–1.2 mg/day	• Oxidation of carbohydrates • Nerve conduction **Athletic performance: conflicting study results**	Deficiency: beriberi (heart disease, weight loss, neurological failure)	Seeds, legumes, pork, and enriched/ fortified grains and cereals
Riboflavin (also called vitamin B_2) 1.1–1.3 mg/day	• Oxidation of carbohydrates and fats • Normal eye function • Healthy skin **Athletic performance: low-level supplement may be desirable for athletes involved in low-intensity, high-endurance sports**	Deficiency: swollen tongue, sensitivity to light, cracked lips, fatigue	Milk, liver, and whole and enriched grains and cereals
Niacin 14–16 mg/day	• Oxidation of carbohydrates and fats • Electron transport (energy reactions) **Athletic performance: conflicting study results**	Deficiency: pellagra (diarrhea, dermatitis, dementia)	Amino acid tryptophan (60:1 conversion ratio), and enriched grains and cereals

TABLE 6.12 FAT-SOLUBLE VITAMINS

Vitamin and Adult Requirement	Functions	Deficiency/Toxicity	Food Sources
Vitamin A (retinol) ~1,000 retinol equivalents 700–900 mg/day (This vitamin is potentially highly toxic taken in large amounts)	• Vision • Growth • Reproduction • Immune function • Healthy skin **Athletic performance: no evidence that supplementation aids performance**	Deficiency: night blindness, eye disease, growth failure, unhealthy skin, susceptibility to infections Toxicity: headache, vomiting, hair loss, bone abnormalities, liver damage, death	Fish liver oils, liver, butter, vitamin A + D-added milk, egg yolk Pro-vitamin A (β-carotene) in dark-green leafy vegetables yellow vegetables and fruits, and fortified margarines
Vitamin D (ergocalciferol and cholecalciferol) Requirement difficult to establish because of variations in sunlight exposure 5 mg/day (This vitamin is extremely toxic taken in high amounts)	• Calcium absorption • Phosphorus absorption • Mineralization of bone **Athletic performance: no studies**	Deficiency: rickets in children, osteomalacia in adults, poor bone mineralization Toxicity (this is the most toxic of the vitamins): renal damage, cardiovascular damage, high blood calcium, calcium deposits in soft tissues	Fish liver oils, fortified (A & D) milk, skin synthesis with exposure to light; small amounts found in butter, liver, egg yolk, and canned salmon and sardines
Vitamin E (α-tocopherol) 15 mg/day	• Powerful antioxidant • Involved in immune function **Athletic performance: antioxidant properties may be useful in preventing oxidative damage**	Deficiency: premature breakdown of red blood cells, anemia in infants, easy peroxidative damage of cells	Vegetable oils, green leafy vegetables, nuts, legumes (foods of animal origin are *not* good sources) and/or in muscle recovery
Vitamin K (phylloquinone K$_1$, menaquinone, menadione) 90–120 mg/day	Involved in blood clotting (referred to as the antihemorrhagic vitamin) **Athletic performance: athletes taking Erythropoietin (EPO) could be at serious risk taking vitamin K supplements**	Deficiency: longer clotting time	Green leafy vegetables and intestinal bacterial synthesis

Adapted from Manore M, Thompson J. *Sports Nutrition for Health and Performance*. Champaign (IL): Human Kinetics; 2000; Williams MH. *Nutrition for Health, Fitness & Sport*. 6th ed. Boston: McGraw-Hill; 2002; and Benardot D. *Nutrition for Serious Athletes: An Advanced Guide to Foods, Fluids, and Supplements for Training and Performance*. Champaign (IL): Human Kinetics; 2000.

people should avoid single-nutrient supplementation unless this has been specifically recommended by a physician to treat an existing nutrient deficiency disease. If a nutrient supplement is warranted because of an obviously poor-quality food intake, people should try a multivitamin, multimineral supplement that provides no more than 100% of the Dietary Reference Intakes (DRI) for each nutrient. The scientific literature suggests that vitamin and mineral deficiencies are uncommon for most people. When deficiencies exist, they are most likely for vitamin B$_6$ and other B-complex vitamins, iron, and calcium, especially when caloric intake is too low to meet energy demands (5).

WATER-SOLUBLE VITAMINS

Water-soluble vitamins, including vitamins B and C, are vitamins for which we have limited storage capacity. These vitamins are typically associated with carbohydrate foods, such as fresh fruits,

TABLE 6.13	MINERALS		
Minerals and Adult Requirement	**Functions**	**Deficiency/Toxicity**	**Food Sources**
Calcium 1,000 mg/day	• Structure of bones and teeth • Blood coagulation • Nerve impulse transmission • Muscle contraction • Acid–base control **Athletic performance: Particularly critical in athletes to ensure adequate bone density to reduce the risk of stress fractures**	Deficiency: Reduced bone density, osteoporosis, stress fractures	Milk and other dairy foods, dark green leafy vegetables, canned fish (with bones), calcium-fortified orange juice
Phosphorus 700 mg/day	• Structure of bones and teeth • Component of adenosine triphosphate (ATP) and other energy-yielding compounds • Part of many vitamin B coenzymes • Part of DNA and RNA • Acid–base control	Deficiency (rare) may occur with large, long-term intakes of magnesium-containing antacids	Meats, cereals, grains, and dairy products
Iron 700 mg/day	• Involved in oxygen transfer to cells (hemoglobin in blood; myoglobin in muscle) • In numerous oxidative enzymes **Athletic performance: Commonly inadequate in athletes, resulting in poor performance and other health problems**	Deficiency: microcytic anemia, leading to weakness, loss of energy, easy fatigue (this is the most common mineral deficiency)	Most absorbable iron: meats, poultry, fish, egg yolk Less absorbable iron: dark-green vegetables, legumes, peaches, apricots, prunes, raisins
Zinc 8–11 mg/day	• Immune system • Wound healing • In more than 70 enzymes involved in energy metabolism	Deficiency: Growth retardation, poor wound healing, frequent infections, muscle weakness	Seafood, organ meat, meat, wheat germ, yeast (most plant foods are not good sources)
Magnesium 320–420 mg/day	• Energy metabolism of carbohydrate and fat • Protein synthesis • Water balance • Muscle contractions	Deficiency: Muscle weakness	Available in many foods, but highest in meats, whole-grain cereals, seeds, and legumes

Adapted from Manore M, Thompson J. *Sports Nutrition for Health and Performance.* Champaign (IL): Human Kinetics; 2000; Williams MH. *Nutrition for Health, Fitness & Sport.* 6th ed. Boston: McGraw-Hill; 2002; and Benardot D. *Nutrition for Serious Athletes: An Advanced Guide to Foods, Fluids, and Supplements for Training and Performance.* Champaign (IL): Human Kinetics; 2000.

breads and cereals, and vegetables. The B vitamins are needed for the metabolism of carbohydrates, proteins, and fats and so are critical to the higher energy requirements of athletes. Luckily, good-quality foods that are high in carbohydrates are typically also foods that provide B vitamins (e.g., enriched breads, enriched cereals, and pasta) (4).

Vitamin C is a water-soluble vitamin that is often the focus of supplements taken by most people. Although vitamin C is critical to good health, people should be reminded that the DRI for vitamin C is only 75–90 mg and that level is 2 standard deviations above the average human requirement. Most supplements contain between 250 and 500 mg of vitamin C or more, providing a good deal more than is needed. On top of the vitamin C intake from foods, which is typically well above the DRI for this vitamin, you can see how easy it is for people to get too much. Although the potential toxicity of vitamin C is relatively low, even an excess of this relatively nontoxic vitamin can increase the risk of kidney stones. People should be encouraged to have a balanced exposure to all the vitamins, a strategy that will help encourage good health and avoid problems associated with excess intake and deficiencies.

FAT-SOLUBLE VITAMINS

Fat-soluble vitamins are those vitamins that are delivered with fats and oils. For instance, milk is fortified with the fat-soluble vitamins A and D, which are in the fat component (cream) of the milk. Vegetable and cereal oils are excellent sources of vitamin E, an important antioxidant that can help protect cells from becoming damaged through oxidation. This is important because physical activity increases the amount of oxygen pulled into cells, thereby increasing the risk for oxidative damage.

Supplements of vitamins A and D should be taken only under the advice of a physician because of their high potential toxicity. Other vitamins such as vitamin B_6 have also been shown to produce toxicity if taken in excess. As a general rule, it is generally better to derive vitamins through the consumption of a wide variety of foods rather than supplements, as supplementation may more easily result in toxicity and may also give individuals the wrong impression that a good quality diet is unnecessary because supplements are consumed.

Minerals

Minerals are inorganic substances that are involved in water balance, nerve impulse stimulation, acid–base balance, and energy reactions (see Table 6.13). Iron and zinc are critically important for energy metabolism but are also among the nutrients of which people may not be consuming enough. This is particularly true of vegetarians, because the best source of these minerals is red meat.

The most common nutrient deficiency in most industrialized countries is a deficiency in iron. Because of the prevalence of this deficiency, people (especially females) should periodically have a blood test to determine iron status. This test should include an assessment of hemoglobin, hematocrit, and ferritin. An assessment of iron status is particularly important for vegetarians or people who are on weight loss diets.

The most common nutrient deficiency in most industrialized countries is a deficiency in iron.

Fluid and Hydration

Water carries nutrients to cells and carries waste products away from cells. It serves as a body lubricant and, through sweat, helps maintain body temperature. Lean tissue (muscles and organs) is more than 70% water, and about 60% of total body weight is water (26). A failure to supply sufficient water is more likely to cause quick death than a failure to supply any other single nutrient.

We lose water through breathing (breath is moist), the skin (this happens even if there is no obvious "sweat"), and urine, sweat, and feces. It is critically important to consume sufficient fluid to maintain body water stores, yet most people rarely stay optimally hydrated (Fig. 6.7). In fact, many people commonly wait until they become extremely thirsty (indicating a state of dehydration) before they consume fluids. Weight stability before and after exercise is a good indication that water needs have been met during an exercise program. People who experience significant weight (i.e., water) loss during practice should learn how to drink more fluid to stabilize weight, because a 2% body weight loss is associated with reduced performance.

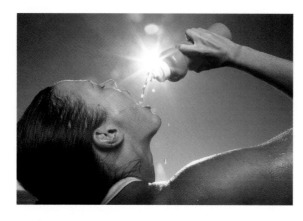

FIGURE 6.7. Fluid and hydration—athlete sweating profusely drinking beverage.

MEETING FLUID NEEDS

A key to athletic success is *avoidance* of a state of underhydration. This is not as easy as it may seem, because many people rely on "thirst" as the alarm bell for when to drink. Thirst, however, is a delayed sensation that does not occur until the person has already lost 1 to 2 liters of fluid. Because of this, people should learn to consume fluids on a fixed time interval rather than relying on thirst for when to drink. Staying optimally hydrated and fueled during exercise has multiple benefits, including (19):

> *People should learn to consume fluids on a fixed time interval rather than relying on thirst for when to drink.*

- A less pronounced increase in heart rate
- A less pronounced increase in core body temperature
- Improvement in cardiac stroke volume and cardiac output
- Improvement in skin blood flow (enabling better sweat rates and improved cooling)
- Maintenance of better blood volume
- A reduction in net muscle glycogen usage (improving endurance)

Fluid intake recommendations are to (1,13):

- Drink as much as needed to match sweat losses
- Not rely on thirst as a stimulus to drink (the thirst sensation will occur only after 1 to 2 liters—1%–2% of body weight—has already been lost)
- Sweat rates are often 1 to 2 liters per hour, and it is difficult to consume and absorb enough fluid to match these losses
- Consumption of large volumes of fluid increases the risk of gastrointestinal distress, thereby affecting performance
- Ingestion of large volumes of dilute, low- (or no-) sodium fluid may increase the risk of hyponatremia
- If left on their own, athletes will often develop dehydration even when there are sufficient fluids nearby for them to consume
- To ensure better athlete compliance, fluids should be cool, should taste good, and should be readily available

FLUID CONSUMPTION GUIDELINES

The National Athletic Trainers' Association guidelines (7) are useful for avoiding dehydration, but the type of fluids consumed is also important for achieving optimal performance. In general, studies have shown that a 6% carbohydrate solution, such as that found in some sports beverages, is ideal from the standpoint of gastric emptying and intestinal absorption for reducing mental and physical fatigue during both stop-and-go sports and endurance sports, for encouraging drinking during physical activity, and for improving performance. Studies comparing a 6% carbohydrate solution

TABLE 6.14	WARNING SIGNS OF DEHYDRATION, HEAT EXHAUSTION, AND HEAT STROKE: WHAT TO DO?
Dehydration with loss of energy and performance	Drink carbohydrate- and electrolyte-containing sports drinks; avoid beverages with carbonation, which can cause gastrointestinal distress
Dehydration with muscle cramps	Immediately stop exercising and massage the cramping muscle(s); consuming a sports beverage that contains sodium may help relieve the cramp
Heat exhaustion with dizziness, light-headedness, and cold, clammy skin	Immediately replace fluids while in a cool, shaded area until the dizziness passes; stretching may improve circulation and prevent fainting; lying with the legs elevated will improve blood circulation to the head, thereby alleviating the dizziness
Heat exhaustion with nausea/headaches	Rest in a cool place until the nausea passes; drinking fluids to rehydrate is critical; lying down may help relieve headaches
Heat stroke with high body temperature and dry skin	Immediately get out of the heat and seek immediate medical treatment; feeling chilly with arms tingling and with goose bumps means skin circulation has shut down and heat stroke is imminent; this is an extremely serious condition that must be immediately treated
Heat stroke with confusion or unconsciousness	Confusion strongly suggests, and unconsciousness confirms, heat stroke. This is a medical emergency that calls for fast cooling with ice baths or any other available means to lower body temperature

Adapted from Casa DJ, Armstrong LE, Hillman SK, et al. National Athletic Trainers' Association position statement: fluid replacement for athletes. *J Athl Train.* 2000;35(2):212–24.

with water and solutions with a higher carbohydrate concentration have consistently found that the 6% carbohydrate solution is best (1).

WATER VERSUS SPORTS DRINKS

There are clear advantages for sports drinks over water for most exercising adults (7):

➤ Water provides no flavor or electrolytes, which cause people to want to drink. Beverages that cause people to *want* to drink help them stay well hydrated. Studies show that people drink 25% more sports drink than water, and young children will drink 90% more sports beverage than water (3,11).

➤ Water has no energy whereas sports beverages contain carbohydrate. The carbohydrate helps provide muscles with needed fuel to avoid early fatigue and poor performance.

➤ The sodium provided by sports beverages helps maintain blood volume, a factor that is critical to maintaining sweat rates and performance. Sweat contains sodium that water alone does not replace (Table 6.14).

Dietary Supplements and Ergogenic Aids

Dietary supplements are concentrated sources of vitamins, minerals, and energy substrates that are taken to "supplement" the nutrients derived from foods. Ergogenic aids are substances that enhance a person's athletic ability, through either improvement in power or enhanced endurance. The terms dietary supplements and ergogenic aids often are used interchangeably, but they are not the same (Fig. 6.8).

Ergogenic aids are substances that enhance a person's athletic ability, through either improvement in power or enhanced endurance.

Dietary supplements may be used to conveniently intervene in a known dietary deficiency, whereas ergogenic aids are often taken for the sole purpose of improved performance whether or not there is a known deficiency. It is common, for instance, for people with iron deficiency anemia to be prescribed iron supplements to help them complement the

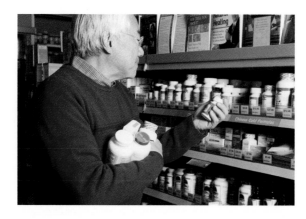

FIGURE 6.8. Dietary supplements and ergogenic aids.

iron they are getting from the food they eat and build up their iron stores. The proven effectiveness for many nutritional supplements, in the face of a nutrient deficiency disorder, has been demonstrated in numerous clinical trials. However, there is no evidence that it is useful or warranted to take high doses of dietary supplements in the absence of a known nutrient deficiency. An example of the overuse of dietary supplements is protein and/or amino acids (the building blocks of protein). In fact, excess nutrients may cause toxicity or, at the very least, create the need to expel the excess nutrients. People wishing to take a nutrient supplement without the diagnosis of a specific nutrient deficiency should limit their intake to multivitamin, multimineral supplements that provide no more than 100% of the recommended daily allowances.

Ergogenic aids, on the other hand, have typically not been tested for either effectiveness or safety. There are two ergogenic aids that have been clearly shown to improve a person's capacity to perform better: carbohydrates and water. With the exception of these, there is little consistent evidence to suggest that other substances touted as having an "ergogenic benefit" actually do anything to improve performance (Table 6.15). When ergogenic aids do work, it is usually because they help meet energy or nutritional requirements as a result of poor eating behaviors. It is clearly healthier and less costly to eat better foods than to rely on substances that are often of unknown origin and unknown quality and untested for safety or effectiveness.

PRACTICAL CONSIDERATIONS

One Day before a Competition

Although athletes often focus on the food consumed immediately before competition, it is actually important to start preparing in advance. Suggested considerations for the day prior to competition include the following:

➤ Avoid high-fat foods such as fried food, chips, cake, and chocolate
➤ Eat a good breakfast (e.g., toast, oatmeal, cereal, milk, and fruit)
➤ Have sandwiches, rolls, pasta, or rice for lunch (Fig. 6.9)
➤ Have rice, pasta, noodles, or potatoes plus vegetables and lean meat, chicken, or fish for dinner and yogurt and fruit for dessert
➤ Eat a carbohydrate snack at dinner
➤ Drink an extra 16 oz (475 mL) of fluid throughout the day

Immediately before Exercise or Competition

The preexercise meal should focus on providing carbohydrates and fluids. Ideally, people should consume a high-carbohydrate, low-fat meal 3 hours before exercising or competition. Light-carbohydrate snacks (e.g., crackers) and carbohydrate-containing beverages can be consumed after the meal and

TABLE 6.15	SAMPLES OF PRODUCTS COMMONLY SOLD AS ERGOGENIC AIDS
Supplement	**Facts**
Androstenedione	Advertised as useful for increasing muscular strength and size. It is a hormone that is used to synthesize the hormone testosterone. (Testosterone is a male anabolic steroid hormone that is known to aid in the development of muscle mass.) There may be negative side effects (increased body hair and cancer are established problems) similar to those of testosterone, but studies on efficacy and safety have not been published. This substance is banned by the IOC, IPC, NCAA, USOC, NFL, and NHL.
Caffeine	Advertised as useful for improving endurance by enabling more effective fat metabolism during exercise. It is a central nervous system stimulant but has a reduced dose effect (people adapt to it, so increasingly higher doses are needed to obtain an ergogenic benefit). In high doses, caffeine may have a diuretic effect, thereby increasing the chance for dehydration. Although in the past caffeine was on the banned substance list by the IOC, it was removed from this list early in 2004.
Creatine	Creatine is synthesized from three amino acids and is part of phosphocreatine, which is a fuel used anaerobically to initiate high-intensity activity. However, stored phosphocreatine suffices to support activity for only several seconds and must be resynthesized for use in similar subsequent activities. It is hypothesized that supplemental creatine aids in this resynthesis, and some studies have shown that creatine supplementation is effective in maintaining strength/power for repeated bouts of short-duration, high-intensity activities. However, creatine supplementation is associated with weight increases (from muscle or water or both), and studies have not evaluated its effectiveness in athletes who are known to be consuming sufficient energy. In addition, the safety of creatine supplementation has not been adequately studied.
Ephedrine	This is a central nervous stimulant that is sold over the counter as a decongestant. Its use is banned by the NCAA and the IOC, and it has undesirable side effects when taken in frequent and/or large doses. (The Food and Drug Administration recommends a maximum of no more than 8 mg/dose provided three times daily for a maximum of 7 days when used as a decongestant.) The side effects associated with ephedrine include increased heart rate, increased blood pressure, and nervousness, all of which are associated with strokes, seizures, and heart attacks. Caffeine consumption appears to increase the effect of ephedrine. It is theorized that ephedrine improves athletic performance and reduces body weight. Its chemical similarity to amphetamine suggests that it may lower appetite and thus have an impact on weight, but there is no evidence that it improves athletic performance.
Ginseng	There are numerous claims for ginseng, ranging from a cure for all ills to improving energy to enhancing immune function. However, it has been difficult to do athletic performance studies with ginseng because concentrations of the active ingredient(s) vary widely within and between brands. Therefore, there is no good evidence to support supplemental ginseng as an ergogenic substance. Luckily, it also appears that ginseng consumption has little risk of producing negative side effects, with the possible exception of causing insomnia in some subjects.
L-Carnitine	This is a substance produced by the body and used to transport fat into cell mitochondria so it can be used as energy. It is theorized that taking carnitine supplements will increase the amount of fat that is moved into mitochondria, thereby increasing the total amount of fat burned and helping reduce body fat levels. There is no solid evidence that supplementary carnitine has this effect.

(continued)

TABLE 6.15	SAMPLES OF PRODUCTS COMMONLY SOLD AS ERGOGENIC AIDS (*Continued*)
Medium-chain triglycerides (MCT oil)	MCT oil is sold as a substance that can improve muscular development and increase the loss of body fat by increasing metabolic rate. Although there is no evidence of these effects, MCT oil may be an effective means of increasing total caloric intake in athletes with high-energy requirements who are having difficulty meeting energy needs. It is metabolized more like a carbohydrate than a fat but has a higher energy density than carbohydrates. Large intakes may be associated with gastrointestinal disturbances.
Omega-3 fatty acids (fish oils, canola oils)	It is hypothesized that omega-3 fatty acids stimulate the production of growth hormone (somatotrophin), thereby enhancing the potential for muscular development. It is well established that omega-3 fatty acids reduce red-cell stickiness, thereby reducing the chance for a blood clot leading to a heart attack. Omega-3 fatty acids are also associated with a reduced inflammatory response in tissues through the production of specific prostaglandins. One of these prostaglandins (E1) may be associated with the production of growth hormone. Although supplemental intake of omega-3 fatty acids may not be warranted, there is sufficient evidence of some beneficial effects that athletes should consider consuming cold-water fish (salmon, tuna) twice weekly.
Pyruvic acid (pyruvate)	Pyruvate is produced from carbohydrates as a result of anaerobic metabolism and is a principal fuel leading into aerobic metabolism. It has been hypothesized, therefore, that supplemental pyruvate will enhance aerobic metabolism and promote fat loss. However, because carbohydrate intake adequately satisfies the entire need for pyruvate, it makes little sense that supplementation of pyruvate will improve performance.

Adapted from Manore M, Thompson J. *Sports Nutrition for Health and Performance*. Champaign (IL): Human Kinetics; 2000; Williams MH. *Nutrition for Health, Fitness & Sport*. 6th ed. Boston: McGraw-Hill; 2002; and Benardot D. *Nutrition for Serious Athletes: An Advanced Guide to Foods, Fluids, and Supplements for Training and Performance*. Champaign (IL): Human Kinetics; 2000.

IPC, International Paralympic Committee; IOC, International Olympic Committee; NCAA, National Collegiate Athletic Association; USOC, United States Olympic Committee; NFL, National Footbal League; NHL, National Hockey League.

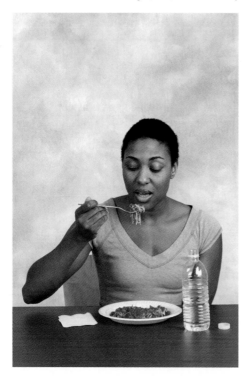

FIGURE 6.9. One day before a competition, an athlete eating pasta (should be relatively small portion).

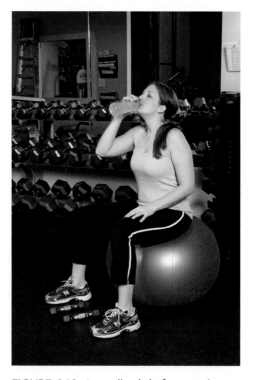

FIGURE 6.10. Immediately before exercise or competition, an athlete sipping on sports beverage.

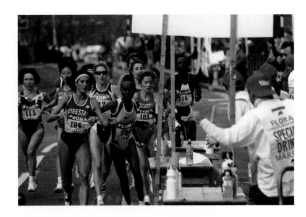

FIGURE 6.11. During exercise or competition, an athlete grabbing drink at fluid station during race (marathon).

before exercise, provided that large amounts are not consumed at one time (Fig. 6.10). There are several goals for the preexercise meal, including (4):

➤ Making certain that athletes obtain sufficient energy to see them through as much of the exercise bout as possible
➤ Preventing feelings of hunger (hungry people may be letting blood sugar get low, which is not a good way to start an exercise bout)
➤ Consuming enough fluids to begin exercise in a fully hydrated state
➤ Consuming only familiar foods
➤ Avoiding foods high in fiber or foods that cause gas (e.g., broccoli, cauliflower)
➤ Drinking 5-7 mL/kg body weight (2–3 mL/lb) of water or sports beverage at least 4 hours before practice or competition
➤ Drinking an additional 7–10 oz (200–300 mL) of fluid 10 to 20 minutes before practice or competition

During Exercise or Competition

There is evidence that people involved in stop-and-go sports of relatively short duration benefit from consumption of carbohydrate-containing drinks (see fluid consumption guidelines). For long-duration activities that allow for consumption of solid foods (e.g., cycling, cross-country skiing), some people prefer to periodically consume bananas, breads, and other easy-to-digest carbohydrate foods. If solid foods are consumed, there should still be ample consumption of carbohydrate-containing beverages (Fig. 6.11). Drink 28–40 oz of fluid (sports beverages containing a 6%–7% carbohydrate solution and electrolytes are preferred) per hour. This corresponds to about 7–10 oz (200–300 mL) every 10–15 minutes, but this amount may need to be adjusted on the basis of body size, sweat rate, exercise intensity, and environmental conditions (Box 6.2). Two main goals are to avoid dehydration and to avoid the mental and muscular fatigue that can be caused by inadequate carbohydrate (4).

After Exercise or Competition

Muscles are receptive to replacing stored glycogen following exercise. Because of this, people should consume 200–400 calories from carbohydrates immediately following activity and then an additional

---

BOX **6.2**	**Practical Suggestion for Assessing Fluid Intake During Exercise**

Weigh an athlete before and after exercise. If the weight difference is more than 1 lb (0.45 kg), the person did not consume enough fluid during exercise to maintain an optimal hydration state. Approximately 20 oz (600 mL) of fluid should be consumed for each pound (0.45 kg) of body weight lost during exercise.

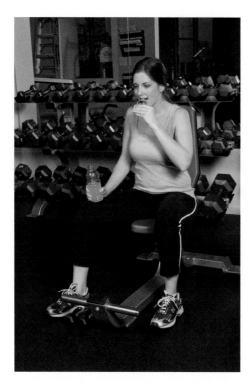

FIGURE 6.12. After exercise or competition, an athlete eating energy bar with bottle of fluid in hand.

200–300 calories from carbohydrates within the next several hours (Fig. 6.12). People who have difficulty eating foods immediately following exhaustive exercise should try high-carbohydrate liquid supplements (4). Some examples of high-carbohydrate foods are included in Table 6.16.

After exercise, people should drink at least 20 oz (600 mL) of fluid per pound of body weight that was lost during the exercise session (25). This should be consumed within 2 hours of finishing the practice or competition, with the goal of returning body weight to near preexercise weight before the next exercise bout.

Eating on the Road

Although it may take a little more effort to maintain a proper diet while traveling, it is well worth the effort.

Although it may take a little more effort to maintain a proper diet while traveling, it is well worth the effort. These suggestions should help your clients maintain a diet that will keep up their level. Try the

TABLE 6.16	EXAMPLES OF HIGH-CARBOHYDRATE FOODS	
Food	Calories	Carbohydrate (%)
1 bagel	165	76
2 slices of bread	135	81
1 Gatorade energy bar	250	75
1 cup of plain pasta	215	81
3 cups of popcorn	70	79
1 baked potato	100	88
1 apple	80	100
1 orange	65	100
1 cup of vegetable juice	55	93

following strategies recommended by the Department of Nutritional Sciences, Cooperative Extension, of the University of Arizona (9).

> **Try to pack nutrient-dense foods for the trip.** Many foods can be packed easily in a gymnastic bag or suitcase. By bringing your own food, you can eat familiar foods. This is especially important when traveling to a foreign country, where familiar foods may be harder to find. Foods such as sports bars, dried fruits, granola bars, bagels, and canned tuna are nutrient dense and travel easily.
>
> **Upon arriving at your destination, make a trip to the local store to pick up some essentials.** Picking up some basic foods can allow some meals to be eaten in the hotel, especially if there is a microwave and refrigerator available. Some of these items may include fresh fruits and vegetables, applesauce, cheese, breads, and soups.
>
> **If eating in hotel rooms or packing foods is an impossibility, it is still possible to eat for performance at restaurants.** Most restaurants have lower-fat items from which to choose. In some cases, finding these lower-fat items may take some detective work, but in other instances the restaurant may have some healthier items already indicated on the menu. In either case, it is important to know what to look for. The following are some general guidelines.

BREAKFAST

➤ Order pancakes, French toast, muffins, toast, cereal, fruit, and juices. These are all higher in carbohydrate and lower in fat than traditional egg and bacon breakfasts.

➤ Request that toast, pancakes, etc., be served without butter or margarine. Use syrup or jam but no butter or margarine to keep carbohydrate high and fat to a minimum.

➤ Choose low-fat dairy products (e.g., skim or 1% milk, low-fat yogurt, low-fat cheese).

➤ Fresh fruit may be expensive or difficult to find. Carry fresh and/or dried fruits.

➤ Cold cereal can be a good breakfast or snack; carry boxes in the car or on the bus. Keep low-fat milk in cooler or purchase at convenience stores.

LUNCH

➤ On sandwiches, look for lower-fat meats such as turkey and chicken. Remember that most of the fat in sandwiches is found in the spread. Prepare or order without the "mayo," "special sauce," or butter. Use ketchup or mustard instead.

➤ Choose foods that are broiled, baked, microwaved, steamed, or boiled rather than fried, and try to avoid breaded items. Salad bars can be lifesavers, but watch the dressing, olives, fried croutons, nuts, and seeds—you could end up with more fat than any super-burger could hope to hold!

➤ Choose low-fat salad dressings. If low-fat dressings aren't available, pack your own.

➤ Baked potatoes should be ordered with butter and sauces "on the side." Add just enough to moisten the carbohydrate-rich potato.

➤ Soups and crackers can be good low-fat meals; stay away from cream soups.

➤ Juices, low-fat milk, and low-fat milk shakes are a more nutritious choice than soda pop.

DINNER

➤ Go to restaurants that offer high-carbohydrate foods such as pasta, baked potatoes, rice, breads, vegetables, salad bars, and fruits.

➤ Eat thick crust pizzas with low-fat toppings such as green peppers, mushrooms, Canadian bacon, and onions. Avoid fatty meats such as pepperoni or sausage, extra cheese, and olives.

➤ Eat breads without butter or margarine—use jelly instead. Ask for salads with dressing "on the side" so that you can add minimal amounts yourself. Ask for low-fat salad dressings.

SNACKS

Whole-grain breads, muffins, bagels, tortillas, fruit, fruit breads, low-fat crackers, pretzels, unbuttered popcorn, oatmeal raisin cookies, fig bars, animal crackers, fruit juice, carrot sticks, cherry tomatoes, breakfast cereal, canned liquid meals, and dried and fresh fruits

DON'T FORGET ABOUT FLUIDS

To prevent dehydration, you should keep well hydrated at all times, even on the road, by drinking frequently before, during, and after exercise.

➤ Do not drown your thirst in calories! Drink plenty of water.
➤ In restaurants, including fast food ones, ask for water in addition to other beverages. Request that a pitcher of water be left at your table.
➤ You can buy bottled water or mineral water at grocery stores and convenience stores.
➤ Carry squeeze bottles of water, sports drinks, and fruit juices with you, especially on long airplane flights.
➤ Limit caffeinated or alcoholic beverages. Caffeine and alcohol are diuretics and cause fluid loss.

UNDERSTANDING A FOOD LABEL (FROM THE US FOOD AND DRUG ADMINISTRATION, CENTER FOR FOOD SAFETY AND APPLIED NUTRITION)

Each food label contains basic information on food components that have the potential of being bad for you, such as total fat, saturated fat, cholesterol, and sodium, and also has information on nutrients that people generally need more of, such as dietary fiber, vitamin C, calcium, and iron.

Food labels can help you understand the nutritional content of a food by serving size. Each food label contains basic information on food components that have the potential of being bad for you, such as total fat, saturated fat, cholesterol, and sodium, and also has information on nutrients that people generally need more of, such as dietary fiber, vitamin C, calcium, and iron.

Serving Size

The serving size listed is different for each type of food to make it easier for people to understand. A typical serving size is in familiar serving size units, such as cups or pieces, and also includes the weight of the serving size in grams. In the example given here for Macaroni and Cheese (Fig. 6.13), the serving size is 1 cup, which for this food has a weight of 228 g. You can also see that the label indicates that there are two servings (i.e., 2 cups) in the container.

Calories

The unit of measure for energy in a food is "calories," and the total calories provided by a single serving (i.e., 1 cup) of this food is 250. Because it is unhealthy for humans to chronically consume more than 30% of total calories from fat, the food label also indicates the calories from fat provided by one serving of food, which in this case is 110 calories. You wouldn't make a decision to eat or avoid a food based on this value, but by helping you understand if the food is relatively low or high in fat, you can make logical decisions about the other foods you consume.

% Daily Value

Each of the nutrients on a label has a recommended "Daily Value" (DV). A DV of 100% represents the recommended upper limit for total fat, saturated fat, cholesterol, and sodium, whereas 100% of

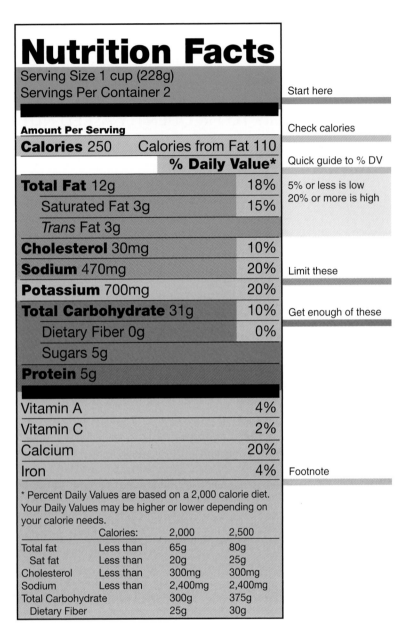

Nutrition Facts

Serving Size 1 cup (228g)
Servings Per Container 2

Amount Per Serving

Calories 250   Calories from Fat 110

% Daily Value*

Total Fat 12g	18%
Saturated Fat 3g	15%
Trans Fat 3g	
Cholesterol 30mg	10%
Sodium 470mg	20%
Potassium 700mg	20%
Total Carbohydrate 31g	10%
Dietary Fiber 0g	0%
Sugars 5g	
Protein 5g	
Vitamin A	4%
Vitamin C	2%
Calcium	20%
Iron	4%

* Percent Daily Values are based on a 2,000 calorie diet. Your Daily Values may be higher or lower depending on your calorie needs.

	Calories:	2,000	2,500
Total fat	Less than	65g	80g
Sat fat	Less than	20g	25g
Cholesterol	Less than	300mg	300mg
Sodium	Less than	2,400mg	2,400mg
Total Carbohydrate		300g	375g
Dietary Fiber		25g	30g

Start here

Check calories

Quick guide to % DV

5% or less is low
20% or more is high

Limit these

Get enough of these

Footnote

FIGURE 6.13. The food label (for more information on how to read a food label, visit the following Web sites: www.cfsan.fda.gov/~dms/foodlab.html or www.health.gov/dietaryguidelines/dga2005/healthieryou/html/tips_food_label.html)

total carbohydrate and dietary fiber represents the recommended minimum intake. However, please note that the DV is based on percentage of a nutrient that would be delivered with a 2,000-calorie diet. Many people, particularly those who are physically active, consume diets that are much higher than 2,000 calories. Therefore, the % DV must be considered in the context of the total calories consumed. Typically, 5% DV or less is considered low and 20% DV or more is considered high. Using the label in Figure 6.1, you can determine that consuming 1 cup (i.e., one serving) of macaroni and cheese would provide you with 18% of the DV for fat, which is OK. However, if you were to consume the entire package content, which has two servings, your % DV would be 36%, which is considered high for a single food. Put simply, a 36% DV for fat means that the other foods you planned on consuming on the same day should be much lower in fat so you can meet your goal of not exceeding a % DV of 100% for fat. The easiest way for you to use the % DV is to compare foods that are similar, so you can see which foods have the lowest fat content or the highest nutrient content.

You can use the % DV to determine the relative content of the nutrients listed on the label. The same rules would apply, but in this case you would like to have foods that are relatively high (i.e., a

% DV of 20 or better) in nutrient concentration. For food substances that do not have a % DV, such as trans fats and sugar, use the label to compare similar products when making a purchasing decision for similar products. In general, you should try to avoid foods that contain trans fats, and limit the intake of sugars.

ANSWERS TO FREQUENTLY ASKED NUTRITIONAL QUESTIONS

Should I Take Protein Supplements?

Protein supplements are popular in most sports, at most athletic levels—from beginners to elite athletes and regardless of the goals of the people taking them. Some people take protein supplements to lose weight, some to gain weight, some to gain muscle, some to make them stronger, and some to increase endurance. The fact is that humans are incapable of using protein for anabolic (tissue-building) purposes above the level of approximately 1.5 g of protein per kilogram of body weight. Protein taken in excess of this amount is either burned as a source of energy (calories) or stored as fat. Neither of the latter two options is particularly good, because people rarely wish to put on additional fat weight, and getting rid of excess nitrogenous waste can make you dehydrated.

What About Creatine?

Creatine monohydrate supplements have been shown to help maintain power on repeated bouts of high-intensity activity. However, this benefit may be as a result of an inadequate caloric intake in the tested subjects. As creatine monohydrate use has never been tested for safety (there is beginning evidence that taking supplements may alter the body's synthesis of creatine), it makes sense to avoid taking creatine but begin making certain that energy (calorie) consumption matches need. A good strategy for doing this is to eat small, frequent meals high in carbohydrates.

Should I Consume Sports Drinks or Does Water Work Just As Well?

Sports drinks contain carbohydrate and electrolytes that are useful in maintaining water and energy balance. Studies of endurance athletes, athletes in stop-and-go sports, and athletes in power sports all show that consumption of sports drinks during practice and competition does a better job of enhancing athletic performance than water alone.

Should I Stay Away from Caffeinated Beverages before a Workout?

People adapt to caffeine, so if you are accustomed to having a cup of coffee or a caffeine-containing cola, there should be no problem with consuming it before a workout. You should never increase the consumption of a caffeinated food or beverage before exercise above a level to which you are accustomed. This would likely increase your heart rate and have a diuretic effect that could make you dehydrated.

Should I Skip Lunch If I'm Trying to Lower My Body Fat Level?

Skipping meals is one of the biggest reasons people have high body fat levels. If you are trying to lose body fat, your goal should be to maintain blood sugar levels through the consumption of small, frequent meals. Skipping a meal will cause you to produce excess insulin the next time you eat, which will make *more* fat than if you ate more frequently.

Will a High-Protein, Low-Carbohydrate Diet Help Me Lose Weight?

There is nothing in the literature to suggest that lowering carbohydrate intake is useful for improving exercise performance. On the contrary, inadequate carbohydrate intake is almost always associated with reduced performance. High-protein, low-carbohydrate diets are typically low-calorie diets—the reason for the weight loss. However, dramatic reductions in caloric intake almost always result in a rebounding of weight. The best strategy for weight loss is to consume a little less than is currently needed to maintain current weight (say, about 300 calories less) and to eat small, frequent meals to maintain blood sugar levels.

Should I Eat or Drink Anything during Exercise?

Maintaining a constant flow of carbohydrates to muscles and maintaining blood sugar during competition is an important strategy for success. Your clients should consider sipping on a sports beverage during competition to achieve this result. If there are long breaks during an exercise workout, then consuming a carbohydrate snack (e.g., crackers, bread) might be acceptable provided that fluid is also consumed.

I'm a Profuse Sweater and Occasionally Get Serious Cramps. Is There Anything I Should Be Doing to Avoid This Problem?

Cramps are typically associated with dehydration and sodium loss. Try making certain that sufficient sodium-containing fluids (i.e., sports beverages) are consumed during practice and competition. Unless you have a history of high blood pressure, you should also consider adding a small amount of salt to the food you eat, following with plenty of water.

How Can I Tell If I'm Dehydrated?

The easiest way to tell is that your urine will be dark, and there won't be very much of it. Light-colored or clear urine is a sign of adequate hydration, whereas dark urine suggests dehydration. It takes time to rehydrate, so avoiding dehydration is the appropriate strategy.

SUMMARY

This important chapter on nutrition is not intended to establish the Personal Trainer as a nutritionist or dietitian. There are laws in most states and around the world that protect this important discipline. It was intended, rather, to make the Personal Trainer aware of certain nutrition-related questions that may come up in a typical training session. The Personal Trainer should be aware of the extent of information that can be distributed to clients and when it might be necessary to refer the client to a licensed dietitian. Both disciplines are encouraged to work together when a client has nutrition-related questions and is in need of a special diet for a medical condition or for a balanced weight loss program. Equally important is for the dietitian to understand the scope of practice for Personal Trainers. A team approach with the Personal Trainer prescribing exercise and the dietitian prescribing nutritional strategies is the recommended method to treating a client with nutrition issues.

REFERENCES

1. American College of Sports Medicine. Position statement: nutrition and athletic performance. *Med Sci Sports Exerc.* 2000;32(12):2130–45.
2. American Diabetes Association. Postprandial blood glucose. *Diabetes Care.* 2001;24(4):775–8.
3. Bar-Or O, Wilk B. Water and electrolyte replenishment in the exercising child. *Int J Sport Nutr.* 1996;6(2):93–9.
4. Benardot D. *Nutrition for Serious Athletes: An Advanced Guide to Foods, Fluids, and Supplements for Training and Performance.* Champaign (IL): Human Kinetics; 2000.
5. Benardot D, Clarkson P, Coleman E, Manore M. *Can Vitamin Supplements Improve Sports Performance?* Barrington (IL): Gatorade Sports Science Institute, Sports Science Exchange Roundtable, Publication no. 45; 2001:12(3).
6. Benardot D, Martin DE, Thompson WR. Maintaining energy balance: a key for effective physical conditioning. *Am J Med Sports.* 2002;4(1):25–30, 40.

7. Casa DJ, Armstrong LE, Hillman SK, et al. National Athletic Trainers' Association position statement: fluid replacement for athletes. *J Athl Train.* 2000;35(2):212–24.

8. Cheuvront SN. The "Zone" diet and athletic performance. *Sports Med.* 1999;27:213–28.

9. Department of Nutritional Sciences, Cooperative Extension, The University of Arizona. *Eating on the Road* [Internet]. 2002. [cited 2002 Dec]. Available from: http://ag.arizona.edu/nsc/new/sn/HP-eatonrd.htm

10. Deutz B, Benardot D, Martin D, Cody M. Relationship between energy deficits and body composition in elite female gymnasts and runners. *Med Sci Sports Exerc.* 2000;32(3):659–68.

11. Gatorade Sports Science Institute. Fluids 2000: *Sports Drinks vs. Water.* Barrington (IL): Sports Science Center Topics; 2000.

12. Hawley JA, Burke LM. Meal frequency and physical performance. *Br J Nutr.* 1997;77:S91–103.

13. Horswill CA. Effective fluid replacement. *Int J Sports Nutr.* 1998;8:175–95.

14. Iwao S, Mori K, Sato Y. Effects of meal frequency on body composition during weight control in boxers. *Scand J Med Sci Sports.* 1996;6(5):265–72.

15. Jenkins DJ, Wolever TM, Vuksan V, et al. Nibbling versus gorging: metabolic advantages of increased meal frequency. *N Engl J Med.* 1989;321:929–34.

16. Lamb DR. *Basic Principles for Improving Sport Performance.* Barrington (IL): Gatorade Sports Science Institute, Sports Science Exchange, Publication no. 55; 1995:8(2).

17. LeBlanc J, Mercier I, Nadeau A. Components of postprandial thermogenesis in relation to meal frequency in humans. *Can J Physiol Pharmacol.* 1993;71(12):879–83.

18. Luke A, Schoeller DA. Basal metabolic rate, fat-free mass, and body cell mass during energy restriction. *Metabolism.* 1992;41(4):450–6.

19. Manore M, Thompson J. *Sports Nutrition for Health and Performance.* Champaign (IL): Human Kinetics; 2000.

20. McArdle W, Katch F, Katch V. *Sports & Exercise Nutrition.* Philadelphia: Lippincott Williams & Wilkins; 1999.

21. Metzner HL, Lamphiear DE, Wheeler NC, Larkin FA. The relationship between frequency of eating and adiposity in adult men and women in the Tecumseh Community Health Study. *Am J Clin Nutr.* 1977;30:712–15.

22. Rankin JW. *Glycemic Index and Exercise Metabolism.* Barrington (IL): Gatorade Sports Science Institute, Sports Science Exchange, Publication no. 64; 1997:10(1).

23. Romijn JA, Coyle EF, Sidossis LS, et al. Regulation of endogenous fat and carbohydrate metabolism in relation to exercise intensity and duration. *Am J Physiol.* 1993;265(3):E380–91.

24. USDA Nutrient Data Laboratory, Agricultural Research Service. *USDA National Nutrient Database for Standard Reference Release 17.* Washington, DC: Government Printing Office; 2004.

25. Wilk B, Bar-Or O. Effect of drink flavor and NaCl on voluntary drinking and hydration in boys exercising in the heat. *J Appl Physiol.* 1996;80:1112–17.

26. Williams MH. *Nutrition for Health, Fitness & Sport.* 6th ed. Boston: McGraw-Hill; 2002.

27. Zvolankova K. The frequency of meals: its relation to overweight, hyper-cholesterolaemia, and decreased glucose tolerance. *Lancet.* 1964;614–15.

Behavior Modification

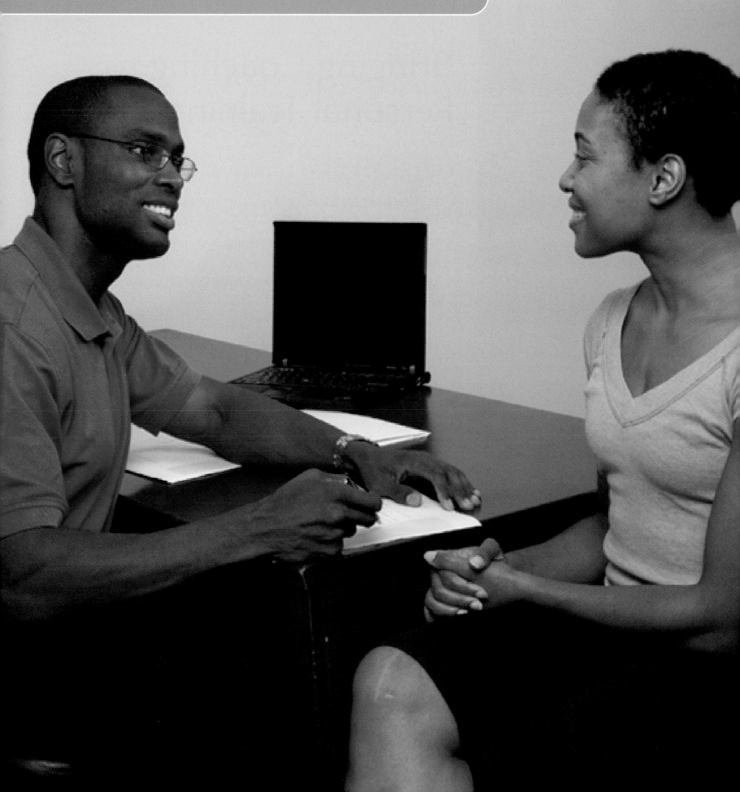

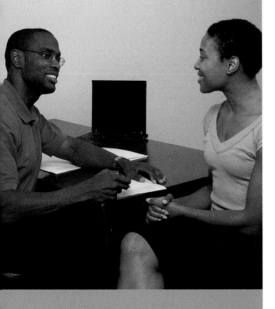

PART III

CHAPTER **7**

Bringing Coaching to Personal Training

OBJECTIVES

- Understand the definition of *coaching* and the distinction between coaching, training, and therapy or psychotherapy.
- Understanding the coaching techniques that will make you a masterful Personal Trainer.
- Understanding how to integrate coaching skills into a personal training session.

Today, much more is expected from Personal Trainers than just an excellent exercise program. You may be the only person in your clients' life who listens to the struggles they have at home and in the office, and their challenges managing their stress and getting proper sleep. They will ask you for advice on nutrition and weight maintenance. You will be best friend, confidant, advisor, cheerleader, sounding board, *and* fitness consultant.

Although you may continually encourage your clients to make positive changes in their health-related behaviors, most will still struggle to find their own motivation. Helping your clients achieve the internal motivation to live a healthy lifestyle will require more than a prescriptive formula.

> *You will be best friend, confidant, advisor, cheerleader, sounding board, and fitness consultant.*

Lifestyle coaching has found its way into the fitness world, and many Personal Trainers have found their jobs more effective and gratifying by implementing strategies and techniques from the coaching world.

WHAT IS COACHING?

Coaching is a relatively new method of support that facilitates personal growth by using evidence-based strategies for behavioral change. Coaching is a process that helps people see where they are, where they want to go, and how to get there (2). Lifestyle coaching is a process of guidance and support for clients who are ready to strategize, plan, and implement self-change and personal improvement programs (1). Lifestyle coaches come from diverse backgrounds and usually specialize in areas such as business and career coaching, transition coaching, executive coaching, and retirement coaching. Wellness coaches and fitness coaches usually have

> *Coaching is a process that helps people see where they are, where they want to go, and how to get there (2).*

a professional background in health and fitness and focus on any health or well-being concerns that can be impacted by lifestyle change: exercise, nutrition, weight loss, stress management, life/work balance, and happiness.

Coaching works with the whole person, connecting his or her core values to their intrinsic motivation for change, and focuses on connecting the client's inner world to his or her outer reality. Inquiry and personal discovery help the clients build awareness, determine solutions, and establish goals (2). It is the coach's job to ask the tough questions that will get clients to come up with their own answers and get in touch with their intuitive sense of what is likely to work for them. Coaches approach their clients with the belief that they are whole, creative, and resourceful and the experts on their own lives. Clients have the answers and know what to do to make the changes they are seeking, but they need the assistance in recognizing and following through.

Coaching is not therapy or counseling. Coaches never diagnose mental or physical health ailments. Therapists often look at the past to ascertain how it is affecting a client's behavior in the present and work on healing these past conflicts, whereas coaches use the past only as a learning tool. The coach's

> *Coaching is not therapy or counseling.*

focus is on actions to be taken in the present that will lead to achieving goals for the future.

HOW WILL ADDING COACHING TECHNIQUES MAKE YOU A MASTERFUL PERSONAL TRAINER?

Traditional Personal Trainers spend most of their time wearing an "expert hat." They are perceived as the experts on exercise and healthy living in general. In a traditional training relationship, the Personal Trainer uses his or her expertise to plan, prescribe, and implement the program that will best suit the client, gathering information from physical assessments and the client's stated goals and preferences. The client is treated as if he or she needs education and guidance, which makes the relationship Personal Trainer–directed and prescriptive in nature. The client is told what to do.

Coaching is client-directed; the focus is on what clients want to achieve. The ultimate goal is for clients to be internally motivated and no longer require Personal Trainers to exercise, eat well, and live a healthy lifestyle. The masterful Personal Trainers help clients gain confidence and a sense of self-efficacy and an understanding of the clients' role in influencing their own health outcomes. Clients ultimately take responsibility to maintain their fitness program for life.

Personal Trainers and wellness coaches share many of the same skills and traits. Both are credible, skilled professionals who are passionate about wellness, preventive medicine, and helping people. Personal Trainers and wellness coaches are knowledgeable about exercise, nutrition, weight management, and stress management. Both are seen as role models for their clients. The personality traits that make for masterful coaches are much the same as for masterful Personal Trainers: both listen well, both are empathetic and nonjudgmental, and both motivate clients with their energy and enthusiasm.

From your first conversation with a prospective client, you can set the stage for growth. You can ask questions and listen to the answers. You can approach clients with the belief that they have their own answers within, and then give them the time and space to figure it out. As you teach your clients how to exercise properly, you also can encourage them to understand their own change process in a safe, nonjudgmental environment.

Boxes 7.1 and 7.2 offer contrasting approaches to a first training session. Notice how much more information the Personal Trainer receives when using the coaching approach than when he uses a

BOX 7.1 Traditional Approach to a First Meeting with a New Client

Peter is a 42-year-old chief executive officer of an international advertising agency. His responsibilities include wining and dining prospective clients, and often he travels internationally to work in the firm's European offices. He lives in the suburbs and commutes an hour back and forth to the office. He is married and has two children, aged 3 and 7, respectively. At his last physical, he was told that his blood pressure was slightly elevated, his cholesterol levels were borderline high, and he was 30 lb above ideal weight. He has a family history of cardiovascular disease and diabetes. The results of an exercise stress test were negative. His physician advised him to "get in shape and lose some weight" to avoid needing medication in the near future. After several attempts on his own, and constant nagging from his wife, he has decided to hire a Personal Trainer to "Get this taken care of once and for all." He joined the fitness center next door to his office and plans to work with his Personal Trainer twice a week from 6 PM to 7 PM before heading home. He does not believe that he is in such a poor shape or that much overweight that it warrants all this concern.

Personal Trainer: So Peter, what is it that you are hoping to accomplish with our working together?

Peter: Well, I need to lose some weight, which hopefully will help bring down my blood pressure and cholesterol levels.

Personal Trainer: That's great. You know, research has shown that exercise can definitely make an impact on both of those profiles. Have you thought about what type of exercise program you would like to do?

Peter: Honestly, I don't really want to do anything. But my doctor and wife are bugging me constantly. I don't know how they think I am going to fit exercise into my life. I barely have time to eat or go to the bathroom during my day. So just tell me what I need to do when we work together that will get me some quick, effective results.

Personal Trainer: Wow, it does sound like you are busy. I assure you, I can create a time efficient program for you. If we get you involved in some cardiovascular exercise, maybe walking on the treadmill or using an elliptical trainer, and do some strength and flexibility training, I'm sure you'll get the results you're after. I can also give you some great tips on changing some of your eating habits, together with the exercise that should really help take the weight off. I have all the results from your assessments, so I've got a pretty good idea of where we are starting. Do you have any questions before we get going?

Peter: Nope, let's just start. I've got to catch the 7:35 PM train or I'll get stuck in the city for another hour.

BOX 7.2   Coaching Approach to First Appointment with a New Client

Personal Trainer: Peter, would it be OK with you if we spent some time before starting your workout to talk and review your background. I want to make sure I have all the information I need to help you create an exercise program that will work for you.

Peter: Sure, as long as we finish by 7 PM, I'll be fine. I need to catch the 7:35 PM train or I'll get stuck in the city for another hour.

Personal Trainer: No problem. I'm sure at the end of a long day, you're anxious to get home. So Peter, what is it that you are hoping to accomplish with our working together? What are your goals and objectives for our training program?

Peter: Well, I need to lose some weight, which hopefully will help bring down my blood pressure and cholesterol levels.

Personal Trainer: Yes, I see in your medical history that your cholesterol and blood pressure are slightly elevated. Can you tell me a bit more about that?

Peter: Sure. The doctor says if I can get it under control, I can avoid going on medication.

Personal Trainer: So, avoiding medication is something you would like to do.

Peter: Yes. I am way too young to be popping pills every morning. It reminds me of my dad, and I certainly don't want to go that route.

Personal Trainer: Go that route?

Peter: My Dad had two heart attacks when he was in his 50s. I can remember my mom lining up his medication on the kitchen table every morning at breakfast.

Personal Trainer: Go on. . . .

Peter: Well as a kid, there was something about that I found really scary. And anytime I asked him to play ball he'd tell me it was no good for his heart. He died when he was 62. He never even got to see my kids.

Personal Trainer: Sounds like it's important to you not to repeat your Dad's history.

Peter: You're not kidding. I want my kids to have a dad who can play with them and is around to watch them grow up and graduate college. It sounds crazy because they are so young now, but I'd like to be around to meet my grandchildren.

Personal Trainer: Doesn't sound crazy to me! Obviously, family is really important to you.

Peter: They are. My kids are fabulous, but I don't get to spend as much time with them as I'd like.

Personal Trainer: Why is that?

Peter: Well, I work really long hours, and sometimes they're in bed before I even get home. I also travel a lot for my job. I didn't even see them yesterday. That's why I want to make that train tonight.

Personal Trainer: Would you tell me more about your work and home routine? How might that affect your getting in shape and losing weight?

Peter: As I explained, I work long hours. So I probably can't get any exercise in besides when you and I are together. And if a last minute meeting comes up and I need to work late, I may have to cancel you at the last minute. When I travel, I'll miss our scheduled sessions, but that I know about in advance.

Personal Trainer: I'll review our cancellation policy with you and make sure you understand it. I will do my best to work around your schedule and try to come up with time slots that will minimize those problems. What else might impact your exercise program and losing weight?

Peter: Part of my job is taking clients out to lunch or dinner. We go to some pretty fancy restaurants. So having a few drinks and eating great meals is expected. When I'm in the office, I usually don't have time to stop for lunch, so I just grab something from the vending machines to hold me over until I get home for dinner.

Personal Trainer: Is there anything else I need to know?

continued >

Box 7.2. Coaching Approach to First Appointment with a New Client, cont.

Peter: Well, if truth be told, it wasn't my idea to hire a Personal Trainer. I just did it to get my wife to stop nagging me. I don't know why she's so crazy about this. I'm not so out of shape, and I'm sure I could take off some of the weight if I really tried.

Personal Trainer: So you hadn't really thought about getting in shape or losing weight before your wife and doctor suggested it?

Peter: Actually I have thought about it in the past. I was really athletic as a kid and in college. I sometimes miss those days. I was in pretty good shape then, and if I must say so myself, I was pretty trim and lean. My wife used to say I had the "best body of all the fraternity brothers!

Personal Trainer (laughing): That must have been great to hear.

Peter: Yup. I used to feel like a million bucks every time she teased me about it.

Personal Trainer: So if I've got this right, some your primary motivator for getting back into shape and losing weight are your concern about your family medical history. You want to stay healthy so that you can play with your kids and watch them grow, and one day even play with grandchildren. You want to avoid medication and live a long healthy life, and not die prematurely as your Dad did.

Peter: Wow, I hadn't even given those things much thought. I just got tired of hearing my wife nag me about this.

Personal Trainer: Is there anything else you can think of that might keep you motivated to stick with a program?

Peter: Well, it's a little embarrassing, but I wouldn't mind feeling better about my body. Sometimes I look in the mirror and I'm not sure who that guy is.

Personal Trainer: No need to be embarrassed. We all like to feel good about ourselves, and how we look does affect that.

Peter: It would be fun to have my wife liking my body again!

Personal Trainer: Peter, I know you want to make that train. So, why don't we spend a few minutes in the gym getting acquainted with the machines and look at some options you'll have for exercise. And next session, would it be OK if we spend a few minutes before we start talking about your time constraints and eating habits?

Peter: Sure, that sounds great. They're pretty bad, so you'll have your work cut out for you!

Personal Trainer: Well, I'll give it my best as long as you do too. Don't worry. Little changes can lead to big results. Let's head for the gym.

more traditional training approach. From this very first conversation, the masterful Personal Trainer is able to get the client (Peter in the example) in touch with some intrinsic motivators for change and connect them with one of his greatest values, his family. The Personal Trainer is able to break through his resistance and defensiveness. Peter will have many challenges ahead, but the Personal Trainer has set up a partnership to strategize ways to overcome them.

When you combine the information from assessments such as the PAR-Q, flexibility and strength testing, $\dot{V}O_{2max}$, and body composition with information gathered from a coaching approach, you will create programs that are far more successful and relevant to the whole person.

INTEGRATING COACHING SKILLS INTO PERSONAL TRAINING SESSIONS

Here are some ways that Personal Trainers can use the skills of coaching within the context of the training relationship.

Help Clients Be Specific about Their Stated Goals

Client goals are often vague and nonspecific. When a client says, "I really want to get in shape," you might ask, "What does being in shape mean to you?" The client then can add richness and depth to her goal: "I want to be able to walk the beach with my husband and not get winded." A goal of "I want to be stronger" can become "I want to be able to pick up and hold my grandson without my back hurting." When you help your clients clarify what they really want, you then have a measurable outcome. This is also the beginning of connecting clients' behaviors to their intrinsic motivation, getting them more in touch with their inner feelings and thoughts.

Connect Stated Goals to Deeper Motivations and Core Values

After a client is able to make a goal more specific, follow up with a question such as "Tell me what makes this important to you?" The woman who wants to walk the beach with her husband may begin to talk about how lonely she feels when her spouse goes walking every evening without her, and how disappointed he seems that she can't share this time. She then begins to talk about how her relationship means everything to her and about her desire to feel closer to her spouse. Suddenly getting in shape becomes more motivating because she can see how this will lead to her feeling more connected to the man she loves, and ultimately happier.

Adopt an Attitude of "Being Curious"

Curiosity removes any hint of judgment or disapproval. For instance, if a client returns from the weekend and reports he "felt out of control with food all weekend," you might ask: "I'm curious, was there anything different about this past weekend from others?" Perhaps you learn that because of a deadline at work, he needed to cancel his plans, leading to feelings of disappointment and frustration at not getting a night out. If you listen, rather than give advice, your client might begin to connect how negative emotions lead to his overeating. From there you might explore other ways to deal with these emotions rather than with eating.

Stop Telling Clients What They Should Do, and Begin Asking What They Are Willing to Do

Any professional Personal Trainer knows exactly what his or her clients need to do to achieve success. The traditional Personal Trainer sends his or her clients off between sessions with words of encouragement and assignments for getting aerobic activity, not skipping meals, and getting to bed early. Although clients leave with the best of intentions, most Personal Trainers have experienced the clients who report at the start of a session, "I was so bad this week!" or "You're going to be so disappointed in me!"

This weekly conversation can be an opportunity for inquiry. "What might you do this week to help you get in some cardiovascular training?" "You have told me you're struggling to eat breakfast before leaving the house each day. How could you make this easier?" The question "How can you add more movement into this upcoming week?" is much less intimidating than asking them to come to the gym twice on their own. Clients then become more creative in their thinking and begin to solve problems for themselves. They begin to have successes between sessions, which, however small, build confidence.

> *This weekly conversation can be an opportunity for inquiry.*

Help Clients Create Small, Manageable Weekly Goals to Work on in between Exercise Sessions

Using ideas generated by your clients helps them set small, achievable goals. One small healthy habit will build on others, leading to lasting change. Teach clients to change the statement "I'm going to increase my aerobic exercise this week" to "I will go to the gym Monday and Thursday directly from work, and use the treadmill for 20 minutes." "I'm really going to eat breakfast this week" will become "I will set out a bowl of cereal at night before bed, and set my alarm for 15 minutes earlier so I eat a good breakfast on Monday, Wednesday and Friday this week." Always ask the clients whether there is anything they can think of that might stand in the way of being successful with this goal so they may anticipate and plan for possible challenges.

Help Clients Focus on What Is Working in Their Wellness Plan, Rather Than What's Not Working

Achieving lifestyle change that leads to improved health and well-being requires both commitment and confidence. Most clients have experienced failed attempts in the past. When they slip up, it confirms their feeling that they are unable to stick to a plan. When you begin a session with a brief discussion about what worked *well* in the previous week, clients can acknowledge their successes and their confidence begins to grow. You will promote success by encouraging clients to do more of what is working and learning from what is not working. Clients should feel good about every little step they master, and that you are their partner—not their judge and jury. Your confidence must exceed the clients' doubts.

> *Most clients have experienced failed attempts in the past. . . . Clients should feel good about every little step they master, and that you are their partner—not their judge and jury.*

SUMMARY

Traditional training is prescriptive, whereas using coaching skills in personal training relies more on clients' expertise. From the first contact with a client, your open dialogue and skillful listening can set the stage for clients' personal growth and success. Remember that your clients will always have deeper motivations for getting fit than it may at first appear. Your openness and curiosity will help your client connect with these powerful motivators.

REFERENCES

1. Gavin J. *Lifestyle Fitness Coaching.* Champaign (IL): Human Kinetics Publishing; 2005.
2. Wellcoaches Corporation. *Fitness Coaching Skills Manual.* Wellesley (MA): Wellcoaches Corporation Publishing; 2003.

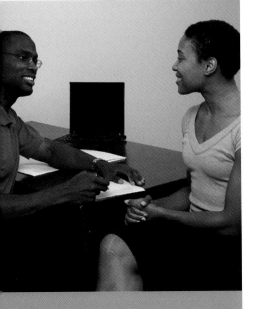

CHAPTER 8

How We Change: Behavior Change and Personal Training

OBJECTIVES

- Understand the distinct, predictable stages of behavior change.
- Determine the stage your client is in for a particular behavior.
- Match training approach to different stages of change.

t is natural to think that when a client comes to you, she or he must be ready to change and commit to regular exercise—clients have paid their money and are ready to get started! Often, however, clients are there to please someone else and may not be ready for a new lifestyle. For example, the client whose husband wants her to "get in shape" and has given her 10-session package training with you as a Christmas present. Or, a client may begin enthusiastically enough, embracing everything you say, but fail to honor commitments to exercise and eat right between sessions. Another client may soon cancel more appointments than he shows up for and eventually disappears altogether. It is easy to take this personally, or worse, to blame your clients and become frustrated with them. Although you can't force clients to show up for their appointments, you can take a step toward improving the current abysmal dropout rate during the first year of personal training by learning to assist clients in making positive changes, not just in their exercise habits, but in other areas of their life as well. Understanding the process of change is the first step toward improving the noncompliance rate.

> *Understanding the process of change is the first step toward improving the noncompliance rate.*

The good news is that it is not your role to change the client. Behavior change is self-change. As a Personal Trainer, your job is to facilitate change by understanding where your client is in the process of change and to encourage forward movement. An exceptional Personal Trainer understands that adding exercise to a client's daily regimen is part of a process that extends far beyond the personal training session. This chapter will describe what is known about behavior change and how it evolves. Subsequent chapters in this section will provide you with tools to recognize, facilitate, and support your clients' positive lifestyle changes.

THE CONTEXT FOR LASTING CHANGE

Relationship

Change occurs best in the context of a supportive and encouraging relationship. The Personal Trainer–client relationship can provide this context when a client wishes to develop a healthier lifestyle. You and your client share a common goal: your client's health and well-being. You both understand that the goal of the relationship is to assist the client in achieving what she or he sets as her or his wellness and fitness goal(s). A skilled Personal Trainer allows the process of change to unfold with ease by offering a profound level of encouragement and willingness to accept and meet the clients

> *A skilled Personal Trainer allows the process of change to unfold with ease by offering a profound level of encouragement and willingness to accept and meet the clients "where they are."*

"where they are." Chapter 9 will discuss in detail the very important elements of the client–Personal Trainer relationship.

Accountability

The Personal Trainer–client relationship provides a structure of accountability for both parties. The Personal Trainer must be accountable to his client. He must show up on time, be professional, and always have the best interests of the client in mind. Conversely, when clients share commitments to achieve goals with Personal Trainers they respect and who believe in them, they are likely to stay motivated and keep their commitments. Accountability is a powerful tool. When the Personal Trainer is encouraging and challenging—without blaming or shaming when a goal is not met— every challenge can be a learning opportunity.

BEHAVIOR MODIFICATION THEORY

Understanding behavior change requires a brief review of the principles of "behaviorism," one of the major theories of psychotherapy. Behaviorism, endorsed by John Watson, Ivan Pavlov, and B. F. Skinner, argues that human behavior is dictated by the environment, primarily the antecedents and consequences of the behavior (5). In a meta-analysis of more than 100 physical activity interventions, behavior modification strategies had greater effects on increasing exercise adherence than all other approaches (2).

Two types of conditioning illustrate the principles of behaviorism: classical and operant conditioning (4,5). Classical conditioning (Pavlov) states that a response (behavior) can be modified by changing the stimulus (antecedent). The most famous example of classical conditioning was "Pavlov's dog," which would salivate when a bell was rung because it had repeatedly been paired with the presentation of food. Accordingly, if we want to change people's behavior, we must change the cues that occur just before the behavior. Operant conditioning (Skinner) is the philosophy that behavior is shaped by consequences or rewards (4,5). If we are given something that we enjoy or like after a behavior, then we will be more likely to repeat that behavior. If we are punished or injured, then we will be less likely to repeat the behavior.

Behavioral Change as a Staged Process

Several decades after Skinner published his major works on behaviorism, Dr. James Prochaska and his colleagues at the University of Maryland were looking for a unifying, or "transtheoretical," model to describe behavior change. After studying the processes of change used in all of the major psychotherapeutic methods, including behaviorism, Prochaska made a startling and revolutionary observation: all of the major psychological theories utilized similar processes at different times during the evolution of change. With this information, Prochaska developed a unifying model describing five Stages of Readiness to Change (7). According to this model, there are five distinct and recognizable stages one goes through when successfully changing a behavior. This model has been tested, revised, and improved over the years, and has produced a paradigm shift in the way healthcare providers have since dealt with high-risk behaviors in their clients. It can be immensely useful for Personal Trainers who wish to better understand and assist their clients to make positive changes.

> *There are five distinct and recognizable stages one goes through when successfully changing a behavior.*

The Stages of Behavior Change

There are five stages of readiness to change, defined as (7):

➤ Precontemplation
➤ Contemplation
➤ Preparation
➤ Action
➤ Maintenance

PRECONTEMPLATION (I WON'T, I CAN'T)

Individuals who are "precontemplators" are in one of two categories: "I won't" or "I can't." Generally speaking, the "I won'ts" are disinterested in change, whereas the "I can'ts" are dispirited and cannot imagine being able to make a change. The "I won't" precontemplators have no interest in changing a behavior because they do not believe they have a problem. When your clients come to you, they are not likely to be in this stage about exercise, but they may be about another behavior. For example, they may still smoke and have no interest in quitting or think that exercising negates the ill effects of smoking.

The "I can't" precontemplators do not believe that they are capable of changing. They are defeated. They are demoralized by previous failures and have sunk into hopeless acceptance of their situation. They often believe that even thinking about trying to change again is too risky, because they cannot take another failure. Some are so broken that they will find any excuse as a setup for failure. Basically, "they have given up on themselves and given in to their problems, which, in turn becomes more dominant" (7). This type of client may come to you to exercise because he or she wants to lower his or her blood pressure but has tried and failed to lose weight before and has no hope of doing that successfully.

CONTEMPLATION (I MIGHT)

The next stage in the evolution of behavioral change is the "contemplation" stage. This stage is often referred to as "I might." As the name suggests, during this stage, clients are "thinking about" changing an unhealthy behavior and are considering taking action within the next 6 months. At this stage, individuals are well aware that a particular behavioral change would benefit them, and they are becoming more dissatisfied with the results of not changing. Yet, they need to resolve their ambivalence before their actions will be successful and sustainable.

In a personal training setting, this is exemplified by clients who may be thinking about adopting a healthy diet to accompany their new exercise regimen. They may be well aware of the benefits of doing so, yet they are still weighing the benefits of this change against the effort it will take. They may be very expressive about this ambivalence, describing feelings of doubt or even impossibility in achieving a change in eating patterns that are well established.

PREPARATION (I WILL)

The next step on the path of change is the "preparation" stage. This is the "I will" stage and is defined as the stage where the client has consciously decided to take action within the next month and is actively planning to do so. The motivators are defined and strong, and feelings of ambivalence have largely been handled. Interestingly, a characteristic behavior at this stage is "experimenting" with the change of concern. The boundary between this stage and the next stage is somewhat fluid, especially early on. It is very common for someone to move back and forth between planning to do something routinely and actually doing it routinely.

Many of your clients may actually still be working through this stage. Given that they are in your gym, it is reasonable to think they have passed the preparation stage and are now in "action." Yet, they may be experimenting with this new exercise behavior. These are the clients who don't always show up or who suddenly just stop coming to see you. When you are able to observe their behavior nonjudgmentally and help them recognize that they are not failing, you can help keep them from slipping back into contemplation and assist their progression to the next stage.

ACTION (I AM)

The "action" stage is where many of your clients will reside. By definition, this is the stage where a client is committed to a new behavior, and she or he is doing it consistently, building up to the target level. This is the busiest stage because people are concentrating and working very hard practicing a new behavior, refining it, and incorporating it consistently into their lives. This stage begins when a client is consistently acting on changing a behavior and ends when they have been doing it consistently for 6 months.

In the action stage, there is a high risk of slipping back to preparation; therefore, techniques to avoid this or recover and learn from this are extremely important. While it may appear to you that the client is breezing through this stage, you must understand and positively reinforce his or her efforts, because this process of establishing a new healthy behavior is not easy.

MAINTENANCE (I STILL AM)

The "maintenance" stage is achieved when someone has adopted a new behavior and done it consistently for 6 months. It is referred to as "I still am!" This is when the new behavior is a firmly established habit and the client is absolutely confident in his or her ability to maintain the behavior. Although this is a time to celebrate, challenges arise that are specific to this stage. Overconfidence, boredom, stress, and negative emotions are all capable of producing slips during the maintenance stage. If recognized early, you can provide the support needed for your client to overcome these common issues.

Effective Use of the Stages of Behavior Change Model

To use this model successfully, you must first determine what stage a client is in for a particular behavior. The "stages of change" model refers to specific behaviors, not general concepts, and your clients will frequently be in different stages of readiness to change for different behaviors. For example, a client may be motivated and ready to walk on a treadmill daily, but very hesitant and unsure about the utility of lifting weights. A savvy Personal Trainer will develop the ability to discern readiness for the different behaviors and then use appropriate strategies for each of the behaviors given the stage of readiness. In some cases, using an inappropriate process can be detrimental. For example, encouraging someone to make a formal commitment to do something before they have worked through their ambivalence about it is a setup for failure. This failure will detract from the client's self-efficacy, which will then make change even more difficult.

The "stages of change" model refers to specific behaviors, not general concepts, and your clients will frequently be in different stages of readiness to change for different behaviors.

Remember that change is uncomfortable and difficult, especially in the early stages. It is common for a client to slip back and forth between adjacent stages. This is not a sign of failure but instead is indicative that more time and efforts need to be placed in appropriately moving through one stage to the next. Also, life events occasionally intervene, and the process may need to start over again. You can help by reminding clients that slips are a normal part of the process of change, and encouraging them to stay positive and not to give up.

DIFFERENT STRATEGIES FOR DIFFERENT STAGES: AN OVERVIEW

To apply the Stages of Change Model to the real world, you first need to discern the stage your client is in for a specific behavior. You can do this in a couple of ways. You might use simple tools such as those shown in Tables 8.1 and 8.2 during your initial meeting with your client. The "Readiness Summary" (Table 8.1) assists both you and your client to understand how the different components of fitness can be addressed separately. The "Am I Ready to Change" tool (Table 8.2) can then help them understand and plan for their change process. After reviewing the summary and readiness quiz with

TABLE 8.1	SAMPLE READINESS SUMMARY				
Stage of Readiness		**Aerobic**	**Strength**	**Flexibility**	**Balance**
PCN = I WON'T					
PCB = I CAN'T					
C = I MAY					
P = I WILL					
A = I AM					
M = I STILL AM					

A, action; C, contemplation; M, maintenance; P, preparation; PCB, precontemplation believer; PCN, precontemplation nonbeliever.

TABLE 8.2	CLIENT HANDOUT

Client Handout—Am I Ready to Change?

Am I ready to change?

Research has shown that self-change is a staged process. We move from not thinking about changing a behavior to thinking about it, to planning to change, and then to testing out ways to do it before we actually start. A number of techniques can help you move from not thinking, to thinking, to planning, to doing, and to continue doing.

When we think about changing a behavior, questions we ask ourselves are:

Why do I want to change the behavior (the "pros")?
Why shouldn't I try to change the behavior (the "cons")?
What would it take for me to overcome my cons and change the behavior (what's my strategy)?

To move forward, we need to have our "pros" outweigh our "cons" and develop realistic strategies to overcome our "cons."

Behavioral scientists recognize five stages of readiness to change behavior:
- Precontemplation (I won't or I can't in the next 6 months)
- Contemplation (I may in the next 6 months)
- Preparation (I will in the next month)
- Action (I'm doing it now)
- Maintenance (I've been doing it for at least 6 months)

We want to help you determine how ready you are to change a behavior so that we can best help you make that change. To help you understand your stage of readiness, we ask that you complete the short questionnaire below.

Your Personal Trainer will discuss your answers with you, and make suggestions to help you move through the stages of change and reach your goals.

1. The goal or behavior I want to work on first is:
2. My reasons for wanting to accomplish this goal (same as change this behavior) are:
3. The obstacles standing in the way of my changing this behavior are:
4. The efforts I made toward changing this behavior in the last week are:
5. My goal for next week with respect to this behavior is:
6. My readiness to change this behavior is (type *yes* beside the level that best describes where you are):
   - I won't do it
   - I can't do it
   - I may do it
   - I will do it
   - I am doing it
   - I am still doing it

your client, you will be better positioned first to help them understand their readiness stages, and then to use thoughtful strategies for each different component of exercise.

> *By observing behavior and listening carefully to what is said in response to your skillful questioning, you can accurately determine a client's stage of readiness and then use appropriate strategies to facilitate forward progress.*

The other way of understanding what stage your client is in is using the observational skills that you will develop over time. By observing behavior and listening carefully to what is said in response to your skillful questioning, you can accurately determine a client's stage of readiness and then use appropriate strategies to facilitate forward progress. See Boxes 8.1 and 8.2 for descriptions of cognitive and action-based change processes to use with your clients as they progress through the stages of change.

Precontemplation

Precontemplators have not yet discovered enough "pros" to outweigh the discomfort and difficulty of change. These clients need information. They need to understand all of the benefits of a positive change, and they need to find the ones that matter to them. They also must be receptive to the

---

BOX **8.1**   **Cognitive Change Processes (Thinking and Feeling)**

Consciousness raising: Includes information gathering, either by learning new facts about a subject or by discovering previously unknown feelings, values, etc. Health education is an important consciousness-raising technique for Personal Trainers to utilize. For example, when doing fitness assessments, clients can discover exactly what their fitness levels are in relation to healthy norms.

Self-image (self-reevaluation): A positive self-image should be aligned with the new behavior. Clients are excited when they consider how they will look, feel, and act, and how their life will be better as their changed self, they are drawn to the target behavior.

Dramatic release: Dramatic release is similar to consciousness raising but works at a deeper, emotional level. For example, when a client's close friend has a sudden heart attack, this may motivate him or her to start running again.

Social norms: Social norms reflect the relationships between individuals and provide support and reinforce new behavior. Groups such as Weight Watchers are very helpful in early stages of change. In these settings, group expectations reinforce the new healthy behavior. There is a palpable collective empathy for the "changer," and at the same time, numerous role models are present to provide tips and encouragement.

Role modeling: The process of role modeling involves considering how our behaviors affect those whom we love. For example, parents who begin to question what they are teaching their children about health and wellness may take up exercise or quit smoking. This process is helpful in the early stages of change when finding the pros of a behavior change is occurring.

BOX **8.2**   **Behavioral Change Processes (Action Oriented)**

Commitment: Making a formal commitment connotes a full acceptance of responsibility for changing. An example of this change strategy is called a contingency contract (1), an agreement between you and your client that details goals, time frames, measures of success, and rewards. The more specific a commitment, the more effective it is.

Environmental control: In environmental control, the client identifies and eliminates the cues that produce the problem behavior from the environment. They then develop new cues that signal the healthy behavior. For example, they can be reminded to exercise by strategically placing notes to themselves, by getting e-mails from you, or by putting exercise clothes in their car to encourage going to the gym after work.

Substitutions (counterconditioning): Countering, or substituting healthy behaviors in the place of unhealthy ones, can be called the "instead of" process. When exercising is the target behavior, you can encourage stairs "instead of" elevators, or biking to work "instead of" driving, or substituting a short walk for zoning out in front of the television.

Social support (helping relationships): This process is important in all stages of change. You can provide a very important element of social support for your client as they traverse the stages of change. Other sources of support can come from family close friends and should be encouraged. For example, suggest a client walk with a friend, because it is much more likely that they will keep their promise to walk if they are meeting someone.

Rewards (reinforcement): In this process, the target behavior is rewarded to help increase its frequency (4). The reinforcement could come from you, by rewarding a client for completed exercise sessions and/or for accomplishing specific goals. The clients can come up with their own reward system and make it part of their formal commitments (see above).

BOX **8.3**   **Peter in Precontemplation for Weightlifting**

Peter: Boy, was I ever sore from our first session! It's embarrassing to know that just learning how to use the machines would make me sore. I've got to tell you, I'm not so sure about this weightlifting stuff. I've always hurt myself when I've tried to do this in the past, and I can't afford an injury with all the traveling I do. I'd rather just focus on the treadmill. I know I need to do that to lose this weight, and since my time is so limited, let's just stick to that.

[*"Peter equates weightlifting with pain and injury. He has not been successful with a resistance training program in the past and does not trust that he can do it without injuring himself. He also does not understand how weightlifting will benefit his weight management issue. He is a bit of an "I won't/I can't" hybrid. Notice below that the Personal Trainer responds with empathy and a nonjudgmental attitude and builds Peter's confidence in his own ability."*]

Personal Trainer: It is definitely amazing how sore you can get a day or two after lifting. I hate to go down any stairs 24 hours after I do squats, and I've been doing this for years! I'm sorry you were injured, though. What happened?

Peter: Oh, it was so stupid. I was trying to show off for my wife when she finally convinced me to go to her gym. I remembered that back in college I could bench my weight easily, so I tried it without remembering that my weight is 30 lb heavier now than it was then. Anyway, I tweaked my shoulder just taking the weight off the rack, and vowed I would never do that again. My shoulder ached for weeks!

Personal Trainer: Ouch! I can understand your hesitancy to try again, but I'm pretty sure I can help you start up without any injuries. How about this: I'll give you an article I read just last night about how resistance training benefits weight loss. Then we can talk about it next time, OK? Let's go get on the treadmill. By the way, good job getting in 20 minutes twice this week! That is quite a change from not doing any exercise at all.

---

information. The discerning Personal Trainer will know the right time to provide this essential information to their clients in a nonjudgmental way, understanding that information alone will not change their behavior (Box 8.3).

Contemplation

This stage may last awhile. The highlight of this stage is ambivalence. This is the time to listen, to be empathetic, and to understand that your clients need to work through these issues on their own timetables. With your careful help, they will find their own compelling reasons to change and build their own self-confidence (Box 8.4).

Preparation

This stage is recognizable by your clients' commitment to change. With ambivalence behind them, this is the time when potentially all of the cognitive and behavioral processes could be appropriate. This would be a good time to create a written contract, with your client including some rewards for goals met. You can also help your clients decide how to best use the processes of substitution and use of cues (Boxes 8.2 and 8.5) to increase compliance with their commitment to exercise. Specific motivational techniques are discussed in Chapter 10.

Action

The action stage is typically 6 months long and is hard work for your client. Don't be deceived into thinking that they are coasting along easily and do not need your support and encouragement. The

| BOX 8.4 | **Peter in Contemplation for Nutritional Changes** |

Peter (on treadmill): I know we said we'd talk about my eating habits today. I really wish I could figure out how to eat better. I know it would probably be good for me, but I just don't see how to do it when I have to take all these clients out to eat rich food and drink all night.

Personal Trainer: How do you think eating better would improve your life?

Peter: Well, for one thing, I would probably lose this extra 30 pounds I'm carrying around. My doctor seems to think I could lower my cholesterol by changing how I eat, but he has no idea how difficult that would be for me!

Personal Trainer: So, you could lose some weight and lower your health risks. How else would your life be different if you changed the way you eat?

Peter: I know I'd have more energy in the morning if I cut out the after-dinner brandy . . . and probably the martini before dinner. I would also be able to wake up early and actually call my kids before they leave for school when I'm overseas. The desserts are killing me, I just know it . . . but I feel like I have to order something so the client doesn't feel bad when they do.

Personal Trainer: I can see it is a complex issue. Maybe it would help if you made a list of all of the benefits you would get from not eating dessert or drinking brandy after dinner while you are traveling. Then make a list of all of the costs you are paying by continuing to eat and drink in excess. See if those two lists outweigh the list of benefits you get from the desserts and brandy plus the costs to you of giving them up.

Peter: That's a good idea. It sounds like something I would have my employees do . . . a cost/benefit analysis. I like that!

use of cues, substitutions, and rewards is still of great value, as is social support and ongoing commitment. Continue to enhance your clients' internal motivation by reminding them of how far they have come. Use assessments to show objective proof of their gains. Have them review their pros and cons occasionally to remind them why they want to keep up with their efforts. Give them the support and understanding they need to overcome occasional slips (Box 8.6).

| BOX 8.5 | **Peter in Preparation for Nutritional Changes** |

Peter (in the next session): You know, I did that cost/benefit thing that you suggested, and I am now convinced that I need to stop eating desserts and drinking anything other than water after dinner. I've been kidding myself that I do it for the clients . . . I do it because it's a habit, and I can change a habit.

Personal Trainer: Great. Tell me more about why you've made this decision.

Peter: Well, first of all, I figured that by cutting out on just those two things, I'll be halfway to my goal weight by summer, and I'll feel more comfortable swimming with my kids without such a huge spare tire! I just know I'll have more energy to play with them when I lose this weight . . . and if I don't do it soon, they'll be too old to want to hang out with their dad.

Personal Trainer: It sounds like being fun for your kids while they are young is important . . . maybe more important than what your clients think if you don't order dessert with them? What will you do, then, the next time you are out with clients and they order dessert?

Peter: I haven't thought about that yet. Hmmm, I guess I could order some decaf coffee or tea. Or, I could even suggest we go outside for a walk after dinner instead. That would be a surprise to them. They wouldn't dare say no!

Peter in Action: Six Weeks into Exercise Program

Peter: I can't believe how difficult it can be to convince people to walk around the block a few times after dinner! My wife will do it without any problems, but when I'm overseas, I can't convince anyone to go with me! They just want their brandy and cigars. When I was gone last week, I didn't feel safe going alone, so I just went back to the hotel and went to bed.

Personal Trainer: It is definitely hard to convince others to make healthy choices when they aren't ready. But, at least you didn't join them! It would be a shame to go to all that work of developing this great habit, and then lose it due to travel. Especially when you are so close to your goal . . . do you realize how far you have come? Last week you weighed in nine pounds lighter than when you started! That spare tire is shrinking fast. It'll be gone by summer for sure, at this rate, and you will be playing in the pool with pride. Can you think of a safer way to walk after dinner if you have to be alone?

Peter: Definitely! There is always a treadmill in the hotels where I stay. What a good idea! I don't have to let other people constrain me. I always sleep so much better when I walk at night, too. I'm on a roll now!

Maintenance

Even though clients in maintenance have completely accepted the importance of the new behavior, there is always a risk of a slip back to unhealthy behaviors. One of your most important tasks when working with clients in this stage is to be vigilant and recognize the beginning of a lapse. When a lapse is handled appropriately, chances are good that your client will not slip far. Another big challenge at this stage is the avoidance of boredom. You can help alleviate this problem by keeping workouts fresh and fun. Encourage the use of new equipment or change environments. Suggest that your clients try new classes or cross train. Early recognition, followed by corrective adjustments, will usually turn a lapse into a learning experience (Box 8.7).

PROGRESSION THROUGH STAGES IS SPIRAL, NOT LINEAR

Both you and your clients should understand that it is extremely rare to progress in a linear fashion from one stage directly to the next, with no overlap and no slips. Most people slip up at some point and return to contemplation (or even precontemplation) before they successfully move

BOX **8.7**   **Peter in Maintenance**

Peter: I'm really feeling good lately. I can't believe now that exercise wasn't a part of my life. Traveling is still tough, though, and the last trip I took, I was so tired after long meetings every day I just went to bed every night instead of walking.

Personal Trainer: It sounds exhausting! When you know you'll have meetings all day, is there another time you can schedule for exercise?

Peter: Well, I could go in the morning.

Personal Trainer: How would that improve the way you felt the rest of the day?

Peter: Actually, it would be tough getting up in the morning, but I believe my energy would be better. I really noticed my lack of energy on the days I didn't exercise.

Personal Trainer: What if you tried that a couple times and see how you feel? Would you be willing to jot down how you felt after and we can talk about it after your next trip?

Peter: Great. Why not?

> *Most people slip up at some point and return to contemplation (or even precontemplation) before they successfully move forward.*

forward. The entire process takes work and continued application of appropriate processes of change. You must help your clients avoid feeling demoralized by a relapse, but instead, learn how to do better the next time.

Relapse is common, and the feelings that it evokes are unpleasant. As Prochaska et al. point out (7), "A successful self-change is like climbing the Leaning Tower of Pisa: First, you walk up, but as you approach the lower part of each floor, you begin to head down. A few steps later you resume your ascent" (p. 48). The result is that even though your clients may feel as if they are going in circles, the good news is that the circles are spiraling upward. Each time they slip, they learn something that makes the next approach easier.

> *A lapse is a temporary phenomenon. It may occur for a number of reasons, some preventable, many not. A relapse is defined as abandoning the positive behavior with a resulting loss of benefits.*

There is a difference between a lapse and a relapse. A lapse is a temporary phenomenon. It may occur for a number of reasons, some preventable, many not. A relapse is defined as abandoning the positive behavior with a resulting loss of benefits. All relapses begin with a slip or a lapse away from the healthy behavior. However, a lapse does not necessarily lead to relapse. The key to prevention of relapse is to catch a lapse early and to be ready for it with a plan of action.

Lapse leads to relapse due to a number of conditions. One problem is emotional in nature, and the other is environmental. Clients often have an all-or-nothing attitude about behavior change. When they lapse, they feel guilt and self-blame. These feelings do not support the change process, and indeed, guilt alone can turn a lapse into a relapse (7).

The environmental conditions that can lead to a lapse and subsequent relapse include social pressures, work pressures, travel, and boredom. One way to identify "high-risk" situations for relapse is for your client to perform self-monitoring (1). This process can uncover patterns of thoughts, feelings, and situations that have led to skipping a workout. This additional information can then be used to design coping strategies and prevent relapse. For example, many people will forgo exercise when they are stressed about work or their personal life, so it may be helpful for the clients to learn some stress management skills such as progressive relaxation, meditation, or time management skills. Clients who travel frequently face additional challenges to maintenance. They need to have a plan set in place before they leave that will keep them on the fitness path. This may include e-mail reminders from you, with constant encouragement and empathy. Finally, they may be doing a great job and then hit a plateau of interest that no periodization scheme can fix. Boredom can be dealt with effectively by having your clients set new goals, try new activities, or sign up for a competitive event.

SUMMARY

Successful behavior change follows five distinct, predictable stages. A skilled Personal Trainer can facilitate positive change by understanding where his or her client is in the process of change and by encouraging forward progress by using strategies tailored to the specific stage of readiness to change. Cognitive processes are generally more useful in early stages of change, whereas later stages are facilitated by both cognitive and action-based processes. Understand that lapse is a common and temporary phenomenon. A relapse is marked by abandonment of the positive behavior with a resulting loss of benefits. All relapses begin with a lapse; however, a lapse does not necessarily lead to a relapse.

REFERENCES

1. Clark NM, Becker MH. Theoretical models and strategies for improving adherence and disease management. In: Shumaker SA, Schron EB, Ockene JK, McBee WL, editors. *Handbook of Health Behavior Change.* 2nd ed. New York: Springer; 1998. p. 5–32.

2. Dishmam RK, Buckworth J. Increasing physical activity: a quantitative synthesis. *Med Sci Sports Exer.* 1996;28(6):706–19.

3. Highsteen GR, Silverio G. Behavior change. In: *Wellcoaches Training Manual.* 4th ed. Wellesley (MA): Wellcoaches Corporation; 2006. p. 43–52.

4. Lox CL, Martin-Ginis KA, Petruzzello SJ. *The Psychology of Exercise: Integrating Theory and Practice.* 2nd ed. Scottsdale (AZ): Holcomb Hathaway; 2006.

5. Mazur JE. *Learning and Behavior.* 3rd ed. Prentice Hall Englewood Cliffs (NJ): 1994.

6. Moore M, Claps F, Highsteen GR, Larsen K, Graddy LT, Lavin TJ. Exercise psychology, motivation, and behavior change. In: Thompson WR, Baldwin KE, Pire NL, Niederpruem M, editors. *ACSM's Resources for the Personal Trainer.* 2nd ed. Baltimore: Lippincott Williams & Wilkins; 2006. p. 208–237.

7. Prochaska JO, Norcross JC, Diclemente CC. *Changing for Good.* New York: William Morrow; 1994.

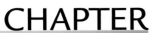

9

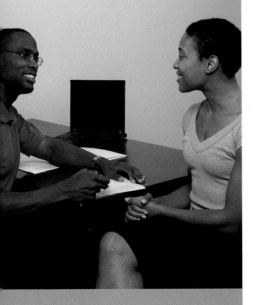

Personal Trainer–Client Relationship: Partnership for Growth

OBJECTIVES

- Understand that a supportive Personal Trainer–client relationship sets the context for successful and lasting change.
- Learn how to build a strong relationship on trust, excellent communication skills, and a nonjudgmental approach.
- Learn the importance of being fully engaged with a client during a training session through managing your energy and focus.

The ability to build quality relationships with your clients is essential for an exceptionally rewarding career as a Personal Trainer. You will need to delicately balance guiding your clients and holding them accountable, a challenging task. As a Personal Trainer, you will build on your clients' strengths and promote positive action to foster lasting change.

The Personal Trainer–client relationship is a partnership that is dedicated to the client's fitness needs and goals (4). When someone hires a Personal Trainer, he or she is making a serious financial, physical, and emotional commitment and desires a program created specifically for him or her. You can and should feel honored that he or she sought your expertise and guidance. Your interactions with a client could be life changing for him or her. Taking relationship building very seriously honors your client's trust in you. This chapter will describe elements for an effective Personal Trainer–client relationship.

BE PROMPT AND PREPARED

Your first impression will set the stage for a successful and potentially long-standing Personal Trainer–client relationship. Always being prompt respects your client's time. Also, when you come into a consultation prepared and organized, you are presenting yourself professionally. Starting and ending training sessions on time is essential. Starting late or ending early does not make good use of the allotted training time. Being professional means being on time.

> *Always being prompt respects your client's time.*

ESTABLISH CREDIBILITY

Establish credibility at the beginning of your training program. It is helpful to have developed a system for the initial consultation including:

➤ A practiced, brief introduction, describing your education, experience, and reasons for becoming a Personal Trainer
➤ A one-paged typed biography
➤ A business card with your contact information

Convey that you are committed to helping your clients achieve their best possible fitness level. If you have a success story with a client in a similar situation, it would be appropriate to share it (maintaining confidentiality, of course). If you are comfortable, share your passion for your own fitness lifestyle as well as for those of your clients.

Tip #1: CREATE A POSITIVE FIRST IMPRESSION

How do you create a positive first impression? To get some ideas, ask the people around you, "What was your first impression of me?" How can you use their answers?

MAINTAIN CONFIDENTIALITY

When words spoken in confidence are shared with others, trust is compromised and you risk irreparable damage to the Personal Trainer–client relationship. Reassure your clients that what they say to you will be held in strictest confidence, and then keep this promise. Some clients will be initially uncomfortable with personal disclosures. As you continue to provide a safe atmosphere of nonjudgment, curiosity, and encouragement, they will begin to open up. Make sure that if a client is sharing something personal with you in a public place, such as the gym, privacy can be maintained. Also, depending on where you work, confidentiality (especially regarding a client's medical history) is a requirement of the job.

DEVELOP TRUST

Trust can be defined as the willingness of your clients to be vulnerable based on their confidence in your benevolence, honesty, openness, reliability, and competence (6). The development of trust begins when you prove to be reliable by following through on promises. Trust is the foundation for strong rapport, which then facilitates positive change in your clients. When your clients trust you, they feel safe and confidant that they can confide in you and that you have their best interests at heart. Trust takes time to develop, but if you meet your commitments to them, maintain strict confidentiality, and are on time, your clients will grow secure with you and with your program for them.

> *The development of trust begins when you prove to be reliable by following through on promises.*

Trust will further grow as your client feels confident in your knowledge and expertise. Continuing to increase your skills and knowledge about exercise prescription and technique, physiology, anatomy, and biomechanics demonstrates your commitment to your career development. Clients will appreciate this and trust your expertise as a result.

Tip #2: ESTABLISH TRUST IN RELATIONSHIPS

How have you established trust in other relationships? What qualities do you have that make it easy for people to trust you? Do you trust yourself and your instincts? If applicable, what has hindered your capacity to trust yourself?

BE PRESENT

Complete focus on your clients lets them know that you care about them and that they are important to you. To build a strong relationship, this focus and mindfulness should exist in a context of true interest in your client and his or her well-being. Your attention is demonstrated both verbally (with questions and feedback) and with body language (turning your body to fully face them). Body language, facial expressions, and tone of voice often tell the clients much more than the actual words you choose.

Mindfulness is the nonjudgmental awareness of what is happening in the present moment. When both the Personal Trainer and client are fully present, the Personal Trainer–client relationship can flourish. Being mindful and in the moment will keep the training session alive and fresh for both of you and will enhance your relationship. For example, as you work with a client, there are many possible external distractions, including people who wish to carry on conversations with you or your client, loud music, watching others, etc. In the presence of external distractions, asking open-ended questions and maintaining eye contact helps to keep you present and engaged with your client.

> *Being mindful and in the moment will keep the training session alive and fresh for both of you and will enhance your relationship.*

Helping your clients develop mindfulness during exercise will actually enhance the experience for them. Clients who claim that they "hate exercise" can be encouraged to focus on one or two actual sensations that occur while exercising. Taking their focus off their judgments about exercise engages them in the experience of exercise.

BE INTERESTED

You demonstrate interest when you begin each session with your clients by asking how their week went and being sincerely concerned about all aspects of their lives. When you understand completely the whole picture of your clients' life, you will have a greater understanding of their potential barriers to change. Demonstrate empathy and be nonjudgmental when conversing about these issues.

PRACTICE ACTIVE LISTENING

The strength of any relationship hinges on superior communication skills, and listening well is an art. When you practice active listening, you not only listen for content, but you also tune into your client's tone, mood, feelings, energy, hesitations, and concerns.

People seldom have the undivided attention of others. You have a unique opportunity to offer this gift to your clients. To convey to clients that you are listening, periodically summarize and restate what you have heard. Ask whether you have understood them correctly. Reflecting what you have heard back to the clients assures them that you are listening, that you care, and that you are working to understand them. When you demonstrate that you appreciate their perspective and concerns, you encourage further dialogue.

> *Reflecting what you have heard back to the clients assures them that you are listening, that you care, and that you are trying to understand them.*

Tip #3 EXAMINE YOUR ACTIVE LISTENING SKILLS

In your next session, pay attention to your "active listening" skills. Do you interrupt? Are you waiting for the chance to say your piece? Are you maintaining eye contact? Are you listening for underlying feelings and concerns? Are you trusting your instincts?

GIVE AND RECEIVE FEEDBACK

Feedback to your client should be nonthreatening, objective, clarifying, reflective (restating what the client says), and supportive. When it is corrective in nature, it should be in the moment, and demonstration may be useful. When appropriate, gentle humor can lighten the moment. However, be sure that your clients do not misinterpret your humor for laughing at them.

Receiving feedback will require an open mind and the maturity to accept criticism in a healthy manner. Do not assume their continued satisfaction with you. Keep asking questions and fine-tuning their program. Remember that your goal in asking for feedback is to serve your client in the best way possible. Letting your clients know that you care about what is working and what is not working can only strengthen your rapport with them.

SHOW POSITIVE REGARD

Benevolence, or unconditional positive regard, is demonstrated by being completely accepting toward your clients. You want your clients to feel safe with you and know that you are in their corner. Judgment, criticism, and arrogance—spoken or unspoken—do not motivate positive behavior change. When we believe in and support our clients, we establish a relationship that bolsters self-esteem (4).

ACCEPT CLIENTS WHERE THEY ARE

As a Personal Trainer, your job is promoting change. Therefore, the idea of "accepting clients as they are" may seem like a paradox. However, giving your clients permission to be as they are promotes self-acceptance and encourages them to feel competent, confident, and effective. When you withhold judgment and focus on their strengths, clients will feel empowered and invigorated.

For example, you have not seen your client for a few days, and she has not done the exercises to which you agreed. She feels guilty and ashamed. Your negative judgment would further diminish positive performance and self-efficacy. Instead, you might ask her questions about the obstacles she had to face: Did she feel the goal was unrealistic? What did she learn from this experience? What could she have done differently? This is also a good time to switch the focus from the negative to the positive. You could ask, "What went well for you?" Or "What are you feeling good about?" By shifting the focus to her victories, she will now begin the session with feelings of optimism rather than inadequacy.

> *Be mindful that the praise and encouragement you offer is genuine and based in reality.*

Regardless of the condition in which a client comes to you, keep an upbeat attitude. Praise your clients for their efforts and focus on their progress. Begin each session by commenting on all the things they are doing well. Be mindful that the praise and encouragement you offer is genuine and based in reality. Being grandiose can be perceived as insincere.

PRACTICE EMOTIONAL INTELLIGENCE

Emotional intelligence describes the competencies and skills that underlie successful relationships (1). There are four main emotional intelligence constructs:

➤ *Self-awareness.* The ability to read one's emotions and recognize their impact while using gut feelings to guide decisions
➤ *Self-management.* Controlling one's emotions and impulses and adapting to changing circumstances
➤ *Social awareness.* The ability to sense, understand, and react to other's emotions while comprehending social networks
➤ *Relationship management.* The ability to inspire, influence, and develop others while managing conflict

Emotional intelligence is the ability to monitor one's own and others feelings to discriminate among them and to use this information to guide one's own thinking and action.

For example, you have planned a challenging workout for your client. However, when she arrives, you can see by her eyes, body language, and tone of voice that she tired, drained, and stressed. You can then tune into your own feelings and emotions and trust your instincts. State your observations with compassion and ask open-ended questions: "You seem tired and stressed. What is going on for you today?" Or "Tell me about your day—how are things going for you?" By conveying your perceptions and understanding, you let your client know you are attentive to her present state, which creates a greater connection with her. On the basis of the outcome of this initial conversation, you are better able to assess whether to stay with your original plan or to modify the workout.

MODEL A HEALTHY LIFESTYLE

Remember that clients are always watching you. Set a positive example by exercising regularly, eating well, and following your own self-care program. Modeling a healthy lifestyle enables clients to see that you are "walking the talk." If you believe it is appropriate and helpful to your client, feel free to discuss your healthy lifestyle. However, be wary of giving anecdotal advice. If you do this, make sure your motivation is sincere and in the best interest of your client. Your discussion of both your successes and failures may help your client relate to you on a more human level.

BE FULLY ENGAGED

When you are fully engaged, you are at your best because you are physically energized, emotionally connected, mentally focused, and spiritually aligned. Managing your energy level well can lead to increased optimism and joy and actually can create greater overall energy (2). When you are more energetic, you connect more effectively with your clients and manifest more joy in your career.

Clients deserve and are paying for your full attention. Many factors can influence your capacity to be fully engaged with them. Eating well, getting plenty of sleep, exercising regularly, and maintaining a balance between work and play are elements of good self-care that optimize your energy and attention. On the other hand, procrastination, multitasking, and other energy drains can pull your attention away from your client. To be a masterful Personal Trainer, you must be focused. Your clients will notice and appreciate your attention to them.

Tip #4 ENGAGE FULLY WITH YOUR CLIENTS

What does being fully alive and present mean to you? How does taking care of yourself help you be fully engaged with clients? What energizes you? What are you feeling right now?

SUMMARY Personal training is a rewarding and challenging profession. As a Personal Trainer, you have a wonderful opportunity to enrich other people's lives. Be willing to cultivate your own personal growth to enhance your ability to connect with your clients. Emulate someone you admire—become the trainer you would like to have train you. Learn, practice, learn, practice—these are constant in the life of a Personal Trainer. Developing and cultivating favorable Personal Trainer–client relationships will enhance your experience and increase the longevity of your personal training career.

REFERENCES

1. Goleman D. *Working with Emotional Intelligence*. New York: Bantam Books; 1998.
2. Loehr J, Schwartz T. *The Power of Full Engagement*. New York: Free Press Publishing; 2003.
3. Moore M, Claps F, Highsteen GR, Larsen K, Graddy LT, Lavin TJ. Exercise psychology, motivation, and behavior change. In: Thompson WR, Baldwin KE, Pire NL, Niederpruem M, editors. *ACSM's Resources for the Personal Trainer*. 2nd ed. Baltimore: Lippincott Williams & Wilkins; 2006. p. 208–37.
4. Moore M. *Wellcoaches Training Manual*. Wellesley (MA): Wellcoaches Corporation; 2006.
5. Moore M, Tschannen-Moran R. *Coaching Psychology Manual*. Philadelphia: Lippincott Williams & Wilkins; 2010.
6. Tschannen-Moran M. *Trust Matter: Leadership for Successful Schools*. San Francisco: Jossey-Bass; 2004.

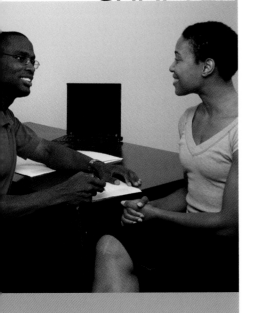

CHAPTER 10

Motivational Tools

OBJECTIVES

- Understand factors that motivate people to change their behaviors.
- Differentiate extrinsic motivators from intrinsic motivators.
- Identify the "5 Ds" of appreciative inquiry and their relevance to personal training.
- Define motivational interviewing and discuss how it can be used by Personal Trainers.
- Define change talk and resistance talk, and discuss how each impacts behavior change.
- Define the four OARS skills and how they can be used in personal training sessions.
- Explain how using a client's strengths and positive experiences can help facilitate successful behaviors.
- Discuss the impact of self-esteem and self-efficacy on clients' motivation and adherence to exercise programs.

lients who seek out Personal Trainers usually have come to a point in their lives where they realize that they want to make fitness and exercise a part of their life. They are willing to invest the extra time and money to hire a professional who can help them attain more than they could do alone. You will need to identify and understand the factors that motivate each individual to achieve what he or she may not be able to achieve alone. Good Personal Trainers will work to keep their clients motivated during each and every session. Great Personal Trainers, however, will not only motivate their clients during each and every session but keep them motivated between sessions as well. Sustaining change is the goal. There are several approaches and theories that have been shown to be helpful in maintaining clients' motivation.

APPRECIATIVE INQUIRY

Largely because of its successes in the business world, appreciative inquiry (AI) has been adopted by professionals who work with health behavior change (14,22). Simply put, AI assists clients in moving beyond obstacles to behavior change by building on past successes and visualizing great possibilities. Appreciative inquiry relies on the relationship and communication between the client and the Personal Trainer, focusing on the Personal Trainer's powerful and positive questions. This in turn unleashes energy, knowledge, and images that invoke change.

> *Appreciative inquiry assists clients in moving beyond obstacles to behavior change by building on past successes and visualizing great possibilities.*

Appreciative inquiry is based on five principles that interact with and build upon one another. Together, they generate positive actions on the part of clients to achieve and maintain their goals.

➤ *The Constructionist Principle*: You and the client construct the positive environment desired for change by applying lessons from past successes to current challenges.
➤ *The Simultaneity Principle*: Inquiry and change are interrelated. When you ask questions in a positive frame, it plants the seed for positive change.
➤ *The Anticipatory Principle*: Without vision, clients may wander without focus. By creating a vision for the future, clients become more purposefully driven and make more mindful choices in the present.
➤ *The Poetic Principle*: Clients can change and influence their story at any time. Regardless of clients' experiences with exercise, there is always the opportunity to influence the future to become more hopeful.
➤ *The Positive Principle*: When you and client are bonded by positive emotion and inspiration for the future, positive change will be lasting and successful.

The 5-D Cycle of Appreciative Inquiry

Appreciative inquiry's true potential is realized through the conversations between the Personal Trainer and client. Appreciative inquiry builds on the aspirations, ideas, and values of the individual (14). Often referred to as the 5 Ds, the core AI approaches and processes are as follows (7,22):

➤ *Define*: Through conversation and questions, you and your client agree on the focus of training and the best way to get there.
➤ *Discover*: You and your client explore the forces, strengths, and values that have been a part of the client's past.
➤ *Dream*: You and your client work together to identify realistic yet challenging goals that will allow the client to grow and improve. Your questions and dialogue invite the client to think great thoughts and possibilities for his or her future.

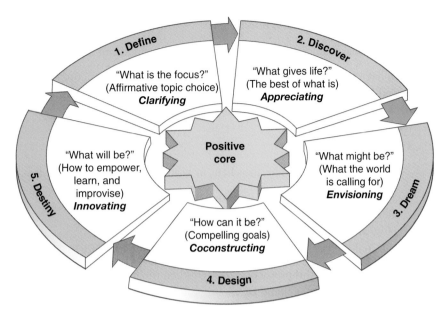

FIGURE 10.1. The 5 Ds. (From Moore M, Tshannen-Moran B. *Coaching Psychology Manual.* Philadelphia: Wolters Kluwer/Lippincott Williams & Wilkins; 2010.)

➤ *Design:* You and your client begin to develop the plans that will allow the client to reach agreed-upon goals, and the client's dream begins to grow wings.

➤ *Destiny:* Here the dreams become a set of manageable actions, steps that propel clients toward their desired goals.

By developing the skills of the 5-D cycle, clients will learn to approach their fitness and wellness with a positive eye and see obstacles more as opportunities. Figure 10.1 demonstrates the Five-D cycle (22) of AI.

Appreciative Interview Protocol

The Appreciative Interview Protocol can be adapted by Personal Trainers for their specific programmatic needs (22). Below are some questions to initial AI dialogue (22):

BEST EXPERIENCE

In this part of the discovery process, the past is mined for successes:

➤ Tell me about a time when you felt you were the fittest or you truly enjoyed exercising?
➤ Describe a time when you followed a healthy lifestyle.
➤ What did you appreciate most about this time in your life?
➤ Who else was part of this experience with you and what role did they play?

CORE VALUES

Using these questions, the Personal Trainer helps the client discover his or her deeper motivation:

➤ Tell me about what is really important to you?
➤ What do you value? How does becoming more physically fit relate to your values?

GENERATIVE CONDITIONS

The Personal Trainer and client can explore the conditions that fostered past successes.

➤ What are some of the things (internal and external) that encouraged you to be at your best health and fitness?
➤ What enabled you to have fun experiences?

THREE WISHES

The Personal Trainer guides the client in visioning his or her future dreams:

➤ Tell me about your dreams for your future.
➤ Tell me about your dreams related to your health and fitness.
➤ How are all of these dreams connected?
➤ If I could grant you three wishes, what would you wish for?

The purpose of this protocol is to strengthen the positive energy and enhance the self-confidence and self-esteem of the client. By identifying with their strengths and experiences in their past, they will begin to gain confidence and motivation that will assist them in achieving lasting change. Box 10.1 is an example of AI in action.

BOX **10.1** **Appreciative Inquiry in Action**

Susan started gaining significant weight in college. When she went home for visits, her mother nagged about watching what she eats and getting more exercise. Susan would go to the fitness center to exercise. There she felt out of place among the thinner members and endured rude comments made behind her back. She eventually cancelled her membership and has done minimal exercise since.

Personal Trainer: Describe a time when you were your fittest? Who was important in your life at that time?

Susan: Well, in high school I was part of my high school volleyball team. Our team was pretty good and I played a fair amount. My good friend and I played together and had a great time. Our coach was really supportive, but made us work very hard.

Personal Trainer: What did you really like about that time in your life? How did being on the team with your friend support you?

Susan: We really had fun together, but we pushed each other hard, too. So I guess you could say we worked hard and played hard! I really liked the way I felt back then. I was fit, I slept great, and I was happy.

Personal Trainer: That sounds great. Imagine yourself feeling now like you did back then. How would that change things for you?

Susan: I'd be happier because I wouldn't feel so alone in this challenge and I'd have somebody there to support me. That would feel really great.

Personal Trainer: That does sound motivating and happy. Can you picture doing that now with someone?

Susan: I could get my sister to come to the gym with me. She is hilarious and we have a great friendly rivalry going. We're pretty competitive but have grown beyond beating each other up!

Personal Trainer: That's great. How could you get her on board?

Susan: Well, actually, she has been wanting to do something with me since she gained weight after her pregnancy, but I was always busy. But now, I don't remember why I thought I was too busy to get together with her! And the gym has childcare!

Personal Trainer: Great. Do you think she'd be interested in doing some group training with us?

Susan: That would be awesome, and help us each stay on our budgets! And we have always talked about running the local Race for a Cure. We could train together for that.

Personal Trainer: Great! How would you like to begin?

Susan: I'll talk to her today, and call you tomorrow morning.

The length of time of the AI dialogue can fit well into the training session. Within the first 5 to 8 minutes, a Personal Trainer using AI can usually inquire about the client's stories (discover phase). Another 5–8 minutes will allow the Personal Trainer to learn about what the client is hoping to accomplish (dream phase). During the course of a 30-minute training session, it is highly likely that the client could easily move through most of the 5-D cycle. Obviously, with all of the other teaching that is taking place over the course of a training session, it may be difficult to work AI into the initial training session. However, during the course of the training relationship, Personal Trainers can work with their clients to incorporate AI into the sessions. Regardless of how AI is worked into the training session, remember the distinctive features of AI (14):

- AI is affirmative.
- AI is based in dialogue and positively framed questions (inquiry).
- AI is highly individualistic and based on the client's story.
- AI focuses on positive change rather than on fixing what is wrong.

A good Personal Trainer might think that the process of AI comes to an end with the achievement of the goal or dream. The great Personal Trainer knows that the process of growing, learning, and goal setting does not end; rather, the great Personal Trainer teaches and works with the client to create the cycle, the dream, and desire to continue to work toward the positive. The possibilities of what the client might achieve are seemingly endless; one achievement motivates the client to accomplish another, thus creating a momentum of motivation.

CONCEPT CHECK FOR APPRECIATIVE INQUIRY

- Appreciative inquiry builds on clients' past successes and helps them visualize future possibilities.
- The 5-D cycle—define, discover, dream, design, destiny—brings out the best aspirations, ideas, and values of the individual.
- Success breeds success.

MOTIVATIONAL INTERVIEWING

Motivational interviewing (MI) was developed 25 years ago as a counseling methodology for the treatment of alcohol abuse. Since then it has been used successfully in a variety of settings by a range of practitioners and is now recognized as an effective way to facilitate behavior change of many kinds. Motivational interviewing can be a valuable tool for Personal Trainers as they help clients adopt healthy behaviors that extend beyond the training session itself.

> MI "is not something that one does to people; rather, it is fundamentally a way of being with and for people."

Miller and Rollnick (12), the principal architects of MI, define it as "a client-centered, directive method for enhancing intrinsic motivation to change by exploring and resolving ambivalence" (p. 25). They expand this definition to explicitly acknowledge MI's spirit: MI "is not something that one does to people; rather, it is fundamentally a way of being with and for people."

A Client-Centered Conversation: The Heart of MI

The heart of MI is a conversation between a Personal Trainer and a client shaped by a shared vision and collaborative spirit. Reflecting this spirit, it is not your job to cajole, persuade, or coerce a client to change; rather, MI conversations facilitate behavior change by creating a partnership of equals. As equals, you and your client each bring a recognized expertise to the training relationship. Your expertise is obvious and acknowledged by your clients. But they are experts in their own lives and understand better than anyone their perspectives, values, and goals.

By assuming a client-centered approach, you respect the clients' expertise and their capacity for self-direction. After all, the power and choice to change are theirs alone. This can be challenging if you are accustomed to being the authority in the training relationship but it is, nonetheless, a valuable lesson to learn.

Client-centered relationships reduce confrontation and lower client resistance to change because they are inherently nonmanipulative. The ability to help clients adopt healthy behaviors ultimately depends on the clients' choice to move beyond their present circumstances—not your ability to craft their argument for them.

TIP #1: Change talk is the client's own argument for changing his or her behavior. It will always be more powerful to the client than your argument!

Acknowledge and Encourage Change Talk

When clients talk about adopting a new behavior in their own words, they clarify for themselves why the desired behavior is important to them. This is change talk, the fuel of an MI conversation. Change talk expresses readiness to change (the time is now), willingness to change (the change is important to me), and ability to change (I am confident). Learning to hear clients' change talk is the first step in engaging them in a conversation that increases the likelihood that change will occur. Here is what to listen for:

➤ *Disadvantages of the current behavior.* Clients may state that they are unhappy or discontent with "the way things are" right now. Statements can begin with "I want to" or "I really need to" or "There are good reasons to." Other examples are "I hate it that I have no energy." or "It really bothers me that I can't keep up with my spouse when we walk."

➤ *Advantages of change.* Clients may wistfully remark how much better "things" would be if present circumstances changed, and refer to a future behavior they are considering: "It might be better if . . ." or "It would be so nice to . . ." or "It will be great when . . . ." Change talk may also sound like "I'd probably be able to run a 5k" or "I'd feel a lot better." Note the unspoken word "if" or "when" at the end of these two sentences. When you hear a statement like this, prompt your client to examine the future more closely by asking, "What would have to happen in order to . . .?" or "What would you need to do in order to . . .?"

➤ *Optimism for change.* Clients may make confident or hopeful statements about change beginning with the words "I could" or "I can." The clients are stating that (a) change is possible and (b) they are the persons who can make it happen. Other examples might be "I can do it if I set my mind to it" or "I'm really determined this time."

➤ *Intention to change.* These statements can range from the committed language of "I will" to the more tentative "I may" or "I could consider" or "I think it's time."

TIP #2: When you hear a client's change talk, don't just stand there! Acknowledge it! Your client is exploring behavior change and inviting you to join them.

Harness the Power of Intrinsic Motivation

Clients who hire Personal Trainers are often motivated by extrinsic or outside factors. One client may want to wear a special outfit to a high school reunion. Another may be interested in lowering blood pressure and reducing medication dosage. Both these clients are extrinsically motivated: their rationale for exercise is logical and supported by their desire to attain a future goal or reward.

There is nothing wrong with extrinsic motivators. In fact, they are often important incentives. At the same time, extrinsic motivators have limited power and, by themselves, can not usually support lasting behavior change. Think about what happens to a client's motivation to lose weight after they have attended that special occasion.

All personal training clients are intrinsically motivated as well, although they often can't articulate it at first. Some clients may hire a Personal Trainer to help them lose a dress size (extrinsic) and grow to love exercise because it makes them feel strong and accomplished (intrinsic). Others may hire a Personal Trainer because they are worried about developing diabetes (extrinsic) and discover that being stronger permits them to play with the grandchildren they adore (intrinsic). Intrinsic motivators will remain important to clients long after they achieve the extrinsic goal they initially hired a Personal Trainer to help them accomplish. Such is the power of intrinsic motivation. Motivational interviewing uses this power to help move people beyond ambivalence, that place where your clients "sit on the fence" and debate with themselves about whether or not they will change.

Help Clients Explore and Resolve Ambivalence

Ambivalence is "sticky." It holds people in stasis and makes it difficult to change behavior. Motivational interviewing considers ambivalence a normal part of human nature and a natural component of change. Indeed, it's difficult to imagine a person who is 100% certain about everything 100% of the time, and this includes your clients! As frustrating as your ambivalent clients can be, remember that their wishy-washiness is a rich source of change talk. Asking them to explore it will help them resolve it. Motivational interviewing's four principles, along with the OARS communication skills, help create a collaborative environment (12).

Four MI Principles

The following four principles foster behavior change and maximize the power of change talk.

➤ *Empathy: Accept clients where they are.* Empathy flows naturally from a client-centered approach. When you accept clients' perceptions, values, and concerns without judgment or blame, you facilitate understanding. Empathy does not imply agreement, however, and you can empathize with clients without endorsing their beliefs and actions. Showing empathy will permit you to express your own opinions within an environment of mutual respect.

➤ *Self-efficacy: Believe in your clients.* Self-efficacy, discussed later in this chapter, is your clients' belief in their ability to succeed. This belief is both a good predictor of whether or not change will occur and a powerful motivator. Confidence can reignite enthusiasm when clients doubt their ability. Encouragement can help them retain focus during challenging times.

➤ *Rolling with resistance (Box 10.2):* Resistance talk is the opposite of change talk; it moves a person away from change. A client's resistance is a clear signal for you to respond differently. When you roll with resistance, you do not argue or directly oppose the client even if the science is supportive. The Personal Trainer's role is to honor the clients' perspective as valid for them even if there is disagreement with their position. When appropriate, invite the clients to consider other perspectives.

TIP #3: When you encounter resistance from a client, stop talking! Listen! Put yourself into the client's shoes and hear things from his or her perspective!

➤ *Developing discrepancy (Box 10.3):* Help your clients explore the gap between where they are now and their vision for the future. Developing discrepancy stimulates behavior change because it creates internal discomfort. The greater the gap between the status quo and the desired future, the harder it becomes to justify the current behavior, the more attractive change becomes, and the less ambivalence a person feels. When the discrepancy becomes untenable, people will choose to change. They will become unstuck and move past their ambivalence in order to close the gap.

| BOX 10.2 | **Rolling with Resistance** |

Your client wants to lose weight. She is willing to exercise with you, but she says that discussion of her diet is off limits. You believe that this will make it more difficult for her to achieve her weight loss goal. To share your knowledge in a way that is nonconfrontational and honors her beliefs, ask your client whether she is willing to discuss general nutritional guidelines. Chances are good she will agree. If she doesn't, let it go and reassure her that if she ever wants to discuss this topic with you, you are willing. If she agrees, however, you now have permission to share nutrition information and you can even voice your opinion. When you do this nonjudgmentally and in the spirit of helpfulness, you will not put your client on the defensive.

When you are finished, ask your client how she wants to use the information. Be ready to accept what she tells you as the truth for her in that moment. If she asks for additional information and/or feedback, acknowledge her receptiveness and provide it. If not, simply thank her for listening and express your confidence in her ability to use the information if and when she's ready.

Linking the gap to an intrinsic motivator—like a personal goal or value—is a powerful way to foster behavior change, and it is in this way that MI is directive.

TIP #4: MI deliberately develops discrepancy to widen the gap between clients' present behaviors and the future they want. Exploring this gap reduces ambivalence and encourages clients to move forward.

These four principles (empathy, self-efficacy, rolling with resistance, and developing discrepancy) create an environment for conversations that are client-centered and directive. The skills below provide the nuts and bolts of these conversations to generate and sustain change talk.

OARS: Crafting an MI Conversation

The four skills of OARS—open-ended questions, affirmations, reflections, and summary—are the primary communication skills of MI. Collectively, they provide a framework for acknowledging and responding to a client's change talk (12).

➤ Open-ended questions presume no specific answer and encourage clients to look deeper into their own experience and remain engaged in change talk. They are not "yes or no" questions, nor

| BOX 10.3 | **Developing Discrepancy in Action** |

To develop discrepancy, you must be curious about the gap—not just the benefits of the new behavior, but the costs as well. The following sets of questions ask a client to examine and articulate the pros and cons of both adopting the new behavior and maintaining the status quo.

"Sue, how will exercise impact your life?" and "What if you didn't begin to exercise. What would life be like for you in 5 years?"

"Dave, what are the things you like best about strength training? What makes them of value to you?" and "What are some of the not-so-great things? What makes them a concern?"

"Lisa, why is losing 20 pounds important to you?" and "Why now?"

Your interest and curiosity will help your clients identify and explore both sides of the gap and weigh the pros and cons, enabling them to choose their own path and be confident in their choice.

do they elicit specific data in response (e.g., "When was the last time you exercised?"). Such questions shut the door to the clients' self-exploration. In contrast, consider asking, "How did you feel the last time you exercised?" This open-ended question invites your clients to describe the experience in any way they choose.

➤ Affirmations are compliments or statements of appreciation and understanding that show interest and respect for the client. How clients respond to an affirmation tells a lot about what they value. When clients are acknowledged for a value that is special to them, they will "glow" as if you have shown a spotlight on a part of their character in which they take pride. For example, when a client makes a special effort to fit a workout into his or her busy schedule, you can acknowledge his or her commitment: "I know it took some extra planning to get your workouts in this week. You're really committed to improving your health!" Notice that you are doing more than complimenting *what* your client did. You are recognizing something about him or her *as a person*—in this case your client's willingness to take responsibility for his or her own health. This is what makes acknowledgments so powerful.

➤ Reflections mirror clients' statements back to them (Box 10.4). They allow clients to hear their own words and intentions a second time. They reinforce the original message and encourage them to elaborate and amplify their original intention. Try to use reflections twice as often as open-ended questions because they keep the client "in the experience." Reflections are declarations. Your voice should not rise at the end of the statement as if asking a question. Begin a reflection by saying: "So you feel. . . . It sounds like you. . . . You're wondering if. . . ."

➤ Summarizing provides a way for you to make sure that you have heard your clients correctly. And, like reflections, summaries let the clients hear their words one more time. A summary statement might be "It sounds like you're pleased with your progress thus far and I really appreciate your commitment!" or "You're consistently exercising twice each week on your own, and you feel stronger and look forward to your workouts."

The heart of MI is a conversation of equals infused with a collaborative spirit. Fueling this conversation is the clients' own change talk. Accept the client wholly—including their perceptions, their ambivalence, and their resistance. Hear and respond to the clients' change talk, and help them explore the discrepancy between the present they experience now and the future they want to create. Listen for and help clients distinguish their intrinsic motivators, those motivators that support long-term, sustainable behavior change.

BOX **10.4**   **Reflections in Action**

Reflections can range from a simple statement that repeats an element of what the speaker has said to a guess about an unspoken meaning. In the examples below, the Personal Trainer (1) acknowledges the client's words, (2) his or her emotion, and (3) makes a guess about future actions.

Client: I'm definitely going to walk 3 miles 3 times this week.

Personal Trainer (1): Great! You'll walk 3 miles 3 times this week.

Personal Trainer (2): You're really excited that you can walk 3 miles 3 times this week! or
    You sound hesitant about walking 3 miles 3 times this week. What's up?

Personal Trainer (3): Three miles, 3 times this week. . . . You're thinking about the 5k this fall!

    Reflections need not be wholly accurate to be effective. If you miss the mark, your client will acknowledge your statement, offer a correction, and move on in the conversation. The important thing is that you are inviting additional exploration and stimulating change talk. Trust that when you do this, your client will know what to do.

Concept Check for MI

➤ MI is a client-centered approach that respects a client's expertise in his or her own life.

➤ Change talk is fundamental to behavior change because it is the client's own argument for change.

➤ Intrinsic motivators are more powerful and more lasting than extrinsic motivators. A masterful Personal Trainer will help the clients link their intrinsic motivators to their goals.

➤ The four OARS skills are open-ended questions, affirmations, reflections, and summaries. These skills provide a framework for acknowledging and responding to clients' change talk.

BUILDING ON POSITIVE EXPERIENCE

Help clients identify and use their intrinsic motivators by building on their positive experiences, present and past.

Intrinsic motivators are important to long-term behavior change; these factors make it easier for clients to maintain momentum, recover from lapses, and learn from their past successes. Help clients identify and use their intrinsic motivators by building on their positive experiences, present and past. In this section, we will examine three avenues.

➤ *Personal strengths.* Everyone has personal strengths, and creating a life that uses our strengths makes us happy and fulfilled. Both you and your clients bring a set of strengths to your training sessions and to your relationship. Acknowledging yours will elevate the level of service you provide. Reinforcing your clients' strengths will help them stay true to their goals.

➤ *Generative moments.* Personal Trainers continually have the opportunity to ask clients what they are learning about themselves and how they can apply this learning to their lives. This kind of growth and learning is empowering to clients because it builds self-awareness and self confidence.

➤ *Self-efficacy and self-esteem.* Building self-efficacy and self-esteem are critical components to behavior change and are covered in detail later in this chapter. By identifying and discussing a client's past successes with self-change, you can begin the process of confidence building, a foundation for the development of self-esteem and self-efficacy.

Your Personal Strengths

Using personal strengths feels natural and easy because they are innate characteristics. When you bring your strengths to a training session, you will function at your best.

Positive psychology is the study of positive emotion, positive character, and positive institutions (19). This relatively new field has provided many significant developments in the understanding of what makes people happy and fulfilled as human beings. One such development is the concept of *signature strengths.* There are 24 character strengths (16), each describing a specific aspect of positive human character. The strengths are grouped into six categories or virtues. Virtues are prized among most religious and philosophical traditions (19), and collectively they "capture the notion of good character." The characteristics of character strengths are:

➤ moral traits and can be developed and strengthened by choice

➤ valued for themselves rather than as a means to an end

➤ using a strength elevates rather than diminishes others

➤ ubiquitous

Each person has the capacity to exhibit any of the 24 character strengths (Box 10.5) and tends to rely on some more than others. The Web site www.authentichappiness.com offers a free, online survey called the VIA (Values in Action) Signature Strengths Questionnaire, which ranks individual strengths in order of importance to the individual completing the questionnaire. The top five

---

BOX 10.5   Values in Action Signature Strengths

Wisdom and knowledge—*Cognitive strengths that entail the acquisition and use of knowledge*
Curiosity: taking an interest in all of ongoing experience
Love of learning: mastering new skills, topics, and bodies of knowledge
Open-mindedness: thinking things through and examining them from all sides
Creativity: thinking of novel and productive ways to do things
Perspective: being able to provide wise counsel to others
Courage—*Emotional strengths that involve the exercise of will to accomplish goals in the face of opposition, external or internal*
Bravery: not shrinking from threat, challenge, difficulty, or pain
Persistence: finishing what one starts
Authenticity: speaking the truth and presenting oneself in a genuine way
Zest: approaching life with excitement and energy
Humanity—*Interpersonal strengths that involve "tending and befriending" others*
Kindness: doing favors and good deeds for others
Love: valuing close relationships with others
Social intelligence: being aware of the motives and feelings of self and others
Justice—*Civic strengths that underlie healthy community life*
Fairness: treating all people equitably
Leadership: organizing group activities and seeing that they happen
Teamwork: working well as a member of a group or team
Temperance—*Strengths that protect against excess*
Forgiveness: forgiving those who have done wrong
Modesty: letting one's accomplishments speak for themselves
Prudence: being careful about one's choices; not saying or doing things that might later be regretted
Self-regulation: regulating what one feels and does
Transcendence—*Strengths that forge connections to the larger universe and provide meaning*
Appreciation of beauty and excellence: appreciating beauty, excellence, and/or skilled performance in all domains of life
Gratitude: being aware of and thankful for the good things that happen
Hope: expecting the best and working to achieve it
Humor: liking to laugh and tease; bringing smiles to other people
Spirituality/religiousness: having coherent beliefs about the higher purpose and meaning of life

---

strengths are the Signature Strengths. These are the qualities a Personal Trainer naturally brings to the work and other life activities. Identifying Signature Strengths is the first step to using them effectively.

USING YOUR STRENGTHS

Look at Box 10.5. Which of the strengths resonate most? How do you use your strengths? Which strengths do you use when you are with clients? Which could you use more fully? How do your strengths impact the way you view your job? How do they influence which clients you attract?

TIP #5: Consider. . . . Do you love the creativity of designing new training programs for your clients? Do you naturally bring humor onto the fitness floor and into your training sessions? Do open-mindedness and love of learning make you the perfect Personal Trainer for novice exercisers?

Are you the Personal Trainer who is both kind and authentic—the one who attracts "high maintenance" clients because you know exactly what to say to keep them engaged and committed to their program? Choose a strength you would like to use more effectively (it needn't be a Signature Strength). Make a list of ways you can use it. Practice using it and, as you do, notice the impact it has on your effectiveness as a Personal Trainer and your satisfaction with your job. Keep in mind that while all strengths are desirable and good, you may find that some will serve you better in certain situations. Fortunately, you can develop any strength you choose.

TIP #6: Consider. . . . How does practicing modesty by attributing a client's progress to his or her hard work—rather than to your skills—alter your relationship? What happens when you remain curious about your client's habitual noncompliance rather than labeling him or her (to yourself) as lazy or a sloth? What client attributes bring you zest? What strengths are missing when you stop listening and cease to be empathetic?

The Personal Trainer's ability to impact the health of clients depends on more than your knowledge and experience. Just as education is fundamental to success, self-awareness serves equally as well. Character strengths shape the content and quality of interactions with people. They are a fundamental piece of who you are as a Personal Trainer, what you bring to your work, and how you impact your clients. As you consciously apply your strengths, you will find new ways to include them into your work. The reward is a practice that gives you greater fulfillment and becoming the best Personal Trainer you can be.

YOUR CLIENTS' STRENGTHS

Even if you do not use the Signature Strengths Questionnaire with your clients, your awareness of their strengths and values will be helpful as you facilitate their development of new healthy behaviors. For example, your client's family is the linchpin of her life and every session includes a story about her grandchildren and their antics. In fact, she hired you to elevate her level of self-care so that she could be a good role model for her children and lives long enough to play with her grandchildren. Her love of family is a powerful intrinsic motivator, one that you can acknowledge by regularly asking questions that tie your client's growing strength and capacity to her ability to lead the life she wants. Listening to clients for clues about other strengths can help you key into untapped sources of motivation for them.

Generative Moments

Most Personal Trainers have heard clients repeatedly grumble how their hectic lives make it difficult to schedule time to keep fit. Some have experienced the thrill of seeing clients arrive for training sessions literally glowing with the sense of accomplishment after completing their first 10K race. Others have watched frustration build as clients repeatedly fail to achieve their weekly workout commitments or weight loss goals. Although the circumstances vary, these examples have something in common. They all present an opportunity for the client to learn from their behavior and choose a new course of action. They all are the "stuff" of generative moments.

> Generative moments "are moments when clients are stimulated by the prospect of change. Such moments can often be recognized by the strength of their emotional charge, either positive or negative" (20).

Generative moments "are moments when clients are stimulated by the prospect of change. Such moments can often be recognized by the strength of their emotional charge, either positive or negative" (p. 3) (20). Circumstances or experiences that carry an emotional charge connect people with their values and intrinsic motivators. In short, it's difficult for us to get excited or agitated about things we don't care about. When we are emotionally invested, the opposite is true.

BOX **10.6**	**Making the Most of Generative Moments**

Ultimately, generative moments help your client learn about himself or herself and grow as an individual. You can help him or her by asking the following questions. Notice that they are all open-ended questions, and give your client space to look for an answer that suits them:
- "What did you learn from this experience [or discussion]?"
- "How can you use this knowledge going forward?"
- "How might this learning affect your future?"
- "What would you like to do now?"
- "What is the next step for you?"

The answers your client provides to these questions will reinforce what has been learned and how it will be applied in his or her life. This is what makes generative moments such powerful learning experiences for your client and rewarding experiences for you. They are cocreated by you and your client, and they confirm a relationship built on trust, respect, and common goals.

During generative moments, clients are often able to examine the factors that give the experience value and meaning. Because of this new information and awareness, they may be more receptive to taking action that applies this learning in some way. Personal Trainers who are able to recognize these moments can offer their clients a special gift that extends beyond their more traditional role.

Each generative moment begins with a story or theme. A client's story could be: "My first 10k was such an amazing experience. It was so much fun and I really felt like an athlete!" Themes usually link a series of experiences: "I'm frustrated because I'm not making any progress. I weigh myself every day and the scale doesn't move." As your client provides the details of his or her experience, listen with curiosity, reflection, and empathy.

When his or her energy is positive, you can ask your client to identify what made the experience so great. This will help clients acknowledge their values and determine why the experience was meaningful. You can then help your client integrate this knowledge into a fitness regimen. For example, maybe your client is willing to train more intensely when his schedule is related to a local road race. He is driven by the competition along with the new sensation of feeling like an athlete.

When the client's energy is negative, help him or her realize that lack of success is also an opportunity to learn if he or she is willing to explore the experience and his or her behavior with you. You can help him or her do this with open-ended questions like "What troubles you the most about your lack of progress?" or "What do you think your biggest obstacles are?" or "What do you have to do more [or less] of to achieve your goals?" Your client's answers to these questions will point to some aspect of his or her behavior that will benefit from further exploration.

For example, maybe your client states that her biggest obstacle is consistently measuring and weighing her food as she promised to do. You investigate further and learn that she regularly guesses the quantity of what she's eating. Now that you know this, the two of you can brainstorm other options that are more acceptable and your client can choose one that works for her. She might choose to cook a prepackaged healthy meal once each day and supplement it with a salad. The two of you agree that she can have unlimited vegetables (no measuring) and she is willing to limit the salad dressing to two capfuls (easy, convenient measuring). When you brainstorm with your clients, be creative and willing to think outside of the box (see Box 10.6).

Concept Check for Positive Experience

> Personal Trainers can help clients build on their own powerful intrinsic motivators by exploring character strengths, capturing generative moments, and increasing self-efficacy.

➤ Consciously using your own character strengths in your work will enhance your sense of fulfillment and joy. Identifying your clients' strengths will help them stay connected to the values that drive their goals and nourish their self-efficacy.

➤ A generative moment is identified by a strong emotional charge, either positive or negative. An exceptional Personal Trainer can transform the client's emotion into positive change talk.

Self-Efficacy and Self-Esteem

TIP #7: Henry Ford once said: "If you think you can do a thing, or think you can't do a thing, you're right."

Self-efficacy and self-esteem are different but related constructs (Box 10.7). Whereas self-efficacy has more to do with initiating and sustaining positive behavior outcomes, self-esteem relates to overall happiness, self-worth, self-respect, and an internal sense of well-being. Personal Trainers work to improve both. Nothing is more personal than our bodies, our feelings, and how we perceive ourselves; consequently clients must become physically and emotionally comfortable with the process and the pursuit of personal change. The impetus for change becomes motivational only when it involves the whole person; how we feel about the process of change impacts our ability to make the changes. The cause-and-effect relationship goes both ways: physiological states affect self-efficacy and vice versa (1).

> *Whereas self-efficacy has more to do with initiating and sustaining positive behavior outcomes, self-esteem relates to overall happiness, self-worth, self-respect, and an internal sense of well-being.*

SELF-EFFICACY

Self-efficacy describes the circular relationship between belief and action: the more you believe you can do something, the more likely it is that you will do it; the more you do something successfully, the more you believe that you will be able to do it again. The opposite is also true: the more you believe that you cannot do something, the less likely you will do it; the more you do something unsuccessfully, the less you believe that you will be able to do it again. In other words, adapting an old adage, "nothing succeeds like success," and "nothing breeds failure like failure." Your clients' sense of self-efficacy will influence the choices they make, the amount of effort they exert, whether they will persist when they are confronted with obstacles, and how they perceive their ability to positively affect their own lives.

A strong sense of self-efficacy enhances accomplishment in many ways. People with high self-efficacy are more inclined to attempt new behaviors, set challenging goals, and maintain a strong commitment. They recover their confidence quickly after a setback or relapse. They have a more positive outlook, which enhances accomplishments, lowers stress, and decreases the occurrence of depression. People with low self-efficacy are less likely to try new things. They tend to give up easily when faced with difficult tasks and often have little motivation or commitment. They are slow to recover confidence after a setback or relapse and are more prone to suffer from stress and depression (1).

BOX 10.7 Self-Efficacy and Self-Esteem

Self-Efficacy = the belief that one has the capability to initiate and sustain a desired behavior (the exercise of control)

Self-Esteem = the belief that one has value and self-worth (the evaluation of self)

SELF-ESTEEM

Self-esteem concerns one's sense of personal value, self-worth, and overall happiness and positive feelings. Although high self-esteem does not necessarily predict that a client will be successful in taking positive action, it does impact two areas of which Personal Trainers and clients can leverage self-efficacy. First, high self-esteem can increase a client's initiative—those with high self-esteem are more likely to participate in activities that will make them feel good (conversely those with low self-esteem are less likely to make the connection between positive actions and feeling good). Second, clients with high self-esteem will be more resilient in the face of failure. For example, a person with high self-esteem is more likely to return to the gym and "try again" after a particularly challenging workout or to get back to positive eating habits after a lapse. In short, they rebound move quickly than do clients with lower self-esteem (4). High self-esteem can be used by Personal Trainers and clients in the development of self-efficacy. When that happens in an area that matters greatly to the client, self-efficacy helps bolster self-esteem and the two concepts work hand in hand.

Many of the tools and techniques covered in this chapter, including AI, MI, and setting SMART goals (Box 10.8), serve to enhance both self-efficacy and self-esteem. As umbrella concepts, self-efficacy and self-esteem encompass these various approaches and serve to illuminate the best coaching has to offer.

FOSTERING SELF-ESTEEM AND SELF-EFFICACY IN CLIENTS

In the course of training clients, Personal Trainers will have many opportunities to help them grow their self-esteem and self-efficacy.

Tune in to the Client's Self-Image. The chances of getting someone who really believes that he or she is a "couch potato" to start to exercise are slim. This inconsistent self-image is something that

---

BOX 10.8   How to Set SMART Goals?

Help your clients develop goals that are specific, measurable, action-based, realistic, and time-constrained.

Specific
Goals should be specific and well-defined, with clear actions that will be taken. Details of how and when your client will accomplish each specific behavior can be detailed in a contingency contract.

Measurable
Goals should be objective and measurable so that it is clear to both the client and the Personal Trainer when they have been achieved.

Action-based
Your clients' goals should be things they will actually do. For example, losing 2 lb is an outcome, not an action. Doing cardiovascular exercise for 30 minutes each day and eating a healthy breakfast every day are actions.

Realistic
Your clients' goals must be possible to achieve, given the time and resources available.

Time-constrained
Goals must have a deadline. If there is no time frame set, there is no sense of urgency.
   Here are examples of SMART goals. Notice that each meets all the criteria a SMART goal requires:
   I will do my strength training routine at the club on Tuesday and Friday evening of this week.
   On Monday, Wednesday, and Friday morning I will walk at a pace of 3.5 mph on my treadmill at home for 30 minutes.

must be confronted for change to begin; the "couch potato" must truly begin to believe that change is possible. Overcoming negative thoughts and staying positive help a client reestablish positive self-talk and, as a result, positive self-image. So, for example, you might encourage your client to take a negative statement ("I cannot possibly do push-ups; push-ups hurt my wrists.") and rephrase it into a positive one ("I can do five push-ups against the wall.") The client can then begin to associate the desired behavior with a positive self-image, leading to increased performance and adherence. Encouraging appropriate expectations ("I will exercise 3 days next week" instead of "I will lose 20 pounds this month") will prevent clients' disappointment and frustration.

Using positive reinforcement also assists clients in changing negative self-concept. A simple tool to use is to have the clients write positive notes after each workout about their efforts. Maintaining a workout journal, tracking how they felt about themselves after each workout, gives them an accurate record of their own attempts, the Personal Trainer's comments, and a tool for personal reflection.

Be Mindful of the Client's Mood. Mood can also greatly affect a client's estimation of his or her own personal efficacy. A positive mood will improve a client's perception of self-efficacy, whereas a depressed mood will lessen it. Feelings of stress and tension may affect a client's expectation of his or her performance. In areas of strength and endurance, clients may interpret fatigue or aches and pains as

> *A positive mood will improve a client's perception of self-efficacy, whereas a depressed mood will lessen it.*

signs of weakness. When a client presents with an exhausted or stressed appearance, the Personal Trainer might begin with a simple warm-up and gradually add intensity as the client's mood improves. Psychologically, exercise causes a boost in self-esteem, improved self-image, confidence, and feelings of accomplishment—as well as a break from other aspects of life.

Partner with the Clients in Planning and Decision Making. The greater the sense of ownership clients have over their exercise program, the greater will be their confidence and sense of control. Encouraging client participation in the planning process can be a balancing act. You want them to be involved, but you, as an exercise professional, should be aware of potential outcomes of different workout regimens and intensities. Your honesty in explaining this to your clients will help them make the right choices and increase your worth in their eyes.

Use Sincere and Authentic Verbal Persuasion. Effective verbal persuasion communicates to clients a confidence in their ability to achieve their goals. It is not about convincing them to do something they are not ready to do. Such persuasion hinges on the credibility of the Personal Trainer and the quality of the client–Personal Trainer relationship. Verbal persuasion can bolster clients' self-change when it is based on a realistic assessment of their abilities. Your clients can be persuaded that they are able to master given tasks when you sincerely believe that they are able to do so. Clients

> *Verbal persuasion can bolster clients' self-change when it is based on a realistic assessment of their abilities.*

are more likely to put forth and sustain greater efforts than if they harbor self-doubts and dwell on their own personal deficiencies. For example, a client may balk at adding more to her program, believing that she is at her maximum effort. But you notice that she is finishing the final set at the current weight with ease and rebounding quickly, and sincerely believe that she can safely and successfully increase the weight. Your expressing your confidence that she can indeed lift the heavier weight may convince her to try. On the other hand, if your client is dragging at the end of her final set and struggling with the last few repetitions, attempting to persuade her that she can do it is likely to backfire and affect your credibility.

Encourage the Client to Identify Positive Role Models. People want to identify with other people. We often look to others to emulate a desired behavior. This is called modeling, and these experiences are not only highly effective in learning new behaviors but also a vital factor in building self-efficacy. The Personal Trainer is the role model, which comes with both great opportunity and responsibility! Clients will notice how fit you look, what you relate to them about your nutrition, and how they perceive you treating them and others. Clients will observe and copy your technique until they internalize these skills and can consequently manage each desired exercise protocol successfully.

> *The more success stories clients have in their repertoire, and the more they tell those stories both to their Personal Trainer and to others, the more likely it becomes that they will see themselves as able to achieve their desired outcomes.*

Sharing and telling stories are other ways to help clients build self-efficacy. Tell stories from your own life experience (taking care not to sound boastful). It is even more effective to encourage clients to find their own success stories. For example, you might encourage a client who wants to participate in a 5K race to first attend a local race and watch others compete. This will increase your clients' self-efficacy, especially if they are watching people similar to themselves. The greater the perceived similarity, the greater the impact this vicarious experience will have on self-efficacy. The more success stories clients have in their repertoire, and the more they tell those stories both to their Personal Trainer and to others, the more likely it becomes that they will see themselves as able to achieve their desired outcomes.

Facilitate the Client's Mastery Experiences. For the client, a mastery experience is the feeling he or she gets when achieving a goal. It is both a powerful source and the ultimate outcome of self-efficacy. Positive outcomes lead to increased self-efficacy, whereas negative outcomes lead to decreased self-efficacy. Setting small achievable goals (e.g., SMART goals; Box 10.8) is effective because it facilitates early and ongoing mastery experiences.

SUMMARY

These motivational tools have proven invaluable to a range of healthcare professionals in facilitating behavior change; however, they are not a one-size-fits-all approach. Every client will come with his or her own set of traits, troubles, desires, and dreams. The Personal Trainer's ability to effectively listen to them, discover and amplify their strengths, help them uncover their intrinsic motivators, and work together with them to build their sense of accomplishment is the difference between being a good Personal Trainer and being a masterful Personal Trainer. Self-efficacy is the belief that you have the capability to initiate and sustain a desired behavior. Self-esteem is the belief that one has value and self-worth. Appreciative inquiry, MI, and setting SMART goals serve to enhance both self-efficacy and self-esteem. Setting and achieving SMART goals encourage early mastery experiences, which foster adherence and further success.

REFERENCES

1. Bandura A. *Self-Efficacy: The Exercise of Control*. New York: W.H. Freeman and Company; 1997.
2. Bandura A. Self-efficacy. In: Ramachaudran VS, editor. *Encyclopedia of Human Behavior*. Vol. 4. New York: Academic Press; p. 71–81. (Reprinted in Friedman H, editor. *Encyclopedia of Mental Health*. San Diego (CA): Academic Press; 1994.)
3. Bandura A. *Social Foundations of Thought and Action: A Social Cognitive Theory*. Upper Saddle River (NJ): Prentice Hall; 1986.
4. Baumeister RF, Campbell JD, Krueger JI, Vohs KD. Does high self-esteem cause better performance, interpersonal success, happiness or healthier lifestyles? *Psychol Sci Public Interest*. 2003;4(1):1–44.
5. Berg-Smith S. *The Art of Health Behavior Change Counseling: An Introduction to Motivational Interviewing*. San Francisco (CA): Berg-Smith Training and Consultation; 2006.
6. Biswas-Diener R, Dean B. *Positive Psychology Coaching*. Hoboken (NJ): John Wiley & Sons, Inc.; 2007.
7. Cox R. Effecting positive change through appreciative inquiry [Internet]. 2004 [cited 2008 Sept 8]. Available from: www.executiveforum.com. Bernard J. Mohr. *25th Anniversary Management Forum Series*. Portland, OR; 2004 Oct 27.
8. Duskey H, Lincoln G. Making your job work for you—Cultivating your personal strengths. *NEHRSA E-News* [Internet]. [cited 2008 March]. Available from: http://www.nehrsa.org/Files/Library/ENews_March08_Full.pdf
9. Duskey H. Get out of sales and go fishing! *ACSM's Certified News*. Vol. 17, Issue 5. Indianapolis (IN): American College of Sports Medicine; 2007;17(5):7.
10. Fredrickson BL. The value of positive emotions. *Am Sci*. 2003;91:330–5.
11. Highsteen G, Silverio G. Coaching behavior change. In: *Wellcoaches Training Manual*. Wellesley (MA): Wellcoaches Corporation; 2004. p. 7–30.

12. Miller WR, Rollnick S. *Motivational Interviewing*. 2nd ed. New York (NY): The Guilford Press; 2002. p. 25.

13. Moore M, Claps F, Highsteen GR, Larsen K, Graddy LT, Lavin TJ. Exercise psychology, motivation, and behavior change. In: Thompson WR, Baldwin KE, Pire N, Niederpruem, M, editors. *ACSM's Resources for the Personal Trainer*. 2nd ed. Baltimore (PA): Lippincott Williams & Wilkins; 2006. p. 208–37.

14. Moore SM, Charvat J. Promoting health behavior change using appreciative inquiry: moving from deficit models to affirmation models of care. *Fam Community Health*. 2007:30 S64–74.

15. Orem S, Binkert J, Clancy A. Building dialog for effective change: coaching with the five principles of appreciative inquiry [Internet]. 2005. [cited 2008 Sept 8]. International Coach Federation Research Symposium, San Jose, CA. Available from: www.coachfederation.org

16. Peterson C. *A Primer in Positive Psychology*. New York: Oxford University Press; 2006.

17. Rhode R. Introduction to motivational interviewing for health, fitness & wellness coaches. In: *Wellcoaches Training Manual*. Wellesley (MA): Wellcoaches Corporation; 2004. p. 1–21.

18. Seligman MEP, Steen A, Park N, Peterson C. Positive psychology progress: empirical validation of interventions. *Am Psychol*. 2005;60(5):410–21.

19. Seligman MEP. *Authentic Happiness*. New York (NY): Free Press; 2002. p. 129–37.

20. Tschannen-Moran B, Jackson E. Generative moments in coaching. In: *Wellcoaches Training Manual*. Wellesley (MA): Wellcoaches Corporation; 2004. p. 1–17.

21. Tschannen-Moran B, Moore M. Coaching presence. In: *Wellcoaches Training Manual*. Wellesley (MA): Wellcoaches Corporation; 2004. p. 1–22.

22. Tschannen-Moran B. Appreciative inquiry in coaching. In: *Wellcoaches Training Manual*. Wellesley (MA): Wellcoaches Corporation; 2004. p. 1–18.

23. Tschannen-Moran B. Motivational interviewing in coaching. In: *Wellcoaches Training Manual*. Wellesley (MA): Wellcoaches Corporation; 2004. p. 1–17.

24. Wellcoaches Corporation. Self efficacy and self esteem. In: *Wellcoaches Training Manual*. Wellesley (MA): Wellcoaches Corporation; 2004. Chapter 5.

25. Whitworth L, Kimsey-House H, Sandahl P. *Co-Active Coaching*. Mountain View (CA): Davies-Black Publishing; 1998.

11

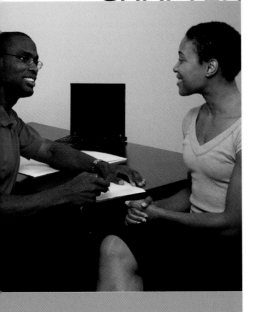

Training the Whole Client: Putting It All Together

OBJECTIVES

- Understand the concept of the expert paradox and how it can impact your effectiveness as a Personal Trainer.
- Describe the five levels of the Behavior Change Pyramid and discuss how clients might progress from the base to the peak.
- Put the motivational tools into context by thinking about in which stages you would employ different techniques.
- Discuss relapse prevention and specific ways you can help your client anticipate and avoid relapses.

Change is not a linear process. In these chapters, we have investigated the science of behavior change and have provided you with the tools to consider, assess, and address the complex interactions that make up your clients' change. It may seem a little less straightforward than originally thought: A potential client decides to get in shape, chooses you to help her, and works diligently to achieve the outcomes and rewards you both envision.

Indeed, you may occasionally have a client for whom this linear path applies. But for the most part, you will be partnering with unique individuals with intricate sets of thoughts, feelings, attitudes, and issues, all of which impact how they show up in your life on any given day. Your successful navigation of these issues, and your sensitivity to how they impact your clients' performance, will make you a successful Personal Trainer. In the process, you will learn and grow yourself in ways that enhance both your career and your life. In the following chapter, we present a way for you to pull together all you have learned in Chapters 7–10.

> *You will be partnering with unique individuals with intricate sets of thoughts, feelings, attitudes, and issues, all of which impact how they show up in your life on any given day.*

THE BEHAVIOR CHANGE PYRAMID

Just as MapQuest (www.mapquest.com) outlines each step between our home and our destination, the Behavior Change Pyramid (Fig. 11.1) helps the Personal Trainer and the client move forward toward the client's fitness goals (3). The Pyramid draws on the Transtheoretical model for behavior change developed by Prochaska et al. (4) discussed in Chapter 8, which describes how people move through stages of change. Using the stages of change outlined in this work, the Pyramid provides a systematic "roadmap" through the change process beginning with the all-important step of imagining the change—the cognitive work that supports any change. You and your clients can use this roadmap to work together to help them stay on course throughout their journey, building self-efficacy and a sense of accomplishment.

> *The Pyramid provides a systematic "roadmap" through the change process beginning with the all-important step of imagining the change—the cognitive work that supports any change.*

THE EXPERT PARADOX

As a Personal Trainer, you (like other healthcare professionals) will give advice and instruction based on your expertise and experience, and clients will come to you because you are an expert. But paradoxically, research has shown that this relationship also can encourage the lack of confidence people already feel—the sense that they are not really "in charge" (2). Feelings of low self-efficacy ("I can't really do this") eventually win out over behaviors as the newness wears off and people find it difficult to find the time to exercise or the desire to make healthy food choices. You may find that they begin not to show up for training appointments or not to honor the commitments they made about their behaviors between sessions.

So what do you do? Climbing the Pyramid with your clients, you can

1. facilitate the connections between their behaviors with their own deeper motivation (Vision);
2. help them make a commitment and plan for the support they need to act (Preparation);
3. help them set appropriate goals and rewards for achieving them (Action);
4. help them brainstorm relapse prevention strategies (Results); and
5. celebrate their achievement (The New Me).

Climbing the Pyramid does not require abandoning the critical role of providing expert guidance, but rather recognizing that people change from within—not simply in response to information (if this

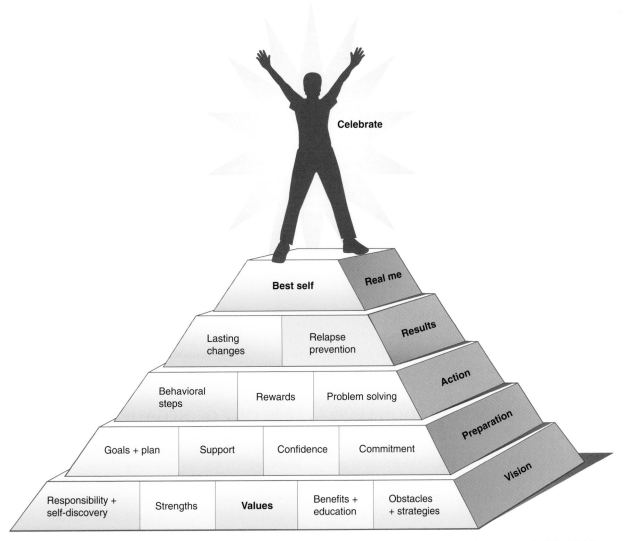

FIGURE 11.1. The behavior change pyramid. (From Moore M, Tshannen-Moran B. *Coaching Psychology Manual*. Philadelphia: Wolters Kluwer/Lippincott Williams & Wilkins; 2010.)

were the case, everyone who now smokes would quit after he or she reads the Surgeon General's notice on a pack of cigarettes). Helping clients climb the Pyramid requires a challenging shift from telling to asking, from knowing (the facts) to being comfortable not knowing (the client's thoughts), from drawing conclusions for struggling clients to letting them find their own way, and from trying to get clients to build new and unfamiliar strengths to recognizing and building on strengths they already possess.

THE VISION LEVEL—DEVELOP A SOLID BASE FOR CHANGE

The all-important vision level builds self-awareness of the benefits of change, the obstacles to change, and the opportunity for your client to explore why he or she wants to change in the first place. Your being interested in and curious about clients' readiness to change in initial sessions can help them look internally and do some of this work. For example, you may, as one seasoned Personal Trainer does, encourage clients to get at their core values by asking them to write down 15 reasons why they want to get in shape (Goldman E, personal interview, 2006). After listing each one, she instructs them to answer the question "What's so great about that?" The client who has made a New Year's resolution may eventually get down to the very real wish of wanting to be healthy enough to play with her growing grandchildren, which connects her with her key life values. Eventually, your clients will get a little deeper and begin to draw on their motivation—or find out they are not all that motivated right now.

Connecting clients with their strengths can help them overcome the negative self-talk that often accompanies their efforts to change. Harvard psychologist Kauffman (1) recommends shifting your clients attention "away from pathology and pain and direct it toward a clear-eyed concentration on strength, vision, and dreams" (p. 220). Similarly, when you can encourage clients to come up with their own solutions, it has an immediate impact on their sense of self-efficacy. You may have a client who routinely asks and then fails to follow your advice about what to eat on the weekend. Consider asking the same client what challenges she might encounter over the weekend and how she might plan to meet that challenge. Clients also can be prompted to think about what they have done successfully. If they are reminded that they have successfully completed graduate school or raised a family or achieved careers goals, they are more likely to see healthy behavior change as less daunting. They will identify that they do indeed have the power to accomplish difficult tasks.

> **When you can encourage clients to come up with their own solutions, it has an immediate impact on their sense of self-efficacy.**

When clients see that they do have the skills and the motivation to accomplish their fitness goals, they will see themselves as less dependent on you—and take on the responsibility for their own change. Whereas many people will look to professionals to constantly keep them motivated, those who take responsibility for their change will find that motivation within.

THE PREPARATION LEVEL—CLIMB OUT OF NEGATIVITY

In the preparation level, you may hear negative statements like "I'm lazy," "I'll never be able to get to my goal weight," "I've been this way for years," or "It's easy for you—you do this for a living." While your immediate response might be to encourage and cheer on your clients, that might sound hollow and pro forma. Instead, try focusing the clients on what they want—the positive outcomes of their behavior change—not what they don't want (e.g., "I don't want to get diabetes, I don't want to stay the way I am"). This technique can help them inch up the Pyramid.

You can also encourage your clients to plan and get support for their new behavior. When they can actually make the time in their schedules for working out and preparing healthy food, it is far likelier to happen and be integrated into their daily life. When they have the support of their friends and family, they will not constantly be tempted to return to old, unhealthy behaviors. This will increase their confidence that the change truly is within their power.

THE ACTION LEVEL—SET GOALS AND REWARD ACHIEVEMENT

The third level depicts the doing process (specific behavioral goals) with early wins and constant fine-tuning. The action level is where you will encounter many of your clients. Their motivation and commitment seem so strong that lapsing seems impossible to them. Be aware of the pitfalls of the action phase and assist clients in setting reasonable, measurable goals that can be completed in a short period of time—and detail these SMART goals (see Chapter 10) in a written plan. Measuring and recording short- and long-term successes help document the change and provide a record of how far your client has come.

Problem solving is often the neglected step in clients' behavior change efforts. Integrating new behaviors into a life that hasn't made room for them is next to impossible for even the most committed person. You can ask clients simple questions to help them think about how they will integrate new behaviors in their already busy and hectic lives. When they fall short of their goals because their

> *Integrating new behaviors into a life that hasn't made room for them is next to impossible for even the most committed person.*

busy lives got in the way, you can help them brainstorm other options, other times, and use your good humor, curiosity, and creativity to help them make mid-course corrections and move on.

Rewarding and celebrating healthy new behaviors are essential. You can ask your clients how they will reward themselves when they reach their goal, and keep track of their goal so that you can acknowledge and celebrate with them. Rewards should reinforce new behaviors, rather than old ones. For example, if your client wants to celebrate her 5-lb (2.3 kg) weight loss by splurging on a burger, you might suggest an alternative, such as a new piece of clothing, a CD, or a massage. You can also encourage clients to notice the qualitative benefits of their new behavior, for example, better sleep, increased energy level, or simply feeling happier.

THE RESULTS LEVEL—PLAN FOR RELAPSE

The saying goes: "If you fail to plan, you plan to fail." People who have successfully integrated a healthy new behavior are often torn between two poles: either believing they will inevitably relapse and fail or being so overconfident about their new path that they believe relapse is impossible. Often, they prefer not to think about relapse for fear of jinxing the process! But by addressing it explicitly, you can remove the shroud of fear and superstition from relapse and treat it as simply another aspect of the change process. Planning for times of relapse prevents being taken by surprise, and you can help clients brainstorm how they will respond to lapses. You can also take note, for example, when someone hasn't been in the gym for a week and call to provide support and nonjudgmental feedback for clients who have lapsed.

Celebrate Clients' "Best Self"

Clients believe that achieving their wellness goals will make their lives different and, in many cases, that does happen. But aside from the physical changes and the increased self-esteem associated with behavior change, making it through the change process itself is a feat to be celebrated. Encouraging clients' celebration of their determination and willingness to meet challenges helps open a window into their best selves. Linking their

> *Encouraging clients' celebration of their determination and willingness to meet challenges helps open a window into their best selves.*

changes back to their original motivation, values, and vision can help them expand that view and keep it fresh and current.

SUMMARY

The "expert paradox" fails to acknowledge individuals' own expertise about themselves and their desires and actually lowers their sense of self-efficacy. Mount Lasting Change provides a useful model for the Personal Trainer who is ready to use coaching skills to help clients overcome this problem. The foundation of lasting change includes client self-awareness of the benefits of change and the obstacles to change, and rigorous exploration of why they want to change in the first place. Setting and achieving SMART goals then help a client build on early successes. Relapse is simply another stage in the change process. When the Personal Trainer helps clients prepare for them, lapses are less likely to become long-term relapses of old, unhealthy behaviors.

REFERENCES

1. Kauffman C. Positive psychology: the science at the heart of coaching. In: Stober DR, Grant AM, editors. *Evidence Based Coaching Handbook: Putting Best Practices to Work for Your Clients*. Hoboken (NJ): John Wiley & Sons; 2006. p. 219–53.
2. Moore M, Boothroyd L. *The Obesity Epidemic: A Confidence Crisis Calling for Professional Coaches*. Wellesley (MA): Wellcoaches Corporation; 2006.
3. Moore M, Tschannen-Moran R. *Coaching Psychology Manual*. Baltimore: Lippincott Williams & Wilkins; 2009.
4. Prochaska JO, Norcross JC, Diclemente CC. *Changing for Good*. New York: William Morrow; 1994.

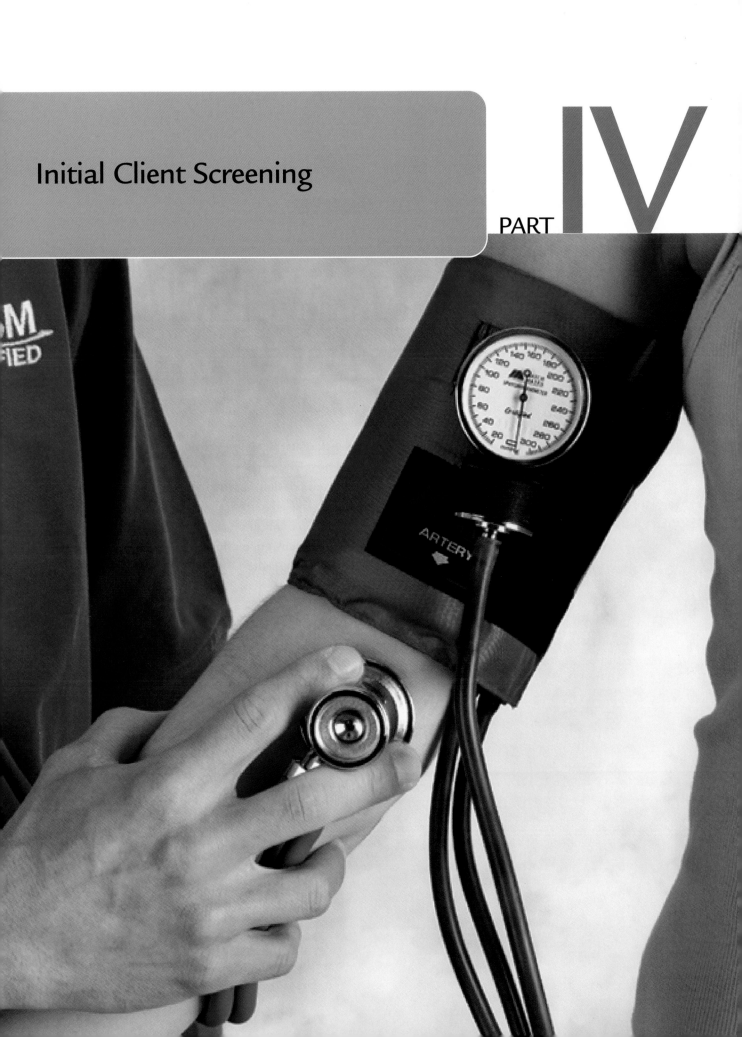

Initial Client Screening

PART IV

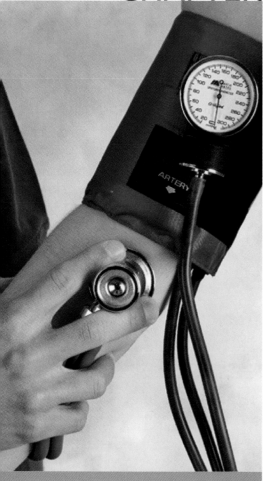

 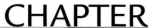
The Initial Client Consultation

OBJECTIVES

- Understand the critical attributes for providing exceptional customer service and hospitality
- Learn the attributes of relationship marketing and how it pertains to the initial and ongoing appointments with the client
- Learn the nonverbal communication skills needed to successfully engage the client during any appointment
- Become familiar with client-centered approach to health and fitness coaching
- Understand the elements and value of the initial client contact as a precursor to the initial client consultation
- Understand the components of the initial client consultation, how to structure the appointment, and the precedence it sets for the duration of the client–Personal Trainer relationship
- Learn strategies for recommending and selling appropriate personal training packages and obtaining client commitment

t is within the initial client consultation that the Personal Trainer establishes a precedence for the type of working relationship that will ensue. Therefore, it is critical that a sound foundation is built to facilitate a trusting, respectful, and mutually rewarding professional relationship. This chapter is designed to expose the Personal Trainer to both behavioral and business aspects of communication that should be utilized in the initial meeting with the client and beyond. Specific attributes for the initial client contact and initial client consultation are detailed, along with the rationale for why these appointments are structured in a systematic and comprehensive manner. There are likely program and process differences between Personal Trainers who work in a commercial club, private gym, or corporate fitness facility yet there are more commonalities that exist in the profession. Although the chapter is written to address universal professional themes, at times differentiating between settings, each Personal Trainer is encouraged to adapt the content accordingly to the work environment and the relationship built with the client.

ASPECTS OF SUCCESSFUL CLIENT RELATIONS

The profession of personal training is centered on a strong relationship between the client and the Personal Trainer. Although relationship dynamics vary from client to client, there are some behaviors that the Personal Trainer should exhibit as a foundation for business development. For example, customer service and hospitality are essential to demonstrate continuously to garner client trust and respect. Incorporating relationship marketing concepts will further enhance the Personal Trainer's communication style and assist in conveying to the client that the relationship is of extraordinary value and importance. Additionally, being aware of nonverbal communication skills and using a client-centered approach to coaching are important. Collectively, the Personal Trainer can and should create a strong framework for attracting and retaining long-lasting client–Personal Trainer relationships.

> *The Personal Trainer can and should create a strong framework for attracting and retaining long-lasting client–Personal Trainer relationships.*

Customer Service and Hospitality

Personal Trainers, similar to a variety of healthcare providers, are in the service management industry. Clients seek out a Personal Trainer because they desire a service that will assist and guide them in a direction that is compatible with their health and fitness goals. Similar to those who seek out a clergy member who can assist with spiritual goals or call on a financial advisor to be guided in monetary matters, so too do people seek out the services of a Personal Trainer. The Personal Trainer should recognize this entrusted opportunity—to guide and to make a direct positive impact on another person's life, as an honor and a special privilege. To reciprocate for the trust that the client wants to give to the Personal Trainer, customer service and hospitality should always be exhibited. Author and restauranteur Danny Meyer firmly espouses that it takes both great customer service and hospitality to rise to the top of any service field, and distinguishing between the two is critical for success (7).

Meyer refers to customer service as the delivery of technical processes or preplanned behaviors that are to be performed in a certain manner toward the client. In other words, these actions can be described as a monologue between the business provider and the customer (7). Customer service is exhibited by simply delivering a standard of service that meets the client's needs and expectations. However, it should be noted that clients do not seek or expect only mediocre service (5). Therefore, it is recommended that the Personal Trainer continually perform at a higher level than expected to accommodate the discerning client.

Examples of customer service include the following:

- Be on time, or early, for appointments
- Be 100% prepared for all appointments
- Respond to phones and e-mail messages promptly and courteously
- Demonstrate organization and reliability, and always follow up on what has been promised
- Provide fitness training programs that are based on science or credible resources
- Answer client questions concisely and accurately within the scope of practice
- Refer clients to appropriate professionals when the issue is outside of the scope of practice
- Listen to client concerns, respond with sincerity, and solicit feedback
- Speak respectfully to the client and of others
- Dress appropriately and professionally

A commitment to customer service should be a consistent practice to establish the Personal Trainer's reputation as a business professional. Consistently performing these actions will undoubtedly make an impression on the client and set the groundwork for a successful personal training business.

The principle of hospitality is also centered in customer service (5), while further providing a "holistic approach to meeting customers' needs within the context of a personal relationship and experience." Where customer service focuses on meeting the client's rational needs and expectations, hospitality also addresses the client's emotional needs by demonstrating graciousness, caring, and thoughtfulness toward a guest (7). This emotional element is what creates an "experience" and is what will establish true client loyalty.

Although most commonly associated with the hotel or restaurant industry, hospitality is a focal point for companies in the health and fitness industry as well (1). One such fitness management company sees caring and serving the client so vital that it is stated as one of four operating missions of the organization. In conjunction, the company offers a hospitality-based employee training program that has proven to be a distinguishing factor among competitors and is a key component in attracting and retaining world-class clients. Addressing hospitality outside of the hotel and restaurant industry, a business consultant who assists organizations in enhancing their customer experience aptly titled a recent article "No Matter What Business You're in, You're in the Hospitality Business" (1).

By many definitions, hospitality is centered on the intangible and emotionally driven behaviors that demonstrate to the clients that they are special and cared for by the Personal Trainer. Where customer service is a monologue, hospitality is a dialogue, conveying that the client's needs are the priority in an interactive communication (7). Warmth, friendliness, kindness, and the instinct to want to do the right thing for the client are ultimately at the core of hospitality. These emotional skills are difficult to find in individuals, and even more difficult to train, but if demonstrated can pay big dividends. Exhibiting hospitality often equates to clients thoroughly enjoying themselves, and as a result they yearn to have the experience again and will share it with others. The net result of sharing with others, known as word-of-mouth advertising, cannot be understated because it leads to client loyalty and referrals that are paramount to the success of a Personal Trainer in business.

> *Hospitality is centered on the intangible and emotionally driven behaviors that demonstrate to the clients that they are special and cared for by the Personal Trainer.*

According to Meyer (7), professionals who create a hospitality experience typically possess the following traits:

- *Optimistic warmth*: Genuine kindness, thoughtfulness, and a sense that the glass is always at least half full
- *Intelligence*: Open-mindedness and an insatiable curiosity to learn
- *Work ethic*: A natural tendency to do something as well as it possibly can be done

➤ *Empathy*: An awareness of, care for, and connection to how others feel and how the individual's actions affect others

➤ *Self-awareness and integrity*: Understanding what makes you tick and a natural inclination to be accountable for doing the right thing

A Personal Trainer possessing the traits above will innately be able to exhibit the following examples of hospitality:

➤ Greet the client with a strong handshake, authentic smile, and eye contact
➤ At the end of a session, sincerely thank the client for his or her time
➤ Address client requests and do anything possible to make them happen
➤ Convey that the client's best interest is in mind under any circumstance
➤ Make follow-up calls/e-mails to see how the client feels after a personal training session
➤ Send a hand-written card to thank the client after an initial appointment or when a significant goal has been reached
➤ Search for opportunities to go above and beyond what is expected

The Personal Trainer should strive to embrace and exhibit both customer service and hospitality. Establishing a habit of providing consistent and reliable service, as well as taking the extra steps to demonstrate to the clients that they are cared for, will make an indelible impression. Many clients are more interested in knowing how much the Personal Trainer cares than how much the Personal Trainer knows. Conveying this will allow the Personal Trainer to experience not only the joy of giving and the pride that accompanies it but certainly the rewards of client satisfaction and allegiance as well.

Relationship Marketing

The principle of marketing is central to any successful business and incorporates many of the concepts from customer service and hospitality. Considered a future trend in marketing, relationship marketing is a vital component in the service industry and encourages thinking and acting like the customer to secure and retain a trusting and loyal long-term relationship (5). It should be noted that although similar, hospitality and relationship marketing are not mutually exclusive and in fact should be carried out simultaneously. The primary goal of marketing is to bring the buyer (client) and the seller (Personal Trainer) together, the strategies of which are worthy of the Personal Trainer's attention leading into the initial client consultation.

What differentiates this new paradigm of relationship marketing from conventional marketing is that first, a personal relationship with the customer should take precedence and sales will follow; and second, retaining existing clients should take precedence over seeking new customers (Box 12.1). In contrast, traditional marketing places great emphasis on the constant hunt for new sales to new customers. Although traditional marketing has its place in the business of personal training, relationship marketing concepts certainly have notable implications for the Personal Trainer as well.

BOX **12.1**   **Principles of Relationship Marketing**

- A personal relationship with the customer should take precedence and sales will follow.
- Retaining existing clients should take precedence over seeking new customers.

Adapted from Kandampully JA. *Services Management: The New Paradigm in Hospitality*. Upper Saddle River (NJ): Pearson Education, Inc.; 2007, p. 378.

The first premise of relationship marketing is to emphasize the personal relationship with the client, which is supported by the idea that customers have a deep desire to trust the business provider and are inherently loyal (5). Customers have also been found to be loyal to those who trust them, so it is crucial that the Personal Trainer interact with the client in a way that reinforces this trust. As a result, the Personal Trainer will be rewarded with the client's desire to maintain the working relationship. On the other hand, even though clients resist changing business providers, as is the case with dentists or doctors, they will seek another provider if this trust is abused (5). Thinking and acting like the client will facilitate this mutual desire to have a trusting, loyal, and long-lasting working relationship.

> *Thinking and acting like the client will facilitate this mutual desire to have a trusting, loyal, and long-lasting working relationship.*

The second premise of relationship marketing is to focus on retaining existing clients as opposed to only seeking new clients. Research indicates that retained customers are very profitable over time for reasons including increased purchases, referrals, and lower operating costs (to maintain existing clients vs. marketing for new clients). It is common for businesses to lose an average of 15%–20% of its customers each year; however, businesses can double business growth if those customer defections are cut in half (11). Additionally, traditional business research estimates that it costs five times more to attract a new client than it does to keep an existing one (2,4). As such, it is in the best interest of the Personal Trainer to survey departing clients in order to understand the reasons for leaving. If they are controllable factors, the Personal Trainer should take action with existing clients to minimize these defections in the future.

The Personal Trainer should pay close attention to relationship marketing as a means to success. Perhaps the most cost-effective marketing strategy in business, favorable word-of-mouth advertising, has the opportunity to flourish if the Personal Trainer is meeting expectations and nurturing the client relationship. Furthermore, when the broader business concepts of customer service, hospitality, and relationship marketing are integrated, the Personal Trainer will be better equipped to face the challenges that inherently exist in the business world. Considering that 25%–50% of business operating costs stem from poor service, or not performing up to par the first time, it behooves the Personal Trainer to be attentive to the facets that enhance service quality right from the start (4). When putting these conceptual tools into action prior to and during the first client meeting, the Personal Trainer will have a greater capacity to not only survive but excel in attracting and retaining clients as well.

The Power of Nonverbal Communication

Because the client–Personal Trainer relationship is crucial for success, every facet of relationship building is important and the spoken word is only part of the communication puzzle. In fact, much can be learned about people by observing their nonverbal cues, because most people are not good at concealing emotions (8). In some cases, watching nonverbal cues is believed to be more reliable and essential to understanding another person than listening to speech (8). For example, if there seems to be a discrepancy between one's speech and body language, the listener will likely place more value in the body language of the communicator. Therefore, knowledge of body language is invaluable for success in both personal and professional relationships. Not only can a Personal Trainer learn to become a more effective nonverbal communicator but learning these cues will enhance the ability to understand the client as well.

> *Watching nonverbal cues is believed to be more reliable and essential to understanding another person than listening to speech.*

Body language such as posture, eye contact, and facial expressions speak volumes about an individual's thoughts and emotional state. For example, posture and stance are strong indicators of how engaged a person is in a job and if he or she believes in the product or service being sold. Simply observing a person's stance can quickly determine his or her energy, confidence, and sense of power in a position (9). Facial expressions may provide the best body language clues though. In particular, a person is said to lack sincerity or truthfulness if there is a contradiction between words and facial expressions. Additionally, facial expressions from emotional responses come and go quickly; therefore, a person who holds an expression for an extended period of time may not be exhibiting a genuine emotion (10).

Although a powerful tool, interpreting body language is a science that has evolved over time and still holds some disagreement among experts. For example, it has been thought that people who stand while holding their hands behind their back exude power; however, it has also been found that observers think these people are untrustworthy instead. Additionally, individuals who are unable to make eye contact have been thought to be lying, yet this can also be interpreted as nervousness (8).

These and other body language distinctions can be used to provide the Personal Training client with tailored customer service and hospitality. For example, the Personal Trainer should be observant of the client when he or she is walking into the facility, office, or on the exercise floor. Upon meeting, if the client has slouching posture, crossed arms, and shifty eye contact, this may indicate nervousness and insecurity. The Personal Trainer should take extra steps to maintain a warm and patient demeanor while explaining what to expect during the meeting and give the client opportunities to express concern or ask questions. In another scenario, if the client's facial expression indicates confusion while hesitantly performing a new exercise, he or she may not verbalize the need for assistance. In response, the Personal Trainer should take the initiative to demonstrate the exercise again, reiterate movement cues, and provide positive reinforcement of what the client is doing correctly to increase confidence of the skill.

On the other hand, the Personal Trainer must be aware that his or her nonverbal communication is being observed and equally has an impact. For example, imagine a client enthusiastically describing how he or she felt after the last training session while the Personal Trainer is leaning against the exercise machine looking off in another direction. How would this make the client feel? Similarly, imagine a client performing an exercise and inquiring if the movement is being done correctly, only to discover that the Personal Trainer is preoccupied with watching television. How would this make the client feel? Apathy and divided attention are not attributes of customer service, hospitality, or the client-centered approach, and should be avoided at all costs, or trust will diminish. The Personal Trainer must exercise self-awareness at all times when working with clients to ensure that positive nonverbal communication is being expressed. Pagers, cell phones, and other personal communication devices should be left in the locker room as your first priority must be the client with whom you are working.

Exhibiting positive body language can certainly be a powerful business tool. Consider that the actions a business person exhibits within the first 15 seconds of walking into a room will likely make or break a sale even before talking begins (9). Regardless of the type of business, this type of influence is very valuable and has been shown to be a function of a person's body language attractiveness. All else being equal, those who have attractive body language tend to be more successful. Below are some behaviors that increase one's body language attractiveness and can improve nonverbal communication skills (9):

➤ *Eye contact*: The more frequent eye contact the better, although staring for more than a few seconds at a time can be uncomfortable for the client and may be construed as flirtatious. Frequent blinking conveys a wandering mind or one that wants to interrupt; therefore, blink less.
➤ *Facial expressions*: Smile often and appear interested. Widening the eyes and raising eyebrows express interest and surprise. On the contrary, narrowing the eyes or lowering the eyebrows can mean disgust, anger, or sadness.
➤ *Head movements*: Keep chin up and nod "yes" to show interest.
➤ *Gestures*: Be expressive with hands and body movements without exaggeration.
➤ *Posture*: Sit and stand erect, and lean forward to show interest. Leaning back is perceived as informal. Keep arms and legs uncrossed to convey a secure and welcoming demeanor.

> *Proximity and orientation*: Be as close as possible without crowding the client. A comfortable range is between 1.5 and 4 feet (0.46–1.22 meters), yet it is important to read the client's body language to adjust accordingly.

> *Appearance and physique*: Maintain good hygiene along with a healthy and fit appearance. Clothing colors are also influential. For example, these are the specific messages that some colors can convey: red (power, danger, force, passion), orange (excitement, encouragement), yellow (happiness, energy, intelligence), green (harmony, safety), blue (trust, confidence, peace), purple (luxury, creativity), white (safe, purity), black (power, mystery, aggressive, unsafe) (3). Depending upon the kind of message the Personal Trainer wants to convey to a client on any particular day, uniform colors can have a powerful influence on the relationship with the client.

> *Timing and synchronization*: Speed up activities, but not to the point of ineffectiveness.

> *Nonverbal aspects of speech*: Balance the need to listen with the need to talk.

These categories of behavior increase the attractiveness of a person to others, which can assist in enhancing communication between two people. In short, possessing enthusiasm can quickly lead to all the behaviors listed without consciously having to focus on each point. Conscious awareness can not only enhance the Personal Trainer's ability to exhibit these traits but also improve the ability to identify them in others.

The Client-Centered Approach to Coaching

In conjunction with exhibiting acts of customer service and hospitality, there are health coaching skills that will further enhance the client–trainer relationship if taken into account. These fundamental skills will increase the trainer's understanding of the client; therefore, increase the trainer's ability to affect behavior change. Referred to as the "client-centered approach," the counseling skills of rapport building, exhibiting empathy, and active listening are central to keeping the client's perspective at the forefront (15). Although this style of relationship building takes more time in the initial client consultation and beyond, the nonjudgmental approach will likely yield more positive results. For example, when used by physicians, the results include higher client satisfaction and improved compliance along with reduced concerns and physical symptoms (13). Contrary to the style of many Personal Trainers, this approach does not encourage giving unsolicited advice. Although under some circumstances it is beneficial, Rollnick et al. have found that advice giving can hinder behavior change because it can be perceived as condescending and undermines the client's intelligence and sense of independence (12). Telling a client what to do may lead to resentment, so it is important for the Personal Trainer to think twice before attempting an unwelcome verbal monologue of directions. Clearly a client seeks a Personal Trainer for motivation and advice, but the way in which it is done should be considered, and the client-centered approach provides the context for such communication.

> *Referred to as the "client-centered approach," the counseling skills of rapport building, exhibiting empathy, and active listening are central to keeping the client's perspective at the forefront (15).*

RAPPORT BUILDING

The first element of the client-centered approach is establishing rapport, which is developed by building a trusting and respectful relationship with the client. Starting the working relationship in this manner is critical and can readily be accomplished by asking open-ended questions (Box 12.2). For example, simply asking the client to describe a typical day will give the Personal Trainer information that may be useful in guiding the client to more healthful eating or exercise habits (12). For this type of rapport building to be effective, the Personal Trainer must keep in mind that open-ended

| BOX **12.2** | **Summary of Client-Centered Techniques** |

- Ask simple, open-ended questions (i.e., questions that elicit details instead of yes-or-no responses).
- Listen and encourage with verbal and nonverbal prompts.
- Clarify and summarize. Check your understanding of what the client said and check to see whether the client understood what you said.
- Use reflective listening. This involves making statements that aim to bridge the gap between what the client is saying and the meaning behind the statements.

From Rollnick S, Mason P, Butler C. *Health Behavior Change. A Guide for Practitioners.* New York (NY): Churchill Livingstone; 1999. p. 225.

questions are meant to gather information rather than be an interrogation. This process should take approximately 3–5 minutes and can start by simply asking, "Can you tell me about a recent typical day for you from beginning to end, so I can get a clearer picture of what it looks like?" If the clients feel that they are being judged, they will be less likely to elaborate, so it is important to allow the clients to speak freely without interrupting to point out problem areas. Ideally, the Personal Trainer will be speaking 10%–15% of the time and be focused on pacing the conversation—asking the clients to elaborate when necessary (12).

EXHIBITING EMPATHY

Another way of establishing rapport is to demonstrate empathy by earnestly listening and expressing understanding. Individuals often feel a kinship with others who can relate to them or who have had similar experiences. One way of demonstrating empathy is to listen, repeat what was said, and clarify what was said in the form of a question (15). As an example, a client may volunteer information about his exercise habits over the years and state that he is reluctant to get in shape for fear of experiencing more injuries. In this case, the Personal Trainer may ask: "So that I understand you, fear of injuries has kept you from engaging in a regular exercise routine. Is that correct?" This reaffirms to the client that the Personal Trainer was listening intently and understands.

ACTIVE LISTENING

Attempting to understand the underlying meaning of what a client is saying is referred to as active listening. Although requiring more skill and practice, this technique further enhances rapport and demonstrates empathy through the use of reflective statements (15). Using the example above, the Personal Trainer may say: "It sounds like you are hesitant to exercise regularly at this time (reflective statement). Many people are hesitant to exercise after an injury (empathetic statement). Can you tell me about your specific concerns (open-ended question)? This nonjudgmental style of communication tells the client that the Personal Trainer understands the emotions that the client may be experiencing, while providing an additional opportunity for the Personal Trainer to learn more about the client. This process will help garner mutual trust, enhance the client's self-awareness in the client, and provide the Personal Trainer with more insight as to what will help facilitate healthful behavior change.

Building rapport, exhibiting empathy, and listening actively will help build an effective communication bridge between the client and the Personal Trainer. A summary of the three techniques can be seen in Box 12.2, whereas Box 12.3 lists the indicators that the client-centered approach is being used.

BOX 12.3	Indicators That the Client-Centered Approach Is Being Used

- The Personal Trainer is speaking slowly.
- The client is talking more than the Personal Trainer.
- The client is talking about behavior change.
- The Personal Trainer is listening intently and directing the conversation when appropriate.
- The client appears to be making realizations and connections not previously considered.

From Rollnick S, Mason P, Butler C. *Health Behavior Change. A Guide for Practitioners.* New York (NY): Churchill Livingstone; 1999. p. 225.

PRECEDING THE INITIAL CLIENT CONSULTATION

Generating Clients

Certainly one of the pressing issues in any business is attracting new customers or clients. Some Personal Trainers may have the luxury of working in a facility where clients are continually being referred, in which case the Personal Trainer has to focus only on client retention, utilizing concepts stated previously. However, in many cases the responsibility is on the Personal Trainer to not only retain clients but seek and secure new ones as well. Below are strategies to generate new clients that can be applied to corporate, private, or commercial club settings.

WORD-OF-MOUTH ADVERTISING

As previously discussed, one of the most cost-effective and powerful methods of marketing is word-of-mouth referrals from satisfied clients. Oftentimes these referrals will be unsolicited without any effort needed on behalf of the Personal Trainer. On the other hand, the Personal Trainer may also want to express to existing clients that new clients are desired and that referrals are appreciated. In this case, the Personal Trainer may want to advertise a client referral program in which the existing client receives a complimentary fitness assessment or receives a discount on future sessions for each referred new client.

FITNESS FLOOR EXPOSURE

Personal Trainers working with clients on the floor are a walking advertisement of their style and services. For this reason, it is important to consistently exhibit professionalism and provide focused attention while training an existing client. Potential clients will likely not be attracted to Personal Trainers who appear distracted, disinterested, or not respectful of the client being trained. However, keeping an approachable disposition and making friendly eye contact with other members between exercises are certainly encouraged. If not working with a client, Personal Trainers may want to walk the fitness floor and make themselves available for questions, which may additionally lead to more interest and personal training inquiries.

COMPLIMENTARY CONSULTATIONS

Although some may be of the opinion that offering free services devalues a service overall, occasionally marketing complimentary initial client consultations may be a strategy that can differentiate one Personal Trainer or club over another and lead to more clients.

FRONT DESK CONTACTS

Depending on the size of the club and member inquiry process, the front desk staff or receptionist may be the first individual to field a question about personal training services. The process may dictate that staff refer member inquiries to the Personal Trainer directly or to a Personal Training Director first. In either case, it is important for the Personal Trainer to develop a strong working relationship with the "gatekeeper" staff and routinely communicate if new clients are desired. Stating availability, training style, and desired client special populations of interest may also be valuable reminders to the staff.

PROFESSIONAL NETWORKING AND REFERRALS

Personal trainers should be part of an integrated community network of mutually referring healthcare professionals including but not limited to doctors (medical, chiropractic, naturopathic), physical therapists, certified athletic trainers, exercise physiologists, massage therapists, acupuncturists, wellness coaches, and registered dieticians. Retail fitness, nutrition, and health food stores are viable referral points, as well as local service professionals such as real estate and insurance agents and accountants. The Personal Trainer may want to join a professional networking group to facilitate these relationships in the community or make personal office visits and ask whether it is possible to display business cards or brochures while providing referrals in return.

ACTIVE MARKETING

Increasing the number of exposure points will certainly enhance the consistency of new client interest. An internet Web presence is a necessary and powerful tool—whether it be the Personal Trainer's personal Web site, the club's Web site, or both. Creating and maintaining a Web site Blog is also recommended, which may help not only attract but retain clients by facilitating a continual dialogue. Brochures and promotional flyers should also be displayed whenever possible. At all marketing points, both Web and paper, particular attention should be given to professional design and layout as it is all a professional reflection on the Personal Trainer.

Initial Client Contact

It is advisable for the Personal Trainer to have a process by which to screen and take new clients. This will not only assist the Personal Trainer in gathering and organizing critical information about a potential client but perhaps more importantly it is the first opportunity to make an impression on the client by demonstrating organization, care, and professionalism. A flowchart of the recommended initial client contact process is shown in Figure 12.1. This process may occur in person, over the phone, or via e-mail. Regardless of the communication method, great care should be taken to ensure that all elements of customer service, hospitality, and the client-centered approach are being incorporated when interfacing with the client (Fig. 12.2).

INITIAL CLIENT CONTACT PROCESS

A more detailed description of the initial client contact process (Fig. 12.1) is outlined below:

➤ Assess compatibility and refer as needed
  - Discuss the client's health and fitness goals and specific health conditions/limitations, and ensure experience and scope are sufficient to meet the client's needs.
  - State the fee structure and ensure that it is agreeable to the client.
  - Discuss experience, style, and educational background and ensure that it is both adequate and appealing to the client.
  - Discuss the client's schedule preferences and assess compatibility for ongoing appointments.
  - Refer to an alternate Personal Trainer or other healthcare professional if goals and interests are not compatible or if outside scope of practice or expertise (see Chapter 14 for detailed guidance on the professional referral process).
➤ Exchange contact information
  - Exchange phone numbers and e-mail addresses, while identifying the preferred method of communication.

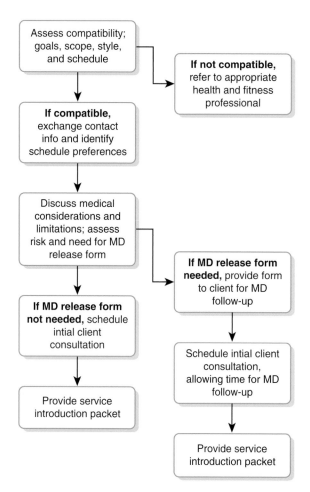

FIGURE 12.1. Initial client contact process.

➤ Evaluate need for medical release form
  • Inquire with the client if there is any reason why a doctor would restrict him or her from performing fitness testing or light/moderate exercise. Explain that a more thorough health history evaluation and/or physical activity readiness questionnaire will be required for the initial client consultation (see Chapter 14 for detailed guidance on the use of a health history evaluation and/or PAR-Q Form).
  • Provide the client with Medical Clearance Form to be completed by his or her physician if there are clear restrictions to light/moderate exercise (see Chapter 14 for detailed guidance on the use of a Medical Clearance Form).
➤ Schedule the initial client consultation
  • Schedule a mutually agreeable appointment for the initial client consultation if there is clear compatibility and interest between both parties to proceed.

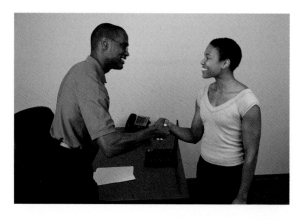

FIGURE 12.2. Greeting a client.

- Explain clearly what to expect and how to prepare for the initial client consultation in terms of appropriate dress and what the appointment will include.
➤ Provide a service introduction packet
  - Present the client with a service introduction packet to be reviewed prior to the initial client consultation.
  - Provide additional information on a Web site dedicated to the service introduction, which may contain supporting marketing materials such as client testimonials, healthcare professional endorsements, and Personal Trainer publications or press clippings.
  - Contents of the packet intended for review may include business card, Personal Trainer bio and welcome letter, facility brochure, and training services pricing structure.
  - Contents of the packet intended to be returned prior to the next appointment may include Health History Evaluation Form, Informed Consent Waiver, and Medical Clearance Form if necessary (see Chapter 14 for sample forms). Additionally, the Client–Personal Trainer Agreement (Fig. 12.4) should be given to the client to be completed and returned at the next appointment. These forms may be distributed directly or blank forms can be sent electronically to the client. Completed forms will be gathered at the next meeting.

CLIENT INTAKE FORM

The above process should be used in conjunction with the client intake form, which is used to obtain the critical client contact information (Fig. 12.3).

ARRANGING AND PREPARING FOR THE NEXT MEETING

The initial client contact is the precursor to the initial client consultation and is a valuable springboard for the next meeting when set up correctly. First, it is important that the Personal Trainer remind the client the day and time of the next meeting and the time allotted for the appointment. Next, it should be clearly articulated what the next appointment will include, the recommended attire, necessary equipment, and if a hydration bottle is needed. The client should also be reminded to complete and return the necessary forms and to contact the Personal Trainer if any questions or concerns arise. The Personal Trainer should take exceptional care in departing with the new client by making eye contact and shaking hands, walking the client to the door, and then thanking him or her by name while genuinely expressing that the next visit is eagerly awaited. Ideally, if the Personal Trainer exhibits traits of outstanding customer service, hospitality, and relationship building in this initial meeting, the client will be motivated and inspired to return for the next visit.

> *The Personal Trainer should take exceptional care in departing with the new client by making eye contact and shaking hands, walking the client to the door, and then thanking him or her by name while genuinely expressing that the next visit is eagerly awaited.*

INITIAL CLIENT CONSULTATION

Up to this point, much of the groundwork has been laid in preparation for the initial client consultation. Indeed, some of the most important work in a Personal Trainer's profession is in establishing rapport, creating a comfortable and welcoming environment, and stimulating motivation in a client. What remains are the more technical elements that a consultation may include.

Consultation Location and Confidentiality

Of utmost importance is the location of the client consultation, as it sets the tone for information sharing and relationship building. The Personal Trainer must view this experience through the eyes of a new client and create a hospitable and private environment accordingly. Of primary importance, discussion of personal and confidential health information must be held in the

New Client Intake Form

Contact Information

Date: _____   ☐ Phone   ☐ In-Person

Name: _____

Address: _____

Phone (home): _____

Phone (cell): _____

Email: _____

Training Schedule Interest (circle all that apply):

Sunday	Monday	Tuesday	Wednesday	Thursday	Friday	Saturday
am	am	am	am	am	am	am
midday	midday	midday	midday	midday	midday	midday
pm	pm	pm	pm	pm	pm	pm

Health & Fitness Information

General Health & Fitness Goals (check all that apply):

☐ Strength   ☐ Disease Management

☐ Endurance   ☐ Stress Management

☐ Sport Performance   ☐ Weight Management

☐ Physical Appearance   ☐ Energy/Vitality

Health or Fitness Professional(s) treating client: _____

_____

Medical Considerations/Limitations: _____

_____

MD Release Form Needed: Y   N

MD Name/Phone Contact (if necessary): _____

Action Items

If not compatible:
Referral to Health or Fitness Professional: Y   N
        Referral:_____

If compatible:
MD Release Form (if necessary) Date Sent: _____   Rec'd: _____

Initial Client Consultation Date: _____

Service Introduction Packet Delivered: In-Person   Email   Mail

Comments: _____

_____

_____

FIGURE 12.3. New client intake form.

strictest confidence and taken seriously. Additionally, it is common for new clients to feel uneasy about themselves and their health and fitness status and a fitness center environment may exacerbate those insecurities. Although not all clients will externally exhibit such sensitivities, it is best to err conservatively. Therefore, creating a welcoming and nonjudgmental atmosphere in a private space should be a priority.

Specifically, the consultation and assessment areas should be in an enclosed room or remote space within the facility such that verbal communication is not clearly discernible to other clients. The space should be absent of distracting background noise or music, along with any visual distractions that could hinder a focused conversation between client and Personal Trainer. The area should be clean and organized, comfortably accommodate two to four chairs, and have a desk or table wide enough for the Personal Trainer to review or explain documents. The area should have good lighting and proper ventilation. In accordance with ACSM recommendations, the assessment area should maintain a comfortable temperature between 68°F and 72°F (20°C–22°C), with humidity below 60% (14). If it is not possible to have a separate room to conduct the initial consultation, sitting with the client facing away from other clients may be advisable to maximize privacy and prevent voices from carrying.

Introduction and Consultation Agenda Review

As previously discussed, the Personal Trainer should warmly welcome the client upon first sight with a handshake and smile and engage in light conversation to put the client at ease. Next, the Personal Trainer should lead the client to the private consultation area and review the sequence and content of the initial client consultation. Even though the Personal Trainer has previously outlined the process in the initial client contact, it is recommended that a step-by-step review of the process again be provided at this point. For example, the Personal Trainer may say:

> *I'm very glad that you have taken this step toward enhancing your health and fitness and I'm eager for us to get started. First, I'd like to outline what this appointment will include so that you know what to expect and to see if you have any questions or concerns. Does that sound alright with you?*

If concerns are expressed, address them and then continue.

> *We will begin by reviewing the paperwork that you were asked to complete (Client–Personal Trainer Agreement, Health History Evaluation Form (and/or PAR-Q), Informed Consent Waiver, and Medical Clearance Form as needed). Then, I'd like to hear more about your health and fitness goals and interests. This will help me get to know you better and help us determine which fitness assessments we should perform. Finally, we will conduct the fitness assessments, discuss the results, and discuss an action plan together. Do you have any questions before we begin?*

Not only does clearly defining the structure of the appointment lessen anxiety, but it provides an opportunity for the client to express his or her concerns or feelings about performing a given part of the assessment. For example, a client may be uncomfortable with the prospect of a caliper body-fat composition test if he or she is self-conscious about a weight problem. This provides the Personal Trainer an opportunity to empathize with the client and modify or eliminate a test as appropriate. If a client expresses any trepidation about a test, the Personal Trainer should immediately honor the request without any pressure. During this trust-building time, the benefit of expressing understanding will far outweigh the cost of convincing a client to do something with which he or she is uncomfortable.

Detailed Consultation Components

Once the stage has been set for the appointment, the Personal Trainer can continue with carrying out the key components of the consultation. This includes reviewing the documents that were given to the client during the initial client contact. Ideally, the client will have already completed the forms so that more time can be spent on getting to know the client, performing assessments, and goal setting; otherwise, it is important to note that these elements may be provided over the course of one or two appointments, depending on the time availability and appointment structure of the Personal Trainer's club or facility. Either way, the following elements should be included.

CLIENT–PERSONAL TRAINER AGREEMENT

It is very important to review expectations between the client and the Personal Trainer before joining in a business relationship. For example, cancelled or no-show appointments have financial ramifications for both parties, so ensuring mutual understanding is critical from the start. The document can be adapted to include other essential business expectations (Fig. 12.4). Be sure to retain a copy of this document for yourself and give a copy to the client.

Personal Training Client Agreement

I, _____, have read and agree to the following:
  (Client's Name-Please Print)

• Appointments will be scheduled directly through my assigned Personal Trainer and can be scheduled on days and times that are mutually agreed upon.

• I have exchanged contact information with my Personal Traininer and have indicated my preference for being contacted. I understand that the facility staff is not authorized to give out my Personal Trainer's personal contact information.

• I may not bring an outside Personal Trainer into the facility to train with me.

• Private personal training sessions are one hour.

• I understand that I am expected to arrive for my appointments on time, dressed and ready to train. If I arrive late for my appointment, I understand that my training session will end at the previously scheduled time.

• Cancellation Policy: I understand that appointments must be cancelled by contacting my Personal Trainer directly, within 24 hours of my scheduled time, in order to avoid being charged for the full session.

• No Show Policy: I understand that if I do not show up for my scheduled training session, I will be charged for the full session.

• In the event that my Personal Trainer fails to contact me within 24 hours of our scheduled session, or does not show up, he/she will schedule an additional session at no cost to me.

• I understand that I may communicate any customer service issue and/or acknowledge excellent performance to the Facility Manager.

Client Signature: _____ Date: _____

Personal Trainer (Print): _____ Date: _____

FIGURE 12.4. Example of personal training client agreement. (Adapted from PlusOne Fitness, New York, New York, 2008.)

HEALTH HISTORY EVALUATION FORM AND/OR PAR-Q

Discussing the client's current health status and history is imperative in getting to know his or her areas for improvement as well as limitations. This information will further assist the Personal Trainer in assessing risk and whether a Medical Clearance Form is necessary to proceed (see Chapter 14 for more detailed guidance on the use of a Health History Evaluation Form and/or PAR-Q).

INFORMED CONSENT

It is important that the client understand the risks and benefits of performing assessments and engaging in a guided exercise program. The informed consent serves as a document of understanding and should be signed by the client (see Chapter 14 for more detailed guidance on the use of an informed consent waiver).

MEDICAL CLEARANCE FORM

If determined through the use of the health history evaluation or PAR-Q that the client should see a physician before starting either a moderate- or high-intensity exercise routine, it is imperative to have this document signed by both the client and the physician. It may provide important restriction information that should be taken into account during program testing and design (see Chapter 14 for more detailed guidance on the use of a Medical Clearance Form).

CLIENT GOALS

The Personal Trainer should ask additional questions about the client's goals to get more specific responses as well as timelines that the client seeks for achievement.

Using the information from the client intake form (Fig. 12.2) as a guide, the Personal Trainer should ask additional questions about the client's goals to get more specific responses as well as timelines that the client seeks for achievement (see Chapter 10 for more detailed guidance on goal setting).

HEALTH AND FITNESS ASSESSMENT

Once any health limitations or restrictions are ascertained and goals identified from the process above, it is time to perform the fitness assessment. Even though a general overview of the tests to be performed is explained at the beginning of the consultation, it is advised to thoroughly explain and demonstrate each assessment immediately prior to it being performed to further minimize any anxiety or confusion that the client may have (Fig. 12.5). Selecting and explaining tests that emphasize a balanced program is important and may include resting heart rate and blood pressure, as

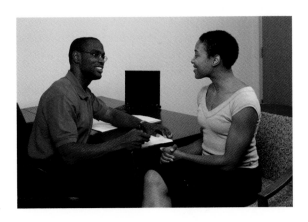

FIGURE 12.5. Client consultation.

well as body composition, cardiovascular fitness, strength, endurance, range of motion, anthropometric, and postural measures (see Chapter 14 for more detailed guidance on health and fitness assessments).

ASSESSMENT RESULTS AND ACTION PLAN

Upon the completion of any assessment, most clients are eager to receive the results. If the results can be given immediately after the tests, it enables the client and the Personal Trainer to begin taking action toward mutually identified goals. It is important to share the results in a positive manner, emphasizing that the results are a baseline with which to measure progress over time.

Recommending Appropriate Personal Training Packages

At this time, based on the findings of the assessment and verbalized goals, the Personal Trainer should detail a recommended action plan for training with the client. The appointment frequency and number of sessions purchased should be determined by the client's needs and goals. For example, if an experienced client wants to learn new exercise movements to supplement his or her current routine of 4 days per week, then the Personal Trainer likely should recommend meeting only once a week. On the other hand, a new client who is unfamiliar with exercise not only needs to learn how to perform exercise movements safely and with good form but may also need assistance in establishing an exercise habit. In this case, to facilitate learning and encourage an active lifestyle, the Personal Trainer may want to suggest training two to four times per week for 4–16 weeks. This will help the client begin to perfect and memorize the movement patterns and build the foundation for habitual exercise.

Unfortunately, a problem occurs when the beginning exerciser purchases too few sessions. As a result, the sessions occur so infrequently that the client does not have the opportunity to memorize and perform the movement patterns correctly. The disappointed client then feels that the Personal Trainer or training itself is not successful. For this reason the Personal Trainer must be clear with the client at the beginning and recommend the exercise program that the client needs to succeed. Otherwise, it does the client a disservice if the Personal Trainer is making recommendations solely on monetary concerns versus what will help the client reach individual goals. Thus, the importance of clarity when recommending personal training packages during the initial client consultation becomes apparent and will ultimately help the Personal Trainer succeed in being truthful and realistic about progress.

Obtaining Client Commitment

Obtaining client commitment through the act of purchasing a package of training sessions can be an act fraught with anxiety for many Personal Trainers. Making recommendations is one part of the equation, yet "landing the sale" is another aspect that does not always come easily. Ideally, the selling process at this point of the initial client consultation should be a positive one for both parties. After developing rapport during the initial client contact, along with a thoughtful, caring, and educational approach to the initial client consultation, the client's purchase of a personal training package will be a natural step in the process of obtaining exercise and fitness training.

> *After developing rapport during the initial client contact, along with a thoughtful, caring, and educational approach to the initial client consultation, the client's purchase of a personal training package will be a natural step in the process of obtaining exercise and fitness training.*

The Personal Trainer should keep in mind that the client needs the help of a personal training professional and that this is the primary reason that the client has sought out personal training services. The Personal Trainer should focus the client's attention on the service, instruction, motivation, guidance, enthusiasm, safety, and education that he or she will receive from the personal training experience. The Personal Trainer may also remind the client of the value of personal training by the increased sense of self-esteem and the benefits of feeling healthier and being in better shape to actively enjoy life.

One approach to the sale of training sessions is to review the personal training packages that the facility offers and to point out the most commonly purchased package by clients and why. For example, the Personal Trainer can tell the client that most of his or her beginning training clients purchase package A and train 2 days per week. The Personal Trainer could ask, "Would you like to purchase that package?" or "How would you like to proceed?" This approach can help move the client toward purchasing a package of sessions.

Common objections to personal training package purchases may arise from the client because of money, time, procrastination, and/or other conflicts. Thus, the Personal Trainer should be prepared to respond and anticipate possible objections. It is important to remember that pressuring a client into an exercise program to which he or she is not willing or is unable to commit could be a pitfall rather than a success story for both the client and the Personal Trainer. On the contrary, the Personal Trainer should maintain a positive attitude, relax and listen to what the client has to say, and then evaluate the objection and respond with empathy and truthfulness.

When the client commits, the Personal Trainer should not act surprised with the sale, but rather show appreciation by thanking the client and have the client review and sign all required agreements or contracts. If a commitment is not obtained from the client, the Personal Trainer should maintain a positive perspective and remember that not everyone is going to seek services after the initial client consultation. Demonstrating professionalism, the Personal Trainer should recommend other sources to the client to enhance health and fitness. Based on this customer-focused behavior, the client may likely refer friends or family members or decide to give personal training another chance in the future.

Leading into the Next Client Appointment

The Personal Trainer should express gratitude to the client for his or her time and display eagerness for the next visit.

Ideally, throughout both the initial client contact and consultation, the Personal Trainer will have exhibited outstanding customer service and hospitality, along with positive nonverbal communication. In addition, behaviors to enhance the concepts of relationship marketing and the client-centered approach to coaching should have been conscientiously demonstrated.

After the initial client consultation is complete, all the necessary paperwork has been reviewed and a goal-setting action plan has been discussed, the next appointment should then be confirmed. At that time, the Personal Trainer should express gratitude to the client for his or her time and display eagerness for the next visit. As an example of hospitality, the Personal Trainer should send a follow-up note or phone call to the client to compliment him or her on the successful step toward health and fitness, while reminding the client of the next appointment and how to prepare.

As was discussed in the section on relationship marketing, it is important for businesses to continually evaluate success in order to minimize the percentage of "defections" or those clients who do not return. Appropriately at this time, the Personal Trainer should reevaluate how the meeting went. Whether it ended in a large package purchase or not, the Personal Trainer should spend time mentally reviewing and then write down the positives and negatives that occurred in the consultation. He or she should work on the areas of communication skills or approach that may need improvement. All these actions combined will certainly help facilitate a successful beginning to a long-lasting client relationship and set the standard for future client interactions.

SUMMARY

There are several points of client contact leading up to the initial client consultation appointment that set the groundwork for a successful client–Personal Trainer relationship. This includes contact when attempting to generate new clients, the initial client contact when identifying compatibility, and the initial client consultation itself. Every stage of the relationship is critical, so attention to detail should be paid to effective communication throughout the process. Demonstrating exceptional customer service, hospitality, and positive nonverbal cues from the onset not only communicates pride in professionalism but speaks to the respect and high regard placed in the client as well. Furthermore, a focus on relationship marketing coupled with a client-centered approach engenders trust between both parties. Finally, the Personal Trainer should demonstrate professionalism during the initial client consultation by using appropriate information-gathering tools and testing protocols, while communicating skillfully about health and fitness results and the respective personal training action plan.

REFERENCES

1. Capek F. No matter what business you're in, you're in the hospitality business. *Customer Innovations—Driving Profitable Growth* [Internet]. November 2007 [Cited 2008 July 19]. Available from http://customerinnovations.wordpress.com/2007/11/14/no-matter-what-business-youre-in-youre-in-the-hospitality-business/

2. Gummesson E. Making relationship marketing operational. *Int J Serv Industry Manag*. 1994;5(5):5–20.

3. Hagen S. *The Everything Body Language Book: Master the Art of Nonverbal Communication to Succeed in Work, Love, and Life*. Cincinnati (OH): Adams Media Publishing; 2008. 289 p.

4. Holmund M, Kock S. Relationship marketing: the importance of customer-perceived service quality in retail banking. *Serv Ind J*. 1996;16(3):287–304.

5. Kandampully JA. *Services Management: The New Paradigm in Hospitality*. Upper Saddle River (NJ): Pearson Education, Inc.; 2007. 378 p.

6. Kandampully J. Service quality to service loyalty: a relationship which goes beyond customer services. *Total Qual Manag*. 1998;9(6):431–43.

7. Meyer D. *Setting the Table: The Transforming Power of Hospitality in Business*. New York (NY): HarperCollins Publishers; 2006. 320 p.

8. Morgan N. The truth behind the smile and other myths. In: *The Results-Driven Manager: Face-to-Face Communications for Clarity and Impact*. Boston: Harvard Business School Publishing Corporation; 2004. p. 73–81.

9. Morgan N. Are you standing in the way of your own success. In: *The Results-Driven Manager: Face-to-Face Communications for Clarity and Impact*. Boston: Harvard Business School Publishing Corporation; 2004. p. 82–5.

10. Morgan N. What your face reveals and conceals. In: *The Results-Driven Manager: Face-to-Face Communications for Clarity and Impact*. Boston: Harvard Business School Publishing Corporation; 2004. p. 86–94.

11. Reichheld FF, Sasser WE Jr. Zero defections: quality comes to services. *Harv Bus Rev*. Sept–Oct 1990:105–11.

12. Rollnick S, Mason P, Butler C. *Health Behavior Change. A Guide for Practitioners*. New York (NY): Churchill Livingstone; 1999. 225 p.

13. Stewart M, Brown JB, Weston WW, et al. *Patient-Centered Medicine: Transforming the Clinical Method*. 2nd ed. Abingdon, Oxfordshire (UK): Radcliffe Medical Press Ltd.; 2003. 360 p.

14. Whaley MH, Brubaker PH, Otto RM, et al., editors. *ACSM's Guidelines for Exercise Testing and Prescription*. 7th ed. Baltimore: Lippincott Williams & Wilkins; 2006. 56 p.

15. Whiteley JA, Lewis B, Napolitano MA, Marcus BH. Health counseling skills. In: Kaminsky LA, et al., editors. *ACSM's Resource Manual for Guidelines for Exercise Testing and Prescription*. 5th ed. Baltimore: Lippincott Williams & Wilkins; 2006. p. 588–97.

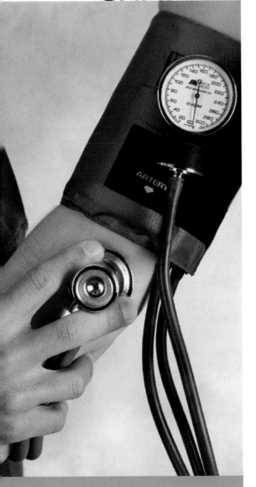

 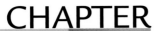

Screening and Risk Stratification

OBJECTIVES

- To communicate the importance of standardized screenings for clients
- To identify and describe appropriate screening components and processes
- To provide resources and templates for the screening process

Guidelines for preparticipation health screening and risk that occur during the initial client consultation with the Personal Trainer are presented within this chapter. The American College of Sports Medicine (2–6), the American Heart Association (2,9), and the American Association of Cardiovascular and Pulmonary Rehabilitation (1) provide published guidelines, in addition to other professional organizations. The exercise professional should review these and other guidelines for additional direction. In addition, the Personal Trainer should assess the guidelines when establishing policies for preparticipation health screening and medical clearance.

WHY SCREEN?

The exercise professional should screen clients before beginning an exercise program, because, despite all of the health, fitness, and functional benefits that come from regular exercise participation, exercise can acutely and transiently increase a client's risk of sudden cardiac death (7,8,15,16) and acute myocardial infarction (heart attack) (11,12). The Personal Trainer must remember that exercise usually provokes cardiovascular events only in clients with preexisting heart disease. Exercise typically does not promote cardiac events in clients with normal cardiovascular systems. However, many clients are unaware of their risk of cardiovascular disease (CVD) or of how other health conditions may be affected by exercise training.

> *Many clients are unaware of their risk of cardiovascular disease (CVD) or of how other health conditions may be affected by exercise training.*

Purposes of Screening

To optimize safety during exercise participation, Personal Trainers should screen all new clients for risk factors and/or symptoms of cardiovascular, pulmonary, and metabolic diseases, as well as for conditions (e.g., pregnancy, orthopedic injury) that may be aggravated by exercise. Even more specifically, the purposes of this preparticipation health screening include the following (4):

➤ Identification and exclusion of clients with medical contraindications to exercise
➤ Identification of clients at increased risk for disease because of age, symptoms, and/or risk factors who should undergo a medical evaluation and exercise testing before starting an exercise program
➤ Identification of clients with clinically significant diseases who should participate in a medically supervised exercise program
➤ Identification of clients with other special needs
➤ Identification of the Personal Trainer best suited to work with the client based on his or her risk factors and/or medical conditions

In addition, the screening process can begin the communication process between the Personal Trainer and the client's healthcare provider while providing opportunities for immediate client education.

THE SCREENING PROCESS

Because Personal Trainers work individually with clients, they are able to develop a more in-depth profile of a client than that typically performed by a client exercising independently outside a clinical program or by a typical health club. The process can be broken down into three distinct, but related, phases:

1. Risk stratification
2. Health history evaluation and related assessments
3. Medical clearance or referral

The screening process should be followed by a discussion of the results with the client, a description of any additional fitness assessments that he or she will perform, and completion of an informed consent. The Personal Trainer can adopt this process by following these steps:

Step 1: Determine the number of risk factors, based on Table 13.1, "Atherosclerotic Cardiovascular Disease Risk Factor Thresholds for Use with ACSM Risk Stratification," and the number of signs and symptoms, based on Table 13.2, "Major Signs or Symptoms Suggestive of Cardiovascular, Pulmonary, or Metabolic Disease."

Step 2: Determine whether the client is at low, moderate, or high risk, based on Figure 13.5, "ACSM Pre-Participation Screening Logic Model."

Step 3: Determine whether a medical evaluation or exercise testing is necessary on the basis of Figure 13.6, "Exercise Testing and Test Supervision Recommendations Based on Risk Stratification"

Step 4: Conduct a health history evaluation (Figs. 13.1 and 13.2).

Step 5: Obtain a medical clearance if indicated by steps 3 or 4 (Figs. 13.3 and 13.4).

Step 6: Complete an informed consent (Fig. 13.8).

Step 7: Conduct appropriate assessments (see Chapter 15).

Step 8: Refer the client to a physician or other healthcare provider if warranted.

Risk Stratification

The ACSM risk stratification process has been widely used to identify clients who should undergo a medical examination and exercise testing before beginning a moderate or vigorous exercise program. The process is based on the client's risk factors for cardiovascular, pulmonary, or metabolic disease; signs and symptoms suggestive of disease; and diagnoses of diseases. This procedure provides recommendations for both medical clearance and physician involvement in submaximal or maximal cardiovascular fitness testing.

> *The ACSM risk stratification process has been widely used to identify clients who should undergo a medical examination and exercise testing before beginning a moderate or vigorous exercise program.*

This important process is frequently not quite as straightforward as described within this chapter. Some Personal Trainers prefer to embed the ACSM risk stratification information into the health history evaluation so they are not two separate pieces. Nothing is wrong with doing this as long as the process to determine risk stratification is followed correctly. Potential musculoskeletal problems can also be assessed through the health-history evaluation. Medical clearance (if necessary) should be obtained after the Personal Trainer has conducted both the risk stratification and a thorough health-history interview with the client. This eliminates the aggravation of contacting the healthcare provider multiple times if medical clearance becomes necessary.

Self-administered questionnaires such as the Physical Activity Readiness Questionnaire (PAR-Q) (Fig. 13.1) and the AHA/ACSM Health/Fitness Facility Pre-Participation Screening Questionnaire (2) can be used as screening/educational tools in both health/fitness facilities and unsupervised fitness facilities (Fig. 13.2). The PAR-Q focuses on symptoms of heart disease, while also identifying musculoskeletal problems that should be evaluated prior to participation in an exercise program. The one-page AHA/ACSM questionnaire is more extensive than the PAR-Q and uses history, symptoms, and risk factors to direct clients to either participate in an exercise program or contact their healthcare provider before participation. Although providing great value to independent exercisers or fitness facilities providing general supervision, self-administered questionnaires are not as useful for Personal Trainers who require a more extensive health profile of their clients.

Personal Trainers, who work in health clubs, should not assume that because clients have been cleared for a membership based on either of these screening tools or based on more in-depth assessments collected previously, they do not require further evaluation or medical clearance. Many

Physical Activity Readiness
Questionnaire - PAR-Q
(revised 2002)

PAR-Q & YOU

(A Questionnaire for People Aged 15 to 69)

Regular physical activity is fun and healthy, and increasingly more people are starting to become more active every day. Being more active is very safe for most people. However, some people should check with their doctor before they start becoming much more physically active.

If you are planning to become much more physically active than you are now, start by answering the seven questions in the box below. If you are between the ages of 15 and 69, the PAR-Q will tell you if you should check with your doctor before you start. If you are over 69 years of age, and you are not used to being very active, check with your doctor.

Common sense is your best guide when you answer these questions. Please read the questions carefully and answer each one honestly: check YES or NO.

YES	NO		
☐	☐	1.	Has your doctor ever said that you have a heart condition <u>and</u> that you should only do physical activity recommended by a doctor?
☐	☐	2.	Do you feel pain in your chest when you do physical activity?
☐	☐	3.	In the past month, have you had chest pain when you were not doing physical activity?
☐	☐	4.	Do you lose your balance because of dizziness or do you ever lose consciousness?
☐	☐	5.	Do you have a bone or joint problem (for example, back, knee or hip) that could be made worse by a change in your physical activity?
☐	☐	6.	Is your doctor currently prescribing drugs (for example, water pills) for your blood pressure or heart condition?
☐	☐	7.	Do you know of <u>any other reason</u> why you should not do physical activity?

If you answered

YES to one or more questions

Talk with your doctor by phone or in person BEFORE you start becoming much more physically active or BEFORE you have a fitness appraisal. Tell your doctor about the PAR-Q and which questions you answered YES.

- You may be able to do any activity you want — as long as you start slowly and build up gradually. Or, you may need to restrict your activities to those which are safe for you. Talk with your doctor about the kinds of activities you wish to participate in and follow his/her advice.
- Find out which community programs are safe and helpful for you.

NO to all questions

If you answered NO honestly to <u>all</u> PAR-Q questions, you can be reasonably sure that you can:
- start becoming much more physically active — begin slowly and build up gradually. This is the safest and easiest way to go.
- take part in a fitness appraisal — this is an excellent way to determine your basic fitness so that you can plan the best way for you to live actively. It is also highly recommended that you have your blood pressure evaluated. If your reading is over 144/94, talk with your doctor before you start becoming much more physically active.

DELAY BECOMING MUCH MORE ACTIVE:
- if you are not feeling well because of a temporary illness such as a cold or a fever — wait until you feel better; or
- if you are or may be pregnant — talk to your doctor before you start becoming more active.

PLEASE NOTE: If your health changes so that you then answer YES to any of the above questions, tell your fitness or health professional. Ask whether you should change your physical activity plan.

<u>Informed Use of the PAR-Q</u>: The Canadian Society for Exercise Physiology, Health Canada, and their agents assume no liability for persons who undertake physical activity, and if in doubt after completing this questionnaire, consult your doctor prior to physical activity.

No changes permitted. You are encouraged to photocopy the PAR-Q but only if you use the entire form.

NOTE: If the PAR-Q is being given to a person before he or she participates in a physical activity program or a fitness appraisal, this section may be used for legal or administrative purposes.

"I have read, understood and completed this questionnaire. Any questions I had were answered to my full satisfaction."

NAME _____

SIGNATURE _____   DATE _____

SIGNATURE OF PARENT _____   WITNESS _____
or GUARDIAN (for participants under the age of majority)

Note: This physical activity clearance is valid for a maximum of 12 months from the date it is completed and becomes invalid if your condition changes so that you would answer YES to any of the seven questions.

CSEP
SCPE © Canadian Society for Exercise Physiology   Supported by: [Canada flag] Health   Santé
                                                                        Canada   Canada   continued on other side...

FIGURE 13.1. PAR-Q & You. (Used with permission from the Canadian Society for Exercise Physiology. Physical Activity Readiness Questionnaire [PAR-Q]. 2002. www.csep.ca.)

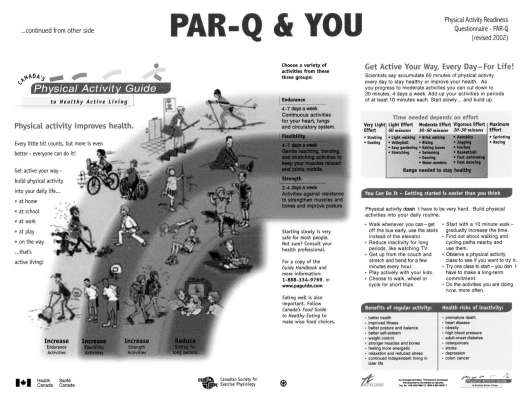

...continued from other side

PAR-Q & YOU

Physical Activity Readiness
Questionnaire - PAR-Q
(revised 2002)

Source: Canada's Physical Activity Guide to Healthy Active Living, Health Canada, 1998 http://www.hc-sc.gc.ca/hppb/paguide/pdf/guideEng.pdf
© Reproduced with permission from the Minister of Public Works and Government Services Canada, 2002.

FITNESS AND HEALTH PROFESSIONALS MAY BE INTERESTED IN THE INFORMATION BELOW:

The following companion forms are available for doctors' use by contacting the Canadian Society for Exercise Physiology (address below):

The **Physical Activity Readiness Medical Examination (PARmed-X)** – to be used by doctors with people who answer YES to one or more questions on the PAR-Q.

The **Physical Activity Readiness Medical Examination for Pregnancy (PARmed-X for Pregnancy)** – to be used by doctors with pregnant patients who wish to become more active.

References:
Arraix, G.A., Wigle, D.T., Mao, Y. (1992). Risk Assessment of Physical Activity and Physical Fitness in the Canada Health Survey
    Follow-Up Study. **J. Clin. Epidemiol.** 45:4 419-428.
Mottola, M., Wolfe, L.A. (1994). Active Living and Pregnancy, In: A. Quinney, L. Gauvin, T. Wall (eds.), **Toward Active Living: Proceedings of the International
    Conference on Physical Activity, Fitness and Health**. Champaign, IL: Human Kinetics.
PAR-Q Validation Report, British Columbia Ministry of Health, 1978.
Thomas, S., Reading, J., Shephard, R.J. (1992). Revision of the Physical Activity Readiness Questionnaire (PAR-Q). **Can. J. Spt. Sci.** 17:4 338-345.

For more information, please contact the:

Canadian Society for Exercise Physiology
202-185 Somerset Street West
Ottawa, ON K2P 0J2
Tel. 1-877-651-3755 • FAX (613) 234-3565
Online: www.csep.ca

© Canadian Society for Exercise Physiology

Supported by: Health Canada / Santé Canada

The original PAR-Q was developed by the British Columbia Ministry of Health. It has been revised by an Expert Advisory Committee of the Canadian Society for Exercise Physiology chaired by Dr. N. Gledhill (2002).

Disponible en français sous le titre «Questionnaire sur l'aptitude à l'activité physique - Q-AAP (revisé 2002)».

FIGURE 13.1. *(Continued)*

AHA/ACSM Health/Fitness Facility Preparticipation Screening Questionnaire

Access your health status by marking all *true* statements

History

You have had:
- a heart attack
- heart surgery
- cardiac catheterization
- coronary angioplasty (PTCA)
- pacemaker-implantable cardiac defibrillatory/rhythm disturbance
- heart valve disease
- heart failure
- heart transplantation
- congenital heart disease

Symptoms

- You experience chest discomfort with exertion
- You experience unreasonable breathlessness
- You experience dizziness, fainting, or blackouts
- You take heart medications

> If you marked any of these statements in this section, consult your physician or other appropriate health care provider before engaging in exercise. You may need to use a facility with a **m edically qualified staff.**

Other health issues

- You have diabetes
- You have asthma or other lung disease
- You have burning or cramping sensation in your lower legs when walking short distances
- You have musculoskeletal problems that limit your physical activity
- You have concerns about the safety of exercise
- You take prescription medications
- You are pregnant

Cardiovascular risk factors

- You are a man 45 years or older
- You are a woman 55 years or older
- You smoke, or quit smoking within the previous 6 months
- Your blood pressure is >140/90 mm Hg
- You do not know your blood pressure
- You take blood pressure medication
- Your blood cholesterol level is >200 mg/dL
- You do not know your cholesterol level
- You have a close blood relative who had a heart attack or heart surgery before age 55 (father or brother) or age 65 (mother or sister)
- You are physically inactive (ie, you get <30 minutes of physical activity on at least 3 days/week)
- You are >20 pounds overweight.

> If you marked two or more of the statements in this section, you should consult your physician or other appropriate healthcare provider before engaging in exercise. You might benefit from using a facility with a **professionally qualified exercise staff[†]** to guide your exercise program.

[†] Professionally qualified exercise staff refers to appropriately trained individuals who posses academic training, practical and clinical knowledge, skills and abilities commensurate with the credentials defined in Appendix D of <u>ACSM's Guidelines for Exercise Testing and Prescription 8e.</u>

- None of the above

> You should be able to exercise safely without consulting your physician or other appropriate health care provider in a self-guided program or almost any facility that meets your exercise program needs.

Modified from **American College of Sports Medicine and American Heart Association ACSM/AHA** joint position statement. Recommendations for cardiovascular screening, sta ffing and emergency policies at health fitness facilities. Med Sci Sports Exerc 1998:1018.

FIGURE 13.2. AHA/ACSM Health/Fitness Facility Preparticipation Screening Questionnaire. (Modified from American College of Sports Medicine Position Stand and American Heart Association. Recommendations for cardiovascular screening, staffing, and emergency policies at health/fitness facilities. *Med Sci Sports Exerc.* 1998:1018; American College of Sports Medicine. *ACSM's Guidelines for Exercise Testing and Prescription.* 8th ed. Baltimore: Lippincott Williams & Wilkins; 2010.)

health clubs require absolutely no health paperwork to be submitted before being accepted as a new member. Personal Trainers should always confirm with clients that their risk stratification and health information are accurate and up-to-date before proceeding with exercise training. Signs and symptoms suggesting CVD can appear suddenly, medication changes are frequent, and injuries may occur without warning. A client is possibly seeking the assistance of a Personal Trainer because he or she has begun to experience new or additional signs and symptoms that he or she has not yet communicated to others (e.g., healthcare providers).

Clients transitioning out of cardiopulmonary rehabilitation, physical therapy, or another medically supervised program will still need written medical clearance even if their physicians referred them to a

> *Clients transitioning out of cardiopulmonary rehabilitation, physical therapy, or another medically supervised program will still need written medical clearance even if their physicians referred them to a Personal Trainer or a club or recommended that they continue exercise on their own.*

Personal Trainer or a club or recommended that they continue exercise on their own. The advantage for the Personal Trainer is being able to access the client's exercise records and clinical documentation. This can be accomplished by asking the client to get a copy of his or her file from the healthcare provider or sign a waiver for the Personal Trainer to obtain a copy directly from the healthcare provider (Figs. 13.3 and 13.4).

Coronary Artery Disease Risk Factors

The ACSM risk stratification has been recently updated to include an individual's age, prediabetes, and exposure to environmental tobacco smoke (4). Nevertheless, as the Personal Trainer can tell, this risk stratification is based, in part, on the presence or absence of the CVD risk factors listed in Table 13.1 (4–6,10,11,13,14,17–19). The risk factors in Table 13.1 must not be viewed as an all-inclusive list, but rather as a group with *clinically relevant thresholds* that should be considered collectively when making decisions about the level of medical clearance, the need for exercise testing before initiating participation, and the level of supervision for both exercise testing and exercise program participation. The *scope* of the list and the *threshold* for each risk factor should not be viewed as inconsistent with other risk factor lists that are intended for use in predicting coronary events during long-term follow-up (4), because the intended use for the list in Table 13.1 is to aid in the prediction or identification of as yet undiagnosed coronary artery disease.

SIGNS OR SYMPTOMS OF CARDIOVASCULAR, PULMONARY, AND METABOLIC DISEASES

Table 13.2 presents a list of major signs or symptoms that suggest cardiovascular, pulmonary, and/or metabolic disease, along with additional information to aid in the clarification and significance of each sign or symptom (4). The presence of most of these risk factors can be detected using a questionnaire; however, a few (e.g., shortness of breath while lying down or orthopnea, ankle swelling or edema, heart murmur) require a more thorough medical history and/or examination.

ACSM RISK CATEGORIES

Once the symptom and risk factor information is known, potential clients can be stratified on the basis of the likelihood of events during exercise program participation. Risk stratification becomes progressively more important as disease prevalence increases in the population under consideration.

> *Risk stratification becomes progressively more important as disease prevalence increases in the population under consideration.*

Using health status, symptoms, and risk factor information, potential clients can be classified into one of three risk strata (Fig. 13.5) for referral to other healthcare providers for further screening prior to participation.

Sample medical clearance form

Date: *Insert here*

Dear Dr. Rodriguez,

I am writing to you in regard to your patient, Suzanne Walker-Smith, a 40 year-old female (DOB: December 6, 1969), who indicated you are her primary physician. She would like to begin a moderate to vigorous intensity exercise program under the supervision of a certified Personal Trainer. I have attached her authorization for the release of her medical information, plus her responses to our cardiovascular screening questionnaire.

Please provide your recommendation regarding her exercise participation and any restrictions and/or limitations you suggest for her program. Should you have any questions or concerns, please contact me at the number below. Thank you.

Physician recommendation:

☐ Patient may participate in unrestricted activity.

☐ Patient may participate in light to moderate activities only.

☐ Patient should not participate in activity at this time.

☐ Other: please specify: _____

_____

Please specify any restrictions or limitations you feel appropriate: _____

_____

Physician (print name):_____ Date: _____ Telephone: _____

Signature: _____

Personal Trainer (name):_____ Date: _____ Telephone: _____

Send this form to:

Your first/last name, title
Company Name
Street address
City, State, Zip Code
Fax
Email address

FIGURE 13.3. Sample medical clearance form.

Inherent within the concept of risk stratification is the impression that signs and symptoms (Table 13.2) represent a higher level of concern for decision making than do risk factors (Table 13.1). However, hypertension (high blood pressure) represents a unique risk factor in that it may be aggravated by short-term exercise, such as weight training. Therefore, although it appears within Table 13.1, special consideration should be given to hypertensive clients when screening for exercise testing or training. The Seventh Report of the Joint National Committee on Prevention, Detection, Evaluation, and Treatment of High Blood Pressure (JNC7) (18) recommends a thorough medical history, physical examination, routine laboratory tests, and other diagnostic procedures in the

Release of medical information form

Date: *Insert here*

Dear Dr. Rodriquez,

I, Suzanne Walker-Smith, a 40 year-old female, (DOB: December 6, 1969), hereby authorize the immediate release of a copy of all my medical information to the following person(s):

Your first/last name, Personal Trainer
Company Name
Street address
City, Staty, Zip Code
Fax
Email address

My purpose of disclosing this information is to begin/continue an exercise program with the above Personal Trainer.

Patient's signature: _____ Date: _____ Telephone: _____

FIGURE 13.4. Example of release of medical information form.

evaluation of clients with documented hypertension. Because hypertension is commonly clustered with other risk factors associated with CVD (e.g., dyslipidemia, obesity, diabetes), most hypertensive clients who want to start an exercise program fall into the *moderate-* or *high-*risk category as defined in Figure 13.5. For such clients, the medical examination suggested in Figure 13.6 is consistent with the screening recommendations for hypertensive clients outlined in JNC7 (18). However, in cases of isolated hypertension (i.e., hypertension is the only risk factor from those conditions listed in Table 13.1), prudent recommendations for preparticipation screening should be based on the severity of the hypertension and the desired intensity of exercise. For *low-*risk clients with isolated stage 1 hypertension (<160/100 mm Hg), exercise testing generally is not necessary for clearance to engage in up to moderate-intensity exercise. However, it is advisable for such clients to have physician clearance prior to participation. On the other hand, if the client has documented stage 2 hypertension or if a client with stage 1 hypertension desires to engage in more intense exercise training, an exercise assessment is recommended to quantify blood pressure responses during exercise to aid in establishing prudent guidelines for exercise training (4).

Exercise Testing and Testing Supervision Recommendations

The Personal Trainer must remember that no set of guidelines for exercise testing and participation can cover all situations. Many circumstances, policies, and program procedures vary by location. To provide some general guidance on the need for a medical examination and exercise testing prior to

TABLE 13.1	ATHEROSCLEROTIC CARDIOVASCULAR DISEASE RISK FACTOR THRESHOLDS FOR USE WITH ACSM RISK STRATIFICATION
Risk Factors	**Defining Criteria**
Positive	
Age	Men $\geq$ 45 yr; women $\geq$ 55 yr
Family history	Myocardial infarction, coronary revascularization, or sudden death before 55 years of age in father or other male first-degree relative, or before 65 years of age in mother or other female first-degree relative
Cigarette smoking	Current cigarette smoker or those who quit within the previous 6 months or exposure to environmental tobacco smoke
Sedentary lifestyle	Not participating in at least 30 min of moderate-intensity (40%–60% $\dot{V}O_2R$) physical activity on at least 3 days of the week for at least 3 months
Obesity[a]	Body mass index >30 kg · m^2 or waist girth >102 cm (40 in) for men and >88 cm (35 in) for women
Hypertension	Systolic blood pressure $\geq$ 140 mm Hg or diastolic $\geq$ 90 mm Hg, confirmed by measurements on at least two separate occasions or on antihypertensive medication
Dyslipidemia	Low-density lipoprotein cholesterol $\geq$ 130 mg · dL^{-1} (3.4 mmol · L^{-1}) or high-density lipoprotein (HDL-C) cholesterol <40 mg · dL^{-1} (1.04 mmol · L^{-1}) or on lipid-lowering medication; if total serum cholesterol is all that is available, use $\geq$200 mg · dL^{-1} (5.2 mmol · L^{-1})
Prediabetes	Impaired fasting glucose = fasting plasma glucose $\geq$ 100 mg · dL^{-1} (5.50 mmol · L^{-1}) but <126 mg · dL^{-1} (6.93 mmol · L^{-1}) *or* impaired glucose tolerance = 2-hour values in oral glucose tolerance test $\geq$ 140 mg · dL^{-1} (7.70 mmol · L^{-1}) but <200 mg · dL^{-1} (11.00 mmol · L^{-1}) confirmed by measurements on at least two separate occasions
Negative	
High serum HDL cholesterol[b]	$\geq$60 mg · dL^{-1} (1.6 mmol · L^{-1})

Reprinted from American College of Sports Medicine. *ACSM's Guidelines for Exercise Testing and Prescription.* 8th ed. Baltimore: Lippincott Williams & Wilkins; 2010.

Hypertension threshold based on National High Blood Pressure Education Program. The Seventh Report of the Joint National Committee on Prevention, Detection, Evaluation, and Treatment of High Blood Pressure, 03-5233, 2003. Lipid thresholds based on National Cholesterol Education Program. Third Report of the National Cholesterol Education Program Expert Panel on Detection, Evaluation, and Treatment of High Blood Cholesterol in Adults (Adult Treatment Panel III). NIH Publication no. 02-5215, 2002. Impaired FG threshold based on Expert Committee on the Diagnosis and Classification of Diabetes Mellitus. Follow-up report on the diagnosis of diabetes mellitus. *Diabetes Care.* 2003;26:3160–7. Obesity thresholds based on Expert Panel on Detection, Evaluation, and Treatment of Overweight and Obesity in Adults. National Institutes of Health. Clinical guidelines on the identification, evaluation, and treatment of overweight and obesity in adults—the evidence report. *Arch Intern Med.* 1998;158:1855–67. Sedentary lifestyle thresholds based on U.S. Department of Health and Human Services. Physical activity and health: a report of the Surgeon General, 1996.

[a]Professional opinions vary regarding the most appropriate markers and thresholds for obesity, and therefore, allied healthcare professionals should use clinical judgment when evaluating this risk factor.

[b]It is common to sum risk factors in making clinical judgments. If HDL is high, subtract one risk factor from the sum of positive risk factors, because high HDL decreases CAD risk.

participation in a moderate-to-vigorous exercise program, ACSM suggests the recommendations presented in Figure 13.6 for determining when a medical examination and diagnostic exercise test are appropriate and when physician supervision is recommended during exercise testing. Although the testing guidelines are less rigorous for those clients considered to be at low risk, the information gathered from an exercise test may be useful in establishing a safe and effective exercise prescription for these clients. The exercise-testing recommendations found in Figure 13.6 reflect the notion that the risk of cardiovascular events increases as a function of increasing physical activity intensity. Personal Trainers should choose the most appropriate definition of their setting when making decisions about the level of screening to use prior to exercise training and whether or not it is necessary to have physician supervision during exercise testing.

TABLE 13.2	MAJOR SIGNS OR SYMPTOMS SUGGESTIVE OF CARDIOVASCULAR, PULMONARY, OR METABOLIC DISEASE[a]
Sign or Symptom	**Clarification/Significance**

Pain, discomfort (or other anginal equivalent) in the chest, neck, jaw, arms, or other areas that may result from ischemia	One of the cardinal manifestations of cardiac disease, in particular coronary artery disease
	Key features *favoring an ischemic origin* include:
	  Character: Constricting, squeezing, burning, "heaviness" or "heavy feeling"
	  Location: Substernal, across midthorax, anteriorly; in both arms and shoulders; in neck, cheeks, and teeth; in forearms and fingers; in interscapular region
	  Provoking factors: Exercise or exertion, excitement, other forms of stress, cold weather, occurrence after meals
	Key features *against an ischemic origin* include:
	  Character: Dull ache; "knifelike," sharp, stabbing; "jabs" aggravated by respiration
	  Location: In left submammary area; in left hemithorax
	  Provoking factors: After completion of exercise, provoked by a specific body motion

Shortness of breath at rest or with mild exertion	Dyspnea (defined as an abnormally uncomfortable awareness of breathing) is one of the principal symptoms of cardiac and pulmonary disease. It commonly occurs during strenuous exertion in healthy, well-trained persons and during moderate exertion in healthy, untrained persons. However, it should be regarded as abnormal when it occurs at a level of exertion that is not expected to evoke this symptom in a given individual. Abnormal exertional dyspnea suggests the presence of cardiopulmonary disorders, in particular left ventricular dysfunction or chronic obstructive pulmonary disease.
Dizziness or syncope	Syncope (defined as a loss of consciousness) is most commonly caused by a reduced perfusion of the brain. Dizziness and, in particular, syncope *during* exercise may result from cardiac disorders that prevent the normal rise (or an actual fall) in cardiac output. Such cardiac disorders are potentially life-threatening and include severe coronary artery disease, hypertrophic cardiomyopathy, aortic stenosis, and malignant ventricular dysrhythmias. Although dizziness or syncope shortly *after* cessation of exercise should not be ignored, these symptoms may occur even in healthy persons as a result of a reduction in venous return to the heart.
Orthopnea or paroxysmal nocturnal dyspnea	Orthopnea refers to dyspnea occurring at rest in the recumbent position that is relieved promptly by sitting upright or standing. Paroxysmal nocturnal dyspnea refers to dyspnea, beginning usually 2–5 hours after the onset of sleep, which may be relieved by sitting on the side of the bed or getting out of bed. Both are symptoms of left ventricular dysfunction. Although nocturnal dyspnea may occur in persons with chronic obstructive pulmonary disease, it differs in that it is usually relieved after the person relieves himself or herself of secretions rather than specifically by sitting up.
Ankle edema	Bilateral ankle edema that is most evident at night is a characteristic sign of heart failure or bilateral chronic venous insufficiency. Unilateral edema of a limb often results from venous thrombosis or lymphatic blockage in the limb. Generalized edema (known as anasarca) occurs in persons with the nephrotic syndrome, severe heart failure, or hepatic cirrhosis.

(continued)

TABLE 13.2	MAJOR SIGNS OR SYMPTOMS SUGGESTIVE OF CARDIOVASCULAR, PULMONARY, OR METABOLIC DISEASE[a] (*Continued*)
Palpitations or tachycardia	Palpitations (defined as an unpleasant awareness of the forceful or rapid beating of the heart) may be induced by various disorders of cardiac rhythm. These include tachycardia, bradycardia of sudden onset, ectopic beats, compensatory pauses, and accentuated stroke volume resulting from valvular regurgitation. Palpitations also often result from anxiety states, such as anemia, fever, thyrotoxicosis, arteriovenous fistula, and the so-called idiopathic hyperkinetic heart syndrome.
Intermittent claudication	Intermittent claudication refers to the pain that occurs in a muscle with an inadequate blood supply (usually as a result of atherosclerosis) that is stressed by exercise. The pain does not occur with standing or sitting, is reproducible from day to day, is more severe when walking upstairs or up a hill, and is often described as a cramp, which disappears within 1 or 2 minutes after stopping exercise. Coronary artery disease is more prevalent in persons with intermittent claudication. Patients with diabetes are at increased risk for this condition.
Known heart murmur	Although some may be innocent, heart murmurs may indicate valvular or other cardiovascular disease. From an exercise safety standpoint, it is especially important to exclude hypertrophic cardiomyopathy and aortic stenosis as underlying causes because these are among the more common causes of exertion-related sudden cardiac death.
Unusual fatigue or shortness of breath with usual activities	Although there may be benign origins for these symptoms, they also may signal the onset of, or change in the status of, cardiovascular, pulmonary, or metabolic disease.

Reprinted with permission from American College of Sports Medicine. *ACSM's Guidelines for Exercise Testing and Prescription.* 8th ed. Baltimore: Lippincott Williams & Wilkins; 2010.

[a] These signs or symptoms must be interpreted within the clinical context in which they appear because they are not all specific for cardiovascular, pulmonary, or metabolic disease.

> *The degree of physician supervision may differ, depending on local policies and circumstances, the client's health status, and the experience of the staff conducting the test.*

Medical supervision of exercise tests varies appropriately from physician-supervised tests to situations in which there may be no physician present (5). The degree of physician supervision may differ, depending on local policies and circumstances, the client's health status, and the experience of the staff conducting the test. The appropriate protocol should be based on the age, health status, and physical-activity level of the potential client to be tested. In all situations in which exercise testing is performed, site personnel should at least be certified at a level of basic life support (4,5) (including operation of automated external defibrillators); preferably, one or more staff members should be certified in advanced cardiac life support (2). Because of their knowledge, skills, and abilities, ACSM-certified professionals should, ideally, be the individuals performing exercise testing.

Health-History Evaluation

Conducting a thorough health history will provide the Personal Trainer with valuable information for developing a client's program (Fig. 13.7). Specifically, the purposes of a health history are to identify known disease and risk factors for disease, especially CVD, and to identify conditions that

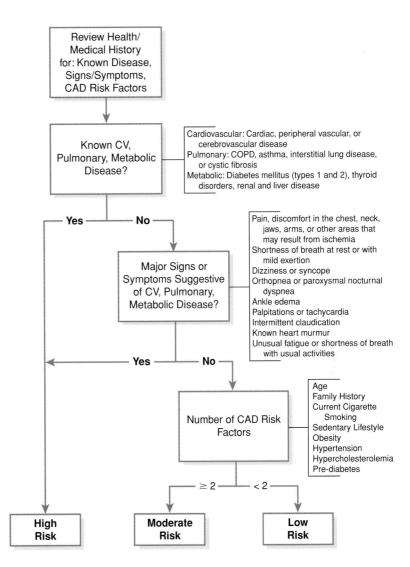

FIGURE 13.5. ACSM preparticipation screening logic model for risk stratification. (Reprinted from American College of Sports Medicine. *ACSM's Guidelines for Exercise Testing and Prescription.* 8th ed. Baltimore: Lippincott Williams & Wilkins; 2010.)

warrant special consideration when developing an exercise program or require referral to a health-care provider.

The Personal Trainer needs to remember, because no standard health-history form exists (because forms often vary depending on the setting), a description of the kinds of information to include on a health-history form is discussed below. A sample self-administered health-history form is shown in Figure 13.2. While traditionally not viewed as health-history information, assessments of physical activity level, dietary habits, and learning style may also be included in the initial client consultation to provide the most complete picture of the client's health. The new ACSM/American Medical Association *Exercise is Medicine*™ Campaign now encourages physicians to ask about patient physical activity level at every visit and treat physical activity level as a vital sign.

➤ **Medical history:** Current and previous medical conditions, injuries, surgical procedures, and therapies are all vital factors that influence the development of an exercise plan. The Personal Trainer should always include dates for each and discuss each one with the client so that there is a full understanding of the extent or severity of any medical condition.

➤ **Medications:** Some medications, such as calcium channel blockers and β-blockers, affect heart rate and/or blood pressure response to exercise, thus altering the exercise prescription. Because

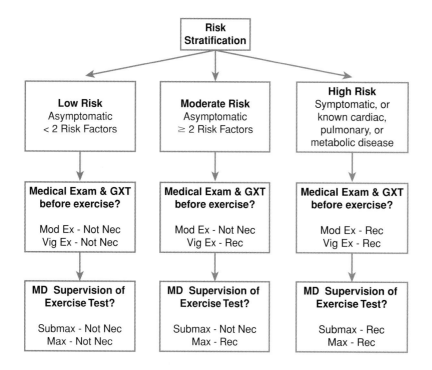

Mod Ex: Moderate intensity exercise; 40-60% of $\dot{V}O_{2max}$; 3-6 METs; "an intensity well within the individual's capacity, one which can be comfortably sustained for a prolonged period of time (~45 minutes)"

Vig Ex: Vigorous intensity exercise; > 60% of $\dot{V}O_{2max}$; > 6 METs; "exercise intense enough to represent a substantial cardiorespiratory challenge"

Not Nec: Not Necessary; reflects the notion that a medical examination, exercise test, and physician supervision of exercise testing would not be essential in the preparticipation screening, however, they should not be viewed as inappropriate

Rec: Recommended; when MD supervision of exercise testing is "Recommended," the MD shold be in close proximity and readily available should there be an emergent need

FIGURE 13.6. Exercise testing and test supervision recommendations based on risk stratification. (Reprinted from American College of Sports Medicine. *ACSM's Guidelines for Exercise Testing and Prescription*. 8th ed. Baltimore: Lippincott Williams & Wilkins; 2010.)

medications change frequently, clients need to be instructed to report any significant alterations in their prescriptions immediately to their Personal Trainer.

➤ **Exercise history:** A client's experience with exercise is an important factor to consider when developing a program, as it could affect his or her ability to advance to more difficult movements, attitude toward exercise, and the kinds of exercise in which he or she is willing to engage.

➤ **Nutrition:** Dietary intake affects many aspects of a client's life, such as weight and body composition, risk for disease, mood, and energy level. Nutrition and dietary aspects related to exercise are discussed in more depth in Chapter 6.

Documentation

Documentation is an important and critical aspect of risk management. Personal Trainers should maintain accurate records of client responses to testing and training, changes in reported health status, and how these are referred to appropriate healthcare providers. Client health information should be updated regularly to document any changes in medications and conditions. The Personal Trainer needs to ensure that this documentation is kept in a safe place to maintain the client's confidentiality. Although no set rule exists for how long records should be maintained, 3–5 years is a typical length of time.

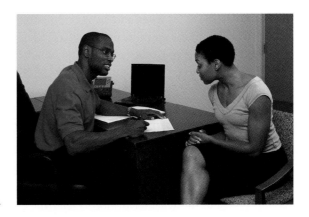

FIGURE 13.7. Consultation with a client.

MEDICAL CLEARANCE AND REFERRAL

Obtaining Medical Clearance

According to the ACSM risk-stratification process, initial clearance to exercise should be obtained from a physician when necessary. This clearance should also be obtained when clients have had any significant or recent change in health status that has not yet been evaluated by a physician. This can be accomplished by sending a medical clearance form (Fig. 13.3) to the physician's office. Also, make sure that the client agrees to release this additional medical information (Fig. 13.4) per the Health Insurance Portability and Accountability Act.

Clients commonly have multiple healthcare providers, such as a general practitioner, specialists (e.g., cardiologist, orthopedist, oncologist, obstetrician), and therapists. As all of these professionals work together as a team, they rely on one another to make decisions that are beyond their scope of practice and expertise. Many times, the general practitioner will defer clearance to the specialist based on specific medical conditions. Although necessary, it can slow down the clearance process, because the Personal Trainer may need to contact multiple providers.

The Personal Trainer should keep in mind, however, that there is a difference between obtaining medical clearance to exercise and obtaining expert opinion that will help create the best possible exercise program for the client. Obtaining medical clearance means that the Personal Trainer will not allow the client to exercise until the physician approves to do so. When seeking an expert opinion, the Personal Trainer typically proceeds with training, even if modified, and incorporates the recommendations of the physician into the program. The Personal Trainer should make sure that communication with healthcare providers clearly explains the intent of the questions. More information on working with healthcare providers is discussed in subsequent sections in this chapter.

> *Obtaining medical clearance means that the Personal Trainer will not allow the client to exercise until the physician approves to do so.*

When to Refer?

> *It is the responsibility of the Personal Trainer to refer clients to other members of the team when problems or potential problems arise or are identified that are beyond the Personal Trainer's scope of practice.*

By screening and assessing a new client, the Personal Trainer becomes a part of the healthcare team, which may include physicians, specialists, clinical exercise physiologists, physical therapists, physical therapy assistants, chiropractors, registered dietitians, athletic trainers, nurses, nurse practitioners, and physician assistants. Therefore, it is the responsibility of the Personal Trainer to refer clients to other members of the team when problems or potential problems arise or are identified that are beyond the Personal Trainer's scope of practice. Referring clients for medical clearance based on the ACSM risk stratification process or information obtained during the health-history evaluation has already been briefly discussed, but referral may take place at any time, such as during the physical assessment process, once exercise training has begun or even several months into training.

REFERRAL DURING SCREENING

The physical assessments described in detail in Chapter 14 are designed to provide the Personal Trainer with more information regarding the client's abilities and potential limitations. Potential problems may be discovered during these assessments. When this occurs, the Personal Trainer must decide whether or not to refer the client to a healthcare provider for a more in-depth assessment. It is certainly advisable to err on the side of caution. If in doubt, the Personal Trainer should refer the client to an appropriate physician or specialist.

For example, a new client reports no joint problems on the health history evaluation but during an initial assessment the Personal Trainer discovers the client's left arm can abduct only 45° while maintaining scapular retraction. Upon questioning the client, the Personal Trainer learns that the client injured his left shoulder when he was in elementary school. The client has not had complete range of motion since that time. However, because it does not cause him pain and he has learned to live with the limitation, he did not feel that it was important enough to report on the health-history form. Given the significant limitation of the shoulder joint and the risk of further damage during upper body strength movements, the Personal Trainer may decide to refer the client to a physician for further assessment. In the meantime, the Personal Trainer proceeds with cardiovascular, lower body, and core exercises so the client can begin training without risking further injury to the shoulder joint.

REFERRAL DURING TRAINING

Personal Trainers are responsible to continually reevaluate the health status of their clients through either formal (direct questions, written or physical assessments) or informal (casual conversation, observation) means, even as the exercise training begins. The onset of new signs and symptoms, aggravation of existing medical conditions, or occurrences of injury may warrant stopping or modifying exercise training until after further consultation with the physician. Recognizing these situations and communicating effectively with the healthcare team will maximize the safety of clients, increase their probability of successfully reaching established health and fitness goals, and raise the stature of the Personal Trainer in the eyes of the medical community. Any incident of a client reporting new signs or symptoms as listed in Table 13.2 requires that the Personal Trainer stop exercise training and initiate an immediate examination by a medical professional. Likewise, any significant change in the frequency, intensity, or nature of a client's existing signs and symptoms should also prompt immediate referral to a physician.

Serious joint injuries or those that do not resolve quickly should, at a minimum, prompt modification of training techniques to protect or minimize strain on the joint and a recommendation to follow up with a healthcare professional. In addition, clients reporting a muscle or joint problem (e.g., redness, swelling, pain, stiffness, burning sensation) that has been either brought on or aggravated by exercise should be referred to a healthcare professional. Sometimes this is an unclear situation that depends on the Personal Trainer's experience and interpretation of the information. Sometimes determining the difference between discomfort associated with exercise and signs of an injury or other orthopedic condition can be difficult. When in doubt, the Personal Trainer should seek the advice of healthcare professionals. The Personal Trainer should encourage the injured clients to use the

When in doubt, the Personal Trainer should seek the advice of healthcare professionals.

RICE (rest, ice, compression, and elevation) method until they can get an appointment with their physicians.

When referring a client for consultation, sending documentation directly to the physician is helpful. The Personal Trainer should be sure to include any measurements taken of the client, such as heart rate and blood pressure before, during, and after exercise, along with any observed signs and symptoms (e.g., sweating, pain). A clear, concise, and accurate description of the situation will allow the physician to make an informed decision as to the best course of action for the client.

Communicating with Healthcare Providers

Communicating with healthcare providers can be intimidating at first, but when done properly and consistently, it can lead to great benefits for both the Personal Trainer and the client. The Personal Trainer can follow these simple guidelines to maximize the effectiveness of communications with healthcare providers:

➤ Always include information that clearly identifies the client, including his or her full name, age, gender, and date of birth.
➤ Be clear and to the point as to the purpose of the communication (physicians, especially, have very little time to read long documents).
➤ Set a response date (if something needs to be turned around quickly, write "URGENT" in big letters at the top of the form).
➤ Provide options that can be checked off easily.
➤ Allow room for additional comments.
➤ Faxing or e-mailing is typically more effective and quicker than the mail system (for a quicker reply, call the office staff and notify them that a fax or an e-mail that needs attention is on the way).
➤ If requesting a release or personal medical information, then automatically include a release of medical information form (Fig. 13.4) signed by your client. Again, include information that will identify your specific client (e.g., full name, date of birth, age, and gender).

Not all communications need to request a response. Simply informing and educating the physician and/or other individuals in the medical community about the Personal Trainer's training, experience, and services can be a valuable marketing tool. Some Personal Trainers find it useful to personally visit medical offices, provide in-service training over lunch hours for medical staff, send introductory packets or letters to physicians of new clients, and provide brief periodic updates on clients.

Informed Consent

Although some locations do not require informed consent for fitness assessments, it is widely accepted within the health/fitness industry to do so. The informed consent form is intended to ensure that the client:

➤ Has full knowledge of what tests are going to be performed.
➤ Understands the relevant risks associated with those tests.
➤ Knows about alternative procedures.
➤ Understands the benefits associated with the assessments.
➤ Is provided with an opportunity for inquiry.

Written consent is preferable to verbal or implied consent. A sample informed consent form is included in Figure 13.8; however, the Personal Trainer should always obtain appropriate legal counsel when creating or adopting an informed consent document.

Informed consent for an exercise test

— Purpose and explanation of the test

You will perform an exercise test on a cycle ergometer or motor-driven treadmill. The exercise intensity will begin at a low level and will be advanced in stages depending on your fitness level. We may stop the test at any time because of signs of fatigue or changes in your heart rate, ECG, or blood pressure, or symptoms you may experience. It is important for you to realize that you may stop when you wish because of feelings of fatigue or any other discomfort.

— Attendant risks and discomforts

There exists the possibility of certain changes occurring during the test. These include abnormal blood pressure, fainting, irregular, fast or slow heart rhythm, and in rare instances, heart attack, stroke, or death. Every effort will be made to minimize these risks by evaluation of preliminary information relating to your health and fitness and by careful observation during the testing. Emergency equipment and trained personnel are available to deal with unusual situations that may arise.

— Responsibilities of the participant

Information you possess about your health status or previous experiences of heart-related symptoms (e.g., shortness of breath with low-level activity, pain, pressure, tightness, heaviness in the chest, neck, jaw, back, and/or arms) with physical effort may affect the safety of your exercise test. Your prompt reporting of these and any other unusual feelings with effort during the exercise test itself is very important. You are responsible for fully disclosing your medical history, as well as symptoms that may occur during the test. You are also expected to report all medications (including non-prescription) taken recently and, in particular, those taken today, to the testing staff.

— Benefits to be expected

The results obtained from the exercise test may assist in the diagnosis of your illness, in evaluating the effect of your medications or in evaluating what type of physical activities you might do with low risk.

— Inquiries

Any questions about the procedures used in the exercise test or the results of your test are encouraged. If you have any concerns or questions, please ask us for further explanations.

— Use of medical records

The information that is obtained during exercise testing will be treated as privileged and confidential as described in the Health Insurance Portability and Accountability Act of 1996. It is not to be released or revealed to any person except your referring physician without your written consent. However, the information obtained may be used for statistical analysis or scientific purposes with your right to privacy retained.

— Freedom of consent

I hereby consent to voluntarily engage in an exercise test to determine my exercise capacity and state of cardiovascular health. My permission to perform this exercise test is given voluntarily. I understand that I am free to stop the test at any point if I so desire.

I have read this form, and I understand the test procedures that I will perform and the attendant risks and discomforts. Knowing these risks and discomforts, and having had an opportunity to ask questions that have been answered to my satisfaction, I consent to participate in this test.

Signature of Patient _____ Date _____

Signature of Witness _____ Date _____

Signature of Physician or _____ Date _____
Authorized Delegate

The following points should be considered for inclusion in such preliminary instructions; however, specific instructions vary with test type and purpose.

- Participants should refrain from ingesting food, alcohol or caffeine or using tobacco products within 3 hours of testing.
- Participants should be rested for the assessment, avoiding significant exertion or exercise on the day of the assessment.
- Clothing should permit freedom of movement and include walking or running shoes. Women should bring a loose-fitting, short-sleeved blouse that buttons down the front and should avoid restrictive undergarments.
- If the evaluation is on an outpatient basis, participants should be made aware that the evaluation may be fatiguing and that they may wish to have someone accompany them to the assessment to drive home afterwards.
- If the test is for diagnostic purposes, it may be helpful for patients to discontinue prescribed cardiovascular medications, but only with physician approval. Currently prescribed antianginal agents alter the hemodynamic response to exercise and significantly reduce the sensitivity of ECG changes for ischemia. Patients taking intermediate- or high-dose β-blocking agents may be asked to taper their medication over a 2 to 4-day period to minimize hyperadrenergic withdrawal responses.
- If the test is for functional purposes, *patients should continue their medication regimen* on their usual schedule so that the exercise responses will be consistent with responses expected during exercise training.
- Participants should bring a list of their medications, including dosage and frequency of administration, to the assessment and should report the last actual dose taken. As an alternative, participants may wish to bring their medications with them for the exerise testing staff to record.
- Drink ample fluids over the 24-hour period preceding the test to ensure normal hydration testing.

FIGURE 13.8. Sample of informed consent form for a symptom-limited exercise test. (From American College of Sports Medicine. *ACSM's Guidelines for Exercise Testing and Prescription.* 8th ed. Baltimore: Lippincott Williams & Wilkins; 2010.)

SUMMARY

The preparticipation health screening that takes place during the initial client consultation is an extremely important process yielding valuable information concerning a client's risk and health status. It is essential that the Personal Trainer obtain as much information as possible about a client's health status to maximize benefit and minimize risk. This information should serve as the Personal Trainer's foundation to developing a safe and effective exercise program.

REFERENCES

1. American Association of Cardiovascular and Pulmonary Rehabilitation. *Guidelines for Cardiac Rehabilitation and Secondary Prevention Programs*. 4th ed. Champaign (IL): Human Kinetics; 2003.
2. American College of Sports Medicine and American Heart Association. ACSM/AHA Joint position statement: recommendations for cardiovascular screening, staffing, and emergency policies at health/fitness facilities. *Med Sci Sports Exerc*. 1998;31:1018.
3. American College of Sports Medicine. *ACSM Fitness Book: A Proven Step-by-Step Program from the Experts*. Champaign (IL): Human Kinetics; 2003.
4. American College of Sports Medicine. *ACSM's Guidelines for Exercise Testing and Prescription*. 8th ed. Baltimore: Lippincott Williams & Wilkins; 2010.
5. American College of Sports Medicine. *ACSM's Resource Manual for Guidelines for Exercise Testing and Prescription*. Baltimore: Lippincott Williams & Wilkins; 2005.
6. American College of Sports Medicine. Position stand: exercise and hypertension. *Med Sci Sports Exerc*. 2004;36:533–53.
7. Corrado D, Migliore F, Basso C, Thiene G. Exercise and the risk of sudden cardiac death. *Herz*. 2006:31:553–8.
8. Durakovic Z, Misigoj-Durakovic M, Vuori I, Skavic J, Belicaz M. Sudden cardiac death due to physical exercise in male competitive athletes. A report of six cases. *J Sports Med Phys Fitness*. 2005;45:532–6.
9. Fletcher GF, Balady GJ, Amsterdam EA, et al. Exercise standards for testing and training. A statement for health care professionals from the American Heart Association. *Circulation*. 2001;104:1694–740.
10. Genuth S, Alberti KG, Bennett P, et al. Follow-up report on the diagnosis of diabetes mellitus. *Diabetes Care*. 2003;26:3160–7.
11. Giri S, Thompson PD, Kiernan FJ, et al. Clinical and angiographic characteristics of exertion-related acute myocardial infarction. *JAMA*. 1999;282:1731–6.
12. Mittleman MA, Maclure M, Tofler GH, et al. Triggering of acute myocardial infarction by heavy physical exertion. Protection against triggering by regular exertion. Determinants of myocardial infarction onset study investigators. *N Engl J Med*. 1993;329:1677–83.
13. National Heart, Lung and Blood Institute, National Institutes of Health, National Cholesterol Education Program. [Internet]. *Third Report of the National Cholesterol Education Program (NCEP) Expert Panel on Detection, Evaluation, and Treatment of High Blood Cholesterol in Adults (Adult Treatment Panel III) Final Report*. NIH Publication no. 02-5215, 2002 [cited 2008 Aug 27]. Available from http://www.nhlbi.nih.gov/guidelines/cholesterol/atp3full.pdf
14. National Institutes of Health. Expert panel on detection evaluation and treatment of overweight and obesity in adults. Clinical guidelines on the identification, evaluation, and treatment of overweight and obesity in adults—the evidence report. *Arch Intern Med*. 1998;158:1855–67.
15. Siscovick DS, Weiss NS, Fletcher RH, et al. The incidence of primary cardiac arrest during vigorous exercise. *N Engl J Med*. 1984;311:874–7.
16. Thompson PD, Funk EJ, Carleton RA, et al. Incidence of death during jogging in Rhode Island from 1975 through 1980. *JAMA*. 1982;247:2535–8.
17. U.S. Department of Health and Human Services, Centers for Disease Control and Prevention, National Center for Chronic Disease Prevention and Health Promotion. [Internet]. *Physical Activity and Health: A Report of the Surgeon General*. Atlanta (GA): U.S. Department of Health and Human Services; 1996 [cited 2008 Aug 27]. Available from http://www.cdc.gov/nccdphp/sgr/contents.htm
18. U.S. Department of Health and Human Services, National Institutes of Health, National Heart, Lung, and Blood Institute. [Internet]. *National High Blood Pressure Education Program Seventh Report of the Joint National Committee on Prevention, Detection, Evaluation, and Treatment of High Blood Pressure (JNC7)*. NIH Publication no. 03-5233, 2004 [cited 2008 Aug 27]. Available at http://www.nhlbi.nih.gov/guidelines/hypertension/
19. Wilson PW, D'Agostino RB, Levy D, et al. Prediction of coronary heart disease using risk factor categories. *Circulation*. 1998;97:1837–47.

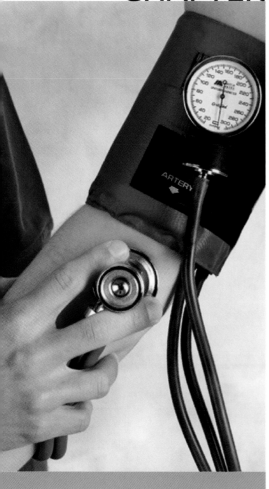

14

Client Fitness Assessments

OBJECTIVES

- Understand selecting the proper sequence of fitness assessments
- Present information on how to perform basic health-related physical fitness assessments common to the field of personal training.
  - Resting heart rate and blood pressure
  - Body composition: height, weight, body mass index, circumferences (waist and hip), skinfolds, and bioelectrical impedance
  - Cardiovascular: field tests, step tests, and submaximal cycle ergometer tests
  - Muscular fitness (muscular strength, muscular endurance, and flexibility): 1-RM chest press, partial curl-up, and sit-and-reach tests

The assessment process can be extremely intimidating to clients, especially those who are self-conscious about their appearance and intimidated by the idea of joining a fitness facility. As their Personal Trainer, it is important that you make your clients feel as comfortable as possible in the assessment process. During this process, share with your clients what you will be doing and how this will be accomplished. Clients may feel uncomfortable during certain parts of the assessment, such as weight assessment, measurement of waist circumference, and skinfold assessment. For example, if a client is overweight and a skinfold measurement at the abdomen site would be unsuccessful, do not attempt to take the abdomen site measurement. If the client is apprehensive about any part of the assessment process, explain the importance of accurately recording the measurements. If this explanation does not alleviate the client's anxiety, record any modifications to the measurement/assessment process for future reference. The success of the Personal Trainer–client relationship is built on a foundation of respect for the client. Respect can be established by providing information about the assessment process, listening to and addressing the client's concerns, and demonstrating competence in the assessment procedures. The Personal Trainer should guide the selection of the assessments (in consultation with the client) and the sequence of these assessments.

> *The success of the Personal Trainer–client relationship is built on a foundation of respect for the client.*

SELECTION AND SEQUENCE OF ASSESSMENTS

A Personal Trainer has many options available to assess a client's health-related physical fitness. Among the considerations are the client's needs/desires, the situation or setting, and the Personal Trainer's training and experience. The exact sequence of assessments is dictated most by the setting and equipment available; however, a few generalizations regarding sequencing can be made. Resting measures (i.e., resting heart rate [HR], resting blood pressure [BP], and body composition) typically should be taken prior to any exertional assessments, such as cardiorespiratory fitness (CRF) and flexibility. The Personal Trainer should perform assessments after the client has completed a health and physical activity questionnaire. One recommended order for performing assessments is the following (1):

1. Heart rate: resting
2. Blood pressure: resting
3. Body composition: height and weight, body mass index (BMI), waist-to-hip ratio, skinfolds, and/or bioelectrical impedance
4. Cardiovascular assessment: Rockport 1-mile walk test procedures, 1.5-mile run test procedures, Queens College Step Test, and/or the Astrand–Rhyming Submaximal Cycle Ergometer test
5. Muscular fitness: muscle strength, muscular endurance, and flexibility

HEART RATE: RESTING, EXERCISE, AND RECOVERY

Heart rate (HR) is the number of times that the heart beats or contracts, usually reported in beats per minute (bpm). Although there are no known or accepted standards for resting HR, resting HR has often been thought of as an indicator of CRF because it tends to decrease as the client becomes more physically fit. There are also no standards for exercise HR, but the HR response to a standard amount of exercise is an important fitness variable and the foundation for many cardiorespiratory endurance tests. Recovery HR is often thought of as an excellent index of CRF and is used as a variable in some CRF tests (e.g., Queens College Step Test). It is important to note that there are certain medications that may affect resting HR and HR response to exercise, so these statements may not always hold true in these cases.

Measurement of Heart Rate

There are many ways to assess or measure HR, including manual palpation at various anatomical sites and use of an HR monitor/watch or the electrocardiogram.

PALPATION OF PULSE

There are three common anatomical sites for the measurement of HR (2):

➤ *Radial*: Lightly press the index and middle fingers against the radial artery in the groove on the anterior surface of the lateral wrist (bordered by the abductor pollicis longus and extensor pollicis longus muscles). The radial palpation site is shown in Figure 14.1.
➤ *Brachial*: Located in a groove between the triceps and biceps muscles on the medial side of the arm, anterior to the elbow, and palpated with the first two fingers in the medial part of this groove (Fig. 14.1). This pulse location is also used for the auscultation of BP.
➤ *Carotid*: May be more visible or easily found than the radial pulse; press fingers lightly along the medial border of the sternocleidomastoid muscle in the lower neck region (on either side). Avoid the carotid sinus area (stay below the thyroid cartilage) to avoid the reflexive slowing of HR or drop in BP by the baroreceptor reflex. The carotid palpation site is shown in Figure 14.1 and should be used only if you or the client fails to feel the pulse in the radial or brachial sites.

When clients experience difficulty in palpating the pulse, the use of an HR monitor as a learning tool to check the accuracy of the palpated HR with the monitor's HR may be desirable. The electrocardiogram is not often used by Personal Trainers to assess HR.

All the above methods, when applied correctly, should yield similar results. The method for HR measurement by palpation of the pulse can be mastered through practice and should be taught to

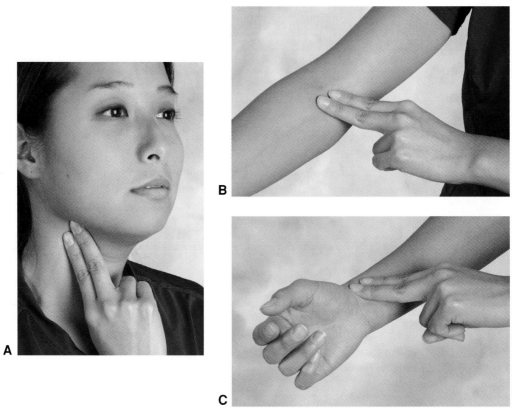

FIGURE 14.1. Locations for pulse determination.

your clients. However, some clients, as a result of anatomical aberrations, are more difficult to palpate (2).

The measurement of HR by palpation of the carotid artery may lead to an underestimation of the true HR because the baroreceptors in the carotid sinus region often become stimulated when touched. This may reflexively reduce the client's HR as the baroreceptors sense a false increase in BP. Therefore, the radial or brachial arteries are the locations of choice for palpation.

> *The radial or brachial arteries are the locations of choice for palpation.*

The baroreceptor reflex becomes a more important issue with HR counts longer than 15 seconds. It is recommended that a full 60-second count be performed for accuracy in resting HR. However, a 30-second time period may be sufficient for the count. "Resting" conditions must be present; for example, the client should be seated for at least 5 minutes with the back supported. Clients should be free of stimulants such as tobacco and caffeine for at least 30 minutes before taking the measurements (similar to resting BP). A resting HR may alternatively be assessed by having clients take their own pulse at home in bed upon waking in the morning. This resting HR may prove to be useful for the calculation of the exercise target HR zone.

MEASUREMENT OF EXERCISE HEART RATE

By the palpation method, measure the number of beats felt in a 15- or 30-second period and multiply by 4 (for 15 seconds) or 2 (for 30 seconds) to convert to a 1-minute value (bpm). Although the 30-second count may be more accurate and less prone to error than a 15-second count, the latter is typically used immediately postexercise because HR may decrease rapidly during recovery. When counting the exercise HR for a time count period less than 1 minute, you should start the count at zero (reference) at the first beat felt and start the time period at that beat (2).

The use of HR monitors has increased in popularity as these monitors have become more available and affordable. Some monitors are prone to error (i.e., not always consistent in measuring HR); however, newer technology has resolved the reliability problem previously associated with many of these monitors. HR monitors that rely on the opacity of blood at the earlobe or fingertip to measure/count flow are generally not as accurate as the monitors that use a chest electrode strap.

BLOOD PRESSURE: RESTING AND EXERCISE

Blood pressure is the force of blood against the walls of the arteries and veins created by the heart as it pumps blood to every part of the body. BP is typically expressed in millimeters of mercury (mm Hg). BP is a dynamic variable with regard to location (i.e., artery vs. vein and the level in an artery). Personal Trainers are most concerned with arterial BP at the level of the heart. This arterial, heart-level BP is the one typically measured at rest and during exercise (2). More discussion concerning the regulation of BP can be found in Chapter 5.

> ➤ Systolic blood pressure (SBP) is the maximum pressure in the arteries when the ventricles of the heart contract during a heartbeat. The term derives from systole or contraction of the heart. The SBP occurs late in ventricular systole. SBP is thought to represent the overall functioning of the left ventricle and is thus an important indicator of cardiovascular function during exercise. SBP is typically measured from the brachial artery at the heart level and is expressed in units of mm Hg.

> ➤ Diastolic blood pressure (DBP) is the minimum pressure in the arteries when the ventricles relax. The term is derived from diastole or relaxation of the heart. The DBP occurs late in ventricular diastole and reflects the peripheral resistance to blood flow in the arterial vessels. DBP is typically measured from the brachial artery at the heart level and is expressed in units of mm Hg.

TABLE 14.1	CLASSIFICATION OF RESTING BLOOD PRESSURE FOR ADULTS	
Classification	Systolic (mm Hg)	Diastolic (mm Hg) (5th phase)
Normal	<120	<80
Prehypertension	120–139	80–89
Hypertension Stage 1 Stage 2	 140–149 >160	 90–99 >100

Reprinted with permission from the National High Blood Pressure Education Program, The Seventh Report of the Joint National Committee on the Prevention, Detection and Treatment of High Blood Pressure; JNC7, 2003.

"Hypertension," or high BP, is a condition in which the resting BP, either SBP and/or DBP, is chronically elevated above the optimal or desired level. The standards for classifying resting hypertension are presented in Table 14.1. "Hypotension" is the term for low BP and there are no accepted standards for a value that classifies an individual with hypotension. Hypotension exists medically if the individual has symptoms related to low BP such as lightheadedness, dizziness, or fainting (2). BP is typically assessed using the principle of indirect auscultation. Auscultation involves the use of a BP cuff, a manometer, and a stethoscope. Measurement of BP is a fundamental skill and is covered in detail in this chapter (12).

Measurement of BP

The measurement of BP is an integral component of a resting health-related physical fitness assessment. BP measurement is a relatively simple technique and may be used in risk stratification, as discussed in Chapter 13. Hypertension cannot be diagnosed from a single measurement; serial measurements must be obtained on separate days. The BP of a client should be based on the average of two or more resting BP recordings during each of two or more visits (2).

Hypertension cannot be diagnosed from a single measurement; serial measurements must be obtained on separate days.

For accurate resting BP readings, it is important that the client be made as comfortable as possible. To accomplish this, take a few minutes to talk to the client after having him or her sit in a chair. Make sure the client does not have the legs crossed. Also, be sure to use the correct size of BP cuff. Choosing the correct cuff size is addressed later in this chapter. As with many other physiological and psychological measures, clients may experience "white coat syndrome" during the measurement of BP. White coat syndrome refers to an elevation of BP resulting from the anxiety or nervousness associated with being in a doctor's office or in a clinical setting (i.e., clinician wearing a white lab coat). Thus, having a client in a relaxed state is important when taking a resting BP measurement.

KOROTKOFF SOUNDS

To measure BP by auscultation, the Personal Trainer must be able to hear and distinguish between the sounds of the blood as it makes its way from an area of high pressure to that of lower pressure as the air is let out of the pumped-up cuff. These sounds are known as Korotkoff sounds. The sounds can be divided into five phases (2):

➤ Phase 1 (SBP)
- The first, initial sound or the onset of sound
- Sounds like clear, repetitive tapping
- Sound approximates the SBP, the maximum pressure that occurs near the end of systole of the left ventricle

➤ Phase 2
- Sounds like a soft tapping or murmur; sounds are often longer than those in the first phase; these sounds have also been described as having a swishing component
- Phase 2 sounds are typically 10–14 mm Hg after the onset or just below Phase 1 sounds

➤ Phase 3
- Sounds like loud tapping; high in both pitch and intensity
- Sounds are crisper and louder than Phase 2 sounds

➤ Phase 4 (also known as the true DBP)
- Sounds like muffling of the sound; sounds become less distinct and less audible; another way of describing this sound is as soft or blowing
- This is often considered the true DBP and is typically recorded as the DBP

➤ Phase 5 (also known as the clinical DBP)
- Sounds like the complete disappearance of sound

The true disappearance of sound usually occurs within 8–10 mm Hg of the muffling of sound, also known as Phase 4. Phase 5 is considered by some to be the clinical DBP. Phase 5 is the reading most often used for resting DBP in adults, whereas Phase 4 is considered the true DBP and should be recorded, if discerned.

INSTRUMENTS USED FOR BP MEASUREMENT

A sphygmomanometer consists of a manometer and a BP cuff. The prefix *sphygmo-* refers to the occlusion of the artery by a cuff. A manometer is simply a device used to measure pressure. Two common types of manometers are available for BP measurement: mercury (see Fig. 14.2) and aneroid (see Fig. 14.3). Mercury is the standard for accuracy; however, because of the toxic nature of mercury, aneroid sphygmomanometers are becoming more common in the workplace.

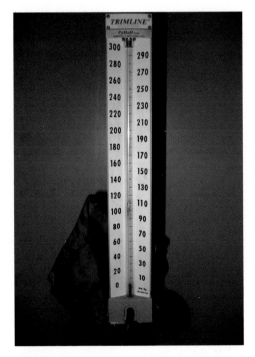

FIGURE 14.2. Sphygmomanometer, gravity mercury. Freestanding pressure manometer of the gravity mercury type, which uses the height of a mercury column in a glass tube to indicate cuff pressure.

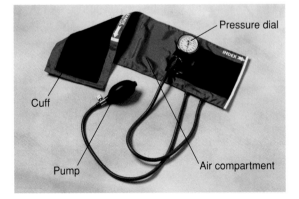

FIGURE 14.3. Aneroid sphygmomanometer and blood pressure cuff.

Position the manometer at your eye level to eliminate the potential for any reflex errors when reading either the mercury level or the needle if using the aneroid manometer. This is very important. Aneroid manometers are usually of a dial type (round), whereas mercury manometers are usually of a straight tube/column type. The cuff typically consists of a rubber bladder and two tubes, one to the manometer and one to a hand bulb with a valve that is used for inflation. The bladder must be of appropriate size for accurate readings. The sizing of a BP cuff should be:

➤ Width of bladder = 40%–50% of upper arm circumference
➤ Length of bladder = almost long enough (~80%) to circle upper arm

Three BP cuff sizes are commonly used in the health and fitness field: a pediatric or child cuff for small arm sizes (13–20 cm; 5–8 in); a normal adult cuff for arm size between 24 and 32 cm (9–11 in); and a large adult cuff for larger arm sizes (32–42 cm; 12–16 in). There are index lines on many of the newer sphygmomanometers cuffs to help "fit" the cuff for a client's arm circumference. In general, the appropriate BP bladder should encircle at least 80% of the arm's circumference. A cuff that is too small in length or width will generally result in a BP measurement that will be falsely high.

The cuff should be positioned at the level of the heart; if below the level of the heart, the BP reading will be falsely high. The cuff must be applied snugly or tightly. If the cuff is too loose, the BP measurement will typically be falsely high.

Equipment used in the measurement of BP is widely available commercially and varies greatly in quality. BP sphygmomanometer units can be purchased in most drug stores, from various health and fitness commercial catalogs and at medical supply stores. Stethoscopes are also widely available and vary in quality. Electric amplification of the sounds is available on some stethoscope models (2).

RESTING BP MEASUREMENT PROCEDURES

1. Position yourself to have the best opportunity to hear the BP and see the manometer scale. Take control of the client's arm while having it supported by some piece of furniture when listening to the sounds. Make sure that your stethoscope is flat and placed completely over the client's brachial artery. The room noise should be at a minimum and the temperature should be comfortable (21°C –23°C; 70°F–74°F). If you have some form of sinus congestion, your ability to hear the BP sounds may be diminished. Clearing your throat before attempting a BP measurement may be helpful. Of course, practice in the skill of resting BP measurement is important for its mastery.

2. The client should be seated, with the feet flat, the legs uncrossed, and the arm free of any clothing and relaxed. The arm you are using for the BP measurement should be well supported by you or resting on a piece of furniture. Your client's back should also be well supported.

3. Measurement should begin after at least 5 full minutes of quiet, seated rest. The client should be free of stimulants (nicotine products, caffeine products, recent alcohol use, or other cardiovascular stimulants) for at least 30 minutes prior to the resting measurement. In addition, your client should not have exercised strenuously for at least the prior 60 minutes.

4. There is no practical difference between a seated and supine resting BP; however, statistically, SBP tends to be higher by about 6–7 mm Hg and DBP by 1 mm Hg in the supine position.

5. It matters little which arm is chosen for the resting BP measurement; however, it is important to use the same arm for both resting and exercise measurements. The American Heart Association recommends that you measure both right and left arm BPs on your client on the initial evaluation and the arm with the higher pressure be chosen. However, if BP is normal in the right arm, it tends to be normal in the left arm. Conventionally, the left arm is typically used.

6. Center the rubber bladder of the BP cuff over the client's brachial artery; the lower border of the cuff should be 2.5 cm (1 in) above the antecubital fossa or crease of the elbow. Be sure to use the appropriate-size BP cuff, as discussed previously. Make sure that you palpate your client's brachial artery to determine its location.

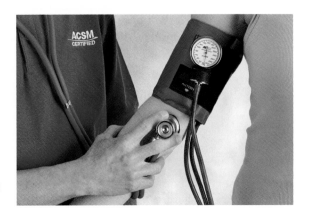

FIGURE 14.4. Position of the stethoscope head and blood pressure cuff.

7. Secure the BP cuff snugly around the arm. Again, be sure to use the appropriate-size cuff. The client should have no clothing on the upper arm to secure the cuff properly. Clothing on the arm where you place the stethoscope will also muffle the intensity of the sound.

8. Position the client's arm so it is slightly flexed at the elbow; support the arm or rest it on some piece of furniture. If the client supports his or her own arm, the constant isometric contraction by the client may elevate the DBP. By having the client support the arm on a table, you can reduce the "noise" heard during the procedure, which may increase measurement accuracy. Figure 14.4 depicts how the client's arm should be positioned with the BP cuff and stethoscope.

9. Position the BP cuff on the upper arm with the cuff at heart level. For every centimeter, the cuff is below heart level, the BP tends to be higher by 1 mm Hg. The reverse is true for a BP cuff that is above heart level.

10. Find the client's brachial artery. This artery, and thus pulse, is just medial to the biceps tendon. Mark the artery with an appropriate marker (water color) to "locate" the artery for the stethoscope bell placement. To best find the client's brachial artery, have the client face the palm upward and rotate the arm outward on the thumb side with the arm hyperextended.

11. Firmly place the bell of the stethoscope over the artery located in the antecubital fossa. Do not place the bell of the stethoscope under the lip of the BP cuff. There should be no air space or clothing between the bell of the stethoscope and the arm. The stethoscope earpieces should be directed facing slightly forward, toward your nose and in the same direction as your ear canal. Do not press too hard with the stethoscope bell on the arm. The earpieces of a stethoscope should be cleaned with rubbing alcohol before use each time.

12. Be sure to position the manometer (either mercury or aneroid) so that the dial or tube is clearly visible and at eye level to avoid any parallax (distortion from looking up or down) error.

13. Choose between any one of the following three accepted methods for BP cuff inflation. Quickly inflate the BP cuff to approximately:
    • 20 mm Hg above the SBP, if known
    • Up to 140–180 mm Hg for a resting BP
    • Up to 30 mm Hg above disappearance of the radial pulse if you palpate for radial pulse first. This is called the palpation method. Many educators favor the palpation method when the technician is first learning BP measurement to "feel" for and then listen to the SBP.

14. Deflate the pressure slowly; 2–3 mm Hg per heart beat (or 2–5 mm Hg per second) by opening the air exhaust valve on the hand bulb. Rapid deflation leads to underestimation of SBP and overestimation of DBP. Slow the deflation rate to 2 mm Hg per pulse beat when in the anticipated range of the systolic to diastolic BP; this will compensate for slow HRs. A falsely low BP tends to result from too rapid deflation of the cuff.

15. Record measures of SBP and DBP in even numbers. Always round off upward to the nearest 2 mm Hg. Always continue to listen to any BP sounds for at least 10 mm Hg below the fifth phase (to be sure you have correctly identified the fifth phase).

16. Rapidly deflate the cuff to zero after the DBP is obtained.

Wait one full minute before repeating the BP measurement. Average at least two BP readings to get a "true sense" of an individual's BP. It is suggested that BP readings on clients be taken on at least two separate occasions to screen for hypertension. Also, the two readings on your client in any given session should be within 5 mm Hg of each other. If they are not, you should take another BP reading.

The norms (13) presented in Table 14.1 for resting BP are for those older than 18 years. To use these norms, individuals should not be taking any antihypertensive medications and should not be acutely ill during the measurement. When SBP and DBP fall into two different classifications, the higher classification should be selected. This classification is based on two or more readings taken at each of two or more visits after an initial BP screening. Generally, these norms are revised periodically. It is generally recommended that all persons older than 30 years have their BP checked annually (11).

BODY COMPOSITION

Body composition can be defined as the relative proportion of fat and fat-free tissue in the body (percent body fat). The assessment of body composition is necessary for numerous reasons. There is a strong correlation (5) between obesity and increased risk of chronic diseases including coronary artery disease, diabetes, hypertension, certain cancers, and hyperlipidemia. There is a frequent need to evaluate body weight and body composition in the health and fitness field. Most often this evaluation is done to establish a target, desirable, or optimal weight for an individual. There are several ways to evaluate the composition of the human body. Body composition can be estimated with both laboratory and field techniques that vary in terms of complexity, cost, and accuracy. For the purposes of this text, the following techniques are reviewed:

> *Body composition can be defined as the relative proportion of fat and fat-free tissue in the body (percent body fat).*

- ➤ Height and weight
- ➤ BMI
- ➤ Waist-to-hip ratio (waist and hip circumference measures)
- ➤ Skinfolds
- ➤ Bioelectrical impedance analysis (BIA)

Height and Weight

Measure the client's height. Instruct the client with shoes removed to stand straight up, the client's heels should be together and their head should be level, they should take a deep breath and hold it, and look straight ahead. Record the height in centimeters or inches.

- ➤ 1 in = 2.54 cm
- ➤ 1 m = 100 cm
- ➤ For example: 6 feet = 72 inches = 183 cm = 1.83 m

Measure the client's weight with his or her shoes removed and as much other clothing removed as is practical and possible. Convert weight from pounds to kilograms when necessary.

- ➤ 1 kg = 2.2 lb
- ➤ For example: 187 lb = 85 kg

Compare the client's height and weight with one of the several height–weight tables that are available. One such source for height–weight tables is the *ACSM's Health-Related Physical Fitness Assessment Manual* (2). With the many criticisms of the validity of the height–weight tables (including using a select group of individuals for development and the imprecise concept of "frame size"), there has been a strong trend recently to discontinue their use. Thus, this chapter discusses more advanced methods of anthropometry and body composition analysis.

Body Mass Index

Body mass index, also called the Quetelet's Index, is used to assess weight relative to height. BMI has a similar association with body fat as the height–weight tables previously discussed. This technique compares an individual's weight (in kilograms) with his or her height (in square meters), much like a height–weight table would. The BMI gives a single number for comparison, as opposed to the weight-to-height ranges located in the tables.

$$\text{BMI } (kg \cdot m^{-2}) = \text{weight (kg)/height } (m^2)$$

For example, an individual who weighs 150 lb and is 5 feet, 8 in tall has a BMI of:

$$5 \text{ ft } 8 \text{ in} = 173 \text{ cm} = 1.73 \text{ m} = 2.99 \text{ m}^2$$
$$\text{and } 150 \text{ lb} = 68.18 \text{ kg}$$
$$\text{BMI} = 68.18/2.99 = 22.8 \text{ kg} \cdot m^{-2}$$

The major shortcoming with using BMI for body composition is that it is difficult for a client to relate to and/or interpret needed weight loss or weight gain. Also, the BMI does not differentiate fat weight from fat-free weight and has only a modest correlation with percentage body fat predicted from hydrostatic weighing (2). Standards and norms for BMI are presented in Table 14.2 and Figure 14.5.

Waist-to-Hip Ratio

The waist-to-hip ratio (WHR) is a comparison between the circumference of the waist and the circumference of the hip. This ratio best represents the distribution of body weight, and perhaps body fat, in an individual. The pattern of body weight distribution is recognized as an important predictor of health risks of obesity. Individuals with more weight or circumference on the trunk are at

TABLE 14.2	**CLASSIFICATION OF DISEASE RISK BASED ON BODY MASS INDEX (BMI) AND WAIST CIRCUMFERENCE**		
	BMI (kg · m^{-2})	**Disease Risk^a Relative to Normal Weight and Waist Circumference: Men < 102 cm; Women < 88 cm**	**Men > 102 cm; Women > 88 cm**
Underweight	<18.5	—	—
Normal	18.5–24.9	—	—
Overweight	25.0–29.9	Increased	High
I	30.0–34.9	High	Very high
II	35.0–39.9	Very high	Very high
III	≥40	Extremely high	Extremely high

Modified from Expert Panel. Executive Summary of the clinical guidelines on the identification, evaluation, and treatment of overweight and obesity in adults. *Arch Intern Med.* 1998;148:1855-67. Reprinted from American College of Sports Medicine. *ACSM's Guidelines for Exercise Testing and Prescription.* 8th ed. Baltimore: Lippincott Williams & Wilkins; 2010.

^{a}Disease risk for type 2 diabetes, hypertension, and cardiovascular disease. Dashes (—) indicate that no additional risk at these levels of BMI was assigned. Increased waist circumference can also be a marker for increased risk, even in persons of normal weight.

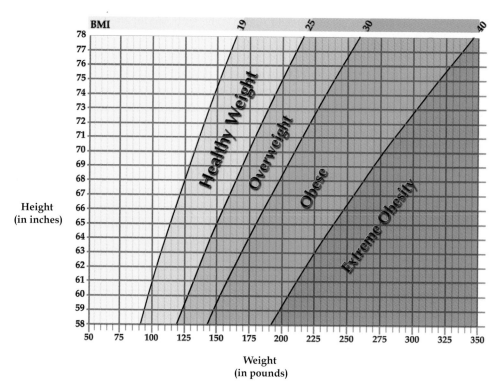

FIGURE 14.5. The risks of obesity. How is body fat measured? Body mass index (BMI) is a measure of weight in relation to a person's height. For most people, BMI has a strong relationship to weight. For adults, BMI can also be found by using this table. To use the BMI table, first find your weight at the bottom of the graph. Go straight up from that point until you reach the line that matches your height. Then look to see what weight group you fall in. (Reprinted with permission from Anatomical Chart Co.)

higher risk of hypertension, type 2 diabetes, hyperlipidemia, and coronary artery disease than individuals who are of equal weight but have more of their weight distributed on the extremities. Some experts suggest that the waist circumference alone can be used as an indicator of health risk (1).

➤ Waist: The waist circumference has been frequently defined as the smallest waist circumference, typically measured 1 in (2.54 cm) above the umbilicus or navel and below the xiphoid process.
➤ Hip: The hip circumference has been defined as the largest circumference around the buttocks, above the gluteal fold (posterior extension).
➤ WHR is a ratio (thus, there are no units).
➤ WHR = waist circumference/hip circumference

Measure the waist and hip circumferences in either inches or centimeters (1 in = 2.54 cm). A quality tape with a spring-loaded handle (i.e., Gulick) should be used to measure circumferences. Take multiple measurements until each is within 5 mm (1/4 in) of each other. For example, if a male client has a waist circumference of 32 in (81.3 cm) and a hip circumference of 35 in (88.9 cm), his WHR is 32/35 = 0.91. Health risk is very high for young men when the WHR is more than 0.95 and for young women when the WHR is more than 0.86.

Waist Circumference Alone

Some experts suggest that the waist circumference alone may be used as an indicator of health risk. For example, the health risk is high when the waist circumference is greater than or equal to 35 inches (88 cm) for women and 40 inches (102 cm) for men. A very low risk is associated with a waist circumference less than 27.5 in (70 cm) for women and 31.5 in (80 cm) for men.

BOX 14.1   Standardized Description of Skinfold Sites and Procedures

Skinfold site

Abdominal	Vertical fold; 2 cm to the right side of the umbilicus
Triceps	Vertical fold; on the posterior midline of the upper arm, halfway between the acromion and olecranon processes, with the arm held freely to the side of the body
Biceps	Vertical fold; on the anterior aspect of the arm over the belly of the biceps muscle, 1 cm above the level used to mark the triceps site
Chest/pectoral	Diagonal fold; one half the distance between the anterior axillary line and the nipple (men), or one third of the distance between the anterior axillary line and the nipple (women)
Medial calf	Vertical fold; at the maximum circumference of the calf on the midline of its medial border
Midaxillary	Vertical fold; on the midaxillary line at the level of the xiphoid process of the sternum. An alternate method is a horizontal fold taken at the level of the xiphoid/sternal border in the midaxillary line
Subscapular	Diagonal fold (at a 45° angle); 1–2 cm below the inferior angle of the scapula
Suprailiac	Diagonal fold; in line with the natural angle of the iliac crest taken in the anterior axillary line immediately superior to the iliac crest
Thigh	Vertical fold; on the anterior midline of the thigh, midway between the proximal border of the patella and the inguinal crease (hip)

Procedures

- All measurements should be made on the right side of the body with the subject standing upright
- Calipers should be placed directly on the skin surface, 1 cm away from the thumb and finger, perpendicular to the skinfold, and halfway between the crest and the base of the fold
- Pinch should be maintained while reading the calipers
- Wait 1–2 seconds (no longer) before reading calipers
- Take duplicate measures at each site and retest if duplicate measurements are not within 1–2 mm
- Rotate through measurement sites or allow time for skin to regain normal texture and thickness

Reprinted with permission from *ACSM's Guidelines for Exercise Testing and Prescription*. 8th ed. Baltimore: Lippincott Williams & Wilkins; 2010. Box 4.2.

Skinfolds

Skinfold determination of the percentage of body fat can be quite accurate if the technician is properly trained in the use of skinfold calipers and the caliper is of high quality. It should be remembered, however, that skinfold determination of percent body fat is still an estimate or a prediction of percentage body fat, not an absolute measurement. This estimate is based on the principle that the amount of subcutaneous fat is proportional to the total amount of body fat; however, the proportion of subcutaneous fat to total fat varies with gender, age, and ethnicity. Regression equations considering these factors have been developed to predict body density and percent body fat from skinfold measurements (7).

Standardized descriptions as well as pictorial descriptions of skinfold sites are provided in Box 14.1 and Figure 14.6.

SKINFOLD MEASUREMENT PROCEDURES

The following procedures help standardize the skinfold measurement (2).

1. Firmly grasp a double fold of skin (a skinfold) and the subcutaneous fat between the thumb and index finger of your left hand and lift up and away from the body. Be certain that you have not grasped any muscle in this procedure and that you have taken up all the fat. You can also have the subject first flex the muscle below the site to help distinguish muscle from fat before you measure. Be sure, however, to have the subject relax the area prior to measurement.

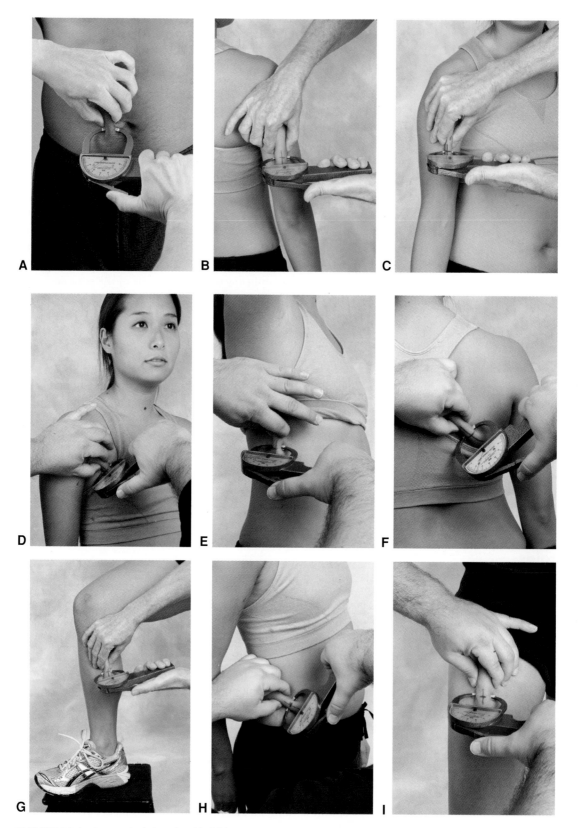

FIGURE 14.6. Anatomical sites for skinfold measurement.

2. You should grasp the skinfold site with your two fingers about 8 cm (3 in) apart on a line that is perpendicular to the long axis of the skinfold site. You should be able to form a fold that has roughly parallel sides. Larger skinfolds (obese individuals) will require separating your fingers farther than 8 cm. All skinfolds should be taken on the right side of the body.

3. Hold the calipers in your right hand with the scale facing up to ease your viewing. Place the contact surfaces of the calipers 1 cm (0.5 in) below your fingers. The calipers should be placed on the exact skinfold site, whereas your fingers should be above the site by 1 cm. Place the tips of the calipers on the double fold of skin and fat. By marking the skin on the specific sites (Fig. 14.6), you will be able to accurately place the caliper head at the correct location. This will allow for measurement at the same site during duplicate measures.

4. Release the scissor grip of the calipers claws with your hand and continue to support the weight of the calipers with that hand. Be sure to maintain a firm hold on the skinfold throughout the entire measurement process.

5. Record the reading on the calipers scale 1–2 seconds (not longer) after releasing the scissor grip lever to allow the jaws of the calipers to measure the skinfold site. Measure the skinfold to the nearest 0.5 mm (if using the Lange brand calipers). Be careful to avoid jaw slippage of the calipers.

6. Measure each skinfold site at least twice. Rotate through the measurement sites to allow time for the skin to regain its normal texture and thickness. If duplicate measurements are not within 1 or 2 mm (or 10%), retest this site.

7. Sum the mean, or average, of each skinfold site to determine percent body fat. You can use specific skinfold equations to determine body density and percent body fat and these equations can be found in other sources (1,7). For the purpose of this text we suggest using the Jackson–Pollock 3-site Skinfold Formula as discussed below. Percentile rankings for percent body fat for men and women can be found in Table 14.3.

JACKSON–POLLOCK 3-SITE SKINFOLD FORMULA FOR PERCENT BODY FAT

Jackson and Pollock (8) have developed several skinfold formulas for the prediction of percent body fat or body composition (often referred to as the Jackson–Pollock formulas). Jackson and Pollock developed two 3-site skinfold formulas in 1980 and 1985, as well as a 7-site skinfold formula (1). The 1980 formula provides percent body fat averages for the skinfold measurement for the chest, abdomen, and thigh (for men) and triceps, suprailiac, and thigh (for women). Sum the means of the three skinfold site measures and use the nomogram provided in this text (Fig. 14.7) for percent body fat estimation or tables published in other resources (7). Using the Jackson–Pollock nomogram provided in Figure 14.7 involves plotting your client's age along the "Age in Years" section and connecting that point with a straight line to a point plotted along the "Sum of three skinfolds" section. Where the line dissects, the "Percent Body Fat" section of the nomogram represents the client's percent body fat.

Bioelectrical Impedance

Bioelectrical impedance analysis is a noninvasive and easy-to-administer method for assessing body composition. The basic premise behind the procedure is that the volume of fat-free tissue in the body will be proportional to the electrical conductivity of the body. Thus, the bioelectrical impedance analyzer passes a small electrical current into the body and then measures the resistance to that current. The theory behind BIA is that fat is a poor electrical conductor containing little water (14%–22%) whereas lean tissue contains mostly water (more than 90%) and electrolytes and is a good electrical conductor. Thus, fat tissue provides impedance to electrical current. In actuality, BIA measures total body water and uses calculations for percent body fat using some assumptions about hydration levels of individuals and the exact water content of various tissues. The following conditions must be controlled to ensure that the subject has a normal hydration level so the BIA measurement is valid.

➤ No eating or drinking within 4 hours of the test
➤ No exercise within 12 hours of the test

| TABLE 14.3 | BODY COMPOSITION (% BODY FAT) FOR MEN AND WOMEN | | | | | | |

| | Age, yr (Men) | | | | | | |
%	20–29	30–39	40–49	50–59	60–69	70–79	
99	4.2	7.0	9.2	10.9	11.5	13.6	
95	6.3	9.9	12.8	14.4	15.5	15.2	VL[a]
90	7.9	11.9	14.9	16.7	17.6	17.8	
85	9.2	13.3	16.3	18.0	18.8	19.2	
80	10.5	14.5	17.4	19.1	19.7	20.4	E
75	11.5	15.5	18.4	19.9	20.6	21.1	
70	12.7	16.5	19.1	20.7	21.3	21.6	
65	13.9	17.4	19.9	21.3	22.0	22.5	
60	14.8	18.2	20.6	22.1	22.6	23.1	G
55	15.8	19.0	21.3	22.7	23.2	23.7	
50	16.6	19.7	21.9	23.2	23.7	24.1	
45	17.4	20.4	22.6	23.9	24.4	24.4	
40	18.6	21.3	23.4	24.6	25.2	24.8	F
35	19.6	22.1	24.1	25.3	26.0	25.4	
30	20.6	23.0	24.8	26.0	26.7	26.0	
25	21.9	23.9	25.7	26.8	27.5	26.7	
20	23.1	24.9	26.6	27.8	28.4	27.6	P
15	24.6	26.2	27.7	28.9	29.4	28.9	
10	26.3	27.8	29.2	30.3	30.9	30.4	
5	28.9	30.2	31.2	32.5	32.9	32.4	
1	33.3	34.3	35.0	36.4	36.8	35.5	VP
n =	1,826	8,373	10,442	6,079	1,836	301	

Total *n* = 28,857

Norms are based on Cooper Clinic patients.

[a]Very lean—no less than 3% body fat is recommended for males.

Women: VL = very lean, E = excellent, G = good, F = fair, P = poor, VP = very poor.

| | Age, yr (Women) | | | | | | |
%	20–29	30–39	40–49	50–59	60–69	70–79	
99	9.8	11.0	12.6	14.6	13.9	14.6	
95	13.6	14.0	15.6	17.2	17.7	16.6	VL[a]
90	14.8	15.6	17.2	19.4	19.8	20.3	
85	15.8	16.6	18.6	20.9	21.4	23.0	
80	16.5	17.4	19.8	22.5	23.2	24.0	E
75	17.3	18.2	20.8	23.8	24.8	25.0	
70	18.0	19.1	21.9	25.1	25.9	26.2	
65	18.7	20.0	22.8	26.0	27.0	27.7	
60	19.4	20.8	23.8	27.0	27.9	28.6	G
55	20.1	21.7	24.8	27.9	28.7	29.7	
50	21.0	22.6	25.6	28.8	29.8	30.4	

(*continued*)

TABLE 14.3	BODY COMPOSITION (% BODY FAT) FOR MEN AND WOMEN (*Continued*)						
	Age, yr (Women)						
%	20–29	30–39	40–49	50–59	60–69	70–79	
45	21.9	23.5	26.5	29.7	30.6	31.3	
40	22.7	24.6	27.6	30.4	31.3	31.8	F
35	23.6	25.6	28.5	31.4	32.5	32.7	
30	24.5	26.7	29.6	32.5	33.3	33.9	
25	25.9	27.7	30.7	33.4	34.3	35.3	
20	27.1	29.1	31.9	34.5	35.4	36.0	P
15	28.9	30.9	33.5	35.6	36.2	37.4	
10	31.4	33.0	35.4	36.7	37.3	38.2	
5	35.2	35.8	37.4	38.3	39.0	39.3	
1	38.9	39.4	39.8	40.4	40.8	40.5	VP
n =	1,360	3,597	3,808	2,366	849	136	

Total *n* = 12,116

Norms are based on cooper Clinic Patients

*a*Very lean—no less than 10%–13% body fat is recommended for females.

Reprinted with permission from The Cooper Institute, Dallas, Texas. For more information, see www.cooperinstitute.org.

Males: S = superior, E = excellent, G = good, F = fair, P = poor, VP = very poor.

➤ Urinate (or void) completely within 30 minutes of the test
➤ No alcohol consumption in the previous 48 hours before test

A summary of the various body composition techniques discussed in this chapter is provided in Box 14.2 (3).

Calculation of Ideal or Desired Body Weight

Along with the determination of percent body fat, it is often desirable to determine an ideal or desired body weight based on a desired percent of fat for the individual (Box 14.3). Obviously, this process can be problematic in that a desirable percent body fat for an individual must be determined. The determination of a desirable body weight is useful in weight loss and weight maintenance (8).

CRF ASSESSMENT

Cardiorespiratory fitness is related to the ability to perform large muscle, dynamic, moderate- to high-intensity exercise for prolonged periods of time and reflects the functional capabilities of the heart, blood vessels, blood, lungs, and relevant muscles during various types of exercise demands. CRF is a synonym for many terms that may be used for the same thing (2). The following is a list of the terms that all mean essentially the same thing:

Cardiorespiratory fitness is related to the ability to perform large muscle, dynamic, moderate- to high-intensity exercise for prolonged periods of time and reflects the functional capabilities of the heart, blood vessels, blood, lungs, and relevant muscles during various types of exercise demands.

➤ Maximal aerobic capacity
➤ Functional capacity
➤ Physical work capacity

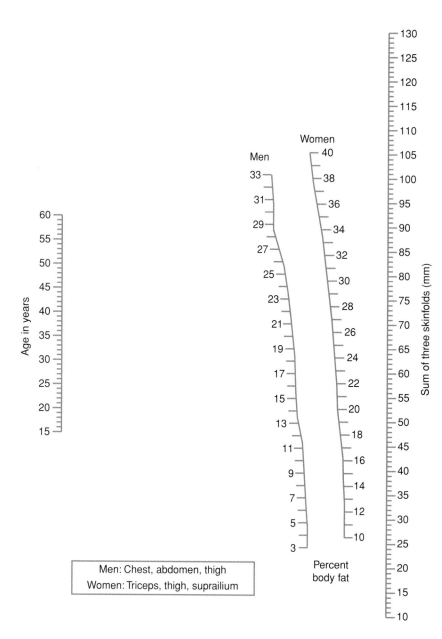

FIGURE 14.7. The Jackson–Pollock nomogram for the estimate of percent body fat. (Reprinted with permission from American Alliance for Health, Physical Education, and Dance, 1900 Association Drive, Reston, VA 20191, taken from Baun WB, Baun MR. A nomogram for the estimate of percent body fat from generalized equations. *Res Q Exerc Sport.* 1981;52(3):382.)

➤ Maximal oxygen uptake ($\dot{V}O_{2max}$) or maximal oxygen consumption or maximal oxygen intake

➤ Cardiovascular endurance, fitness, or capacity

➤ Cardiopulmonary endurance, fitness, or capacity

Cardiorespiratory fitness can be measured or predicted by many methods. This chapter discusses the prediction of CRF by the use of field tests such as the 1.5-mile run test and step tests, as well as laboratory tests such as the submaximal cycle ergometer protocol. The Personal Trainer needs to decide which test may be the most appropriate for CRF determination for a client. The measurement of CRF can be used in:

➤ Exercise prescription and programming

➤ Progress in, and motivation of, an individual in an exercise program (providing both feedback and motivation to keep a client interested in exercise)

➤ Prediction of medical conditions such as coronary artery disease (to further identify or diagnose health problems)

BOX 14.2　Summary of Anthropometry/Body Composition Techniques

Procedure	Comments
Anthropometry: body mass index	Simple technique (only height and weight) and good research to back the normative data for comparison purposes, does not account for differences in weight composition (fat vs. muscle)
Anthropometry: waist-to-hip ratio	Relatively simple-to-perform (some technician training) and good research data to back the normative data for comparison purposes, weight distribution shown to be important to health
Body composition: skinfolds	Highly regarded, many sites and formulas, technician training important, small prediction error (SEE about 3%–4%)
Body composition: bioelectrical impedance	Fairly accurate but many pretest conditions need to be met (hydration of client), technician training minimal, under ideal conditions similar prediction error to skinfolds.

Adapted and modified from American College of Sports Medicine. *ACSM's Resource Manual for Guidelines for Exercise Testing and Prescription*. 5th ed. Philadelphia: Lippincott Williams & Wilkins; 2006. p. 203.

The true measurement of CRF involves maximal exertion as a result of graded exercise testing along with the collection of expired gases during this exercise test. The measurement of expired gases is not always applicable, nor desirable, in many settings such as corporate fitness and wellness programs that wish to measure or quantify CRF; thus, this procedure is likely beyond the scope of practice of many Personal Trainers (2).

Pretest Considerations

It is important to standardize pretesting conditions for all clients who undergo these various tests for CRF. Standardization can also increase the accuracy of prediction of CRF as well as aid in client

BOX 14.3　Ideal Body Weight Calculations

$$\text{Ideal body weight (IBW)} = \frac{\text{LBM (lean body mass)}}{1.00 - (\text{desired \% body fat}/100)}$$

For example, if a man weighs 190 lb (86.4 kg) and is determined to have 22.3% body fat, then

Fat weight = body weight $\times$ (% body fat/100)

$$= 190 \times (22.3/100)$$

$$= 42.37 \text{ lb } (19.25 \text{ kg})$$

LBM = body weight − fat weight = 190 − 42.37 = 147.63 lb (67.1 kg)

$$\text{IBW} = \frac{147.63}{1.00 - (14/100)} \quad (15\% \text{ used for a man; as a guideline})$$

$$= 173.68 \ (78.9 \text{ kg}) \text{ at } 15\% \text{ body fat}$$

Weight loss = body weight − IBW

In this example, 190 − 173.68 = 16.3 lb (7.4 kg) to lose to achieve ideal body weight.

safety. Instructions to clients prior to the test can increase their comfort as well. These general instructions are as follows (1):

- Abstain from prior eating (>4 hours)
- Abstain from prior strenuous exercise (>24 hours)
- Abstain from prior caffeine ingestion (>12–24 hours)
- Abstain from prior nicotine use (>3 hours)
- Abstain from prior alcohol use (>24 hours)
- Medication considerations (if the client's medications affect resting or exercise HR, it will invalidate the test)

Various Field Tests for Prediction of CRF

A field test generally requires the client to perform a task in a nonlaboratory or field setting, such as running 1.5 miles (2.4 km) at near maximal exertion. Thus, field tests, perhaps considered by some to be submaximal, may be inappropriate for safety reasons for sedentary individuals at moderate to high risk for cardiovascular or musculoskeletal complications.

> *Field tests, perhaps considered by some to be submaximal, may be inappropriate for safety reasons for sedentary individuals at moderate to high risk for cardiovascular or musculoskeletal complications.*

Two types of field tests are commonly used for the prediction of aerobic capacity: a timed completion of a set distance (e.g., 1.5-mile run) or a maximal distance for a set time (e.g., 12-minute walk/run). Field tests are relatively easy and inexpensive to administer and thus are ideal for testing large groups of subjects (2,4). Although the particular CRF assessment to select can be a difficult choice, there are criteria you may use to help select the best test for your client:

- What the data will be used for (e.g., exercise programming)
- Need for data accuracy
- Client's age and health status
- Available resources

In general, both walk/run performance tests and step tests are appropriate for a wide range of clients, as long as the appropriate health risk screening has occurred first. One note of importance is that in the performance of a field test (both walk/run and step tests), the client can approach a level of near-maximal exertion and this clearly may not be desirable for all clients.

Walk/Run Performance Tests

There are two common field test protocols that use a walk or run performance to predict CRF. These walk or run tests tend to be more accurate (i.e., less error in prediction) than the step tests discussed next. The performance tests can be classified into two groups: walk/run tests or pure walk tests. In the walk/run test, the subject can walk, run, or use a combination of both to complete the test. In the pure walking test, the subjects are strictly limited to walking (always having one foot on the ground at any given time) the entire test. Another classification for these tests is whether the test is performed over a set distance (e.g., 1 mile or 1.6 km) or over a set time period (e.g., 12 minutes). The first test discussed uses a 1.5-mile (2.4 km) distance and requires the subject to complete the distance in the shortest time possible, either by running the whole distance, if possible, or by combining periods of running and walking to offset the fatigue of continuous running in a less-fit individual. The second test uses a set 1-mile course and requires the subject to walk the entire distance.

1.5-MILE RUN TEST PROCEDURES

1. This test is contraindicated for unconditioned beginners, individuals with symptoms of heart disease, and those with known heart disease or risk factors for heart disease. Clients should be able to jog for 15 minutes continuously to complete this test and obtain a reasonable prediction of their aerobic capacity.

2. Ensure that the area for performing the test measures 1.5 miles in distance. A standard ¼-mile track would be ideal (6 laps in lane 1 = 1.5 miles). For a metric 400-m track, this would be 6 laps (1.49 miles) plus approximately 46 feet to equal 1.5 miles.

3. Inform clients of the purpose of the test and the need to pace themselves over the 1.5-mile distance. Effective pacing and the subject's motivation are key variables in the outcome of the test.

4. Have clients start the test and start a stopwatch to coincide with the start. Give your clients feedback on time throughout the assessment to help them with pacing.

5. Record the total time to complete the test and use the formula below to predict CRF as measured by $\dot{V}O_{2max}$ and recorded in $mL \cdot kg^{-1} \cdot min^{-1}$:

$$\text{For men and women: } \dot{V}O_{2max} \ (mL \cdot kg^{-1} \cdot min^{-1}) = 3.5 + 483/time$$

where time = time to complete 1.5 miles in nearest hundredth of a minute.

For example, if the time to complete 1.5 miles was 14:20 (14 minutes and 20 seconds), then time used in the formula would be 14.33 minutes (20/60 = 0.33).

$$\dot{V}O_{2max} \ (mL \cdot kg^{-1} \cdot min^{-1}) = 3.5 + 483/14.33 = 37.2 \ mL \cdot kg^{-1} \cdot min^{-1}$$

ROCKPORT 1-MILE WALK TEST PROCEDURES

This test may be useful for those who are unable to run because of a low fitness level and/or injury. The client should be able to walk briskly (get the exercise HR above 120 bpm) for 1 mile to complete this test.

The 1-mile walk test requires that subjects walk as fast as they can around a measured 1-mile course. The clients must not break into a run! Walking can be defined as having one foot in contact with the ground at all times, whereas running involves an airborne phase. The time it takes to walk this 1 mile is measured and recorded (9,10).

Immediately at the end of the 1-mile walk, the client counts the recovery HR (or pulse) for 15 seconds and multiplies by 4 to determine a 1-minute recovery HR (bpm). In another version of the test, HR is measured in the final minute of the 1-mile walk (during the last quarter mile). It has been shown that using an HR monitor may give the client more accurate results than manual palpation of HR.

The formula to determine $\dot{V}O_{2max}$ $(mL \cdot kg^{-1} \cdot min^{-1})$ is gender specific (the constant 6.315 is added to the formula for men only). This formula was derived on apparently healthy individuals ranging in age from 30 to 69 years (6).

$$\dot{V}O_{2max} \ (mL \cdot kg^{-1} \cdot min^{-1}) = 132.853 - (0.1692 \cdot WT) - (0.3877 \cdot AGE) + (6.315, \text{for men}) \\ - (3.2649 \cdot TIME) - (0.1565 \cdot HR)$$

where WT = weight in kilograms, AGE = age in years, TIME = time for 1 mile in nearest hundredth of a minute (e.g., 14:42 = 14.7 [42/60 = 0.7]), and HR = recovery HR in bpm.

Step Tests

Step tests have been around for more than 50 years in fitness testing. We will discuss the use of the Queens College Step Test (2) for the prediction of CRF (there are several popular step test protocols). This test relies on having the subject step up and down on a standardized step or bench (standardized for step height) for a set period of time at a set stepping cadence. After the test time period is complete, a recovery HR is obtained and used in the prediction of CRF. The lower the recovery HR, the more fit the individual. Most step tests use the client's HR response to a standard amount of exertion (2).

In general, step tests require little equipment to conduct (a watch, a metronome, and a standardized height step bench). Special precautions for safety are needed for those clients who may have balance problems or difficulty with stepping. It should also be remembered that while step tests may be considered submaximal for many clients, they might be at or near maximal exertion for other clients.

QUEENS COLLEGE STEP TEST PROCEDURES

1. The Queens College Step Test requires that the individual step up and down on a standardized step height of 16.25 in (41.25 cm) for 3 minutes. Many gym bleachers have a riser height of 16.25 in.
2. The men step at a rate (cadence) of 24 steps per minute, whereas women step at a rate of 22 per minute for a total of 3 minutes of exercise. This cadence should be closely monitored and set with the use of an electronic metronome. A 24-steps-per-minute cadence means that the complete cycle of step-up with one leg, step-up with the other, step-down with the first leg, and finally step-down with the last leg is performed 24 times in a minute (up one leg—up the other leg—down the first leg—down the second leg). Set the metronome at a cadence of four times the step rate, in this case 96 bpm for men, to coordinate each leg's movement with a beat of the metronome. The women's step rate would be 88 bpm. Thus, although it may be possible to test more than one client at a time, depending on equipment, it is problematic to test men and women together.
3. After 3 minutes of stepping are completed, the client stops and has his or her pulse taken (preferably at the radial site) while standing and within the first 5 seconds. A 15-second pulse count is then taken. Multiply this pulse count by 4 to determine HR in bpm. Thus, the recovery HR should occur between 5 and 20 seconds of immediate recovery from the end of the step test.
4. The subject's $\dot{V}O_{2max}$ (in $mL \cdot kg^{-1} \cdot min^{-1}$) is determined from the recovery HR using the gender-specific formulas as given in Table 14.4.

Submaximal Cycle Ergometer Tests

CRF may be predicted using several testing methodologies that can vary from submaximal to maximal in nature. We will next discuss the approach of laboratory submaximal exercise testing for the prediction of CRF. Maximal testing is not always a feasible or desirable approach in some settings; thus, the Personal Trainer may need to be able to perform a submaximal exercise test on a client in a laboratory setting.

Per Olaf Åstrand (a famous exercise physiologist from Sweden) along with his wife, Irma Rhyming, developed a simple protocol in the 1950s to be used for the prediction of CRF from laboratory submaximal cycle exercise results known as the Åstrand–Rhyming protocol (Fig. 14.8). This protocol uses a single-stage approach for the prediction of CRF. Although this protocol is not as often used as one developed by the YMCA (4), it is presented in this chapter because it is somewhat simpler to use and thus may represent a good first protocol to use as the Personal Trainer learns how to conduct a laboratory submaximal exercise tests.

TABLE 14.4	CALCULATION OF MAXIMAL OXYGEN CONSUMPTION AS DETERMINED FROM THE RECOVERY HEART RATE	
For Men		**For Women**
$\dot{V}O_{2max}$ (mL · kg^{-1} · min^{-1}) = 111.33/(0.42 × HR)		$\dot{V}O_{2max}$ (mL · kg^{-1} · min^{-1}) = 65.81/(0.1847 × HR)

HR, recovery heart rate (bpm).

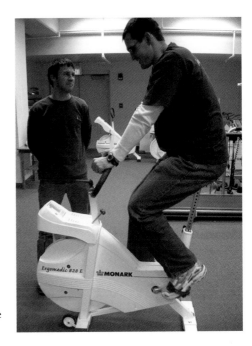

FIGURE 14.8. Submaximal exercise testing on a cycle ergometer.

ÅSTRAND-RHYMING TEST PROCEDURES

In summary, the client performs a 6-minute submaximal exercise bout on the cycle ergometer. Thus, this is typically a single-stage test. The client's HR response to this bout will determine his or her maximal aerobic capacity or CRF by plotting his or her HR response to this one stage on a test-specific nomogram (Fig. 14.9).

1. *Explain the test to your client*: Be sure that you have adequately screened your client via a Health History Questionnaire and/or a PAR-Q and performed ACSM Risk Stratification. Note: Physician supervision is not necessary with submaximal testing in low- and moderate-risk adults. More information on this can be found in Chapter 13 as well as the ACSM Guidelines for Exercise Testing and Prescription (ACSM GETP) (1).

2. *Explain and obtain informed consent*: The safety of this test is reported as >300,000 tests performed without a major complication (1). Informed consent is further discussed in Chapter 13 and ACSM GETP (1). It is very important that the clients understand that they are free to stop the tests anytime, but they are also responsible for informing you of any and all symptoms they might develop.

3. Discuss with your client your general preparedness to handle any emergencies.

4. Take the baseline or resting measures of HR and BP with your client seated.

5. *Adjust seat height*: The knee should be flexed at approximately 5°–10° in the pedal down position with the toes on the pedals. [Another way to check seat height is to have your client place his or her heels on the pedals; with the heels on the pedals, the leg should be straight in the pedal down position. Also, you can align the seat height with you client's greater trochanter, or hip, with your client standing next to the cycle.] Most important is for your client to be comfortable with the seat height. Have your client turn the pedals to test for the seat height appropriateness. While pedaling, your client should be comfortable and there should be no rocking of their hips (you can check on hip rocking by viewing your client from behind). Also, be sure that your client maintains an upright posture (by adjusting the handlebars, if necessary) and does not grip the handlebars too tight.

6. Start the test.

Age	Correction Factor
15	1.10
25	1.00
35	0.87
40	0.83
45	0.78
50	0.75
55	0.71
60	0.68
65	0.65

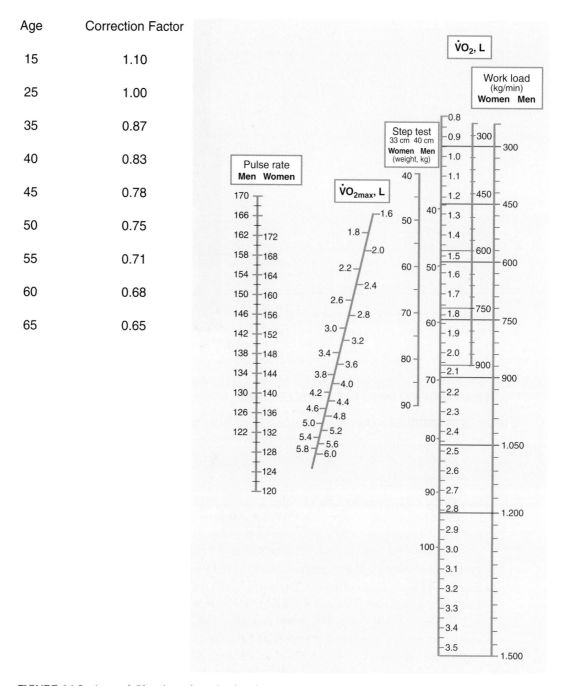

FIGURE 14.9. Astrand–Rhyming submaximal cycle ergometer test nomogram and age-correction factors. (Used with permission from Astrand PO, Rhyming I. A nomogram for calculation of aerobic capacity from pulse rate during submaximal work. *J Appl Physiol*. 1954;7:218–21.)

7. Have your client freewheel, without any resistance (0 kg), at the pedaling cadence of 50 rpm (set the metronome at 100).

8. Remind your client that maintaining 50 rpm throughout the test is essential. The test results will not be valid if there is a large variance in pedaling cadence.

9. Set the first stage's work output according to protocol table (Table 14.5).

10. Start the clock/timer.

11. Measure HR after each minute starting at minute 2. Count the HR for 10–15 seconds. You may wish to use an HR monitor. Record the HR on the data collection sheet.

TABLE 14.5	ASTRAND CYCLE SUBMAXIMAL ERGOMETER TEST INITIAL WORKLOADS
Men	
Unconditioned	300 or 600 kg · m · min^{-1} (50 or 100 W)
Conditioned	600 or 900 kg · m · min^{-1} (100 or 140 W)
Women	
Unconditioned	300 or 450 kg · m · min^{-1} (50 or 75 W)
Conditioned	450 or 600 kg · m · min^{-1} (75 or 100 W)

12. Measure and record the BP after the 3rd-minute HR; ACSM guidelines for test termination and BP are applicable (1).
13. The fifth- and sixth-minute HR will be used in the test determination of $\dot{V}O_{2max}$ as long as there is not more than a 5-beat difference between the two HRs.
14. The following applies for HRs.
    - If there is a difference of less than or equal to 5 bpm, consider the test finished.
    - If there is a difference of greater than 5 bpm, continue on for another minute and check HR again.
15. Regularly check the work output of the cycle ergometer with the pendulum resistance scale on the side of the ergometer and the rpm of subject. For the resistance, do not use the scale on the top front panel for measurement. Adjust the work output if necessary.
16. Regularly check your client's rpm and correct if necessary.

    The Åstrand protocol requires the following for test completion: You need to obtain 5th- and 6th-minute HR (within 5 bpm).

    For the most accurate prediction of $\dot{V}O_{2max}$, the protocol requires the HR be between 125 and 170 bpm.

    If the HR response to the initial work rate is not above 125 bpm after 6 minutes, the test is continued for another 6-minute interval by increasing the work rate by 300 kg · m · min^{-1} (1 kg).

    The HRs at the 5th and 6th minutes, if acceptable to the criteria above, are averaged for the nomogram method (Fig. 14.8).

17. Allow your client to cool down after the protocol is complete. Have your client continue to pedal at 50 rpm and decrease the resistance to 0.5–1 kg for 3 minutes of cool-down or recovery. Take your client's HR and BP at the end of the 3-minute active recovery period. Next, allow your client to sit quietly in a chair for 2–3 minutes to continue the recovery process. Be sure to check your client's HR and BP before allowing your client to leave the laboratory. Hopefully, their HR and BP will approach their resting measures.

PREDICTION OF CRF OR $\dot{V}O_{2max}$ FROM ÅSTRAND–RHYMING RESULTS

There are two methods available:

➤ a popular nomogram technique described in this text (see Fig. 14.8)
➤ a calculation-based formula not described in this chapter; (This method can be found in the *ACSM's Health-Related Physical Fitness Assessment Manual* (2)).

To use Figure 14.8, plot the HR (average for 5th and 6th minutes) on the appropriate gender scale and plot the corresponding work rate in kg · m · min^{-1} on gender-specific workload scale. Connect the two points with a straight line and read off the $\dot{V}O_{2max}$ in L · min^{-1}. Use the correction factor table (Fig. 14.8) to correct the $\dot{V}O_{2max}$ by the person's age (nearest 5 years). Convert absolute $\dot{V}O_{2max}$ in L · min^{-1} to relative $\dot{V}O_{2max}$ (mL · kg^{-1} · min^{-1}) using the client's body weight.

For example, if the estimated $\dot{V}O_{2max}$ (in L · min^{-1}) was 3.65 for a 40-year-old man, the age-corrected $\dot{V}O_{2max}$ would be 3.03 L · min^{-1} [3.65 × 0.83]. If the person weighs 147 pounds (66.8 kg),

TABLE 14.6	PERCENTILE VALUES FOR MAXIMAL AEROBIC POWER (ml · kg^{-1} · min^{-1})				
	Age, yr (Men)				
	20–29	30–39	40–49	50–59	60+
N	2,234	11,148	13,109	5,641	1,244
Percentile					
90	55.1	52.1	50.6	49.0	44.2
80	52.1	50.6	49.0	44.2	41.0
70	49.0	47.4	45.8	41.0	37.8
60	47.4	44.2	44.2	39.4	36.2
50	44.2	42.6	41.0	37.8	34.6
40	42.6	41.0	39.4	36.2	33.0
30	41.0	39.4	36.2	34.6	31.4
20	37.8	36.2	34.6	31.4	28.3
10	34.6	33.0	31.4	29.9	26.7
	Women				
N	1,223	3,895	4,001	2,032	465
Percentile					
90	49.0	45.8	42.6	37.8	34.6
80	44.2	41.0	39.4	34.6	33.0
70	41.0	39.4	36.2	33.0	31.4
60	39.4	36.2	34.6	31.4	28.3
50	37.8	34.6	33.0	29.9	26.7
40	36.2	33.0	31.4	28.3	25.1
30	33.0	31.4	29.9	26.7	23.5
20	31.4	29.9	28.3	25.1	21.9
10	28.3	26.7	25.1	21.9	20.3

Reprinted with permission from The Cooper Institute, Dallas, Texas. For more information, see www.cooperinstitute.org.

Data were obtained from the initial examination of apparently healthy men and women enrolled in the Aerobics Center Longitudinal Study, 1970–2002. The study population for the data set was predominantly white and college educated. Maximal treadmill exercise tests were administered using a modified Balke protocol. Maximal oxygen uptake was estimated from the final treadmill speed and grade using the current ACSM equations found in this edition of the guidelines (1). Development of the original database was supported in part by an NIH grant. The following may be used as descriptors for the percentile rankings: well above average (90), above average (70), average (50), below average (30), and well below average (10).

his or her relative $\dot{V}O_{2max}$ (mL · kg^{-1} · min^{-1}) would be 3.03 L · min^{-1} × 1,000 = 3,030 mL · min^{-1}/ 66.8 kg = 45.4 mL · kg^{-1} · min^{-1}.

Norms for CRF ($\dot{V}O_{2max}$)

Cardiorespiratory fitness is commonly expressed as $\dot{V}O_{2max}$. $\dot{V}O_{2max}$ is expressed as milliliters of oxygen consumed per kilogram of body weight per minute (mL · kg^{-1} · min^{-1}). Table 14.6 shows the norms for $\dot{V}O_{2max}$ for men and women.

MUSCULAR STRENGTH ASSESSMENT: ONE-REPETITION MAXIMUM

Muscular strength is defined as a one-time maximal force that may be exerted and is localized to a joint or muscle group. There are many assessment tests for muscular strength but only one test will

> *A good way of expressing muscular strength is as a ratio to total body weight.*

be covered in this chapter. A good way of expressing muscular strength is as a ratio to total body weight.

The one-repetition maximum (1-RM) stands for a one-time maximum amount of weight lifted. Research has shown that the single best weightlifting test for predicting total dynamic strength is the 1-RM bench press. This test measures the strength of the muscles involved in arm extension: the triceps, pectoralis major, and anterior deltoid. Although determining a 1-RM can be time-consuming and somewhat complicated to perform, the procedures for the 1-RM bench press test are as follows:

1. Allow the subject to become comfortable with the bench press and its operation by practicing a light warm-up of 5–10 repetitions at 40%–60% of perceived maximum.
2. For the test, the subject is to keep his or her back on the bench, both feet on the floor, and the hands should be shoulder width apart with palms up on the bar. It is necessary for the Personal Trainer to ensure that the client is using a closed grip with the thumbs on one side of the bar and the other fingers on the other side encircling the bar. Free weight equipment is preferred over equipment like Universal or Nautilus. A spotter must be present for all lifts. The spotter hands the bar to the subject. The subject starts the lift with the bar in the up position and arms fully extended. The bar is lowered to the chest and then pushed back up until the arms are locked. Be mindful of breathing; avoid a Valsalva maneuver (holding breath).
3. Following a 1-minute rest with light stretching, the subject does three to five repetitions at 60%–80% of perceived maximum.
4. The subject should be close to the perceived maximum. Add a small amount of weight and a 1-RM lift is attempted. If the lift is successful, a rest period of 3–5 minutes is provided. The goal is to find the 1-RM in 3–5 maximal efforts. The process continues until a failed attempt occurs. The greatest amount of weight lifted is considered 1-RM.
5. An interesting way of expressing muscular strength is as a ratio to total body weight. For a ratio determination of the amount of weight lifted compared to the individual's body weight (for normative comparison purposes), divide the maximum weight lifted in pounds by the subject's weight in pounds. Compare the calculated value to the norms (upper body) presented in Table 14.7.

Note: The above procedure can also be utilized for the 1-RM leg press (lower body). The norms for this test are presented in Table 14.8 (1).

MUSCULAR ENDURANCE ASSESSMENT: PARTIAL CURL-UP TEST

Muscular endurance is also joint and muscle group specific and there are many tests available for this component of health-related physical fitness. Muscular endurance denotes the ability to apply a force repeatedly over time. Two common assessments for muscular endurance are the partial curl-up and push-up tests. The partial curl-up test was developed to minimize the criticisms of the traditional and bent-leg sit-up tests but has also come under criticism as being relatively easy to perform (especially for younger and fitter clients).

Box 14.4 presents the procedures for both the push-up and partial curl-up assessments. The normative data for comparison purposes can be found in Table 14.9 for the push-up and Table 14.10 for the partial curl-up tests (1).

FLEXIBILITY ASSESSMENT: SIT-AND-REACH TEST

Although there exists no single best test of overall flexibility, the sit-and-reach test is the most common and most practical to use. Preceded by a proper warm-up, the sit-and-reach test can be easy to administer and interpret. The Personal Trainer should be made aware that this test measures only

TABLE 14.7 · UPPER BODY STRENGTH NORMS

$$\text{Bench press weight ratio} = \frac{\text{weight pushed in lb}}{\text{body weight in lb}}$$

%	<20	20–29	30–39	40–49	50–59	60+	
Males							
99	>1.76	>1.63	>1.35	>1.20	>1.05	>0.94	
95	1.76	1.63	1.35	1.20	1.05	0.94	S
90	1.46	1.48	1.24	1.10	0.97	0.89	
85	1.38	1.37	1.17	1.04	0.93	0.84	
80	1.34	1.32	1.12	1.00	0.90	0.82	E
75	1.29	1.26	1.08	0.96	0.87	0.79	
70	1.24	1.22	1.04	0.93	0.84	0.77	
65	1.23	1.18	1.01	0.90	0.81	0.74	
60	1.19	1.14	0.98	0.88	0.79	0.72	G
55	1.16	1.10	0.96	0.86	0.77	0.70	
50	1.13	1.06	0.93	0.84	0.75	0.68	
45	1.10	1.03	0.90	0.82	0.73	0.67	
40	1.06	0.99	0.88	0.80	0.71	0.66	F
35	1.01	0.96	0.86	0.78	0.70	0.65	
30	0.96	0.93	0.83	0.76	0.68	0.63	
25	0.93	0.90	0.81	0.74	0.66	0.60	
20	0.89	0.88	0.78	0.72	0.63	0.57	P
15	0.86	0.84	0.75	0.69	0.60	0.56	
10	0.81	0.80	0.71	0.65	0.57	0.53	
5	0.76	0.72	0.65	0.59	0.53	0.49	
1	<0.76	<0.72	<0.65	<0.59	<0.53	<0.49	VP
n	60	425	1,909	2,090	1,279	343	

Total *n* = 6,106

%	<20	20–29	30–39	40–49	50–59	60+	
Females							
99	>0.88	>1.01	>0.82	>0.77	>0.68	>0.72	
95	0.88	1.01	0.82	0.77	0.68	0.72	S
90	0.83	0.90	0.76	0.71	0.61	0.64	
85	0.81	0.83	0.72	0.66	0.57	0.59	
80	0.77	0.80	0.70	0.62	0.55	0.54	E
75	0.76	0.77	0.65	0.60.	0.53	0.53	
70	0.74	0.74	0.63	0.57	0.52	0.51	
65	0.70	0.72	0.62	0.55	0.50	0.48	

(continued)

TABLE 14.7 **UPPER BODY STRENGTH NORMS (Continued)**

%	<20	20–29	30–39	40–49	50–59	60+	
			Age, yr				
60	0.65	0.70	0.60	0.54	0.48	0.47	G
55	0.64	0.68	0.58	0.53	0.47	0.46	
50	0.63	0.65	0.57	0.52	0.46	0.45	
45	0.60	0.63	0.55	0.51	0.45	0.44	
40	0.58	0.59	0.53	0.50	0.44	0.43	F
35	0.57	0.58	0.52	0.48	0.43	0.41	
30	0.56	0.56	0.51	0.47	0.42	0.40	
25	0.55	0.53	0.49	0.45	0.41	0.39	
20	0.53	0.51	0.47	0.43	0.39	0.38	P
15	0.52	0.50	0.45	0.42	0.38	0.36	
10	0.50	0.48	0.42	0.38	0.37	0.33	
5	0.41	0.44	0.39	0.35	0.31	0.26	
1	<0.41	<0.44	<0.39	<0.35	<0.31	<0.26	VP
n	20	191	379	333	189	42	

Total n = 1,154

Reprinted with permission from The Cooper Institute, Dallas, Texas. For more information, see www.cooperinstitute.org. VL = very lean, E = excellent, G = good, F = fair, P = poor, VP = very poor. One-repetition maximum bench press, with bench press weight ratio = weight pushed in pounds/body weight in pounds.

TABLE 14.8 **LOWER BODY STRENGTH NORMS**

Percentile	20–29	30–39	40–49	50–59	60+
			Age, yr		
Men					
90	2.27	2.07	1.92	1.80	1.73
80	2.13	1.93	1.82	1.71	1.62
70	2.05	1.85	1.74	1.64	1.56
60	1.97	1.77	1.68	1.58	1.49
50	1.91	1.71	1.62	1.52	1.43
40	1.83	1.65	1.57	1.46	1.38
30	1.74	1.59	1.51	1.39	1.30
20	1.63	1.52	1.44	1.32	1.25
10	1.51	1.43	1.35	1.22	1.16
Women					
90	1.82	1.61	1.48	1.37	1.32
80	1.68	1.47	1.37	1.25	1.18
70	1.58	1.39	1.29	1.17	1.13
60	1.50	1.33	1.23	1.10	1.04
50	1.44	1.27	1.18	1.05	0.99
40	1.37	1.21	1.13	0.99	0.93
30	1.27	1.14	1.08	0.95	0.88
20	1.22	1.09	1.02	0.88	0.85
10	1.14	1.00	0.94	0.78	0.72

One-repetition maximum (1-RM) leg press with leg press weight ratio = weight pushed/body weight.

Reprinted with permission from The Cooper Institute, Dallas, Texas. For more information, see www.cooperinstitute.org. Study population for the data set was predominantly white and college educated. A Universal DVR machine was used to measure the 1-RM. The following may be used as descriptors for the percentile rankings: well above average (90), above average (70), average (50), below average (30), and well below average (10).

BOX **14.4**   **Push-Up and Curl-Up (Crunch) Test Procedures for Measurement of Muscular Endurance**

Push-up

1. The push-up test is administered with male subjects starting in the standard "down" position (hands pointing forward and under the shoulder, back straight, head up, using the toes as the pivotal point) and female subjects in the modified "knee push-up" position (legs together, lower leg in contact with mat with ankles plantarflexed, back straight, hands shoulder width apart, head up, using the knees as the pivotal point).
2. The subject must raise the body by straightening the elbows and return to the "down" position, until the chin touches the mat. The stomach should not touch the mat.
3. For both men and women, the subject's back must be straight at all times and the subject must push up to a straight arm position.
4. The maximal number of push-ups performed consecutively without rest is counted as the score.
5. The test is stopped when the client strains forcibly or is unable to maintain the appropriate technique within two repetitions.

Curl-up (crunch)

1. The individual assumes a supine position on a mat with the knees at 90°. The arms are at the side, palms facing down with the middle fingers touching a piece of tape. A second piece of tape is placed 10 cm apart.[a] Shoes remain on during the test.
2. A metronome is set to 50 beats per minute and the individual does slow, controlled curl-ups to lift the shoulder blades off the mat (trunk makes a 30° angle with the mat) in time with the metronome at a rate of 25 per minute. The test is done for 1 minute. The low back should be flattened before curling up.
3. The individual performs as many curl-ups as possible without pausing, to a maximum of 25.[b]

Adapted with permission from the Canadian Society for Exercise Physiology. *Canadian Physical Activity, Fitness & Lifestyle Approach: CSEP-Health & Fitness Program's Health-Related Appraisal & Counselling Strategy.* 3rd ed. © 2003, Canadian Society for Exercise Physiology.

[a]Alternatives include having the hands held across the chest, with the head activating a counter when the trunk reaches a 30° position and placing the hands on the thighs and curling up until the hands reach the knee caps. Elevation of the trunk to 30° is the important aspect of the movement.

[b]An alternative includes doing as many curl-ups as possible in 1 minute.

TABLE 14.9   **FITNESS CATEGORIES BY AGE GROUPS AND GENDER FOR PUSH-UPS**

| | Age, yr | | | | | | | | | |
| | 20–29 | | 30–39 | | 40–49 | | 50–59 | | 60–69 | |
Category	M	F	M	F	M	F	M	F	M	F
Excellent	36	30	30	27	25	24	21	21	18	17
Very good	35	29	29	26	24	23	20	20	17	16
	29	21	22	20	17	15	13	11	11	12
Good	28	20	21	19	16	14	12	10	10	11
	22	15	17	13	13	11	10	7	8	5
Fair	21	14	16	12	12	10	9	6	7	4
	17	10	12	8	10	5	7	2	5	2
Needs improvement	16	9	11	7	9	4	6	1	4	1

Reprinted with permission from the Canadian Society for Exercise Physiology. *Canadian Physical Activity, Fitness & Lifestyle Approach: CSEP-Health & Fitness Program's Health-Related Appraisal & Counselling Strategy.* 3rd ed., © 2003, Canadian Society for Exercise Physiology.

F, female; M, male.

TABLE 14.10	**FITNESS CATEGORIES BY AGE GROUPS AND GENDER FOR PARTIAL CURL-UP**									
	Age, yr									
	20–29		**30–39**		**40–49**		**50–59**		**60–69**	
Category	**M**	**F**	**M**	**F**	**M**	**F**	**M**	**F**	**M**	**F**
Excellent	25	25	25	25	25	25	25	25	25	25
Very good	24	24	24	24	24	24	24	24	24	24
	21	18	18	19	18	19	17	19	16	17
Good	20	17	17	18	17	18	16	18	15	16
	16	14	15	10	13	11	11	10	11	8
Fair	15	13	14	9	12	10	10	9	10	7
	11	5	11	6	6	4	8	6	6	3
Needs improvement	10	4	10	5	5	3	7	5	5	2

Used with permission from the Canadian Society for Exercise Physiology. *Canadian Physical Activity, Fitness & Lifestyle Approach: CSEP-Health & Fitness Program's Health-Related Appraisal & Counselling Strategy*. 3rd ed., © 2003, Canadian Society for Exercise Physiology.

F, female; M, male.

flexibility of the hamstrings, hip, and lower back. The practical significance of using the sit–and–reach test to measure of flexibility is the significant number of people who complain of low back pain. It is likely that this pain is caused by decreased flexibility, primarily of the hamstrings (which have their anatomical origin in the posterior hip region). For a detailed description of the procedure, see Box 14.5 and Figure 14.10. Percentile rankings for men and women can be found in Table 14.11 (6).

BOX **14.5**	**Trunk Flexion (Sit-and-Reach) Test Procedures**

Pretest: Participant should perform a short warm-up prior to this test and include some stretches for the targeted muscle groups (e.g., modified hurdler's stretch). It is also recommended that the participant refrain from fast, jerky movements, which may increase the possibility of an injury. The participant's shoes should be removed for the assessment.

1. For the Canadian Trunk Forward Flexion test, the client sits without shoes and the soles of the feet flat against the flexometer (sit-and-reach box) at the 26-cm mark. Inner edges of the soles are placed within 2 cm of the measuring scale. For the YMCA sit-and-reach test, a yardstick is placed on the floor and tape is placed across it at a right angle to the 15-in mark. The participant sits with the yardstick between the legs, with legs extended at right angles to the taped line on the floor. Heels of the feet should touch the edge of the taped line and be about 10–12 in apart. (Note the zero point at the foot/box interface and use the appropriate norms.)

2. The participant should slowly reach forward (no bouncing) with both hands as far as possible (to the point of mild discomfort), holding this position approximately 2 seconds. Be sure that the participant keeps the hands parallel and does not lead with one hand. Fingertips can be overlapped and should be in contact with the measuring portion or yardstick of the sit-and-reach box. To assist with the best attempt, the participant should exhale and drop the head between the arms when reaching. Testers should ensure that the knees of the participant stay extended; however, the participant's knees should not be pressed down. The participant should breathe normally during the test and should not hold his or her breath anytime.

3. The score is the most distant point (in centimeters or inches) reached with the fingertips. The better of two trials should be recorded. Norms for the Canadian test are presented in Table 14.11. Note that these norms use a sit-and-reach box in which the "zero" point is set at the 26-cm mark. If you are using a box in which the zero point is set at 23 cm (e.g., Fitnessgram), subtract 3 cm from each value in this table. The norms for the YMCA test are also presented in Table 14.11.

Diagrams of these procedures are available from Golding LA, Myers CR, Sinning WE. *YMCA Fitness Testing and Assessment Manual*. 4th ed. YMCA of the USA, 101 N. Wacker Drive, Chicago, IL 60606, and *Canadian Physical Activity, Fitness & Lifestyle Approach: CSEP-Health & Fitness Program's Health-Related Appraisal & Counselling Strategy* 3rd ed, © 2003, Canadian Society for Exercise Physiology.

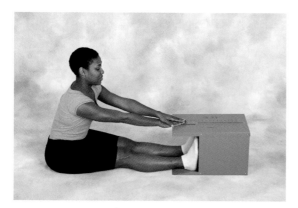
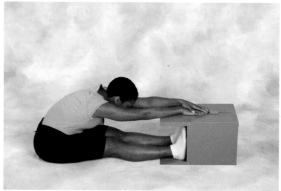

FIGURE 14.10. Client performing a sit-and-reach test.

TABLE 14.11	SIT-AND-REACH NORMS PERCENTILES BY AGE GROUPS AND GENDER FOR YMCA SIT-AND-REACH TEST (INCHES)											
	Age, yr											
	18–25		26–35		36–45		46–55		56–65		>65	
Percentile	M	F	M	F	M	F	M	F	M	F	M	F
90	22	24	21	23	21	22	19	21	17	20	17	20
80	20	22	19	21	19	21	17	20	15	19	15	18
70	19	21	17	20	17	19	15	18	13	17	13	17
60	18	20	17	20	16	18	14	17	13	16	12	17
50	17	19	15	19	15	17	13	16	11	15	10	15
40	15	18	14	17	13	16	11	14	9	14	9	14
30	14	17	13	16	13	15	10	14	9	13	8	13
20	13	16	11	15	11	14	9	12	7	11	7	11
10	11	14	9	13	7	12	6	10	5	9	4	9

Used with permission from the Canadian Society for Exercise Physiology. *Canadian Physical Activity, Fitness & Lifestyle Approach: CSEP-Health & Fitness Program's Health-Related Appraisal & Counselling Strategy.* 3rd ed., © 2003, Canadian Society for Exercise Physiology.

Fitness Categories by Age Groups for Trunk Forward Flexion Using a Sit-and-Reach Box (centimeter)[a]										
	Age, yr									
	20–29		30–39		40–49		50–59		60–69	
Category	M	F	M	F	M	F	M	F	M	F
Excellent	40	41	38	41	35	38	35	39	33	35
Very Good	39	40	37	40	34	37	34	38	32	34
	34	37	33	36	29	34	28	33	25	31
Good	33	36	32	35	28	33	27	32	24	30
	30	33	28	32	24	30	24	30	20	27
Fair	29	32	27	31	23	29	23	29	19	26
	25	28	23	27	18	25	16	25	15	23
Needs Improvement	24	27	22	26	17	24	15	24	14	22

Reprinted with permission from the *YMCA Fitness Testing and Assessment Manual.* 4th ed., © 2000 by YMCA of the USA, Chicago. All rights reserved.

[a]These norms are based on a sit-and-reach box in which the "zero" point is set at 26 cm. When using a box in which the zero point is set at 23 cm, subtract 3 cm from each value in this table.

The following may be used as descriptors for the percentile rankings: well above average (90), above average (70), average (50), below average (30), and well below average (10).

F, female; M, male.

ASSESSMENTS AS A MOTIVATIONAL DEVICE

Health-related physical fitness assessments can serve not only for exercise programming but also for motivational purposes when the results of the various assessments are explained and used in the goal-setting approach. It is important to note that a particular physical fitness assessment that is not used in programming decisions and instilling motivation should be questioned as to its use. In other words, simply testing all clients for all available assessments should be avoided.

Physical fitness assessment should be performed on a regular basis to determine whether established goals have been met. As goals are set, often a time frame for the attainment of those goals is included (e.g., lose 2% body fat in 3 months). For instance, if the individual has a goal to improve his or her overall flexibility in 3 months, then the sit-and-reach test should be performed every 4–6 weeks to measure progress toward that goal. A word of caution about follow-up assessments is that frequent assessments may fail to demonstrate desired changes as some components of physical fitness may take time and effort to change (for instance, significant and lasting body composition changes are not likely to occur in short time intervals). A standard for follow-up may be 4 weeks to 3 months, depending on what is being assessed.

> *Frequent assessments may fail to demonstrate desired changes as some components of physical fitness may take time and effort to change.*

SUMMARY

The results of a health-related physical fitness assessment represent a potential time of change. If a client scores *poorly* or has failed to demonstrate progress in certain areas (such as CRF with the submaximal cycle ergometer test), then answers should be sought as to why the changes were not evident and how the exercise program should be adjusted to produce the desired changes in the future. Once again, the results of the health-related physical fitness assessments should be used with an outcome in mind. As Personal Trainers, we need to realize that not all individuals are going to adapt to our programming suggestions in the same way. Thus, each round of health-related physical fitness assessments calls for a reexamination of the client's goals and objectives. Perhaps new measurable goals may be identified for that individual at some distant time interval.

REFERENCES

1. American College of Sports Medicine. *ACSM's Guidelines for Exercise Testing and Prescription.* 8th ed. Baltimore: Lippincott Williams & Wilkins; 2010.
2. American College of Sports Medicine. *ACSM's Health-Related Physical Fitness Assessment Manual.* 2nd ed. Baltimore: Lippincott Williams & Wilkins; 2008.
3. American College of Sports Medicine. *ACSM's Resource Manual for Guidelines for Exercise Testing and Prescription.* 5th ed. Baltimore: Lippincott Williams & Wilkins; 2006.
4. Golding LA, Myers CR, Sinning WE, eds. *Y's Way to Physical Fitness.* 3rd ed. Champaign (IL): Human Kinetics; 1989.
5. Heyward V. *Advanced Fitness Assessment and Exercise Prescription.* 3rd ed. Champaign (IL): Human Kinetics; 1998.
6. Howley ET, Franks BD. Flexibility and low back pain. In: Bahrke M, Crist R, Washington S, eds. *Health Fitness Instructors Handbook.* 4th ed. Champaign (IL): Human Kinetics; 2003. p. 247–262.
7. Howley E, Franks B. *Health Fitness Instructor's Handbook.* 4th ed. Champaign (IL): Human Kinetics; 2003.
8. Jackson AS, Pollock ML. Practical assessment of body composition. *Physician Sports Med.* 1985;13(5):85.
9. Kline GM, Porcari JP, Hintermeister R, et al. Estimation of $\dot{V}O_{2max}$ from a one-mile track walk, gender, age, and body weight. *Med Sci Sports Exerc.* 1987;19:253–9.
10. Nieman D. *Fitness and Sports Medicine: A Health-Related Approach.* 4th ed. Mountain View (CA): Mayfield; 1999.
11. Perloff D, Grimm C, Flack J, et al. Human blood pressure determination by sphygmomanometry. *Circulation.* 1993;88:5(pt 1): 2460–70.
12. Prisant LM, Alpert BS, Robbins CB, et al. American national standard for nonautomated sphygmomanometry. *Am J Hypertens.* 1995;8:210–3.
13. U.S. Department of Health and Human Services, National Institutes of Health, National Heart, Lung and Blood Institute. [Internet]. National High Blood Pressure Education Program Seventh Report of the Joint National Committee on Prevention, Detection, Evaluation, and Treatment of High Blood Pressure (JNC7). NIH Publication no. 03-5233, 2004 [cited 2008 Aug 27]. Available from http://www.nhlbi.nih.gov/guidelines/hypertension/

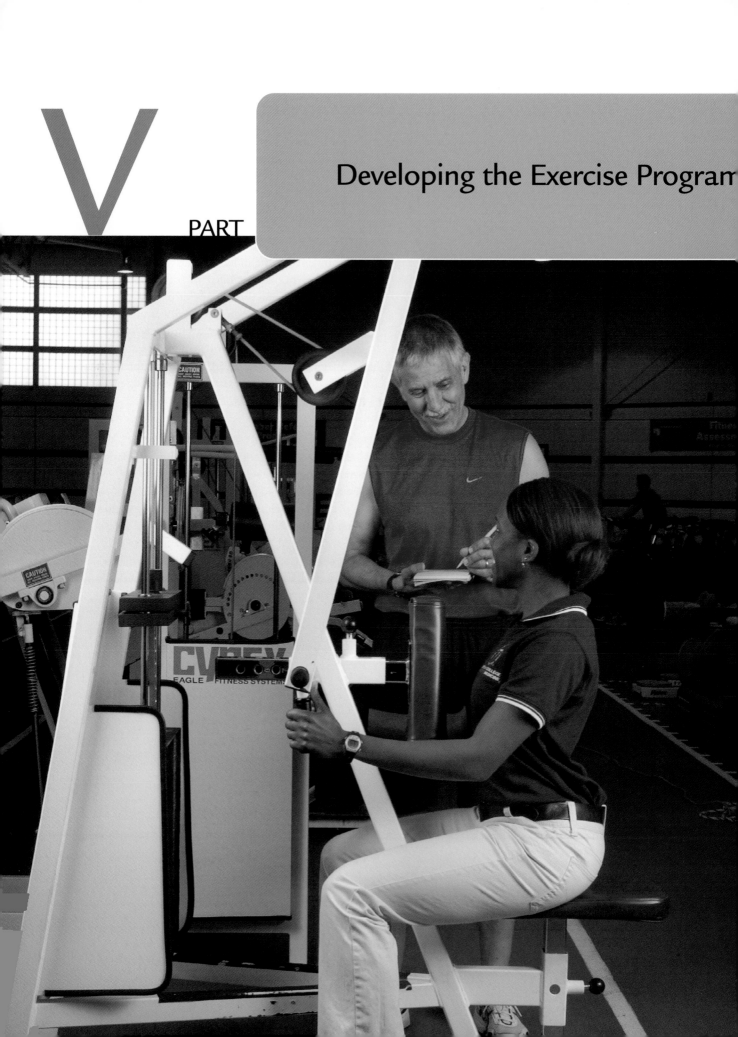

V
PART

Developing the Exercise Program

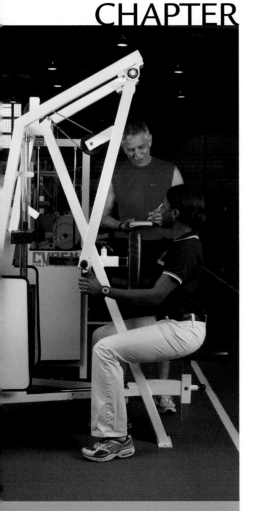

15

Program Design

OBJECTIVES

- Provide the Personal Trainer with the fundamentals needed to safely and effectively design a client exercise program, using principles that are prudent to our field of expertise and within our scope of practice.
- Review the basic physiological systems of the body to better facilitate the client's needs
- Identify the different modes of resistance, cardiovascular, and flexibility training
- Educate the certified Personal Trainer on communication skills and client–trainer relationships
- Prepare the certified Personal Trainer for the first training session as well as subsequent sessions and program variables

This chapter provides the Personal Trainer with the key elements needed to design a safe and effective client exercise program. It provides the Personal Trainer with the tools needed to structure the client exercise program by incorporating a review of basic anatomy, applied physiology, exercise protocol, and program design. This process begins with the initial consultation and the fitness assessment, which are fully explained in Chapter 12. This chapter applies the fundamentals of exercise programming, through the actual personal training session. The core concepts of this chapter are program design, client objectives, and assessment results, the various phases of an exercise program, and methods of strength, resistance, balance, flexibility, and functional training. Other chapters in this book explain, in detail, the physiological responses to the specific types of training programs detailed in this chapter. This chapter briefly addresses the musculoskeletal system, cardiovascular system, and respiratory system, as well as posture and body alignment.

OVERVIEW OF ANATOMY AND PHYSIOLOGY

Musculoskeletal System

This is a brief overview of the structural anatomy of the musculoskeletal system. It is not intended to replace the valuable information in other chapters of this book. In particular, please refer to Chapter 3 for a more detailed explanation and function of each of these components.

➤ There are more than 650 muscles in the human body.
➤ Muscles act as the "movers" for the human body; this movement is caused by the way in which muscles pull on the skeleton.
➤ The muscular system supplies the forces that enable the body to perform physical activity. When a muscle acts (shortens), it moves a bone by pulling on the tendon that attaches the muscle to the bone.
➤ Bones are hard, tough elastic, and compact. Bones provide the support system for soft tissue, providing protection for internal organs, and act as an important source of nutrients and blood constituents. Bones are the rigid levers for locomotion. There are four different types of bones in the body: long bones (diaphysis/epiphysis: centers of ossification)—clavicle, femur; short bones—carpus, tarsus, patellae; flat bones (scapula, skull, and scapula); and irregular bones—vertebrae, maxilla, mandible, and coccyx.

> *The axial skeleton consists of the skull, the vertebral column, sternum, and ribs. The appendicular skeleton is made up of the bones of the upper and lower extremities.*

The axial skeleton consists of the skull, the vertebral column, sternum, and ribs. The appendicular skeleton is made up of the bones of the upper and lower extremities. The major bones of the body are illustrated in Chapter 3.

An outer layer of fibrous connective tissue attaches the bone to muscles, deep fascia, and joint capsules. Just beneath this fibrous outer layer is a highly vascular inner layer that contains cells that provide the creation of a new bone. These outer and inner layers that cover the bones make up the periosteum. The periosteum, along with adjacent articulated structures, anchors the muscles to bone. Tendons are continuous with the epimysium (outer layer of connective tissue that covers muscle). Muscles consist of individual cells, or fibers, connected in bundles. A single muscle is made up of many bundles of muscle fibers, called "fasciculi." Connective tissue runs from end to end of muscle (from the tendon origin to the tendon insertion) and exists within the muscle tissue surrounding the fibers and giving rise to muscle bundles.

The prime mover of a contraction is called the agonist muscle, and the muscle that performs the opposite action is called the antagonist muscle. Muscles are responsible for the following movements: extension, flexion, abduction, adduction, elevation, depression, and rotation.

On the basis of structure and function, muscle tissue is categorized into three types: *smooth, skeletal* (sometimes referred to as striated), and *cardiac*. Refer to Chapter 5 for a full explanation of the muscle fibers and types. Although skeletal muscles are grouped together, they function either separately or along with others (8). Which, and how many, skeletal muscles become involved in a workout depends on which exercises are selected and the techniques used during their execution. For example, the width of stance or grip or the angle and path that a bar is pushed or pulled all have an effect on which muscles (or individual fibers of a muscle) are recruited and to what extent (3).

Skeletal muscles are responsible for creating power and force. However, there are different types of muscle actions; *concentric muscle actions* occur when the muscle fibers shorten. In this case, the muscle force exceeds the resistance, causing the muscle insertion point and point of origin to move closer together. Concentric actions are what are typically thought of as muscle contractions. In contrast, *eccentric muscle actions* are muscle actions in which active muscle fibers elongate. That is, the muscle is generating force, but the resistance exceeds the muscle force, and the muscle point of origin and insertion point move farther apart. Note that eccentric muscle actions occur frequently in daily body movements. Examples include the action of the quadriceps muscles when walking down steps or sitting down into a chair and the action of the forearm flexors when throwing a baseball. Indeed, everyday tasks such as walking or running cause simultaneous actions both concentrically and eccentrically. Finally, *isometric* or static muscle actions refer to a type of muscular activity in which there is tension in the muscle but it does not shorten (or lengthen). The bony attachments are fixed, or the forces functioning to lengthen the muscle are countered by forces that are equal to or greater than those generated by the muscles to shorten. In this case, muscle force and resistance are equal.

ANATOMICAL LOCATIONS AND DEFINITIONS

The following are terms that the Personal Trainer will have to become familiar with to explain anatomical locations (planes of the body) to the client (14):

➤ *Anterior*: to the front of the body
➤ *Anatomical position*: the body is standing erect with feet together and the upper limbs hanging loosely at the sides, with palms of the hands facing forward, thumbs facing away from the body, and fingers extended
➤ *Distal*: farther away from any reference point
➤ *Inferior*: away from the head
➤ *Lateral*: away from the midline of the body
➤ *Medial*: toward the midline of the body
➤ *Posterior*: to the back of the body
➤ *Proximal*: closer to any point of reference
➤ *Superior*: toward the head

COMMON MOVEMENT TERMS AND DEFINITIONS

The following are terms that the Personal Trainer should be familiar with when explaining and demonstrating common movement actions to the client (6) (Fig. 15.1 and Tables 15.1 through 15.4):

➤ *Abduction*: a movement away from the axis or midline of the body when in the anatomical position
➤ *Adduction*: a movement toward the axis or midline of the body when in the anatomical position
➤ *Agonist*: the prime mover—the muscle directly engaged in muscle action as distinguished from muscles that are relaxing at the same time. For example, in a biceps curl, the biceps act as the agonist muscles, whereas the triceps act as the antagonist.
➤ *Antagonist*: a muscle that has an action opposite that of the agonist and yields to the movement of the agonist

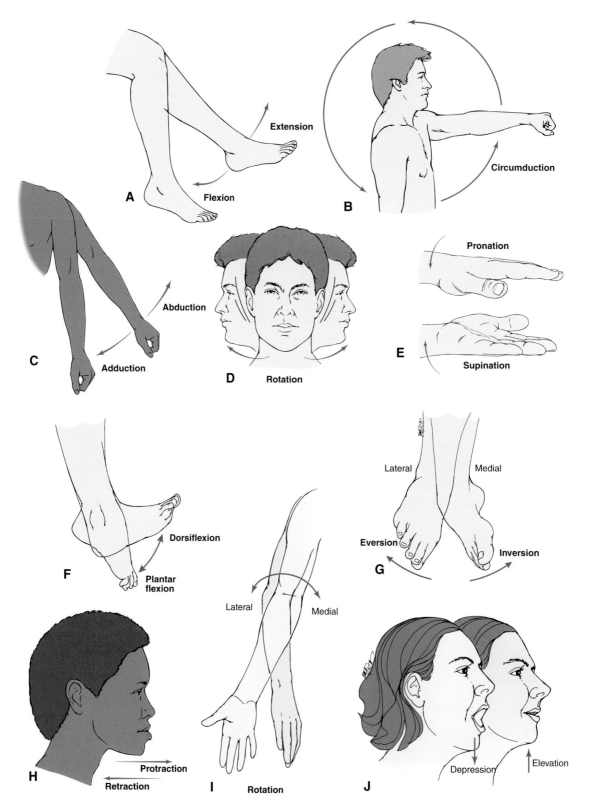

FIGURE 15.1. Joint movements. **A.** Flexion and extension (knee joint). **B.** Circumduction (shoulder joint). **C.** Abduction and adduction (shoulder joint). **D.** Rotation (atlantoaxial joint). **E.** Pronation and supination (elbow joint). **F.** Dorsiflexion and plantarflexion (ankle joint). **G.** Inversion and eversion (ankle joint). **H.** Protraction and retraction (temporomandibular joint). **I.** Medial and lateral rotation (shoulder joint). **J.** Depression and elevation. (From Smeltzer SCO, Bare BG. *Brunner and Suddarth's Textbook of Medical–Surgical Nursing.* 9th ed. Philadelphia: Lippincott Williams & Wilkins; 2002.)

TABLE 15.1   CLASSIFICATION OF JOINTS IN THE HUMAN BODY

Joint Classification	Features and Examples
Fibrous	
Suture	Tight union unique to the skull
Syndesmosis	Interosseous membrane between bones (e.g., the union along the shafts of the radius and ulna, tibia, and fibula)
Gomphosis	Unique joint at the tooth socket
Cartilaginous	
Primary (synchondroses; hyaline cartilaginous)	Usually temporary to permit bone growth and typically fuse; some do not (e.g., at the sternum and rib [costal cartilage])
Secondary (symphyses; fibrocartilaginous)	Strong, slightly movable joints (e.g., intervertebral discs, pubic symphysis)
Synovial	
Plane (arthrodial)	Gliding and sliding movements (e.g., acromioclavicular joint)
Hinge (ginglymus)	Uniaxial movements (e.g., elbow and knee extension and flexion)
Ellipsoidal (condyloid)	Biaxial joint (e.g., wrist flexion and extension, radioulnar deviation)
Saddle (sellar)	Unique joint that permits movements in all planes, including opposition (e.g., the carpometacarpal joint of the thumb)
Ball and socket (enarthrodial)	Multiaxial joints that permit movements in all directions (e.g., hip and shoulder joints)
Pivot (trochoidal)	Uniaxial joints that permit rotation (e.g., humeroradial joint)

Reprinted with permission from *ACSM's Resource Manual for Guidelines for Exercise Testing and Prescription*. 6th ed. Baltimore: Lippincott Williams & Wilkins; 2010. p 19.

TABLE 15.2   MAJOR JOINT MOTIONS AND PLANES OF MOTION

Major Joints	Type of Joints	Joint Movements	Planes
Scapulothoracic	Not a true joint	Elevation–depression	Frontal
		Upward–downward rotation	Frontal
		Protraction–retraction	Transverse
Glenohumeral	Synovial: ball and socket	Flexion–extension	Sagittal
		Abduction–adduction	Frontal
		Internal–external rotation	Transverse
		Horizontal abduction–adduction	Transverse
		Circumduction	
Elbow	Synovial: hinge	Flexion–extension	Sagittal
Proximal radioulnar	Synovial: pivot	Pronation–supination	Transverse
Wrist	Synovial: ellipsoidal	Flexion–extension	Sagittal
		Ulnar–radial deviation	Frontal
Metacarpophalangeal	Synovial: ellipsoidal	Flexion–extension	Sagittal
		Abduction–adduction	Frontal
Proximal interphalangeal	Synovial: hinge	Flexion–extension	Sagittal
Distal interphalangeal	Synovial: hinge	Flexion–extension	Sagittal
Intervertebral	Cartilaginous	Flexion–extension	Sagittal
		Lateral flexion	Frontal
		Rotation	Transverse
Hip	Synovial: ball and socket	Flexion–extension	Sagittal
		Abduction–adduction	Frontal
		Internal–external rotation	Transverse
		Horizontal abduction–adduction	Transverse
		Circumduction	
Knee	Synovial: hinge	Flexion–extension	Sagittal
Ankle: talocrural	Synovial: hinge	Dorsiflexion–plantarflexion	Sagittal
Ankle: subtalar	Synovial: gliding	Inversion–eversion	Frontal

Reprinted with permission from *ACSM's Resource Manual for Guidelines for Exercise Testing and Prescription*. 6th ed. Baltimore: Lippincott Williams & Wilkins; 2010. p. 20.

TABLE 15.3	**MAJOR MOVEMENTS OF THE UPPER EXTREMITY**		
Joint	**Movement**	**Major Agonist Muscles**	**Examples of Resistance Exercises**
Scapulothoracic	Fixation	Serratus anterior	Push-ups
		Pectoralis minor	Parallel bar dips
		Trapezius	Upright rows
		Levator scapulae	Shoulder shrugs
		Rhomboids	Seated rows
Glenohumeral	Flexion	Anterior deltoid	Front raises
		Pectoralis major (clavicular head)	Incline bench press
	Extension	Latissimus dorsi	
		Teres major	Dumbbell pullovers
		Pectoralis major	Chin-ups
		(sternocostal head)	Bench press
	Abduction	Middle deltoid	Lateral raises, dumbbell press
		Supraspinatus	Low pulley lateral raises
	Adduction	Latissimus dorsi	Lats pull-down
		Teres major	Seated row
		Pectoralis major	Cable crossover fly
	Medial (internal)	Latissimus dorsi	Back latissimus pull-downs, bent rows
	rotation	Teres major	One-arm dumbbell rows
		Subscapularis	
		Pectoralis major	
		Anterior deltoid	Rotator cuff exercises
			Dumbbell press, parallel bar dips
			Front raises
	Lateral (external)	Infraspinatus	External rotation exercises
	rotation	Teres minor	Back press, bent-over lateral raises
		Posterior deltoid	
Elbow	Flexion	Biceps brachii	Curls
		Brachialis	Preacher curls
		Brachioradialis	Hammer curls
	Extension	Triceps brachii	Triceps dips, triceps extensions
		Anconeus	Pushdowns, triceps kickback
Radioulnar	Supination	Supinator	Dumbbell supination
		Biceps brachii	
	Pronation	Pronator teres, pronator quadratus	Dumbbell pronation
Wrist	Flexion	Flexor carpi radialis and ulnaris	Wrist curls
		Palmaris longus	
		Flexor digitorum superficialis	
	Extension	Extensor carpi radialis longus,	Reverse wrist curls
		brevis, ulnaris	
		Extensor digitorum	
	Adduction	Flexor and extensor carpi ulnaris	Wrist curls, reverse wrist curls
	(ulnar deviation)		
	Abduction	Extensor carpi radialis longus and	Wrist curls, reverse wrist curls
	(radial deviation)	brevis	
		Flexor carpi radialis	

Reprinted with permission from *ACSM's Resource Manual for Guidelines for Exercise Testing and Prescription.* 6th ed. Baltimore: Lippincott Williams & Wilkins; 2010. p. 22.

➤ *Circumduction*: a movement in which the distal end of a bone inscribes a circle within the shaft rotating

➤ *Extension*: a movement that increases the joint angle between two articulating bones (e.g., extending the elbow joint)

➤ *Flexion*: a movement that decreases the joint angle between two articulating bones (e.g., flexing the knee joint)

TABLE 15.4	MAJOR MOVEMENTS OF THE LOWER EXTREMITY		
Joint	**Movement**	**Major Agonist Muscles**	**Examples of Resistance Exercises**
Intervertebral	Trunk flexion	Rectus abdominis	Sit-ups, crunches, leg raises
		External obliques	Machine crunches
		Internal obliques	High pulley crunches
	Trunk extension	Erector spinae	Back extensions, dead lifts
	Lateral flexion	Rectus abdominis	Roman chair side bends
		External obliques	Dumbbell side bends
		Internal obliques	Hanging leg raises
	Rotation	External obliques	Rotation crunches on exercise ball
		Internal obliques	Machine trunk
			Rotations
Hip	Flexion	Iliacus	Leg raises
		Psoas major	Incline leg raises
		Rectus femoris	Machine crunches
		Sartorius	Leg raises
		Pectineus	Cable adductions
	Extension	Gluteus maximus	Squats, leg presses, lunges
		Hamstrings (semitendinosus, semimembranosus, long head of biceps femoris)	Leg curls (standing, seated, lying) Good mornings
	Abduction	Tensor fasciae latae	Cable hip abductions
		Sartorius	Standing machine abductions
		Gluteus medius	Floor hip abductions
		Gluteus minimus	Seated machine abductions
	Adduction	Adductor longus, brevis, and magnus	Power squats
		Gracilis	Cable adductions
		Pectineus	Machine adductions
	Medial rotation	Semitendinosus	Leg curls (standing, seated, lying)
		Semimembranosus	Floor hip adduction
		Gluteus medius	Machine abductions
		Tensor fascia latae	
		Gracilis	
	Lateral rotation	Biceps femoris	
		Adductor longus, brevis, magnus	
		Gluteus maximus	
Knee	Flexion	Hamstrings	Leg curls (standing, seated, lying prone)
		Gracilis	
		Sartorius	
	Extension	Quadriceps femoris (rectus femoris, vastus lateralis, medialis, and intermedius)	Lunges, squats, leg extensions
Ankle: talocrural	Dorsiflexion	Tibialis anterior	Ankle dorsiflexion against resistance
		Extensor digitorum longus	
		Extensor hallucis longus	
	Plantarflexion	Gastrocnemius, soleus, tibialis posterior	Standing calf raises, donkey calf raises
		Flexor digitorum longus	
Ankle: subtalar	Eversion	Peroneus longus and brevis	Exercises against resistance
	Inversion	Tibialis anterior and posterior	Exercises against resistance

Reprinted with permission from *ACSM's Resource Manual for Guidelines for Exercise Testing and Prescription.* 6th ed. Baltimore: Lippincott Williams & Wilkins; 2010. p. 23.

Cardiovascular System

The cardiovascular system consists of the heart and the blood vessels. The primary function of the cardiovascular system is to act as a transport system that delivers nutrients and removes waste products. The cardiovascular system plays a major role in maintaining homeostasis in the body. The cardiovascular system also assists with maintenance of normal function at rest and during exercise. For a full explanation of the functions of the cardiovascular system, please refer to Chapter 5. As discussed in Chapter 5, the cardiovascular system is responsible for the following specific functions in the body (5,7,13):

> *The cardiovascular system consists of the heart and the blood vessels.*

- Transporting oxygenated blood from lungs to tissues and deoxygenated blood from the tissues to the lungs
- Distributing nutrients (e.g., glucose, free fatty acids, amino acids) to cells
- Removal of metabolic waste products and end-products (e.g., carbon dioxide, urea, lactate) from the periphery for elimination or reuse
- Regulation of pH to control acidosis and alkalosis
- Transportation of hormones and enzymes to regulate physiological function
- Maintenance of fluid volume to prevent dehydration
- Maintenance of body temperature by absorbing and redistributing heat

Respiratory System

The primary function of the respiratory system is the basic exchange of oxygen and carbon dioxide. This will help the certified Personal Trainer better understand the role of this system in exercise selection and programming. Please read Chapter 5 for a full explanation of this system and its components.

TYPES OF TRAINING

Resistance Training

GENERAL TRAINING PRINCIPLES

Resistance training has become an integral part of fitness, wellness, and physical activity programs. Resistance training has been shown to have a positive impact on many health measures, and the collective impact may significantly improve functionality, well-being, and quality of life. When mapping out a plan for an effective resistance training program, the Personal Trainer must follow the following three general training principles: specificity, overload, and progression.

> *When mapping out a plan for an effective resistance training program, the Personal Trainer must follow the following three general training principles: specificity, overload, and progression.*

Specificity. The specificity principle dictates that training a client in a specific way will produce a specific result and that to reach a specific goal the client has to follow a specific type of training program (8). For example, a client whose goal is to strengthen the muscles of the chest must perform exercises such as the bench press or dumbbell flys, to target that area, rather than a lat pull-down, which will work the muscles of the back. The term specificity is also important when the Personal Trainer is designing a "sports-specific" program for a client with specific training goals. For this training method, exercise selection should be based on movements that mimic movements and systems used in competition. For example, a golf-specific training program should focus on exercises that will strengthen the core and trunk muscles, such as swing drills and trunk twists, because they carry over to the specified activity.

Overload. The overload principle states that stress placed on the musculoskeletal system must be greater than normal during a specific workout, and it should exceed the stress during the previous workout. Even the most specifically based training programs will produce only limited results if the client does not experience overload regularly. The degree of overload depends on the load, number of repetitions (refers to the number of times a load is administered), rest between sets, and frequency (number of training sessions per week). To produce strength and endurance gains, resistance training programs should progressively overload the muscular system. This can be done by:

➤ Increasing the resistance or weight
➤ Increasing repetitions
➤ Increasing sets
➤ Decreasing the rest period between sets or exercises
➤ Adding exercises for individual muscle group

Training that incorporates this principle challenges the body to meet and adapt to greater than normal physiological stress. As it does, a new threshold is established that requires an even greater stress to produce an overload (3). The amount of overload clients need to attain their goal is based on their level of muscular fitness. For example, a hockey player requires a different level of overload than a sedentary person. To best determine the load at which your client should be working (either starting from or progressing to), please refer to Chapter 15.

Progression. Progression is defined as an increase in workload to maintain overload. The concept of progression may also include the practice of using very modest weights during the initial sessions of an exercise program. Guidelines for the progression of exercise become a factor in the success of individuals who are beginning exercise programs or who are engaging in specific types of exercise programs. The recommended frequency, intensity, time, type (FITT) framework for the frequency, intensity, and time of aerobic exercise for apparently healthy adults and an example of exercise progression for beginning exercisers (1) is provided in Table 15.5.

GOAL-SETTING

When developing a resistance training program, the most valuable tool that a certified Personal Trainer can have is knowing the client's primary goals. Clients should set short-term and long-term goals. Goal-setting is an essential preliminary step when designing an effective training program. An acronym that can be used to define and quantify goals is S.M.A.R.T. (Specific, Measurable, Attainable, Relevant, Time-bound).

> *Goal-setting is an essential preliminary step when designing an effective training program.*

Goals should be realistic and attainable and focus on attempting to meet the client's medical, emotional, and functional needs, within the limitations of time, interest, and actual physical ability.

The three primary resistance training goals are hypertrophy, muscular strength, and muscular endurance. Explaining the specifics of each of these three primary resistance training goals to the client will not only educate them but also help establish strong client–trainer rapport.

Hypertrophy. Hypertrophy refers to an increase in muscle size or mass. For example, a client who states that he wants to look more "cut" or "wants bigger biceps" is referring to the aesthetic look of the enlarged muscle groups. Physiologically, hypertrophy occurs when there is an increase in size of the existing muscle fibers. Chapter 6 in this text explores the physiology of hypertrophy of the muscle fibers.

Muscular endurance. A client who states that he or she "wants more stamina" or wants to feel "less winded" after a workout is typically looking for a resistance program that will increase his or her muscular endurance. The outcome of training for greater endurance is an enhanced ability of the targeted muscles to perform at a submaximal level for many

TABLE 15.5 RECOMMENDED FITT FRAMEWORK FOR THE FREQUENCY, INTENSITY, AND TIME OF AEROBIC EXERCISE FOR APPARENTLY HEALTHY ADULTS

Habitual Physical Activity/ Exercise Level	Physical Fitness Classification[b]	Frequency		Intensity[a]		Perception of Effort[c]	Time		
		kcal · wk^{-1}	d · wk^{-1}	HRR/$\dot{V}O_2R$	% HR$_{max}$		Total Duration Per Day (min)	Total Daily Steps During Exercise[d]	Weekly Duration (min)
Sedentary/no habitual activity/ exercise/extremely deconditioned	Poor	500–1,000	3–5	30%–45%	57%–67%	Light-moderate	20–30	3,000–3,500	60–150
Minimal physical activity/no exercise/ moderately-highly deconditioned	Poor-fair	1,000–1,500	3–5	40%–55%	64%–74%	Light-moderate	30–60	3,000–4,000	150–200
Sporadic physical activity/no or suboptimal exercise/ moderately to mildly deconditioned	Fair-average	1,500–2,000	3–5	55%–70%	74%–84%	Moderate-hard	30–90	≥3,000–4,000	200–300
Habitual physical activity/regular moderate to vigorous intensity exercise	Average-good	>2,000	3–5	65%–80%	80%–91%	Moderate-hard	30–90	≥3,000–4,000	200–300
High amounts of habitual activity/ regular vigorous intensity exercise	>Good-excellent	>2,000	3–5	70%–85%	84%–94%	Somewhat hard-hard	30–90	≥3,000–4,000	200–300

kcal, kilocalories; $\dot{V}O_2R$, oxygen uptake reserve; HRR, heart rate reserve; %HR$_{max}$, % age-predicted maximal heart rate.

[a]The various methods to quantify exercise intensity in this table may not necessarily be equivalent to each other.

[b]Fitness classification based on normative fitness data categorized by $\dot{V}O_{2max}$.

[c]Perception of effort using the ratings of perceived exertion (RPE) (11,32), OMNI (37,38,48), talk test (33), or feeling scale (17).

[d]Total steps based on step counts from a pedometer.

Note: These recommendations are consistent with the United States Department of Health & Human Services Physical Activity Guidelines for Americans, available at http://www.health.gov/PAGuidelines/pdf/paguide.pdf (October 7, 2008).

Reprinted with permission from ACSM's Guidelines for Exercise Testing and Prescription. 8th ed. Baltimore: Lippincott Williams & Wilkins; 2010. p. 166–7.

repetitions or for an extended period of time. A common example is what the muscles do during an aerobic workout: the lower body muscles contract and relax thousands of times during a 20-minute run (8).

Muscular strength. Many clients will state that they "want to be stronger or 'lift heavier.'" These types of clients generally want to exercise at heavier workloads to enhance their strength and power. Typically, these are athletes who are looking to improve their performance and are already familiar with resistance-based training programs. However, a client who is just starting out should start with a program that emphasizes hypertrophy or a muscle endurance training program first to acclimate his or her body to this type of training.

Cardiovascular Training

Cardiovascular training is often referred to as *aerobic* endurance training or cardiovascular exercise or even more commonly as "cardio" or "aerobics." These terms are synonymous because they all encompass exercise that recruits cardiovascular and respiratory systems (heart, blood vessels, and lungs). This mode of training is an integral part of any exercise session. To effectively and safely design a client's cardiovascular training program, the Personal Trainer must be familiar with the client's current level of fitness, previous fitness history, and, of course, established goals. Commonly, the goal of many people who begin or continue a cardiovascular program is to "burn fat" (i.e., fat loss).

> *Cardiovascular training is often referred to as aerobic endurance training or cardiovascular exercise or even more commonly as "cardio" or "aerobics."*

As with a resistance training program, the same principle of specificity applies to designing a cardiovascular exercise program. Therefore, the results of a cardiovascular-based program will be more specific to aerobic-based training. In other words, resistance training will not significantly improve maximal aerobic power (10,12). In addition, training that involves one mode of aerobic exercise will not necessarily improve a different mode. For example, a client who has a high level of aerobic endurance as a runner may not be able to achieve that same level of endurance as a cyclist. The muscle activation patterns and oxygen requirement vary greatly among different modes of exercise. Therefore, the responses and adaptations will not be equal (4).

As with all types of training programs, cardiovascular training programs are composed of different components. These components are meant to be manipulated in a variety of ways to ultimately produce the desired outcome. These components include the mode of exercise, intensity of exercise, frequency of exercise sessions, and duration of each session. The first logical step is to decide on the mode or type of exercise. Exercise selection plays a major role in all types of training programs. Cardiovascular exercise modes consist of machine- and non–machine-based exercises such as swimming, jump rope, jumping jacks. There are several factors that need to be considered when choosing the mode of cardiovascular exercise for the client. Some of those factors include, but are not limited to, the following:

➤ Availability
➤ Client's ability to perform the specified exercise
➤ Client's preference
➤ Client's goals

It is also important to note that when training athletes, the athletes should choose modes of cardiovascular exercise that most closely mimic their sport or activity. Some of the more popular modes of machine-based cardiovascular exercises include stair stepper, treadmills, rowers, step mills, cycle ergometers, and elliptical trainers. If the Personal Trainer is in a facility that does not have access to equipment, activities such as walking, jogging, running, boxing, swimming, and jumping rope that encompass non–machine-based cardiovascular exercise modes can be utilized. As with resistance training, the mode of exercise should also be based on the client's goals. For example, a client who is preparing to run his or her first 10K will spend the bulk of the session focusing on running, whether on the treadmill or on the track. This may include, but is not limited to, speed and agility drills, running techniques, and running intervals. If you have a client whose goal is to lose body fat, you should implement a cardiovascular program that uses a variety of exercise modes (e.g., 15 minutes on the treadmill; varying intervals, 15 minutes of boxing drills, and 10 minutes of cycling). This type of training is referred to as "cross training" and is very effective in fat loss and caloric expenditure. This also helps the client fight boredom with a specific mode of cardiorespiratory equipment.

EXERCISE INTENSITY

Before the Personal Trainer can establish frequency and duration of the exercise sessions, he or she must determine the appropriate intensity level to attain the client's goals. To design the best aerobic training program for a client, the Personal Trainer must be able to monitor and regulate the exercise intensity. As explained in Chapter 6, a certain threshold of oxygen consumption or heart rate (HR) reserve, which is the difference between a client's resting HR and his or her maximal HR, must be attained during an aerobic exercise session before improvements in the cardiorespiratory system are seen (9). Ultimately, the necessary aerobic exercise threshold depends on the client's initial fitness level. In apparently healthy adults, that threshold for continuous training is generally between 50% and 85% of HR reserve (1).

> **Heart rate.** Heart rate is the number of times the heart beats per minute. Heart rate increases as the work rate and oxygen uptake during dynamic exercise increase. The actual magnitude of the HR increase is related to age, fitness level, medications, body position, blood volume, presence of heart (and other chronic) disease, and environmental factors such as temperature and humidity. Maximum attainable HR decreases with age (7).
> **Stroke volume (SV).** Stroke volume is the amount of blood ejected per heart beat. As explained in Chapter 6, during exercise, SV increases in a curvilinear pattern with the work rate until it reaches near-maximal level equivalent to approximately 50%–70% of aerobic capacity, increasing only slightly thereafter (13).
> **Cardiac output Q̇.** The product of SV and HR determines cardiac output. In apparently healthy adults, the cardiac output increases as the work rate increases. However, like HR, the maximal level of cardiac output depends on factors such as age, posture, body size, level of physical conditioning, and presence of cardiovascular disease (13).
> **Blood pressure.** With increasing levels of exercise comes an increase in systolic blood pressure. Maximal values typically reach 190–220 mm Hg and should not exceed 260 mm Hg. Diastolic blood pressure should decrease slightly or remain unchanged.

Flexibility Training

Proper flexibility and stretching techniques are essential when designing a program to fit a client's needs. Everyone can learn to stretch and improve flexibility, regardless of age, level of fitness, or initial flexibility. The way that the body responds to stretching depends on how the sensory organs respond to the stretch stimulus. When educating the client on the importance of proper stretching techniques, refer to Table 15.6 to discuss the many benefits that are associated with increased levels of flexibility. When starting a stretching or flexibility routine with a client, good communication is essential. Always make sure the client knows that this program will require a lot of hands-on work and always ask questions before the start of the session and throughout the stretching session. This will help build the client–trainer rapport, as well as allow the trainer to understand the client's limitations and preferences.

Everyone can learn to stretch and improve flexibility, regardless of age, level of fitness, or initial flexibility.

TABLE 15.6	THE BENEFITS OF INCREASED FLEXIBILITY
Reduced muscle tension and increased relaxation	
Ease of movement	
Improved coordination through greater ease of movement	
Increased range of motion	
Injury prevention	
Improvement and development of body awareness	
Improved circulation and air exchange	
Decreased muscle viscosity, causing contractions to be easier and smoother	
Decreased soreness associated with other exercise	

Reprinted with permission from *ACSM's Resources for the Personal Trainer*. 1st ed. Baltimore: Lippincott Williams & Wilkins; 2005. p. 44.

It is important that the Personal Trainer learn proper stretching techniques when assisting with or assigning stretching exercises to a client. There is no right or wrong answer as to when is the best time to stretch; it is based on individual preference. Stretching may be performed just before or after exercise (and in between sets as well). When designing an exercise program, the Personal Trainer should allow for stretching exercise to be part of both the warm-up and cool-down phases of the session. As with all exercise programs, there are contraindications and precautions to flexibility training (Tables 15.7 and 15.8).

HOW TO STRETCH?

Table 15.9 outlines the guidelines Personal Trainers should follow for proper stretching techniques.

TYPES OF STRETCHES

There are various ways to gain flexibility through proper stretching programs. The following techniques focus on a different stimulus to elicit a response.

Static stretching. This type of stretching is slow and sustained to increase movement at a particular joint when one segment is manipulated relative to another. The benefits of this type of stretching include the following:
- Decreased possibility of exceeding normal range of motion (ROM)
- Lower energy requirements
- Lower instance of muscle soreness and muscle fatigue
- Decrease in muscle tension

TABLE 15.7	CONTRAINDICATIONS TO FLEXIBILITY TESTING
Motion limited by bony block at a joint interface	
Recent unhealed fracture	
Infection and acute inflammation affecting the joint or surrounding tissues	
Sharp pain associated with stretch or uncontrolled muscle cramping when attempting to stretch	
Local hematoma as a result of an overstretched injury	
Contracture (desired functional shortening) requiring stability to a joint capsule or ligament contracture that is intentional to improve function, particularly in clients with paralysis or severe muscle weakness (e.g., tenodesis of finger flexors to allow grasp in an individual with quadriplegia)	

Reprinted with permission from *ACSM's Resources for the Personal Trainer*. 1st ed. Baltimore: Lippincott Williams & Wilkins; 2005. p. 45.

TABLE 15.8	**PRECAUTIONS FOR FLEXIBILITY TRAINING**
Stretch a joint through limits of normal range of motion (ROM) only.	
Do not stretch at healed fracture sites for about 8–12 weeks postfracture, after which gentle stretching may be initiated.	
In individuals with known or suspected osteoporosis, stretch with particular caution (e.g., men older than 80 years and women older than 65 years, older persons with spinal cord injury).	
Avoid aggressive stretching of tissues that have been immobilized (e.g., cast or splinted). Tissues become dehydrated and lose tensile strength during immobilization.	
Mild soreness should take no longer than 24 hours to resolve after stretching. If more recovery time is necessary, the stretching force was excessive.	
Use active comfortable ROM to stretch edematous joints or soft tissue.	
Do not overstretch weak muscles. Shortening in these muscles may contribute to joint support that muscles can no longer actively provide. Combine strength and stretching exercise so that gains in mobility coincide with gains in strength and stability.	
Be aware that physical performance may vary from day to day.	
Set individual goals.	

Reprinted with permission from *ACSM's Resources for the Personal Trainer*. 1st ed. Baltimore: Lippincott Williams & Wilkins; 2005. p. 45.

Passive stretching. Passive stretching requires assistance from another person. This form of stretching is widely used by Personal Trainers during the client exercise session. To obtain optimal results when performing a passive stretch, the person being stretched must remain relaxed and refrain from any reflexive movements.

Active/dynamic stretching. During an active stretch, the muscle being stretched is actively moved through its ROM. This particular technique requires greater energy than passive or static stretching.

Active assistive stretching. In this type of stretch, the muscle being stretched may require some assistance to go through its ROM, because of muscular weakness or restricted movement due to injury or intervention. This is what is considered a "partner stretch."

Proprioceptive neuromuscular facilitation. Proprioceptive neuromuscular facilitation stretching is an effective and fast way known to increase static–passive flexibility. Technically, this method utilizes a technique of combining passive stretching and isometric stretching to achieve maximum static flexibility. PNF refers to any of several *postisometric relaxation*

TABLE 15.9	**GUIDELINES FOR PROPER STRETCHING**
Determine posture or position to be used. Ensure proper position and alignment prior to the stretch.	
Emphasize proper breathing. Inhale through the nose and exhale through pursed lips during the stretch. One may stretch with the eyes closed to increase concentration and awareness.	
Hold end points progressively for 30–90 seconds and take another deep breath.	
Exhale and feel the muscle being stretched, relaxed, and softened so that further range of motion is achieved.	
Discomfort may increase slightly, but continue to focus on breathing.	
Repeat the inhale–exhale–stretch cycle until the end of the available range for the day.	
Do not bounce or spring while stretching.	
Do not force a stretch while holding the breath.	
Increased stretching range during exhalation encourages full-body relaxation.	
Slowly reposition from the stretch posture and allow muscles to recover at natural resting length.	

Reprinted with permission from *ACSM's Resources for the Personal Trainer*. 1st ed. Baltimore: Lippincott Williams & Wilkins; 2005. p. 45.

stretching techniques in which a muscle group is passively stretched and then contracts iso-metrically against resistance while in the stretched position and then is passively stretched again through the resulting increased ROM. PNF stretching is usually performed with a partner to provide resistance against the isometric contraction and then later to passively take the joint through its increased ROM. It may be performed, however, without a partner, although it is usually more effective with a partner's assistance.

There are different types of PNF stretching that can be performed to elicit the best response to the stretch stimulus. These types include the contract–relax (hold–relax) and the contract–relax–contract (hold–relax–hold). When performing the contract–relax stretch, the muscle is contracted, relaxed, and then further stretched into its available ROM during the brief relax phase. Contract–relax–contract follows the same procedure; however, a subsequent contraction of the antagonist muscle gains slightly more ROM and should be done only by trained practitioners and used with caution due to increased intensity and risk of client injury from overstretching.

Dynamic, phasic, or ballistic stretching. These terms, when associated with stretching, re-fer to quick jerking and often bounce-like movements such as bouncing when trying to touch the toes. Generally it is thought that the disadvantages of this type of stretching far outweigh the benefits. Performing these jerking movements can predispose the muscles to injury. When educating the client on the different types of stretches, the Personal Trainer should provide some flexibility exercises that will help the client gain more flexibility.

Plyometrics and Sports Performance

Plyometric exercises are exercises that engage the body in jumping movements or motions. Exam-ples of these exercises can include skipping, trampoline bounding, jumping rope, hopping, split-squats, clap push-ups, and box jumps. Plyometric exercise programming is very similar to resistance and cardiovascular training. For the Personal Trainer to safely design a plyometric-based training program that will enhance the client's sports performance, the client's goals, needs, and preferences must be established. Plyometric training is not for everyone. This method of training is sport-specific and requires the client to be well conditioned. For athletes to achieve optimal performance in their chosen sport, they must train for speed, strength and power, endurance and flexibility, and coordination.

> *For the Personal Trainer to safely design a plyometric-based training program that will enhance the client's sports performance, the client's goals, needs, and preferences must be established.*

Plyometrics was first introduced as jumping exercises for the lower extremities. Now, however, there are a variety of upper-body (and lower-body) plyometric exercises that athletes and trainers are us-ing to improve skills in almost every sporting platform. These upper-body exercises are performed using a multitude of small fitness tools such as weighted balls, bands, and bars. Plyometrics has been described (5) as beginning with rapid stretching (eccentric muscle actions), followed by a shorten-ing of the same muscle (concentric muscle action). This is known as the stretch–shortening cycle. Plyometric training is based on the principle of using the elastic properties of the muscle. These con-ditions will create a greater force.

Balance and Stability

Another, less obvious form of sports performance training is balance or stability training. "Balance" is defined as the ability to maintain a position for a given period of time without moving. There are many sports performance drills that require the athlete to jump, slide, or step in nontraditional movement patterns (i.e., single leg hop or squat hops). These drills rely on the client's proprio-ception and balance to safely and successfully complete the exercise. Working on clients' core muscles will enhance their ability to maintain the balance and stability needed for their sport. There are several balance drills that can be performed, at various fitness levels, to help develop core strength. Some of these drills include standing on one leg at the beginner level or single leg half squat at the advanced level.

FUNCTIONAL TRAINING

Functional training is another variation of sports performance as well as recreational and general training. This technique allows the client to perform movements that imitate those used in their everyday lives. For example, if the client has a career in which lifting heavy boxes is part of every-day activity, a training program that works the muscles of the lower extremities and strengthens the core muscles would be beneficial, as well as doing exercises that will enhance proper-posture lifting techniques. When training an athlete, functional training plays a key role in training the body the way it will be used in competition, making it a very effective training tool for the Personal Trainer.

PROGRAM DESIGN

The process of exercise programming can be divided into three steps. The first step is the pre-screening stage, where the Personal Trainer assesses all health and fitness information. The second step is interpreting that information. The third step is combining the information with the interpreted results as well as the client's goals, to formulate an exercise program. When designing the actual client program, there are certain variables that the Personal Trainer must consider, such as what exercises to include in the program, the sequence of the selected exercises, how often the client wants to train, the load, repetition, and set assignment, as well as rest periods.

Each individual potential client has specific goals related to health and fitness. Being able to understand and identify this range of goals is an essential step in program design and exercise selection. To most efficiently and effectively design a client exercise program, the Personal Trainer must fully assess the needs of the client based not only on goals but also on the results of the fitness assessment. The measurement or assessment of health-related physical fitness is a common practice by most fitness professionals. Most professionals rely on a PAR-Q (Physical Activity Readiness Questionnaire) or HRA (Health Risk Assessment) form to gauge the health and physical activity of their clients. The Personal Trainer should be able to identify and understand the different components of fitness assessment results to do the following (2):

➤ Educate individuals about their current health-related physical fitness
➤ Use data from the assessments to design individualized exercise programs
➤ Provide baseline and follow-up data to evaluate exercise programs
➤ Motivate individuals toward more specific exercises
➤ Assist with clients' risk stratification
➤ Discuss clients' preferences
➤ Discuss clients' goals
➤ Identify need for physician follow-up or further clearance necessity

Before the initial exercise selection process begins, the Personal Trainer must consider the client's physiological capacity for beginning and maintaining an exercise program. "Exercise training" is defined as planned, structured, and repetitive bodily movement done to improve or maintain one or more components of physical fitness. In Chapter 6, the body's response to exercise and the principles of adaptation are fully explained. Each of these principles guides the design of an exercise program. In exercise training, the mode of exercise and the frequency, duration, and intensity of training are critical in achieving fitness, athletic, or health and

> *Exercise training is defined as planned, structured, and repetitive bodily movement done to improve or maintain one or more components of physical fitness.*

lifestyle outcomes (3). When designing a client's exercise program, the mode must be specific to the targeted component of fitness, and the frequency, duration, and intensity must be combined in a systematic overload that will result in physiological adaptations. This concept is commonly referred to as the S.A.I.D. (Specific Adaptations to Imposed Demands) principle.

Anatomy of an Exercise Session

The three basic components to any personal training session are the warm-up, the conditioning (stimulus), and the cool-down. Workouts should always begin with some warm-up exercises so the body is better prepared to meet the challenges that will be presented by the succeeding conditioning stimulus phase.

> *The three basic components to any personal training session are the warm-up, the conditioning (stimulus), and the cool-down.*

Warm-up and cool-down phases are the periods of metabolic and cardiorespiratory adjustment from rest to exercise and exercise to rest, respectively. Therefore, the most appropriate types of warm-up and cool-down are activities similar to the conditioning stimulus activities, performed at approximately 50% of the stimulus intensity (11).

An appropriate warm-up can improve performance and decrease the risk of cardiac disease events (11), as well as aid in injury prevention. Cool-down has these benefits as well as helping clear metabolic waste from skeletal muscle and prevent exercise-induced hypotension. Older individuals and those at risk of cardiac disease events benefit from longer periods of warm-up and cool-down. The conditioning stimulus may contain a period of aerobic conditioning, muscle conditioning, or both. Depending on the allotted session time, this may be as short as 20 minutes or as long as 60 minutes (1).

Exercise Selection

The exercises selected, the resistance or level of stimulus, as well as the order in which the exercises are selected, will determine the intensity of the client's workout. An advanced training program with a client who is an experienced athlete may include as many as 20 exercises, focusing on sports-specific, plyometric, and/or functional exercises as well as total-body conditioning. However, a beginning or basic exercise program may include only one exercise for each large muscle group of the body (1).

> *Alternating upper- and lower-body exercises does not produce as high an intensity level as performing all lower-body exercises first.*

As previously stated, the order of the exercises affects the intensity of the training session and is therefore a very important consideration. For instance, alternating upper- and lower-body exercises does not produce as high an intensity level as performing all lower-body exercises first. Exercises that involve multiple joints and muscles (referred to as multijoint exercises) are more intense than those that involve only one joint (referred to as single-joint exercises) (8). Below you will find the formulas that are most commonly used to determine sequence of exercise selection.

> - Large muscle groups (i.e., bench press, leg press squats) before smaller muscle groups (i.e., wrist curls, calf raises). This method of exercise arrangement is the most widely used.
> - Multijoint exercises before single-joint exercises, alternate push/pull or upper/lower for total body (extension = push, flexion = pull). An example of this would be a triceps extension (push) followed by a biceps curl (pull).
> - Exercise weak areas before exercises for strong areas
> - Perform exercises that are most intense before those that are least intense

The next step to designing a client exercise program, after determining exercise selection and arrangement, is determining workload. Load refers to the weight used or intensity of the exercise. To best determine the load at which the client should be working, please refer to Chapter 16.

SUMMARY

This chapter is designed to provide the Personal Trainer with a solid base of knowledge in all of the variables that create a client exercise program. This chapter serves as a review for previous chapters in the book that discuss anatomy, physiology, exercise science, exercise physiology, and human behavior. This chapter applies the fundamentals of the previously mentioned topics and applies them within the scope of the Personal Trainer.

REFERENCES

1. American College of Sports Medicine. *ACSM's Guidelines for Exercise Testing and Prescription*. 8th ed. Philadelphia: Lippincott Williams & Wilkins; 2010.
2. American College of Sports Medicine. *ACSM's Health-Related Physical Fitness Assessment Manual*. Philadelphia: Lippincott Williams & Wilkins; 2005.
3. Baechle TR, Groves BR. *Weight Training Instruction: Steps to Success*. Champaign (IL): Human Kinetics; 1994.
4. Bressel E, Heise GD, Bachman G. A neuromuscular and metabolic comparison of forward and reverse pedaling. *J Appl Biomech*. 1998;14(4):401–11.
5. Chu D. *Plyometrics*. Livermore (CA): Bittersweet; 1989.
6. Cooper JM, Adrian M, Glassow RB. *Kinesiology*. St. Louis (MO): Mosby; 1982.
7. Dehn MM, Mullins CB. Physiologic effects and importance of exercise in patients with coronary artery disease. *J Cardiovasc Med*. 1977;2:365–7.
8. Fleck SJ, Kraemer WJ. *Designing Resistance Training Programs*. 2nd ed. Champaign (IL): Human Kinetics; 1997.
9. Hickson RC, Foster C, Pollock ML, et al. Reduced training intensities and loss of aerobic power, endurance, and cardiac growth. *J Appl Physiol*. 1985;58(2):492–9.
10. Luthi JM, Howald H, Claasen H, et al. Structural changes in skeletal muscle tissue with heavy-resistance exercise. *Int J Sports Med*. 1986;7:123–7.
11. McArdle WD, Katch FL, Katch VL. *Exercise Physiology*. Baltimore: Lippincott Williams & Wilkins; 1996.
12. McGee D, Jessee TC, Stone MH, Blessing D. Leg and hip endurance adaptations to three weight training programs. *J Appl Sports Sci Res*. 1992;6:92–5.
13. Mitchell JH, Blomqvist G. Maximal oxygen uptake. *N Engl J Med*. 1971;284:1018–22.
14. Spence AP. *Reading: Basic Human Anatomy*. 3rd ed. Redwood (CA): Benjamin/Cummings; 1991.

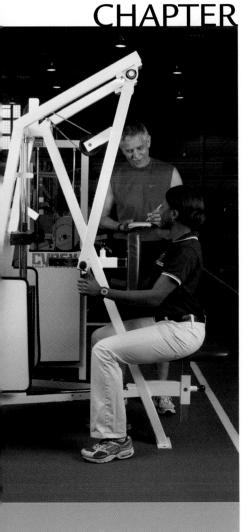

16

Resistance Training Programs

OBJECTIVES

- Define resistance training principles
- Review how and why resistance training should be performed
- Provide direction to the Personal Trainer on how to design, evaluate, and implement resistance training programs
- Provide the fundamental tools to evaluate clients' resistance training needs and progress

R esistance training, also known as strength training or weight training, is now a standard part of a comprehensive personal training program. The benefits of resistance training are numerous and include increases in strength, muscle mass, and bone density, to mention a few. All of these aspects are important to maintain good health in both men and women, and almost every population, from adolescents to senior citizens, can benefit from resistance training.

THE SCIENCE BEHIND RESISTANCE TRAINING

At the end of the second World War, Captain Thomas Delorme, MD, experimented with the use of progressive resistance exercise as a rehabilitation modality for injured soldiers (3). A few years later, DeLorme and A. L. Watkins published the first paper in a scientific journal on the topic of long-term resistance training (4). After the initial work by DeLorme and Watkins, the science of resistance training lay somewhat dormant until the 1980s. Two notable former weightlifters, Dr. Patrick O'Shea from Oregon State University and Dr. Richard Berger from Temple University, became scientists, and their pioneering work in the 1960s and 1970s fueled the eventual explosion in scientific work on this topic (34,35). Prior to that, the most influential personalities in resistance training during the last century were Mr. Bob Hoffman of York Barbell Club, who pioneered the interest in Olympic-style weightlifting and weight training with free weights through his publications and sales of barbells and dumbbells, and Mr. Joe Weider and his brother Ben, who promoted bodybuilding. Since the 1980s, published research on resistance training has grown exponentially in both scientific manuscripts and books on the topic. A resistance training program can affect almost every system in the body and is used in a wide variety of populations, from young children preparing for sports to offsetting the effects of aging. With an explosion of information from books, magazines, and the Internet, a demanding challenge has been placed on the Personal Trainer to study and carefully evaluate information and its scientific rationale as resistance training mythology and marketing ploys remain very common in the field today. Once information has passed a critical evaluation, it is necessary to understand how it can be used in the implementation of a resistance training program that ultimately affects the health, fitness, and performance of a client.

A resistance training program can affect almost every system in the body and is used in a wide variety of populations, from young children preparing for sports to offsetting the effects of aging.

In the later 1980s, the focus of much of the research changed from enhancement of athletic performance to improvement of health and fitness among both men and women in the general population and among special populations (6). Research on resistance training now appears in a wide range of specialized medical and physiological scientific journals such as the American College of Sports Medicine's *Medicine & Science in Sports & Exercise* and the National Strength and Conditioning Association's *Journal of Strength and Conditioning Research*. There are literally thousands of scientific articles examining different aspects of resistance training. This has led to a large and still growing knowledge base of physiological adaptations and mechanisms, gender differences, biomechanical influences, and specificity considerations needed to understand resistance training exercise prescription. As a result, resistance training programs protocols can be guided by scientific facts and not by purely anecdotal evidence or marketing "mythology" as was the case during much of the last century. Today, resistance training is being utilized in a variety of rehabilitation disciplines from orthopedic to cardiac and obesity management based on the work of many contemporary clinicians including Dr. Kerry Stewart (at Johns Hopkins) and Dr. Barry Franklin (at William Beaumont Hospital).

GENERAL RESISTANCE TRAINING PRINCIPLES

The terms resistance exercise and resistance training are often used interchangeably; however, there is an important distinction between the two terms. *Resistance exercise* refers to a single exercise

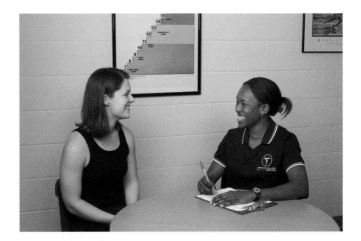

FIGURE 16.1. Exercise prescription in resistance training is an individualized process that requires a series of steps from a needs analysis and goal-setting to evaluations and making changes in the workouts over time.

> *Resistance exercise refers to a single exercise session, whereas resistance training refers to the combination of many consecutive resistance exercise sessions over time.*

session, whereas *resistance training* refers to the combination of many consecutive resistance exercise sessions over time. Thus, a resistance exercise protocol is an exercise prescription for a single session (also called a "workout") and a resistance training program is an overall program guiding the specific exercise parameters chosen for each exercise protocol.

Designing a resistance training program is a very individualized process, and the needs and goals of the client are paramount to the selection of program characteristics (Fig. 16.1). Even though an individual may be training to maximize muscle hypertrophy, the client will also develop some muscular strength and endurance. The general principles of any effective resistance training program are as follows:

1. *Specificity of training*: Only the muscles that are trained will adapt and change in response to a resistance training program. For this reason, resistance programs must target all muscles for which a training effect is desired.
2. *SAID (Specific Adaptations to Imposed Demands) Principle*: SAID relates to the fact that the adaptation will be specific to the demands that the characteristics of the workout place upon the individual. If a high number of repetitions are used, the muscles will increase their ability to perform a high number of repetitions (muscular endurance).
3. *Progressive overload*: As the body adapts to a given stimulus, an increase in the stimulus is required for further adaptations and improvements. Thus, if the load or volume is not increased over time, progress will be limited.
4. *Variation in training*: No one program should be used without changing the exercise stimulus over time. Periodized training is the major concept related to the optimal training and recovery programming.
5. *Prioritization of training*: It is difficult to train for all aspects of muscular fitness. Thus, within a periodized training program, one needs to focus or prioritize the training goals for each training cycle. This technique is often used in athletics paralleling competitive season schedules.

PROGRAM DESIGN PROCESS

The key to improved program design is the identification of specific variables, which need to be controlled to better predict the training outcomes. The most challenging aspect of resistance training exercise prescription is making decisions related to the development and changes of an individual's training goals and program design. One is faced with making appropriate changes in the resistance training program over time. This means that sound "clinical decisions" must be made on the basis of factual understanding of resistance training, the needs of the sport or activity, individual training responses, and testing data. Therefore, planning and changing the exercise prescription are vital for the success of any resistance training program.

An understanding of resistance training exercise prescription allows better quantification of the exercise stimulus. Planning ranges from the development of a single exercise session to the variation of the training program over time. The ability to quantify the workout and evaluate the progress made toward a specific training goal is the basic hallmark of the Personal Trainer who is capable of designing safe and effective programs that lead to optimal physical development.

Training Potential

The gains made in any variable related to muscular performance will ultimately be linked to an individual's genetic potential. If an individual starts to train in a relatively deconditioned state, the initial gains are great because of the large adaptational potential that is available. As training proceeds, gains decrease as an individual approaches his or her genetic potential. At this point, some goals are maintained, whereas other target goals for the resistance training program must be adjusted to prevent the client from losing interest and quitting because of a lack of progress or boredom. Appreciation of this concept is important in understanding the adaptations and changes that occur over time. Furthermore, one can see how almost any program might work for an untrained individual in the early phases of training.

Initial Assessments

When working with a new client, the Personal Trainer should always devote adequate time to evaluate the client's prior resistance exercise experience before beginning any exercise sessions. The initial assessment should include a needs analysis focusing on learning about the client's personal goals and needs, the intended time frame for achieving these goals, targeted areas or muscle groups, health issues (e.g., cardiovascular disease, asthma, diabetes, osteoporosis, osteoarthritis, immune system disorders, neurologic disorders, other), musculoskeletal limitations, recent surgeries, chronic injuries, sites of pain, etc. Furthermore, Personal Trainers should try to understand why these goals are important to the clients as well as the level of support the clients feel they are receiving from their loved ones (see Chapter 10 for additional discussion of social support). Also, Personal Trainers should try to elucidate experiences with resistance training to uncover challenges, barriers, and strategies for motivation that their clients may face. The needs analysis will help the Personal Trainer determine which muscle groups, energy systems, and muscle actions need to be trained and how these and the other acute program variables should be manipulated to meet the specific needs of the training program. Furthermore, the Personal Trainer will be able to develop strategies to help the client overcome potential barriers to resistance training.

Before developing a resistance training program, Personal Trainers should take the time to conduct a baseline fitness assessment, consisting of anthropometric measurements (height, weight, circumferences, skinfolds, etc.), resting hemodynamics (heart rate, blood pressure), body composition, and tests of muscular strength and endurance (see Chapter 14 for more information on evaluations). Initial determination of the level of the different fitness variables can help in the development of an effective training program. Examples of tests of muscular strength include 1 repetition maximum (1RM) testing on a variety of exercises, especially those exercises that involve the major muscle groups such as bench press and squat, but only if tolerable to the client (19). Muscular endurance testing might include 1-minute timed tests of curl-ups, push-ups to fatigue, or maximal amount of repetitions that can be performed at a given percentage of the 1RM load.

Follow-Up Assessments

It is exciting and motivating for clients to see improvements toward reaching their goals. To see these improvements, it is important that Personal Trainers keep records of their clients' progression. Individualized training logs are a useful tool for monitoring progress. These logs should record specific exercises, resistance or load, number of sets, and number of repetitions (consider discussing using an RPE scale or a 0–10 scale rating effort on each exercise). Kept over time, these logs provide the Personal Trainer with a means to examine and evaluate progress and the effectiveness or to identify areas of weakness of the program. Another very important benefit of the training log is that it allows the Personal Trainer to assign the appropriate resistance to be used during an exercise on the basis of the resistance and performance of previous exercise sessions.

Formal reassessment of a client's progress should occur periodically for encouragement, but not so often that there has not been adequate time for noticeable changes to develop. These follow-up assessments should include the same measures as administered at the baseline assessment, including anthropometric measurements and tests of muscular strength, power, and endurance.

Based on these assessments, the concepts of progression, variation, and overload can be applied to the resistance training program to achieve optimal physiological adaptations and to accommodate changing fitness levels and goals of clients. These assessments will give the Personal Trainer a basis for modifying the acute program variables, including choice of exercise, order of exercises, intensity, number of sets, set structure, rest periods, load or resistance, and repetition speed. Variation can be incorporated by altering joint angles and positioning, primary exercises versus assistance exercises, or multijoint exercises versus single-joint exercises to stress the muscles and joints specified by the client's needs analysis. Progressive overload can be accomplished by increasing the intensity and/or volume by increasing the resistance, number of sets, number of repetitions, or number of exercises or by decreasing or increasing the rest intervals.

Individualization

Clients are not replicas of each other. Therefore, skilled and effective Personal Trainers do not give standard programs to multiple clients. Similar training programs provided to different clients will result in varied training responses. Therefore, the exercises that are given to one client may need to be modified to better suit the anatomical characteristics, needs, and abilities of another client. Additionally, the Personal Trainer must make modifications in response to the training adaptations of the specific client. Adjustments to programs should focus on optimizing the individual's physiological adaptations.

Client Feedback

When designing a resistance training program that meets and/or surpasses the needs and expectations of the client, it is critical that the Personal Trainer pay special attention to feedback from the client. This feedback can be openly expressed, clients may request favorite exercises or muscle groups they hope to focus on during the training session, or they may complain of pain or fatigue and require program and exercise modifications. It is important for the Personal Trainer to be alert to this feedback and encourage further feedback to ensure that the program and strategy meet the expectations of the client. This can be accomplished by asking the client for feedback, for example, "How do you think the workout went?" "Did you feel that you worked out hard enough?" "Was the exercise protocol too hard? Just right?" Furthermore, Personal Trainers must learn to recognize physical signs of dizziness and lightheadedness as well as complexion changes, profuse sweating, facial expressions, and muscle exhaustion. Working a client to the point of vomiting or passing out will not leave a good impression with clients or any spectators who are present when medical attention arrives.

Of special concern for Personal Trainers is the careful and proper progression in the resistance training program, especially in beginners or those coming off injury or disease. Too much exercise,

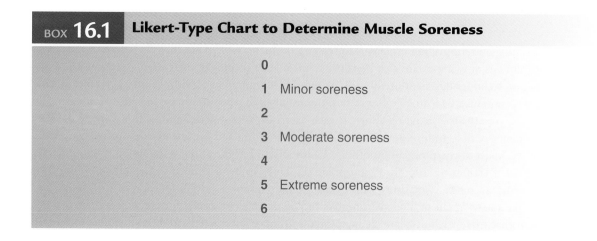

BOX **16.1** **Likert-Type Chart to Determine Muscle Soreness**

0

1 Minor soreness

2

3 Moderate soreness

4

5 Extreme soreness

6

too heavy of exercise, and/or accentuated eccentric exercise can lead to an excessive amount of muscle tissue damage and breakdown. This can result in "rhabdomyolysis" a clinical pathology that promotes the rapid breakdown of muscle tissue resulting in high amounts of breakdown products (e.g., myoglobin, myosin protein) entering into the blood stream that are harmful to kidneys and can cause kidney failure and sometimes death. With exercise, symptoms of delayed onset muscle soreness is a first sign that the individual has done too much too soon. Swelling, pain, and soreness are classical signs of muscle tissue damage, but if an improper workout was used, the damage has already been done. Therefore it is the careful progression to the heavier loads with prudent volume changes over time and the assessment of recovery from each workout that is key not to overshoot an individual's toleration of a resistance stress in a workout. A simple Likert-type (Box 16.1) chart can be used to gauge the level of soreness for the client. Individuals having over a score of 3 should have the resistance intensity and/or volume reduced dramatically and rest allowed in a periodized training program. Again, some muscle soreness is normal but extreme soreness is a sign of physiological overshoot.

> *"Rhabdomyolysis" is a clinical pathology that promotes the rapid breakdown of muscle tissue resulting in high amounts of breakdown products (e.g., myoglobin, myosin protein) entering into the blood stream that are harmful to kidneys and can cause kidney failure and sometimes death.*

Careful attention to hydration levels in a workout with scheduled drinking is vital so as not to augment muscular damage and limit force production capabilities. Medical screening and being aware of medications (e.g., statins, diuretics) the client is taking are also vital to preventing or augmenting muscle tissue damage. There are many nonrelated causes of rhabdomyolysis from disease, infections, metabolic disorders, and drug and alcohol abuse, and even some statins used for the control of cholesterol levels have been linked to muscle tissue damage in some individuals. The main goal of any treatment is to deal with the shock and protect kidney function. Acute renal failure typically develops in 1 or 2 days after tissue trauma and thus it is so important to properly assess workouts and prevent extreme muscle injury from occurring. Within the context of resistance training, the resistance load and the volume of training need to be carefully progressed and monitored to limit muscle tissue damage and develop a physiological toleration to heavier resistance and volumes of exercise stress. Again, paying attention to the basic principle of progression and not doing too much too soon are important to an effective and safe exercise prescription.

Personal Trainers should always explain the muscle group(s) that the exercise is intended to target, and clients should be taught how to differentiate between muscle fatigue and soreness and unintentional pain or injuries. That way, if any pain is felt in any joint or nonsynergistic or stabilizer muscle, the exercise may not be a good match for the client, but it should be kept in mind that new exercises often feel uncomfortable or awkward. Exercises should be stopped immediately if the client complains of pain or the Personal Trainer suspects the client is in pain. The last thing a Personal Trainer wants to do is induce or aggravate an injury.

Feedback from the client can also come from paying close attention to the technique of the client during an exercise. Deterioration in technique often results from fatigue or insufficient flexibility in the range of motion (ROM) involved in the exercise. Proper technique should always be a priority. When the technique is compromised during an exercise, the exercise should be either stopped or modified to reestablish correct technique to avoid injury.

Setting and Evaluating Goals

Personal Trainers encounter an assortment of clients with a plethora of goals including weight loss, weight gain, building strength, building muscle, shaping/toning, improving overall health, improving speed, agility, power, balance, coordination, decreasing blood pressure or cholesterol level, managing diabetes and other chronic diseases, injury rehabilitation, or sport-specific training. Often the desired goals of clients are unrealistic. When improvements do not meet expectations, motivation can be lost, frustration may set in, and nonadherence to the program can occur. Therefore, it is crucial that the Personal Trainer help the client understand what realistic and obtainable goals are, considering the individual's training history and status, fitness level, and genetic potential. The expectations of the client must be realistic and measurable (see Chapter 8), considering the physiological time course of neural and muscle protein adaptations as well as weight loss. Goal-setting and time frame should also be considered, as well as the individual's age, physical maturity, training history, and psychological and physical tolerance. It is important to set measurable goals (such as increase in 1RM or fat mass loss). Progression toward the goals must be gradual to minimize the risk of injury. Resistance training program design and modifications should consider these individualized goals.

Common program goals in resistance training are related to improvements in function, such as increased muscular strength, power, and local muscular endurance or decreased body fat (Fig. 16.2). Other functional gains such as increased coordination, agility, balance, and speed are also common goals of a program. It is becoming clear that such factors as balance may have implications for injury prevention by limiting falls in older individuals. Physiological changes related to increased body mass through muscle hypertrophy and improvement of other physiological functions such as improved blood pressure, decreased body fat, and increased metabolic rate to help burn calories are also goals that may be achieved with resistance training.

For the most part, training goals or objectives should be measurable variables (e.g., 1RM strength, vertical jump height) so that one can objectively judge whether or not gains were made or goals were achieved. Examination and evaluation of a workout log is invaluable in assessing the effects of

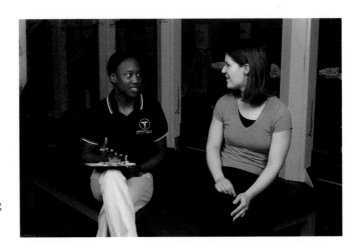

FIGURE 16.2. Setting goals and evaluating progress in a resistance training program are vital to realistic progress and gains.

various resistance training programs. Formal strength tests to determine functional changes in strength can be done on a variety of equipment, including isokinetic dynamometers, free weights, and machines. Using the results of these objective tests can help in modifying the exercise program to reach previous training goals or to develop new goals.

> *Athletic performance and health are not always the same thing.*

It should be noted here that athletic performance and health are not always the same thing. Many elite athletes do things in their training program that far exceed what is recommended for good health (e.g., lifting 7 days a week or running 140 miles in a week or training 4–6 hours a day). Thus, goals in resistance training have to be put in the context of the needed or desired outcome for each individual. Factors such as age, physical maturity, training history, and psychological and physical toleration need to be considered in any goal development process and individual program design. Decisions on the use of the available training time must be made to affect the training goals, which directly influence performance in the sport or activity. This is what makes an optimal program design.

Maintenance of Training Goals

A concept called "capping" may need to be applied to various training situations in which small gains will require very large amounts of time to achieve, and yet in the long run, these small gains are not necessary for success. This may be related to a performance (e.g., bench press 1RM strength) or some form of physical development (e.g., calf size). This is a tough decision that comes only after an adequate period of training time and observation of what the realistic potential for further change is for a particular variable. At some point, one must make a value judgment on how to best spend training time. By not adding any further training time to develop a particular muscle characteristic (e.g., strength, size, power), one decides to go into a maintenance training program. Thus, more training time is available to address other training goals. Ultimately, this decision may result in greater total development of the individual.

Decisions such as capping are part of the many types of clinical decisions that must be made when monitoring the progress of resistance training programs. Are the training goals realistic in relation to the sport or health enhancement for which the client is being trained? Is the attainment of a particular training goal vital to the program's success? These are difficult questions that need to be continually asked in the goal development phase of each training cycle for any program.

Unrealistic Goals

Careful attention must be paid to the magnitude of the performance goal and the amount of training time needed to achieve it. Although scientific studies may last up to 6 months, most real-life training programs are developed as a part of a lifestyle for an individual's sports career or whole life. Goals change and resistance training programs must change to reflect these changing needs.

Too often, goals are open-ended and unrealistic. For most men, the 23-in biceps, the 36-in thighs, the 20-in neck, the 400-lb bench press, and the 50-in chest are unrealistic goals. This is because of genetic limitations most persons have for such extreme muscle size and performance. Women also can have unrealistic goals. Usually this is in an opposite direction from men, in that goals many times include desire for drastic decreases in limb size and body shape. Again, based on genetics, such changes may not be possible in many women because of a naturally larger anatomical structure. Many women mistakenly believe that large gains in strength, muscle definition, and body fat loss can be achieved through the use of very light resistance training programs (e.g., 2- to 5-lb hand-held weights) that attempt to "spot build" a particular body part or muscle. Although one may be able to "spot hypertrophy" a particular body part, it is not done with light resistance.

In addition, the "fear of getting big" has produced unrealistic fears about lifting heavy weights, and thus many women do not gain the full benefits of resistance training. Ultimately, for both men

> *Ultimately, for both men and women, it is a question of whether the resistance training program used can stimulate the desired changes in their body.*

and women, it is a question of whether the resistance training program used can stimulate the desired changes in their body. The desired changes must be carefully and honestly examined.

Unrealistic expectations of equipment and programs also exist when they are not evaluated on the basis of sound scientific principles. In today's "high tech" and "big hype" in marketing products, Internet information, programs, and equipment, unrealistic training expectations can be developed for the average person. In addition, movie actors, models, and elite athletes can also project a desired body image and/or performance level, but for most people such upper levels of physical development and performance are unrealistic. Proper goal development is accomplished by starting out small and making progress and then evaluating where the individual is and what is possible. Most people make mistakes in goal development by wanting too much too soon, with too little effort expended. Making progress in a resistance training program is related to a long-term commitment to a total training program.

In addition to resistance exercise, appropriate cardiovascular conditioning and proper nutrition and lifestyle behaviors can help support training objectives and physical development. Careful evaluation of training goals, objectives, and the equipment needed to achieve these goals and objectives can eliminate wasted time, money, and effort.

RESISTANCE TRAINING MODALITIES

There are many different training tools (e.g., free weights, machines, medicine balls) that can be used in a resistance training programs. All of these tools can be placed into specific categories of training. From the following, it is clear that each category has certain inherent strengths and weaknesses, and therefore, the modality chosen should depend on the needs, goals, experiences, and limitations of the client.

Variable-Resistance Devices

Variable resistance equipment operates through a lever arm, cam, or pulley arrangement. Its purpose is to alter the resistance throughout the exercise's ROM in an attempt to match the increases and decreases in strength (strength curve). Proponents of variable-resistance machines believe that by increasing and decreasing the resistance to match the exercise's strength curve, the muscle is forced to contract maximally throughout the ROM, resulting in maximal gains in strength.

There are three major types of strength curves: ascending, descending, and bell-shaped (Fig. 16.3). In an exercise with an ascending strength curve, it is possible to lift more weight if only the top ½

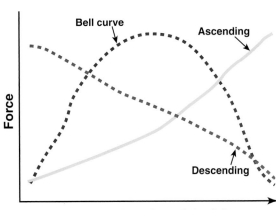

FIGURE 16.3. Three basic strength curves exist for every exercise, with hybrids of them for certain movements.

or ¼ of a repetition is performed than if the complete ROM of a repetition is performed. For example, an exercise with an ascending strength curve is the squat exercise. If an exercise has a descending strength curve, it is possible to lift more weight if only the bottom half of a repetition is performed. Such an exercise is upright rowing. A bell-shaped curve is an exercise in which it is possible to lift more resistance, if only the middle portion of the ROM is performed and not the beginning or end portions of the range of the motion. Elbow flexion has a bell-shaped strength curve. Because there are three major types of strength curves, variable-resistance machines have to be able to vary the resistance in three major patterns to match the strength curves of all exercises. To date, this has not been accomplished. Additionally, because of variations in limb length, point of attachment of a muscle's tendon to the bones, and body size, it is hard to conceive of one mechanical arrangement that would match the strength curve of all individuals for a particular exercise.

Biomechanical research indicates that one cam type of variable-resistance equipment does not match the strength curves of the elbow curl, fly, knee extension, knee flexion, and pullover exercises (8,28). A second type of cam-type equipment has been reported to match the strength curves of females fairly well (12). However, for females, the cam resulted in too much resistance near the end of the knee extension exercise. The cam also provided too much resistance during the first half and too little during the second half of the elbow flexion and extension exercises. The knee flexion machine matched the female's strength curve well throughout the ROM.

Elastic resistance bands have become popular within the fitness world because they are relatively easy to work with and less intimidating to clients. Although very effective as a training modality if the resistance can be heavy enough (20), care must be taken when using elastic bands with certain types of exercises that do not match the ascending strength curve. A possible major drawback to elastic bands is that the resistance increases constantly as the band is stretched, a resistance pattern that only matches an ascending strength curve; thus, at the beginning of a muscle flexion, the resistance is low, and at the end of the flexion, the resistance is very high. This means that only the part of the muscle involved in the latter part of the flexion may be optimally stimulated if the setup is not correct. Thus, proper starting fit and stretch is essential for the training outcome. Also, because of the physics of elastic bands, the resistance during the extension phase will be lower than that during the flexion phase, again reducing the training stimulus. In addition, elastic bands give minimal feedback that may be important to some clients.

Dynamic Constant External Resistance Devices

Isotonic is traditionally defined as a muscular contraction in which the muscle exerts a constant tension. The execution of free-weight exercises and exercises on various weight training machines, though usually considered isotonic, is not by nature isotonic. The force exerted by a muscle in the performance of such exercises is not constant but varies with the mechanical advantage of the joint involved in the movement and the length of the muscle at a particular point in the movement. A more workable definition of isotonic is a resistance training exercise in which the external resistance or weight does not change and both a lifting (concentric) phase and a lowering (eccentric) phase occur during each repetition. Thus, free-weight exercises and exercise machines that do not vary the resistance are isotonic in nature. Because there is confusion concerning the term isotonic, the term dynamic constant external resistance training has been adopted.

The types of devices used for dynamic constant external resistance include dumbbells, barbells, kettle bells, weight machines, and medicine balls; these are generally devices that do not use pulleys or levers. The major disadvantage to this type of device is that it does not stimulate the neuromuscular systems involved maximally throughout the entire ROM. The changes in the musculoskeletal leverage occurring during a movement also change the force requirement and thus the exercise stimulus. However, these types of devices require that muscles other than the primary movers of an exercise are recruited to act as stabilizers, and this increases the total amount of physiological work the body must do to perform the exercise, as well as produce exercise stimuli to the stabilizing muscles that are very important in a real-world setting or for athletic performance. We also call these types of modalities "free form" exercises, as they operate in multiple dimensions of space. Other benefits to most constant external resistance devices include little or no limitation in the ROM allowed and easy adaptation of the exercise to accommodate individual differences such as the clients' body size or physical capabilities. Equipment fit is also not a limiting factor for large and small body sizes and limb lengths.

Static Resistance Devices

Specialized static or isometric contraction devices, in which a person pulls or pushes against an immovable resistance, are rarely used. Pushing an overloaded barbell against the safety racks, or using a wall or partner for an isometric contraction, is occasionally used for an individual to overcome a sticking point, and this form of resistance exercise is called "functional isometrics." Isometrics or static resistance training refers to a muscular action in which no change in the length of the muscle takes place. This type of resistance training is normally performed against an immovable object such as a wall, a barbell, or a weight machine loaded beyond the maximal concentric strength of an individual.

Isometrics can also be performed by having a weak muscle group contract against a strong muscle group. For example, trying to bend the left elbow by contracting the left elbow flexors maximally while resisting the movement by pushing down on the left hand with the right hand with just enough force to prevent any movement at the left elbow. If the left elbow flexors are weaker than the right elbow extensors, the left elbow flexors would be performing an isometric action at 100% of a maximal voluntary contraction.

Review of subsequent studies demonstrated that isometric training leads to static strength gains but that the gains are substantially less than 5% per week (7). Increases in strength resulting from isometric training are related to the number of muscle actions performed, the duration of the muscle actions, whether the muscle action is maximal or submaximal, the angle at which the exercise is performed, and the frequency of training. Most studies involving isometric training manipulate several of these factors simultaneously. It is difficult, therefore, to evaluate the importance of any one factor. Enough research has been conducted, however, to allow some recommendations concerning isometric training. Isometric exercises are thought to strengthen muscle fibers within 15° of the position being held isometrically and therefore clients should perform multiple positions with isometric contraction to ensure full ROM strengthening. Also, isometric training is good for individuals with joint disorders in which pain is elicited by motion (i.e., rheumatoid arthritis).

Other Resistance Devices

Isokinetic devices allow one to maintain a maximum resistance throughout the whole ROM by controlling the speed of the movement. These devices use friction, compressed air, or pneumatics, which often allow for both the concentric and the eccentric component of a repetition, or hydraulics for the concentric component of a repetition. Isokinetic exercises, although popular in the rehabilitation setting, have never caught on as a typical modality used in a weight room. The initial excitement for this training modality was related to the ability to train at fast velocities similar to the high-speed movements seen in sport and real life. Isokinetic refers to a muscular action performed at constant angular limb velocity. Unlike other types of resistance training, there is no set resistance to meet; rather, the velocity of movement is controlled. The resistance offered by the isokinetic machine cannot be accelerated; any force applied against the equipment results in an equal reaction force. The reaction force mirrors the force applied to the equipment by the user throughout the range of movement of an exercise, making it theoretically possible for the muscle(s) to exert a continual, maximal force through the movement's full ROM.

Pneumatic resistance (compressed air) exercise has become relatively popular as it allows both the concentric and eccentric portions of a repetition and can be adjusted during a repetition or a set of exercises with hand-held buttons. This type of device has been popular for working with older populations. In addition, with no deceleration, it can be used effectively to train power with joint exercises not possible with conventional machines. Power is important for older adults to maintain function as well as for athletes. Because of the fixed nature of the configuration for most pneumatic machines, they are unable to address key factors such as balance and control in a multidimensional environment.

Hydraulics equipment has also become more popular with many fitness clubs promoting it as a safe and nonintimidating form of resistance exercise. Although this modality has no deceleration in its repetition range and has been used as a type of power training modality, it also has no eccentric component, which limits its efficiency as twice the number of repetitions may be required to get the same effect as a typical concentric–eccentric repetition (5). The eccentric phase is important to protect the body from injury and also enhance the ability to recover from injury. Furthermore, concentric-only training appears to be less resistant to detraining.

MACHINES VERSUS FREE-WEIGHT EXERCISES

A topic of great debate, especially in the health and fitness world, is the use of free weights versus machine resistance exercises. The two different exercise modalities were covered during the sections on constant external resistance and variable-resistance devices, respectively. Below is a comparison of the two modalities.

> *A topic of great debate, especially in the health and fitness world, is the use of free weights versus machine resistance exercises.*

1. Machines are not always designed to fit the proportions of all individuals. Clients who are obese, have special physical considerations or disabilities, and are shorter, taller, or wider than the norm may not be able to fit comfortably in the machines and use them with ease. Free-weight exercises can easily be adapted to fit most clients' physical size or special requirements.
2. Machines use a fixed ROM; thus, the individual must conform to the movement limitations of the machine. Often, these movements do not mimic functional or athletic movements. Free weights allow full ROM, and the transfer to the real-world movements is greater than that for machines.
3. Most machines isolate a muscle or muscle group, thus negating the need for other muscles to act as assistant movers and stabilizers. Free-weight exercises almost always involve assisting and stabilizing muscles. On the other hand, if the goal is to isolate a specific muscle or muscle group, as in some rehabilitation settings or because of physical disabilities, machine exercises can be used.
4. Although it is never advisable to perform resistance exercise alone, machines do allow greater independence, as the need for a spotter or helper is usually diminished once the client has learned the technique of the exercise. However, there is a misconception of extra safety that may lead to a lack of attention being paid to the exercise. It is still possible to be injured when using machines.
5. Machine exercises may be more useful than free-weight exercises in some special populations. One reason for this is that machines are often perceived to be less intimidating to a beginner. As the resistance training skill and experience level increases, free-weight exercise can gradually be introduced if desired. However, it is important to inform clients of the benefits that free weights have compared with machines (e.g., increased musculoskeletal loading that reduces the risk of developing osteoporosis, improved balance).
6. Certain free-weight exercises (e.g., Olympic-style lifts) and hydraulic and pneumatic machines allow training of power, as no joint deceleration occurs.
7. Rotational resistance accommodates certain body movements (e.g., shoulder adduction) that would be difficult to work through a full ROM with free weights.

From the comparison above, it should be clear that variable resistive devices (machines) in general are at a comparative disadvantage to constant resistance devices (free weights), but machine exercises can still be useful in resistance training when used appropriately. Actually, a safe and optimally effective resistance training program involves a combination of both free-weight and machine exercises, taking into consideration many aspects of the client's needs and the advantages of the different modalities. They can also be used differently to add variation to the training program and as an effective tool in your fitness "tool box" of resistance training devices. To summarize, in general, machines and other variable-resistance devices should be used only as an adjunct to training of mid-level and advanced clients and athletes. For the general population, a combination of free weights and equipment devices is generally most effective.

> *A combination of free weights and equipment devices is generally most effective.*

THE NEEDS ANALYSIS

Before designing a training program, a needs analysis (see Chapter 12) of the client should be performed to design the most effective program (6). Once the needs and goals of the client have been established, the following areas should also be carefully considered so the resistance training program can address questions that will come up when designing the workout using the acute program variables. It is important to keep in mind the general principles of resistance training covered in the beginning of this chapter as one continues with the development of the exercise.

A needs analysis for strength training consists of answering some initial questions that affect the program design components (14). It is important to take time to examine such questions. The major questions asked in a needs analysis are as follows:

1. What muscle groups need to be trained?
2. What are the basic energy sources (e.g., anaerobic, aerobic) that need to be trained?
3. What type of muscle action (e.g., isometric, eccentric actions) should be used?
4. What are the primary sites of injury for the particular sport or prior injury history of the individual?

Biomechanical Analysis to Determine Which Muscles Need to be Trained

The first question requires an examination of the muscles and the specific joint angles designated to be trained. For any activity, including a sport, this involves a basic analysis of the movements performed and the most common sites of injury. With the proper equipment and a background in basic biomechanics, a more definitive approach to this question is possible. With the use of a slow-motion videotape, the coach can better evaluate specific aspects of movements and can conduct a qualitative analysis of the muscles, angles, velocities, and forces involved. The decisions made at this stage help define one of the acute program variables—choice of exercise.

Specificity is a major tenet of resistance training and is based in the concept that the exercises and resistances used should result in training adaptations that will transfer to better performance in sport or daily activity. Resistance training is used because it is often difficult, if not impossible, to overload sports or other physical movements without risk of injury or dramatically altering sport skill technique. Specificity assumes that muscles must be trained similarly to the sport or activity in terms of:

➤ The joint around which movement occurs
➤ The joint ROM
➤ The pattern of resistance throughout the ROM (ascending, descending, or bell-shaped)
➤ The pattern of limb velocity throughout the ROM
➤ Types of muscle contraction (e.g., concentric, eccentric, or isometric)

Resistance training for any sport or activity of daily living should include full ROM exercises around all the major body joints. However, training designed for specific sports or activity movements should also be included in the workout to maximize the contribution of strength training to performance. The best way to select such exercises is to biomechanically analyze, in quantitative terms, the sport or physical activity and match it to exercises according to the above variables. Few such analyses of sports or activities have been done to date. Yet biomechanical principles can be used in a qualitative manner to intelligently select exercises. Ideally, this analysis is followed up with appropriate resistance exercises in the weight room that train the specific muscles and joint angles involved. For general fitness and muscular development, the major muscle groups of the shoulders, chest, back, and legs should be focused on and trained.

> **Biomechanical principles can be used in a qualitative manner to intelligently select exercises.**

Each exercise and resistance used in a program will have various amounts of transfer to another activity or sport. When training for improved health and well-being, such a concept of transfer is related more to its effects on medical variables (e.g., bone mineral density) than to physical performance. The concept of "transfer specificity" is unclear to many Personal Trainers and healthcare/fitness professionals. Every training activity has a percentage of carryover to other activities. Except for practicing the specific task (e.g., lifting groceries or shoveling snow) or sport (e.g., running, basketball) itself, no conditioning activity has 100% carryover. However, some activities have a higher percentage of carryover than others because of similarities in neuromuscular recruitment patterns, energy systems, and biomechanical characteristics. Most of the time, one cannot use the sport or activity to gain the needed "overload" on the neuromuscular system, and this is why resistance training is used in the conditioning process. The optimal training program maximizes carryover to the sport or activity.

Determining the Energy Sources Used in the Activity

Performance of every sport or activity uses a percentage of all three energy sources. The energy sources (see Chapter 5) to be trained have a major impact on the program design. Resistance training usually stresses the anaerobic energy sources (adenosine triphosphate–creatine phosphate [ATP–CP] energy source and glycolytic energy source) more than aerobic metabolism (9). It is very difficult for individuals who have gained initial cardiovascular fitness to improve maximal oxygen consumption values using conventional resistance training alone (23). However, resistance training can be used to improve endurance performance by improving running efficiency and economy (13).

Selecting a Resistance Modality

Decisions regarding the use of isometric, dynamic concentric, dynamic eccentric, and isokinetic modalities of exercise are important in the preliminary stages of planning a resistance training program for sport, fitness, or rehabilitation. The basic biomechanical analysis is used to decide which muscles to train and to identify the type of muscle action involved in the activity. Most resistance training programs use several types of muscle actions. As discussed previously in this chapter, it is important to understand that not all equipment uses concentric and eccentric muscle actions and that this can reduce the training effectiveness (e.g., hydraulics) (5).

Injury Prevention Exercises

It is also important to determine the primary sites of injury in the sport or recreational activity performed along with the prior injury profile of the individual. The prescription of resistance training exercises will be directed at enhancing the strength and function of tissue so that it better resists injury, recovers faster when injured, and reduces the extent of damage related to an injury. The term prehabilitation (the opposite of rehabilitation) has become popular. This term refers to preventing initial injury by training the joints and muscles that are most susceptible to injury in an activity. The prevention of reinjury is also an important goal of a resistance training program. Thus, understanding the sport's or activity's typical injury profile (e.g., knees in downhill skiing or elbows and shoulders for baseball pitchers) and the individual's prior history of injury can help in properly designing a resistance training program.

THE ACUTE PROGRAM VARIABLES

Developed more than 20 years ago, the paradigm of acute program variables allows one to define every workout (15). Every resistance exercise protocol or workout is derived from the five acute program variables. In turn, the choices made for each of these variables define the exercise stimuli and ultimately, with repeated exposure, the training adaptations. Essentially, the choices made for the specific combination of acute program variables create an exercise stimulus "fingerprint" that is specific and unique to that workout protocol. Thus, by making specific choices for the acute program variables that are related to the needs and goals of the client, the Personal Trainer is able to create many different types of workouts (6). The classical acute program variables are choice of exercises, order of exercises, resistance and repetitions used, number of sets for each exercise, and duration of rest period between sets and exercises.

> *The classical acute program variables are choice of exercises, order of exercises, resistance and repetitions used, number of sets for each exercise, and duration of rest period between sets and exercises.*

Choice of Exercises

The choice of exercise will be related to the biomechanical characteristics of the goals targeted for improvement. The number of possible joint angles and exercises is almost as limitless as the body's functional movements. As muscle tissue that is not activated will not benefit from resistance training, the exercises should be selected so they stress the muscles, joints, and joint angles specified by the client's needs analysis. To aid the Personal Trainer in making the correct choices, exercises can be divided into several different categories based on their function and/or muscle involvement.

Exercises can be designated as primary exercises or assistance exercises. Primary exercises train the prime movers in a particular movement and are typically major muscle group exercises (e.g., leg press, bench press, hang pulls). Assistance exercises are exercises that train predominantly a single muscle group (e.g., triceps press, biceps curls) that aids (synergists or stabilizers) in the movement produced by the prime movers.

Exercises can also be classified as multijoint or single-joint exercises. Multijoint exercises require the coordinated action of two or more muscle groups and joints. Power cleans, power snatches, dead lifts, and squats are good examples of whole-body multijoint exercises. The bench press, which involves movement of both the elbow and shoulder joints, is also a multijoint, multimuscle group exercise, although it involves only movement in the upper body. Some examples of other multiple-joint exercises are the lat pull-down, military press, and squat.

Exercises that attempt to isolate a particular muscle group's movement of a single joint are known as single-joint and/or single-muscle group exercises. Biceps curls, knee extensions, and knee curls are examples of isolated single-joint, single-muscle group exercises. Many assistance exercises may be classified as single-muscle group or single-joint exercises.

Multijoint exercises require neural coordination among muscles and thus promote coordinated multijoint and multimuscle group movements. It has recently been shown that multijoint exercises require a longer initial learning or neural phase than single-joint exercises (2); however, it is important to include multiple-joint exercises in a resistance training program, especially when whole-body strength movements are required for a particular activity. Most sports and functional activities in everyday life (e.g., climbing stairs) depend on structural multijoint movements, and for most sports, whole-body strength/power movements are the basis for success. Running, climbing stairs, jumping, as well as activities such as tackling in American football, a takedown in wrestling, or hitting a baseball, all depend on whole-body strength/power movements. Thus, incorporating multijoint exercises in a resistance training program is important for both athletes and nonathletes.

In addition, it is important to consider the inclusion of both bilateral (both limbs) and unilateral (single limb) exercises in a program to make sure that proper balance is seen in the development of the body. Unilateral exercises (e.g., dumbbell biceps curl) play an important role in helping maintain equal strength in both limbs. Bilateral differences in muscle force production can be developed with one limb working harder on every repetition than the other, leading to an obvious force production deficit and imbalances between limbs.

Many multijoint exercises, especially those with an explosive component, involve the need for advanced lifting techniques (e.g., power cleans, power snatches). These exercises require additional technique coaching beyond just the simple movement patterns. An important advantage to multijoint exercises is that they are time efficient, because several different muscle groups are activated at the same time. Therefore they can be especially useful for an individual or a team with a limited amount of time for each training session. In addition, the other benefits of multijoint exercises include enhanced hormonal response and greater metabolic demands. Multijoint exercises also outweigh single-joint exercises. Most workouts should revolve around these types of exercises.

Order of Exercises

The order in which the chosen exercises are performed is an important acute program variable that affects the quality and focus of the workout. It has been theorized that by exercising the larger muscle groups first, a superior training stimulus is presented to all of the muscles involved. This is believed to be mediated by stimulating a greater neural, metabolic, endocrine, and circulatory response, which potentially may augment the training with subsequent muscles or exercises trained later in the workout. This concept also applies to the sequencing of multijoint and single-joint exercises. The more complex multijoint technique-intensive exercises (e.g., power cleans, squats) should be performed initially followed by the less complex single-joint exercises (e.g., leg extension, biceps curls).

The sequencing rationale for this exercise order is that the exercises performed in the beginning of the workout require the greatest amount of muscle mass and energy for optimal performance. This has been observed by Simao et al. (31), who found that performing exercises of both the large and the small muscle groups at the end of an exercise sequence resulted in significantly fewer repetitions in the three sets of an exercise. This decrease in the number of repetitions performed was especially apparent in the third set, when an exercise was performed last in an exercise sequence (31). These sequencing strategies focus on attaining a greater training effect for the large muscle group exercises. If multijoint exercises are performed early in the workout, more resistance can be used because of a limited amount of fatigue in the smaller muscle groups that assist the prime movers during the multijoint exercises. Also, alternating upper and lower body exercises and/or pushing and pulling exercises allows more time for the assisting muscles to recover between exercises.

> If multijoint exercises are performed early in the workout, more resistance can be used because of a limited amount of fatigue in the smaller muscle groups that assist the prime movers during the multijoint exercises.

As the order of exercise affects the outcome of a training program, it is important to have the exercise order correspond to the specific training goals. In general, the sequence of exercises for both multiple and single muscle group exercise sessions should be as follows:

1. Large muscle group before small muscle group exercises
2. Multijoint before single-joint exercises
3. Alternating push/pull exercises for total body sessions

4. Alternating upper/lower body exercises for total body sessions
5. Explosive/power type lifts (e.g., Olympic lifts) and plyometric exercises before basic strength and single-joint exercises
6. Exercises for weak areas (priority) performed before exercises for strong areas of the client
7. Most intense to least intense (particularly when performing several exercises consecutively for the same muscle group)

Resistance and Repetitions Used

The amount of resistance used for a specific exercise is one of the key variables in any resistance training program. It is the major stimulus related to changes observed in measures of strength and local muscular endurance. When designing a resistance training program, the resistance for each exercise must be chosen carefully. The use of either RMs (the maximal load that can be lifted the specified number of repetitions) or the absolute resistance, which allows only a specific number of repetitions to be performed, is probably the easiest method for determining a resistance. Typically, a single training RM target (e.g., 10RM) or an RM target range (e.g., 3–5RM) is used. Throughout the training program, the absolute resistance is then adjusted to match the changes in strength so a true RM target or RM target range resistance continues to be used. Performing every set until failure occurs can be stressful on the joints, but it is important to ensure that the resistance used corresponds to the targeted number of repetitions. This is because performing 3–5 repetitions with a resistance that allows for only 3–5 repetitions or using a resistance that would allow 13 or 15 repetitions produces quite different training results.

> *When designing a resistance training program, the resistance for each exercise must be chosen carefully.*

Another method of determining resistances for an exercise involves using a percentage of the 1RM (e.g., 70% or 85% of the 1RM). If the client's 1RM for an exercise is 200 lb (90.9 kg), a 70% resistance would be 140 lb (63.6 kg). This method requires that the maximal strength in all exercises used in the training program must be evaluated regularly. In some exercises, percent 1RM needs to be used, as going to failure or near-failure is not optimal (e.g., power cleans, Olympic-style lifts). Without regular 1RM testing (e.g., each week), the percentage of 1RM actually used during training, especially at the beginning of a program, will decrease, and the training intensity will be reduced. From a practical perspective, the use of percentages of 1RM as the resistance for many exercises may not be administratively effective because of the amount of testing time required. In addition, for beginners, the reliability of a 1RM test can be poor. It is therefore recommended that the RM target or RM target range be used, as it gives the Personal Trainer the ability to alter the resistance in response to changes in the number of repetitions that can be performed at a given absolute resistance.

As is the case for the acute program variables, the loading intensity should depend on the goal and training status of the client. The intensity of the loading (as a percentage of 1RM) has an effect on the number of repetitions that can be performed, and vice versa. It is ultimately the number of repetitions that can be performed at a given intensity that will determine the effects of training on strength development (10,11). If a given absolute resistance allows a specific number of repetitions (defined as the RM), then any reductions in the number of repetitions without an increase in the resistance will cause a change in the training stimulus. In this case, the change in the stimulus will lead to a change in the motor units recruited to perform the exercise and thus the neuromuscular adaptations. It is also important to understand that differences exist between free weights and machines for percentage of RM used. For example, in a squat exercise, one may be able to perform only 8–10 repetitions, whereas in the leg press, 15–20 repetitions are possible. Differences exist owing to the amount of balance and control that is needed in the exercise, with free weight exercises requiring more neural control and activation of assistance muscle. In addition, the size of the muscle groups used influences this effect as well. With 80% (of 1RM) in an arm curl, a client may be able to do only 6–8 repetitions, so as the muscle group gets smaller, the response to a given percentage of the 1RM gets smaller.

Specific neuromuscular adaptations to resistance training depend in large part on the resistance used. These adaptations follow the SAID principle presented earlier in this chapter. Heavier resistances will produce lower numbers of repetitions (1–6) but will lead to greater improvements in maximal strength (1,32). Thus, if maximal strength is desired, heavier loads should be used. Alternately, if muscular endurance is the goal, a lower load should be used, which will in turn allow a greater number of repetitions (12–15 RM) to be returned (1,32).

Number of Sets for Each Exercise

First, the number of sets does not have to be the same for all exercises in a workout program. In reality, apart from training mythologies, the number of sets performed for each exercise is one variable in what is referred to as the *volume* of exercise equation (e.g., sets × reps × resistance) calculation. As such, one of the major roles of the number of sets performed is to regulate the volume performed during a particular exercise protocol or training program. In studies examining resistance-trained individuals, multiple-set programs have been found to be superior for strength, power, hypertrophy, and high-intensity endurance improvements (24,25). These findings have prompted the recommendation from the American College of Sports Medicine (1) for periodized multiple-set programs when long-term progression (not maintenance) is the goal. No study has shown single-set training to be superior to multiple-set training in either trained or untrained individuals. It appears that both single- and multiset programs can be effective in increasing strength in untrained clients during short-term training periods (i.e., 6–12 weeks). However, some short-term studies (1,32) and all long-term studies (1,32) support the contention that the greater training stimulus associated with the higher volume from multiple sets is needed to create further improvement and progression in physical adaptation and performance. Yet variation in training stimuli, as is discussed in detail later, is also critical for continued improvement. This variation often includes a reduction in training volume during certain phases of the overall training program. The determining factor here is in the "periodization" of training volume rather than in the number of sets, which is only one of the components in the volume equation. Once initial fitness has been achieved, a multiple presentation of the exercise stimulus (three to six sets), with specific rest periods between sets to allow the use of the desired resistance, is superior to a single presentation of the training stimulus. Some advocates of single-set programs believe that a muscle or muscle group can perform maximal exercise only for a single set; however, this has not been demonstrated. On the contrary, studies have found that with sufficient rest between sets, trained individuals can produce the same maximal effort during multiple sets (1).

Exercise volume is a vital concept in resistance training progression, especially for those who have already achieved a basic level of training or strength fitness. As mentioned earlier, the principle of variation in training or more specifically "periodized training" involves the number of sets performed. As the use of a constant-volume program can lead to staleness and lack of adherence to training, variations in training volume (i.e., both low- and high-volume exercise protocols) are important during a long-term training program to provide adequate rest and recovery periods. This concept is addressed later in this chapter under "Periodization of Exercise." Multiple-set programs are superior for long-term progression, but one-set programs are effective for developing and maintaining a certain level of muscular strength and endurance. For some fitness enthusiasts, this given level of muscular fitness may be adequate. Also, one-set programs sometimes result in greater compliance by those who are limited in their time for exercise and also need to perform cardiovascular exercise, flexibility exercise, etc. It may be better for this client to do one set than no sets at all.

> The number of sets performed for each exercise is one variable in what is referred to as the volume of exercise equation (e.g., sets × reps × resistance) calculation.

Duration of Rest Period between Sets and Exercises

The rest periods play an important role in dictating the metabolic stress of the workout and influence the amount of resistance that can be used during each set or exercise. A major reason for this is that the primary energy system used during resistance exercise, the ATP–CP system, needs to be replenished, and this process takes time (see Chapter 5). Therefore, the duration of the rest period significantly influences the metabolic, hormonal, and cardiovascular responses to a short-term bout of resistance exercise, as well as the performance of subsequent sets (21,22). For advanced training emphasizing absolute strength or power (few repetitions and maximal or near-maximal resistance), rest periods of at least 3–5 minutes are recommended for large muscle mass multijoint exercises (such as squat, power clean, or dead lift), whereas shorter rest may be sufficient for smaller muscle mass exercises or single-joint movements (1). For a novice-to-intermediate resistance exercise protocol, rest periods of 2–3 minutes may suffice for large muscle mass multijoint exercises, because the lower absolute resistance used at this training level seems to be less stressful to the neuromuscular system. Performance of maximal resistance exercises requires maximal energy substrate availability at the onset of the exercise and a minimum fatigue level and thus requires relatively long rest periods between sets and exercises.

> *The duration of the rest period significantly influences the metabolic, hormonal, and cardiovascular responses to a short-term bout of resistance exercise, as well as the performance of subsequent sets (21,22).*

Resistance training that stresses both the glycolytic and ATP–CP energy systems appears to be superior in enhancing muscle hypertrophy (e.g., bodybuilding); thus, less rest between sets appears to be more effective in high levels of muscular definition. If the goal is to optimize both strength and muscle mass, both long rest with heavy loading and short rest with moderate loading types of workout protocols should be used. However, it should be kept in mind that the short-rest resistance training programs can potentially cause greater psychological anxiety and fatigue because of the greater discomfort, muscle fatigue, and high metabolic demands of the program (33). Therefore, psychological ramifications of using short-rest workouts must be carefully considered and discussed with the client before the training program is designed. The increase in anxiety appears to be associated with the high metabolic demands found with short-rest exercise protocols (i.e., 1 minute or less). Despite the high psychological demands, the changes in mood states do not constitute abnormal psychological changes and may be a part of the normal arousal process before a demanding workout.

The key to rest-period lengths is the observation of symptoms of loss of force production in the beginning of the workout and clinical symptoms of nausea, dizziness, and fainting, which are direct signs of the inability to tolerate the workout. When such symptoms occur, the workout should be stopped and longer rest periods used in subsequent workouts. With aging, decreased ability to tolerate decreases in muscle and blood pH underscores the need for gradual progression when cutting rest period lengths between sets and exercises (22). Rest periods may be thought of as:

> ➤ Very short rest periods—1 minute or shorter
> ➤ Short rest periods—1–2 minutes
> ➤ Moderate rest periods—2–3 minutes
> ➤ Long rest periods—3–4 minutes
> ➤ Very long rest periods—5 minutes or longer

The more rest that is allowed between sets and exercises, the heavier the resistance. Also, more rest allows for a greater number of repetitions to be performed at a specific RM load (16,22). Improvements take place for a given rest period when the body's bicarbonate and phosphate, blood and muscle buffering systems, respectively, are improved by the gradual use of shorter rest period lengths (16,22).

VARIATION OF THE ACUTE PROGRAM VARIABLES

The acute program variables can be manipulated to develop different workouts for the single-exercise sessions used over time. Also, the number of sets, number of repetitions, relative resistance used, and rest periods do not have to be the same for each exercise in a session. They can all be varied either within an exercise or, more frequently, between different exercises in an exercise protocol. Variation must seek to address the needed change in the demands placed on the neuromuscular system over time, with planned rest a vital part of this principle. It is also important to understand that one can use light exercise to rest higher threshold motor units (i.e., motor neuron and associated muscle fibers). Understanding the "size principle" in this regard is important, as not all motor units are recruited with each resistance loading experience of a muscle, and therefore, different loadings can result in different amounts and types of muscle tissue being used. Heavier loads with adequate volume recruit more muscle tissue and are one reason why women need to have heavy loading cycles in their resistance training programs, regardless of fears related to excessive hypertrophy (6). The use of the size principle is vital for understanding variation in resistance training and ultimately periodized training.

Muscle Actions

Muscles can produce force while performing one of three different actions:

1. When sufficient force is produced to overcome the external load and shorten the muscle, the action is termed *concentric* muscle action or contraction.

2. If the muscle produces force but there is no change in length of the muscle, the action is termed *isometric.*

3. Production of force while the muscle is lengthening (i.e., resisting the movement) is termed *eccentric* muscle action.

In the past, the term *contraction* was used for each of the three muscle actions; however, this use is inappropriate, because only the concentric muscle actions actually involve a muscle contraction in which a classic muscle shortening occurs. An exercise can include one, all, or any combination of the three muscle actions; however, most exercises are performed using either isometric muscle action or both concentric and eccentric muscle actions. The force–velocity curve runs from high- to low-speed eccentric muscle actions to maximal isometric muscle action to slow- to high-velocity concentric muscle contractions, creating a descending hierarchy of force productions. However, the most effective training programs appear to use concentric–eccentric repetitions (5).

The most effective training programs appear to use concentric–eccentric repetitions (5).

True Repetition and Range of Movement

Muscle actions involving movement of a joint are termed *dynamic,* and thus exercises involving joint movements are called dynamic exercises. A full-range dynamic exercise repetition usually contains both a concentric phase and an eccentric phase. The order of the phases depends on the choice of exercise. A squat, for example, starts with the eccentric phase; a pull-up normally starts with the concentric phase. It is important to perform the exercise so that the joints involved move through a large full ROM. For single-joint exercises especially, it is important to move the joint through the full ROM. For example, in the arm curl, a full repetition should start with the elbow almost completely extended, progress until the elbow is maximally flexed, and finish with the elbow almost completely extended again. By using the whole ROM, the whole length of the muscle is stimulated, leading to adaptations throughout the whole muscle and not just in parts of it. However, ROM may need to be carefully monitored and restricted when working with clients who have orthopedic injuries or limitations.

PERIODIZATION OF EXERCISE

Periodization is a concept, and the exact design or workouts used are the program and its application (26). Understanding some of the basic concepts about periodization is important to create workouts and the actual periodized program using the acute program variables. Periodization refers

> *Periodization refers to systematic variation in the prescribed volume and intensity during different phases of a resistance training program.*

to systematic variation in the prescribed volume and intensity during different phases of a resistance training program. A traditional linear periodization program contains four phases:

1. Hypertrophy, consisting of high volume and short rest periods
2. Strength/power, consisting of reduced volume but increased load and rest periods
3. Peaking, consisting of low volume but high load and longer rest periods
4. Recovery, consisting of low volume and load

There is no set formula for how a program should be periodized, as it depends on the specific goals and needs of the clients (29). Table 16.1 presents an example of a traditional four-phase periodized training program aimed at producing maximal power and strength.

The reason for incorporating periodization into the training program is that by systematically varying some of the acute program variables, the muscles are exposed to different stimuli to which they must adapt differently, leading to greater increases in muscle quality, characteristics, and performance. In addition, rest is encouraged at different points in the training program, which allows for recovery and the prevention of both short- and long-term overtraining. Another important benefit to periodization is that it can reduce the potential boredom found with repeating the same resistance exercise program over and over again. This may well affect adherence to a fitness program. Many different models for periodization have been developed; thus, the model to be used should be selected on the basis of the needs and desires of the client.

The popular terms micro-, meso-, and macrocycle refer to different phases of periodization. The largest time frame for a training cycle is the *macrocycle*. In the example used in this chapter, a macrocycle refers to a year, and all phases are included in this cycle. A *mesocycle* refers to the next smaller group of training cycles that make up the macrocycle, usually four to six in a year. Finally, the *microcycle* is the smallest component, which usually ranges in time from 1 to 4 weeks dedicated to one type of workout variable in that phase (e.g., high-volume, low-intensity, power). Anecdotally, it has been found that more mesocycles are more beneficial to the overall training effect, and this leads to the concept that higher degrees of variation in the training stimulus are more effective in producing overall adaptations in the body. In part, this leads to many different variations in the classic periodization model, including nonlinear periodization.

TABLE 16.1	**TRADITIONAL AMERICAN-STYLE PERIODIZATION SCHEDULE**			
Goal	**Hypertrophy**	**Maximal Strength/Power**	**Peak**	**Recovery**
Reps	High	Moderate-low	Low	Moderate
Sets	High	Moderate	Low	Moderate
Rest	Short	Moderate	Long	Moderate
Load	Low	Moderate	Very high	Low
Volume	High-moderate	Moderate	Low	Low

The use of periodized resistance training has been shown to be superior to constant training methods. Periodized training involves the planned variation in the intensity of exercises and in the volume of a workout. Typically, one periodizes large muscle group exercises. However, variation schemes can be created for smaller muscle groups. One must consider the type of periodized program to use. In general, there are two basic types that have been developed, linear and nonlinear periodized protocols for maximal strength development.

Linear Periodization

Classic periodization methods use a progressive increase in the intensity with small variations in each 1- to 4-week microcycle.

Classic periodization methods use a progressive increase in the intensity with small variations in each 1- to 4-week microcycle. An example of a classic four-cycle linear periodized program (4 weeks for each cycle) is presented in Table 16.2.

One can see that there is some variation within each microcycle due to the repetition range of each cycle. Still, the general trend for the 16-week program is a steady linear increase in the intensity of the training program. Microcycle 5 is a 2-week active rest period in which no lifting is done or at best very light, low-volume training is used prior to the next mesocycle. Because of the straight-line increase in the intensity of the program, it has been termed "linear" periodized training. Because most training programs from which periodization evolved were of the single-peaking nature (e.g., track and field, weightlifting), consecutive buildup to the peak was used in this so-called classic method. Now, many more models that are hybrids of this classical model exist.

The volume of the training program will also vary with the classic program, starting with a higher initial volume, and as the intensity of the program increases, the volume gradually decreases. The drop-off between the intensity and volume of exercise can decrease as the training status of the individual advances. In other words, advanced athletes can tolerate higher volumes of exercise during the heavy and very heavy microcycles.

It is important to point out here that one must be very careful not to progress too quickly to train with high volumes and heavy weights. Pushing too hard has the potential for a serious overtraining syndrome. Overtraining can compromise progress for weeks or even months. Although it takes a great deal of excessive work to produce such a long-term overtraining effect, highly motivated individuals can easily make mistakes out of sheer desire to make gains and see rapid progress in their training. So it is important to monitor the stress of the workouts and the total conditioning program. Exercises within a program can interact to compromise each other.

The purpose of the high-volume exercise in the early microcycles is that it has been thought to promote the muscle hypertrophy needed to eventually enhance strength in the later phases of training. Thus, the late cycles of training are linked to the early cycles of training, and they enhance each other as strength gains are related to size changes in the muscle. Programs that attempt to gain strength without the needed muscle tissue are limited in their potential.

The increases in the intensity of the periodized program then start to develop the needed nervous system adaptations for enhanced motor unit recruitment. This happens as the program progresses and heavier resistances are used. Heavier weights demand higher threshold motor units to become involved in the force production process. The subsequent increase in muscle protein from the early

TABLE 16.2	**AN EXAMPLE OF A CLASSIC LINEAR PERIODIZED PROGRAM USING 4-WEEK MICROCYCLES**			
Microcycle 1	Microcycle 2	Microcycle 3	Microcycle 4	Microcycle 5 (2 Weeks)
3–5 sets of 12–15RM	4–5 sets of 8–10RM	3–4 sets of 4–6RM	3–5 sets of 1–3RM	Active rest/Recovery

cycle training enhances force production from the motor units. Here again one sees integration of the different parts of the 16-week training program.

The completion of all of the cycles in this 16-week program would be one mesocycle, and a year training program (macrocycle) is made up of several mesocycles. Again, shorter mesocycles have been used to better delineate the different trainable features of muscle. Each mesocycle attempts to progress the body's musculature upward toward one's theoretical genetic maximum for a given variable. Thus, the theoretical basis for a linear method of periodization consists of developing the body with a sequential loading from light to heavy and from high volume to low volume, thereby addressing the goals of the program for that training cycle while providing active rest at the completion of the mesocycle. This is repeated again and again with each mesocycle, and progress is made in the training program over an entire macrocycle.

Nonlinear Periodized Programs

More recently, the concept of nonlinear periodized training programs has been developed to maintain variation in the training stimulus. However, nonlinear periodized training makes implementation of the program possible because of schedule, business, or competitive demands placed on the individual. The nonlinear program allows variation in the intensity and volume within each week over the course of the training program (e.g., 12 weeks). Active rest is then taken after the 12-week mesocycle. The change in the intensity and volume of training will vary within the cycle, which could be 7–14 days. An example of a nonlinear periodized training program over a 12-week mesocycle is shown in Table 16.3.

> *The nonlinear program allows variation in the intensity and volume within each week over the course of the training program (e.g., 12 weeks).*

The variation in training is much greater within the 7-day period. One can easily see that intensity spans a wide range. This is but just one set of workout options for intensity and volume, and many others can be created. This span in training variation appears to be as effective as linear programs. One can also add a "power" training day in which loads may be from 30% to 45% of 1RM and exercises must not have a high deceleration component, so the choice of exercise and/or equipment used is vital (e.g., Olympic lifts or pneumatic resistance) so that no deceleration exists with the movement of the joint(s), or one can have a plyometric training day of different exercises and intensities (e.g., jumps, bounds, medicine ball exercises).

Unlike the linear programs, one trains the different components of muscle size, strength, and power within the same week. Unlike the linear methods, nonlinear programs attempt to train different features of muscle within the same week (e.g., hypertrophy and power and strength). Thus, one is working at two different physiological adaptations together within the same 7- to 10-day period of the 12-week mesocycle. Such a periodization model may be more conducive to many individuals' schedules, especially when travel, school, competitions, or other schedule conflicts can make adherence to the traditional linear method difficult.

In this program, one just rotates through the different protocols. The workout rotates different workouts with the different training sessions. If one misses the Monday workout, the rotation order is just pushed forward, meaning that one just performs the rotated workout scheduled. For example, if the light 12–15RM workout was scheduled for Monday and you miss it, you just perform it

TABLE 16.3	AN EXAMPLE OF NONLINEAR PERIODIZED TRAINING PROTOCOL		
Monday	**Wednesday**	**Friday**	**Monday**
1 set 12–15RM	3 sets of 8–10RM	4 sets of 4–6RM	Power day 6 sets of 3 at 30%–45% of 1RM in using power exercises (e.g., hang pulls etc.) /plyometrics

This protocol uses a 4-day rotation with 1-day rest between workouts.

on the next training day and continue with the rotation sequence. In this way, no workout stimulus is missed in the training program. One can also say that a mesocycle will be completed when a certain number of workouts are completed (e.g., 48) and not use training weeks to set the program duration.

One of the new advances in periodization is called "unplanned nonlinear periodization." The name is somewhat of a misnomer, as an overall plan is developed for a 12-week mesocycle, but the actual day that a given workout will be performed is based on the readiness to train. In other words, in unplanned nonlinear periodization, a workout plan is set for the mesocycle but deciding what workout is to be done on what day is left to the Personal Trainer, who will base it on the client's fatigue level, psychological state, or fitness, to use only the most optimal workout that can be performed on a given day. In this model, the training session category (e.g., light, moderate, power, or heavy) is prescribed on the basis of the physiological ability or state of the client at the time of the session. Thus, if the client is very fatigued before a particular exercise session, some workouts would not be prescribed (e.g., a power training or plyometrics training day or a high-volume, low-rest training day would not be a good choice because prior fatigue would dramatically reduce the workout quality). After a workout is done, it is checked off in the major planning matrix for the 12-week mesocycle.

In any periodization model, it is the primary exercises that are typically periodized, but one can also use a two-cycle periodization program to vary the small muscle group exercises. For example, in the "triceps pushdown" one could rotate between the moderate (8–10RM) and the heavy (4–6RM) cycle intensities. This would provide not only the hypertrophy needed for such isolated muscles of a joint but also the strength needed to support heavier workouts of the large muscle groups.

In summary, two different approaches can be used to periodize a resistance training program, specifically, linear and nonlinear program workout schedules. The programs appear to accomplish the same effect and appear superior to constant-intensity training programs. This seems to be accomplished by training either the hypertrophy component first and then the neural strength component second in the linear method and both components within a 7- to 14-day time period, depending on the number of workout types one uses in the nonlinear method. The key to workout success is variation, and different approaches can be used over the year to accomplish this training need.

PROGRESSION FROM BEGINNER TO ADVANCED

The level of fitness and resistance training experience of the client is maybe the most important factor to be considered when designing a resistance training program. Resistance exercise can place a large stress on the body, and certain exercises require a high level of technique to avoid injury.

> *Resistance exercise can place a large stress on the body, and certain exercises require a high level of technique to avoid injury.*

The most important aspect for beginners is resistance exercise techniques. At the beginning of the training program, correct technique of the exercises involved should be stressed, and the resistance and volume should be kept low. From a strictly short-term performance-enhancement point of view, a single set per exercise may be enough for beginners to achieve the stimulus needed from an exercise.

Although multiple sets may not lead to greater improvements in performance for beginners in the short term, there may still be benefits to using multiple sets from the onset of the training program (25,30). One reason for this is that more repetitions can lead to faster improvements in the technique of the exercises involved in the training program, especially for multijoint exercises. The squat exercise is an example of an exercise that requires a great deal of technique to be performed correctly. In addition, some studies have found that multiple sets even for beginners create larger improvements than single sets, whereas no study has found that single sets are superior (30).

As the client progresses past the initial few months of training, multisets should be used for each exercise session. As the skill and experience level of the client improves, more technical exercises can be taught. Advanced resistance training can include highly technical exercises such as the clean or the snatch, as well as advanced modalities such as plyometric exercises. The progression will differ among individuals, and the Personal Trainer must evaluate each client extensively and continuously before including more advanced exercises, to ensure that the exercises match the client's skill and experience level.

CLIENTS

Client Interactions

As a Personal Trainer working with clients, it is important to encourage and motivate them as well as to provide innovative, optimal, individualized resistance training programs. Many clients hire Personal Trainers because they feel they need constant guidance. In addition, it provides them with a support system. Most importantly, they are hiring professionals with training and knowledge in conditioning science. They are also hiring professionals to help them perform exercises properly and who understand exercise prescription to allow them to achieve their personal goals and objectives. For some clients, it is an important part of their sports conditioning program. Ultimately, the Personal Trainer must form a special relationship with each and every client that is based on professionalism, trust, and openness (Fig. 16.4).

Clients should feel that their Personal Trainer genuinely cares about them and is personally vested in helping them achieve their goals. Clients expect their Personal Trainer to be a source of knowledge and an educator. Clients expect their Personal Trainer to be able to explain things or answer the question "Why?" Thus, clients appreciate having their Personal Trainer explain why they are doing this exercise or this combination of sets and reps in their program. Personal training has been found to be superior to unsupervised training, even for people who understand resistance training (27).

Personal Trainers should convey the specific benefits of resistance training, including increases in strength, muscle mass, and bone mass, particularly to clients who may be skeptical about why resistance training is important.

Additionally, Personal Trainers should convey the specific benefits of resistance training, including increases in strength, muscle mass, and bone mass, particularly to clients who may be skeptical about why resistance training is important. Many uneducated clients may have false impressions of the outcome from resistance training. In particular, some women often perform programs that are not optimal, excluding a heavy loading workout or cycles because of the "fear of getting big muscles." This misunderstanding of resistance training effects has held many women in particular, back in achieving optimal gains in muscle tissue mass and bone mineral density, which are challenged to a greater extent in women as they age.

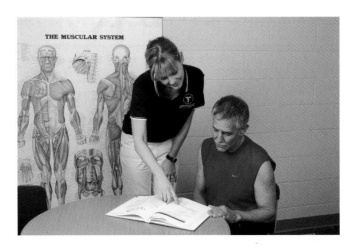

FIGURE 16.4. Having education and being a credible source of knowledge as a fitness expert is part of what Personal Trainers must provide to their clients. This takes continual study and preparation to stay current and up-to-date on basic topics and hot topics of the day.

Clients consider Personal Trainers experts and will often want to hear their opinion on fads facing the fitness industry. Often clients' knowledge of resistance training comes from infomercials and magazine marketing products, which frequently mislead clients by encouraging the sales of the various products. It is important for Personal Trainers to stay educated and ideally current with the scientific literature and know how to do research on topics of interest to their clients. Clients will also ask questions the Personal Trainer cannot answer (nobody knows everything). In these cases, it is best for the Personal Trainer to admit that he or she does not know the answer but will find it from experts in the field, thus showing a broader network of people who can act as resources. This is always a better strategy than conveying potentially incorrect information. Furthermore, Personal Trainers are often required to obtain continuing education credits to maintain their certifications; therefore, staying current is critical to success.

SPOTTING IN RESISTANCE EXERCISE

In comparison with other components of a complete fitness program (such as cardiovascular conditioning), resistance training often requires more physical interaction between the client and the Personal Trainer to ensure proper positioning, fit and setup of a machine, and techniques in both machine and free-weight exercises. It is important for the Personal Trainer to explain to clients the spotting procedures in resistance training and the level of physical interaction required between the client and the Personal Trainer. Always ask your clients before physically touching them, to ensure that they are comfortable with it. For example, when performing elbow extension exercises, it is sometimes helpful for the

Ask your clients before physically touching them, to ensure that they are comfortable with it.

Personal Trainer to place his or her hands on the client's elbows as a reminder to keep the elbow from pointing outward. In these cases, explain to the client, "I am going to put my hands on your elbows to remind you to keep them from pointing outward. Is this okay with you?" In most cases, clients will have no problem with this physical contact, but it is always better to ask than to assume.

Know Proper Spotting Technique

Good spotting technique is vital for a safe resistance training program. It is important for the Personal Trainer to understand proper technique for every exercise and how to position clients for the exercise, whether it is in a machine that may not fit all people or with free weights to get the proper anatomical positioning throughout the exercises. Most important is to understand how to spot each and every exercise in a program. A checklist for the Personal Trainer is:

1. Know proper exercise technique
2. Know proper spotting technique
3. Be sure you are strong enough to assist the lifter with the resistance being used or get help
4. Know how many repetitions the lifter intends to do
5. Be attentive to the lifter at all times
6. Stop lifters if exercise technique is incorrect or they break form
7. Know the plan of action if a serious injury occurs

The goal of correct spotting is to prevent injury. A lifter should always have an exercise spotted, and the Personal Trainer must mediate this process, alone or with additional help.

RESISTANCE EXERCISES

A large number of resistance exercises can be used in a program. It is beyond the scope of this chapter to go through each and every exercise. The reader is referred to a comprehensive list of more than 125 exercise descriptions of both machine and free-weight exercises along with spotting techniques by Kraemer and Fleck (18). Each program should be designed on the basis of the principles outlined in this chapter. Periodization is very important and many Personal Trainers are now using nonlinear methods to keep the clients interested and the programs effective (17). Free weights and machines can be used for each exercise as well as bilateral and unilateral exercises. See Figure 16.5 A–O for examples.

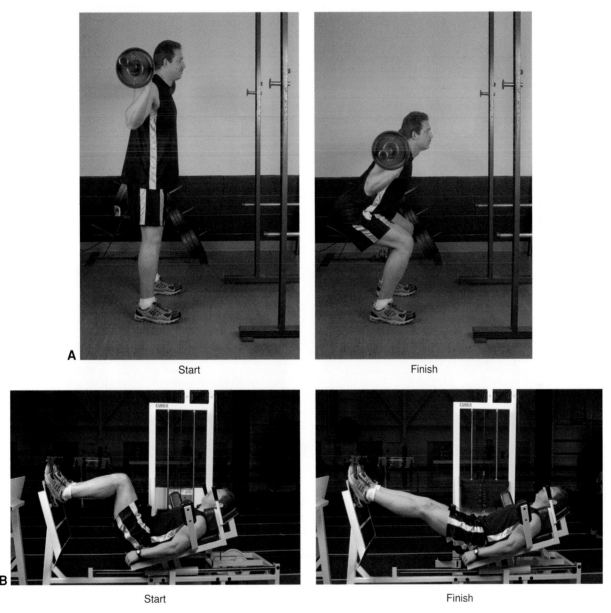

FIGURE 16.5. **A.** Back squat (thighs). Place the barbell on the back of the shoulders and grasp the barbell at the sides, with feet shoulder-width apart, toes slightly out. Dismount bar from rack. Descend until thighs are just past parallel to the floor and then extend the knees and hips until legs are straight, returning you to the starting position. Repeat for the appropriate number of repetitions. Keep the head forward with the chin level, back straight, and feet flat on the floor; keep equal distribution of weight throughout forefoot and heel and either squat within the power rack or have spotter(s). **B.** Supine leg press (thighs). Lie flat on the sled with shoulders against the pad. Place the feet on the platform, making sure that they are securely on the base plate. Extend the hips and knees. Flex the hips and knees until the knees are just short of complete flexion and return to the starting position to complete the repetition. Keep the feet flat on the platform and do not lock the knees. A full ROM should be used; keep the knees in the same direction as the feet.

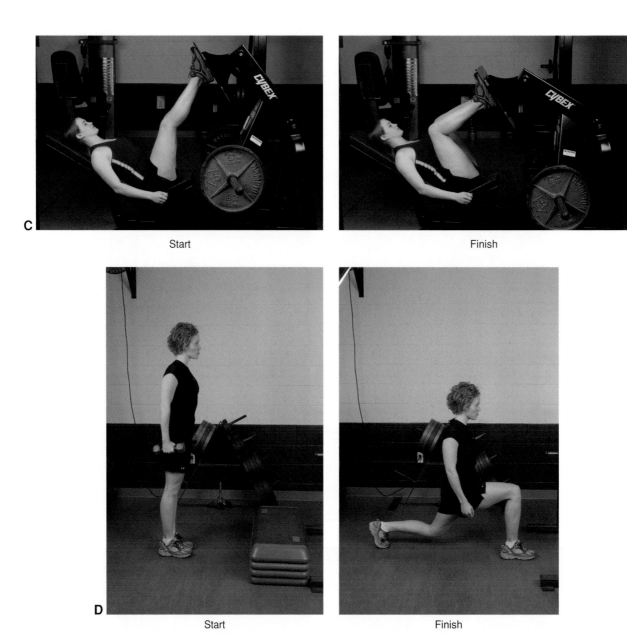

Start

Finish

C

Start

Finish

D

FIGURE 16.5. (*Continued*) **C.** 45° leg press (thighs). Lie down on the machine with the back on the padded supports. Place the feet on the platform. Grasp the handles on the side and release the weight. Lower the weight by flexing the hips and knees until the hips are completely flexed and then extend the knees to complete the repetition. Make sure that the feet are flat on the platform and the knees track over the feet. **D.** Lunge (thighs, unilateral). Standing straight up with feet shoulder-width apart, stand holding the dumbbells at the sides. Lunge forward with one leg at a time, keeping the hips in the middle of the two legs, with the trailing knee just above the ground. Return to the standing position to complete the repetition and then repeat with the opposite leg. Keep the back straight and chin level with the ground.

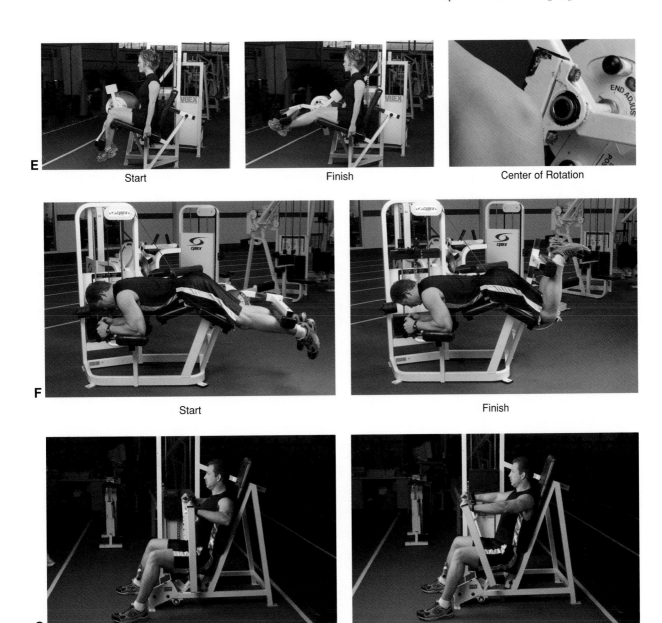

FIGURE 16.5. (*Continued*) **E.** Leg extensions (thighs, bilateral or unilateral). Sit on the machine with the back straight against the back pad or seat and grasp the handles on the side of the machine. Place the legs under the padded lever, making sure that they are positioned just above the ankles. Most machines will allow adjusting the length of the lever. Lift the lever until the legs are almost straight and return to the starting position to complete the repetition. It is important not to "rip" the plates off the stack, as this can add stress to the knees. This exercise can be done with a single leg (unilateral) or with both legs (bilateral). Make sure that the knees are aligned with the machine's center of rotation. **F.** Leg curls (hamstrings, bilateral or unilateral). Lying face down, grab the support handles in the front of the machine with the heels just beyond the edge of the lever pads. Lift the lever arm by flexing the knees until they are straight. Return to the starting position to complete the repetition. Keep the body on the bench and focus on moving only the legs. Many machines are angled so that the user is in a better position for the exercise movement, to reduce stress on the lower back. Other forms of leg curls are standing and seated forms. This exercise can be done with a single leg (unilateral) or with both legs (bilateral). **G.** Vertical machine bench press (chest–triceps, bilateral). Sit on the seat, making sure that the line of the grips is just below the chest. The bar line should be an inch above the chest. Grasp the handles with an overhand grip and make sure that the feet are flat on the ground. Push the lever arm straight out until the elbows are straight. Return to the starting position to complete one repetition.

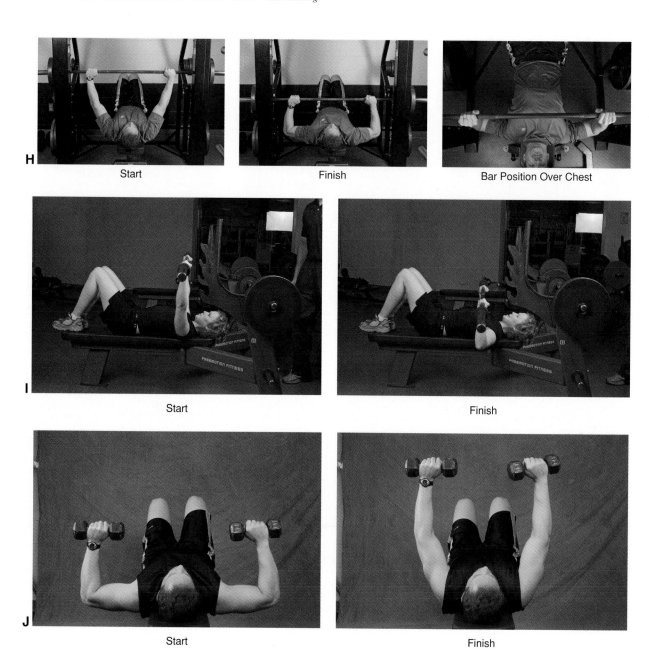

FIGURE 16.5. (*Continued*) **H.** Smith supine bench press (chest–triceps, bilateral). Lie flat on the bench with the upper chest under the bar, as shown in the bar position figure above. Place the feet flat on the floor unless the bench is too high, in which case put them flat on the bench. Keep the shoulders and hips on the bench at all times during the lift. Grasp the bar with elbows at 45° angles. Disengage the bar hooks from the Smith machine. Lower the weight to the chest and then press the bar up until arms are extended to complete the repetition. When completed, rehook the bar to the machine. **I.** Free weight supine bench press (chest–triceps, bilateral). Lie flat on the bench with the upper chest under the bar, as shown in the bar position figure above. Place the feet flat on the floor unless the bench is too high, in which case put them flat on the bench. Keep the shoulders and hips on the bench at all times during the lift. Grasp the bar with elbows at 45° angles. Lower the weight to the chest and then press the bar up until the arms are extended to complete the repetition. When completed, rerack the bar with a spotter's help. **J.** Dumbbell bench press (chest–upper arms–triceps, unilateral). Start in a seated position on the bench with a dumbbell in each hand resting on the lower thigh. Lift the weights to the shoulder and lie back on the bench or have the spotter give you the dumbbells once you are in a position. Position the dumbbells to the side of the upper chest. Press the dumbbells up until the arms are extended and then return to complete a repetition. When completed, return to the seated position with the dumbbells on your thighs or have the spotter take the dumbbells. If heavy weights are used, two spotters may be necessary.

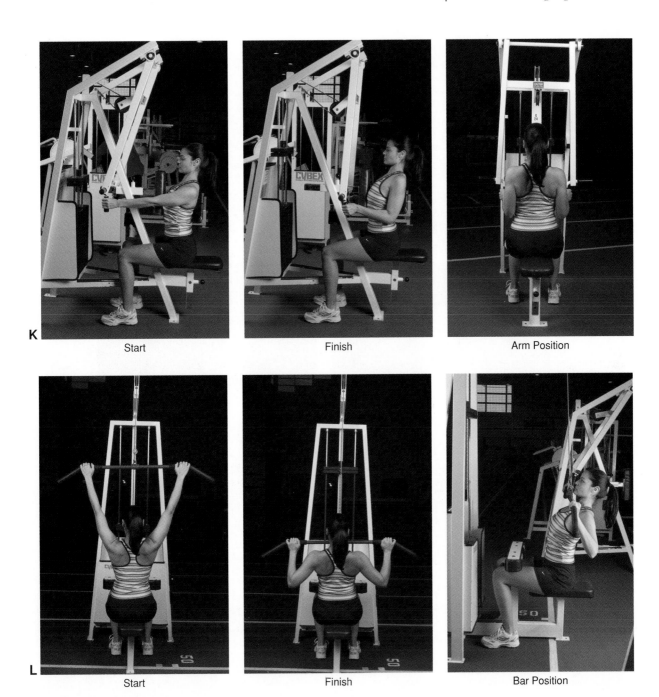

FIGURE 16.5. (*Continued*) **K.** Machine seated rows (upper back, bilateral). Take a seated position with the chest against the pad. Grasp the lever vertical handles with a vertical or horizontal overhand grip. Pull the lever back until the elbows are in line with the upper body and return to complete the repetition. Check the seat height so that the chest is directly in front of the lever handles, and check whether the client is pulling in a straight line parallel to the ground. The client can use an overhand grip as a variation to the movement, using the other horizontal handles. **L.** Front lat pull-down (upper back, bilateral). Use a locked grip (thumb around the bar) and grasp the cable bar with a wide grip. Sit with thighs under machine support. Proceed to pull down the bar to the upper chest. Return to the starting position to complete the repetition.

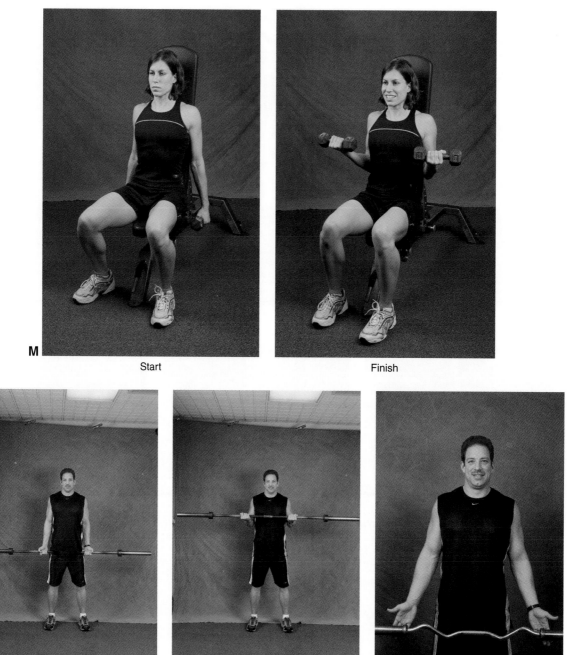

M — Start / Finish

N — Start / Finish / E-Z Bar

FIGURE 16.5. (*Continued*) **M.** Dumbbell arm curls (upper arm–biceps, unilateral). Take a seated position with two dumbbells held at the sides, with the palms facing in and the arms hanging straight down. Raise the dumbbells and rotate the forearm so that the palms face the shoulder. Lower to the original position to complete one repetition. One can also alternate one arm at a time. **N.** Barbell arm curls (upper arm–biceps, bilateral). In the standing position with the feet shoulder-width apart, grasp the straight barbell with an underhand grip and palms facing up. Raise the bar until the forearms are vertical and then lower the bar to the starting position to complete a repetition. One can also perform this exercise with an E-Z bar with the palms facing inward.

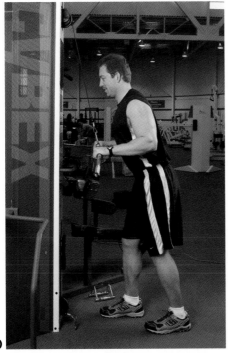 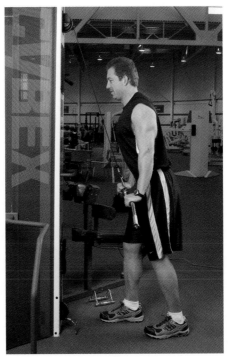

O

Start   Finish

FIGURE 16.5. (*Continued*) **O.** Triceps push down (upper arm–triceps, bilateral). Stand in front of the lat pull station or high pulley station and take an overhand grasp on the bar with your elbows at the sides. Start at chest level and extend the arms down until straight and return to the starting position to complete the repetition. Position the hands above the bar prior to the push-down phase of the repetition.

SUMMARY

Development of a resistance training program is a systematic process in which science and art come together to allow the Personal Trainer to specifically address a client's needs for neuromuscular fitness. A sequence of events in the exercise prescription process consists of getting a client's medical clearance, personal training history, goal generation, a needs analysis, and a general preparation phase of initial training and testing before putting together workouts based on the acute program variables that will be used in a resistance training program. This program is then updated and revised with the same process over time. Education, client interactions, and motivation are vital components of successful resistance training programs that meet each client's goals and objectives.

REFERENCES

1. American College of Sports Medicine Position Stand. Progression models in resistance training for healthy adults. *Med Sci Sports Exerc.* 2002;34:364–80.
2. Chilibeck PD, Calder AW, Sale DG, Webber CE. A comparison of strength and muscle mass increases during resistance training in young women. *Eur J Appl Physiol Occup Physiol.* 1998;77(1/2):170–5.
3. Delorme TL. Restoration of muscle power by heavy resistance exercises. *J Bone Joint Surg.* 1945;27:645.
4. Delorme TL, Watkins AL. Techniques of progressive resistance exercise. *Arch Phys Med.* 1948;29:263–73.
5. Dudley GA, Tesch PA, Miller BJ, Buchanan P. Importance of eccentric actions in performance adaptations to resistance training. *Aviat Space Environ Med.* 1991;62(6):543–50.
6. Fleck SJ, Kraemer WJ. *Designing Resistance Training Programs.* 3rd ed. Champaign (IL): Human Kinetics; 2004.
7. Fleck SJ, Schutt RC. Types of strength training. *Clin Sports Med.* 1985;4:159–69.
8. Harman E. Resistive torque analysis of 5 nautilus exercise machines. *Med Sci Sports Exerc.* 1983;15:113.

9. Hickson JF, Bruno MJ, Wilmore JH, Constable SH. Energy cost of weight training exercise. *Natl Strength Cond Assoc J.* 1984;6:522–3.

10. Hoeger WWK, Barette SL, Hale DF, Hopkins DR. Relationship between repetitions and selected percentages of one repetition maximum. *J Appl Sport Sci Res.* 1990;4(2):47–54.

11. Hoeger WWK, Hopkins DR, Barette SL, Hale DF. Relationship between repetitions and selected percentages of one repetition maximum: a comparison between untrained and trained males and females. *J Appl Sport Sci Res.* 1987;1(1):1–13.

12. Johnson JH, Colodny S, Jackson D. Human torque capability versus machine resistive torque for four Eagle resistance machines. *J Appl Sport Sci Res.* 1990;4:83–7.

13. Johnson RE, Quinn TJ, Kertzer R, Vroman NB. Strength training in female distance runners: impact on running economy. *J Strength Cond Res.* 1997;11(4):224–9.

14. Kraemer WJ. Exercise prescription in weight training: a needs analysis. *Natl Strength Cond Assoc J.* 1983;5(1):64–5.

15. Kraemer WJ. Exercise prescription in weight training: manipulating program variables. *Natl Strength Cond Assoc J.* 1983;5:58–9.

16. Kraemer WJ. A series of studies: the physiological basis for strength training in American football: fact over philosophy. *J Strength Cond Res.* 1997;11(3):131–42.

17. Kraemer WJ, Fleck SJ. *Optimizing Strength Training—Designing Nonlinear Periodization Workouts.* Champaign (IL): Human Kinetics; 2005.

18. Kraemer WJ, Fleck SJ. *Strength Training for Young Athletes.* 2nd ed. Champaign (IL): Human Kinetics; 2005.

19. Kraemer WJ, Fry AC. Strength testing: development and evaluation of methodology. In: Maud P, Foster C, editors. *Physiological Assessment of Human Fitness.* Champaign (IL): Human Kinetics; 1995. p. 115–38.

20. Kraemer WJ, Keuning M, Ratamess NA, et al. Resistance training combined with bench-step aerobics enhances women's health profile. *Med Sci Sports Exerc.* 2001;33(2):259–69.

21. Kraemer WJ, Marchitelli L, Gordon SE, et al. Hormonal and growth factor responses to heavy resistance exercise protocols. *J Appl Physiol.* 1990;69(4):1442–50.

22. Kraemer WJ, Noble BJ, Clark MJ, Culver BW. Physiologic responses to heavy-resistance exercise with very short rest periods. *Int J Sports Med.* 1987;8(4):247–52.

23. Kraemer WJ, Patton JF, Gordon SE, et al. Compatibility of high-intensity strength and endurance training on hormonal and skeletal muscle adaptations. *J Appl Physiol.* 1995;78(3):976–89.

24. Kraemer WJ, Ratamess N, Fry AC, et al. Influence of resistance training volume and periodization on physiological and performance adaptations in collegiate women tennis players. *Am J Sports Med.* 2000;28(5):626–33.

25. Marx JO, Ratamess NA, Nindl BC, et al. Low-volume circuit versus high-volume periodized resistance training in women. *Med Sci Sports Exerc.* 2001;33(4):635–43.

26. Matveyev L. *Fundamentals of Sports Training.* Moscow: Progress; 1981.

27. Mazzetti SA, Kraemer WJ, Volek JS, et al. The influence of direct supervision of resistance training on strength performance. *Med Sci Sports Exerc.* 2000;32(6):1175–84.

28. Pizzimenti MA. Mechanical analysis of the nautilus leg curl machine. *Can J Sport Sci.* 1992;17(1):41–8.

29. Plisk SS, Stone MH. Periodization strategies. *Strength Cond J.* 2003;25(6):19–37.

30. Rhea MR, Ball SD, Phillips WT, Burkett LN. A comparison of linear and daily undulating periodized programs with equated volume and intensity for strength. *J Strength Cond Res.* 2002;16(2):250–5.

31. Simao R, Farinatti Pde T, Polito MD, Maior AS, Fleck SJ. Influence of exercise order on the number of repetitions performed and perceived exertion during resistance exercises. *J Strength Cond Res.* 2005;19(1):152–6.

32. Tan B. Manipulating resistance training program variables to optimize maximum strength in men: a review. *J Strength Cond Res.* 1999;13(3):289–304.

33. Tharion WJ, Rausch TM, Harman EA, Kraemer WJ. Effects of different resistance exercise protocols on mood states. *J Appl Sport Sci Res.* 1991;5(2):60–5.

34. Todd T, Todd J. Dr. Patrick O'Shea: a man for all seasons. *J Strength Cond Res.* 2001;15(4):401–4.

35. Todd T, Todd J. Pioneers of strength research: the legacy of Dr. Richard A. Berger. *J Strength Cond Res.* 2001;15(3):275–8.

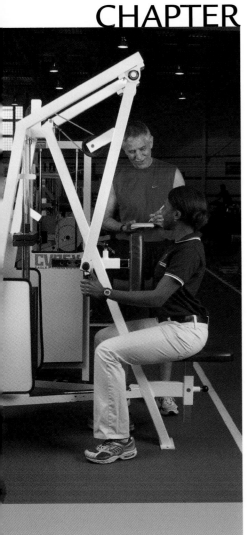

CHAPTER 17

Cardiorespiratory Training Programs

OBJECTIVES

- Identify the components of a cardiovascular training program
- Assess the interaction of frequency, duration, and intensity
- Describe the recommended range of training based on current research

ardiorespiratory training is one of the primary components of a balanced exercise program. The other two major components, resistance and flexibility training, are described in Chapters 16 and 18. The ACSM Position Stand on "The Recommended Quantity and Quality of Exercise for Developing and Maintaining Cardiorespiratory and Muscular Fitness, and Flexibility in Health Adults" (4) emphasizes the importance of these three components.

As a result of specificity of training and the need for maintaining muscular strength and endurance, and flexibility of the major muscle groups, a well-rounded training program including aerobic and resistance training, and flexibility exercise is recommended. (p. 975)

In August 2007, the American Heart Association and the ACSM released two important updates, one focusing on healthy adults aged between 18 and 65 years (5) and the other focusing on adults older than 65 years as well as adults ages 50–64 years with clinically significant conditions or functional limitations affecting physical activity or movement (6). These recommendations were important steps forward in clarifying the type of physical activity recommended. In addition, activities promoting muscular strength and endurance were included in the recommendations (muscular fitness is covered in detail in Chapter 16).

In "Physical Activity and Public Health: Updated Recommendation for Adults from the American College of Sports Medicine and the American Heart Association" (5), the importance of cardiorespiratory training is clearly outlined:

To promote and maintain health, all healthy adults aged 18–65 yr need moderate-intensity aerobic physical activity for a minimum of 30 min on five days each week or vigorous-intensity aerobic activity for a minimum of 20 min on three days each week. . . . Also, combinations of moderate- and vigorous-intensity activity can be performed to meet this recommendation. Moderate-intensity aerobic activity, which is generally equivalent to a brisk walk and noticeably accelerates the heart rate, can be accumulated toward the 30-min minimum from bouts lasting 10 or more minutes. Vigorous-intensity activity is exemplified by jogging, and causes rapid breathing and a substantial increase in heart rate. This recommended amount of aerobic activity is in addition to routine activities of daily living of light intensity (e.g., self care, cooking, casual walking or shopping) or lasting less than 10 min in duration (e.g., walking around home or office, walking from the parking lot).

Similarly, older adults are encouraged to attain similar amounts of physical activity related to days per week and time per session (6). However, the intensity is described on a 10-point scale (6): ". . . sitting is 0 and all-out effort is 10, moderate-intensity activity is a 5 or 6 and produces noticeable increases in heart rate and breathing. On the same scale, vigorous intensity activity is a 7 or 8 and produces large increases in heart rate and breathing." Given the range of fitness levels seen in older adults, the use of this scale allows for appropriate intensity determination. For example, for some older adults, moderate-intensity activity may be a slow walk, whereas for others it may be a brisk walk.

> **For some older adults, moderate-intensity activity may be a slow walk, whereas for others it may be a brisk walk.**

These recommendations (5,6) were reinforced in 2008, when a set of guidelines for physical activity was released by the U.S. Department of Health and Human Services (8). The "2008 Physical Activity Guidelines for Americans" includes messages for all Americans—children and adolescents, adults, older adults, women during pregnancy and postpartum, adults with disabilities, and people with chronic medical conditions. For adults, these guidelines emphasize the health benefits of accumulating at least 150 minutes per week of moderate-intensity physical activity (with additional benefits noted for more physical activity) or 75 minutes per week of vigorous-intensity physical activity (8). Thus, the 2007 recommendations by ACSM/AHA (5,6) are reinforced by the 2008 Guidelines (8) (i.e., moderate-intensity activity for 30 minutes on 5 days per week equals 150 minutes).

GENERAL TRAINING PRINCIPLES

Cardiorespiratory endurance or training refers to the ability of a client to perform large muscle, repetitive, moderate- to high-intensity exercise for an extended period. The goal is to increase heart rate (HR) and respiration in order to place an appropriate physiological stress on the cardiorespiratory system. This required stress is often referred to as "overload." The term overload is most commonly used when referring to resistance or strength training (i.e., lifting a weight heavier than typically done in daily activity to stress the muscle resulting in increases in strength and potential hypertrophy), but also applies to cardiorespiratory training. Overload of the cardiovascular and respiratory systems is required to have beneficial adaptations in cardiorespiratory endurance. Cardiorespiratory fitness is improved by enhanced heart function (i.e., oxygen delivery to the working muscles) and the ability of the working muscles to use the oxygen in metabolic processes allowing for increased energy production (1). Typical measurements used to determine improvements include increases in maximal oxygen consumption and decreases in HR or oxygen consumption in response to a given submaximal workload.

> *Overload of the cardiovascular and respiratory systems is required to have beneficial adaptations in cardiorespiratory endurance.*

The benefits of cardiorespiratory endurance include the following (1):

➤ decreased risk of premature death from all causes and specifically from heart disease,
➤ reduction in death from all causes, and
➤ increased likelihood of increased habitual activity levels that is also associated with health benefits.

More specific benefits are found in Box 17.1 (1). Inclusion of cardiorespiratory endurance provides many benefits and thus is an important element of a balanced exercise program.

The training methods used to bring about these adaptations are quite varied. There is no single exercise program to apply universally. A Personal Trainer must have the knowledge, skills, and abilities to individualize programs based on the client's current health status, risk factors for heart disease, and individual goals.

Different modes, or types, of exercise will bring about specific adaptations as well as more generalized cardiorespiratory fitness gains. The principle of adaptation states that if the cardiorespiratory system is challenged by endurance training of a certain level for a certain period, function (translated as fitness or performance) will improve. Determining how to stress the system for a given individual is one of the roles of a Personal Trainer. This determination is not a one-size-fits-all option. Rather, each client comes with specific health and fitness levels (and risk factors) that should be considered when preparing an exercise program (see Table 13.1 for a list of the risk factors), which must be considered before engaging a client in a fitness program. These risk factors place individuals into general risk classifications, which can be used to determine the need for physician oversight of testing as well as the level of exercise to be prescribed.

To challenge the cardiorespiratory system, an overload must be applied. To overload, activities that increase HR and respiration are prescribed. The minimal amount of overload needed to bring about the desired adaptation is referred to as the "threshold." If the training level exceeds the threshold, then physiological adaptations occur because of the prescribed overload. A properly constructed exercise program includes frequency (number of days per week), duration (minutes per workout), and intensity (how hard the workout is for the client). According to the ACSM Position Stand (4), cardiorespiratory training less than 2 days per week, less than 40%–50% of oxygen uptake reserve (to be described later in this chapter), and for less than 10 minutes will not provide a sufficient overload to develop and maintain fitness in apparently healthy adults.

BOX 17.1   Benefits of Regular Physical Activity and/or Exercise

Improvement in Cardiovascular and Respiratory Function
- Increased maximal oxygen uptake resulting from both central and peripheral adaptations
- Decreased minute ventilation at a given absolute submaximal intensity
- Decreased myocardial oxygen cost for a given absolute submaximal intensity
- Decreased heart rate and blood pressure at a given submaximal intensity
- Increased capillary density in skeletal muscle
- Increased exercise threshold for the accumulation of lactate in the blood
- Increased exercise threshold for the onset of disease signs or symptoms (e.g., angina pectoris, ischemic ST-segment depression, claudication)

Reduction in Coronary Artery Disease Risk Factors
- Reduced resting systolic/diastolic pressures
- Increased serum high-density lipoprotein cholesterol and decreased serum triglycerides
- Reduced total body fat, reduced intra-abdominal fat
- Reduced insulin needs, improved glucose tolerance
- Reduced blood platelet adhesiveness and aggregation

Decreased Morbidity and Mortality
- Primary prevention (i.e., interventions to prevent the initial occurrence)
  - Higher activity and/or fitness levels are associated with lower death rates from coronary artery disease
  - Higher activity and/or fitness levels are associated with lower incidence rates for combined cardiovascular diseases, coronary artery disease, stroke, type 2 diabetes, osteoporotic fractures, cancer of the colon and breast, and gallbladder disease
- Secondary prevention (i.e., interventions after a cardiac event [to prevent another])
  - Based on meta-analyses (pooled data across studies), cardiovascular and all-cause mortality are reduced in postmyocardial infarction patients who participate in cardiac rehabilitation exercise training, especially as a component of multifactorial risk factor reduction
  - Randomized controlled trials of cardiac rehabilitation exercise training involving postmyocardial infarction patients do not support a reduction in the rate of nonfatal reinfarction

Other Benefits
- Decreased anxiety and depression
- Enhanced physical function and independent living in older persons
- Enhanced feelings of well-being
- Enhanced performance of work, recreational, and sport activities
- Reduced risk of falls and injuries from falls in older persons
- Prevention or mitigation of functional limitations in older adults
- Effective therapy for many chronic diseases in older adults

Adapted from U.S. Department of Health and Human Services. *Physical Activity and Health: a Report of the Surgeon General.* Atlanta (GA): Centers for Disease Control and Prevention; 1996. Kesaniemi YK, Danforth Jr E, Jensen MD, et al. Dose-response issues concerning physical activity and health: an evidence-based symposium. *Med Sci Sports Exerc.* 2001; 33:S351–8. Nelson M, Rajeski JW, Blair SN, et al. Physical activity and public health in older adults: recommendation from the American College of Sports Medicine and the American Heart Association. *Med Sci Sports Exerc.* 2007;39(8):1435–45.

Although exceeding the threshold is required for physiological adaptations to occur, excessive overload can result, paradoxically, in diminished performance. When either a single bout or chronic period of excessive stress is placed on the cardiorespiratory system (resulting in a decrease in the physiological capacities), the term retrogression is used (2). The Personal Trainer must carefully balance the frequency, intensity, and duration of the workouts to avoid overchallenging the client beyond an appropriate amount of overload.

Although the desire is for all clients to continue to improve through appropriate levels of overload, there are times when clients stop exercising or decrease the overload below their threshold level. The result will be a loss of physiological adaptations as the person regresses toward preoverload status. This process of losing fitness gains is referred to as regression or de-adaptation (2). Anticipating periods of decreased physical activity (e.g., travel, excessive work obligations) can allow for a planned "reentry" into the exercise program. Chapter 10 includes information on how to keep clients motivated by promoting positive behavior changes.

DESIGN OF CARDIORESPIRATORY TRAINING SESSION

A cardiorespiratory exercise session includes a warm-up, the endurance phase, and a cool-down. The warm-up prepares the person for the focal point of the workout (the endurance phase) when a target intensity is achieved allowing for appropriate overload. The cool-down allows the person to transition back toward resting levels following the endurance phase. Development of the structure of the entire exercise program sequence is presented in Chapter 19.

> *A cardiorespiratory exercise session includes a warm-up, the endurance phase, and a cool-down.*

Warm-Up

A properly constructed exercise program will include a transition period from rest to the target exercise intensity. This transition period is called the warm-up. During the warm-up, the client should gradually increase body temperature by incorporating low-level activity similar to what will be done during the endurance phase. For example, an appropriate warm-up for a brisk walking exercise program would include slow walking. The muscle groups used are similar in the two activities—slow walking being a low-intensity activity, which naturally leads to the brisk walking of the exercise program. The warm-up may also include gentle stretching activities, although stretching should be done only after some activity to warm the muscles. The activities included in a warm-up will vary depending on the target activity to be included in the endurance phase. General recommendations for a warm-up include the following (1):

➤ 5–10 minutes of low-intensity large muscle activity and
➤ intensity progression to the lower end of the target exercise range for the endurance phase.

The intent of a warm-up is to prepare the muscles and cardiorespiratory system for the upcoming workout. It is a time of transition and should provide a gradual (rather than an abrupt) increase in HR, respiration, and body temperature. Taking sufficient time to prepare the body for physical activity increases the safety and enjoyment of the target exercise during the endurance phase. The benefits of completing a warm-up include the following (1):

➤ may reduce the susceptibility of injury to muscles or joints by increasing the extensibility of connective tissue;
➤ improve joint range of motion and function;
➤ improve muscle performance; and
➤ potentially help prevent ischemia (lack of oxygen) of the heart muscle, which may occur in clients with sudden strenuous exertion.

Endurance Phase

The endurance phase is the target of the warm-up. The warm-up has provided the client with a transition from rest to a higher level of intensity. During the endurance phase, the proper overload is implemented to promote beneficial cardiorespiratory adaptations. The Personal Trainer should consider the appropriate mode (i.e., type) of exercise as well as how to balance exercise intensity, duration, and frequency.

EXERCISE MODE

Exercise mode is selected with consideration for the client's fitness, health, and interests. During the consultation with a client, discuss what activities are most enjoyed as well as those that are accessible. Enjoyability and access may seem obvious but are important to consider when selecting an exercise mode for best possible adherence.

Cardiorespiratory exercises involve the use of large muscle groups in a repetitive, or rhythmic, fashion for an extended period. Some activities are weight-dependent, meaning that body weight is moved during the exercise (e.g., walking, running). In other activities, body weight is not a factor because the body is supported (e.g., cycling, swimming). These activities are referred to as weight-bearing and non–weight-bearing exercises, respectively (2). Use of non–weight-bearing exercises may be useful in avoiding injuries of the lower limbs due to overuse (2). Table 17.1 lists a number of cardiorespiratory endurance activities (1). ACSM has classified these activities into four groups. The groups do not necessarily represent an optimal progression but rather present the Personal Trainer with information on important characteristics of the exercise modes when selecting activities.

Group A includes endurance activities that require minimal skill or fitness to perform. Walking would be an example. Group A activities allow for accommodation to individual fitness levels and thus are recommended for all adults (1). Group B activities are those that require minimal skill but, in contrast to Group A activities, are typically performed at a more vigorous intensity. Jogging and running are examples (for others, see Table 17.1). Group B activities are considered for those with regular exercise programs and for those who have at least a baseline level of fitness. Swimming and cross-country skiing are examples of Group C exercises (1). This classification reflects the relationship between skill level and individual energy expenditure. For example, an experienced swimmer may be able to maintain a constant intensity while swimming whereas a person with poor skills would struggle to swim at an appropriate, constant intensity to receive cardiorespiratory benefits.

TABLE 17.1	GROUPING OF CARDIORESPIRATORY EXERCISE AND ACTIVITIES		
Exercise Group	**Exercise Description**	**Recommended for**	**Examples**
A	Endurance activities requiring minimal skill or physical fitness to perform	All adults	Walking, leisurely cycling, aqua-aerobics, slow dancing
B	Vigorous-intensity endurance activities requiring minimal skill	Adults with a regular exercise program and/or at least average physical fitness	Jogging, running, rowing, aerobics, spinning, elliptical exercise, stepping exercise, fast dancing
C	Endurance activities requiring skill to perform	Adults with acquired skill and/or at least average physical fitness levels	Swimming, cross-country skiing, skating
D	Recreational sports	Adults with a regular exercise program and at least average physical fitness	Racquet sports, basketball, soccer, downhill skiing, hiking

From American College of Sports Medicine. *ACSM's Guidelines for Exercise Testing and Prescription.* 8th ed. Baltimore: Lippincott Williams & Wilkins; 2010. Box 7-3.

Recreational sports like basketball, soccer, tennis, and other racquet sports are classified as Group D activities (1). The ability to maintain a constant, controlled intensity is difficult because of the nature of the activities and becomes even more of a challenge when competition is involved. As a result, Group D activities should be used with caution for clients with low fitness or who are at high risk or symptomatic of disease unless modifications to rules are implemented (1). Group D activities are generally recommended for most adults as ancillary physical activities to achieve or maintain health and fitness benefits (1).

The groupings outlined provide the Personal Trainer with guidance on selection of an appropriate exercise mode. Group A activities are very appropriate to use with clients beginning an exercise program. Group B activities are fitting for regular exercisers or those with at least an average fitness level. Group C activities may be included but will require discussion with the client regarding skill levels for the activities in question. Group D activities may best be included as additional activity after a baseline level of fitness is achieved. The Personal Trainer and the client must maintain open lines of communication regarding the selection of exercise modes. In some situations, individuals will be satisfied with continuing with various Group A activities. Other clients may have goals to move to Group B, have the skills or desire to learn new skills to include Group C activities, or enjoy the variety and challenge of Group D activities. See Figures 17.2, 17.3, and 17.4 for different types of activities.

The Personal Trainer should also instruct clients about proper posture and body alignment while conducting cardiorespiratory training. Having a client perform these exercises in a proper biomechanical position is just as important as when clients are performing resistance training exercises, as discussed in Chapter 16. Typical concerns with treadmill exercise include leaning forward and excessive gripping on the handrails. Proper upright posture and body alignment with the use of handrails only for balance should be maintained. Similarly, with stair steppers or other cross-training machines, upright posture should be verified rather than allowing forward head protrusion, rounded shoulders, and poor alignment. The biggest challenge with cycle ergometry is determination of appropriate seat height. Seat height should be adjusted to allow for 5°–10° of knee flexion at the bottom of the pedal stroke (Fig. 17.1).

> *The Personal Trainer should also instruct clients about proper posture and body alignment while conducting cardiorespiratory training.*

EXERCISE INTENSITY

Intensity can be determined using various methods. For a quick overview of the intensity classifications for cardiorespiratory endurance, see Table 17.2 (2). Details on these various methods will be outlined in this section. Some methods require knowledge of maximal oxygen consumption or maximal and/or resting HR. Others rely on estimations of maximal HR based on age. Personal Trainers must use the information available to determine the more appropriate exercise prescription, realizing the shortcomings of the various methods.

When using maximal oxygen consumption, a range of values will be determined. These values can be used to determine the workload for various activities using charts or metabolic calculations. A shortcoming of this technique is the outcome, which is a determination of workload, not the individual's response. For example, determining an outdoor running pace on the basis of oxygen consumption alone may pose the problem of inaccuracy when faced with a hot, humid environment. Factors such as environmental conditions may make the relative intensity higher than prescribed.

> *Factors such as environmental conditions may make the relative intensity higher than prescribed.*

Blindly using workloads can be a concern if physiological responses (such as HR) are not monitored during exercise. Use of HR can be helpful as it represents a client's physiological response but it too has shortcomings. Accuracy can be compromised when estimations of maximal HR are used or when medications are taken, which may influence HR (i.e., β-blockers, a drug that suppresses HR at rest

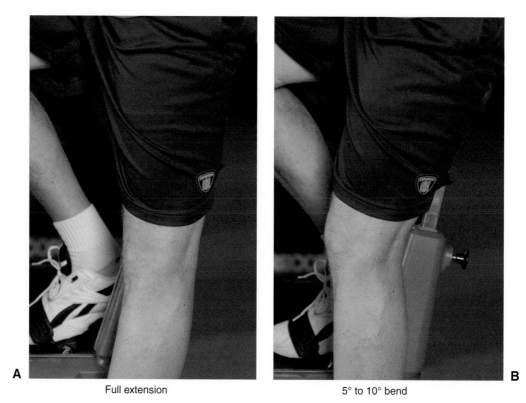

A   Full extension   5° to 10° bend   B

FIGURE 17.1. Personal trainers may instruct clients to adjust seat heights to maintain a 5°–10° bend in the knee before reaching full extension. Full extension of knee while pedaling on the stationary bike is not recommended to reduce compression on the joint structure.

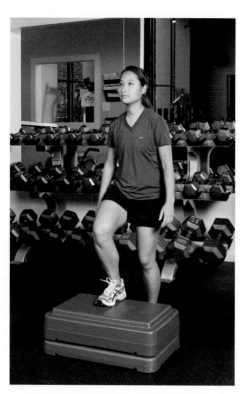

FIGURE 17.2. Stepping activity.

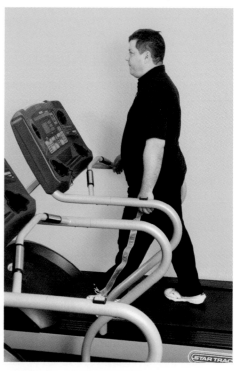

FIGURE 17.3. Walking activity.

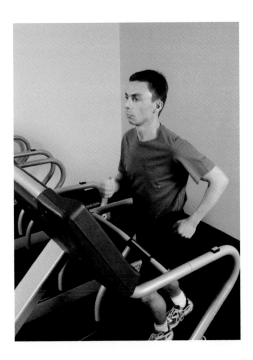

FIGURE 17.4. Jogging activity.

and during exercise). When a measured maximal HR done during a graded exercise test is unavailable, the Personal Trainer commonly uses an age-predicted estimate (220 − age). The concern with this method (1) is the variability for a given single age (1 SD equals ± 10–12 beats per minute). Thus a 20-year-old may not have a maximal HR of 200 as predicted by this formula (could be lower or higher). The role of the Personal Trainer is to use the information available, realizing the shortcomings of the various techniques, to determine an appropriate exercise prescription. A willingness and ability to modify the exercise program to provide an appropriate overload is the sign of a good Personal Trainer.

Oxygen Uptake Reserve. Exercise intensity can be determined from oxygen uptake reserve or HR reserve. ACSM recommends a range of between 40% and 50% up to 85% of oxygen uptake reserve or HR reserve (1). The oxygen uptake reserve (commonly designated as $\dot{V}O_2R$)

TABLE 17.2	CLASSIFICATION OF EXERCISE INTENSITY FOR CARDIORESPIRATORY ENDURANCE		
Intensity	**HRR or $\dot{V}O_2R$ (%)**	**HR_{max} (%)**	**RPE**
Very light	<20	<35	<10
Light	20–39	35–54	10–11
Moderate	40–59	55–69	12–13
Hard	60–84	70–89	14–16
Very hard	>85	>90	17–19
Maximal	100	100	20

HRR, heart rate reserve; $\dot{V}O_2R$, oxygen uptake reserve; HR_{max}, maximum heart rate; RPE, rating of perceived exertion.
American College of Sports Medicine. *ACSM's Resource Manual for Guidelines for Exercise Testing and Prescription.* 5th ed. Baltimore: Lippincott Williams & Wilkins; 2006. Table 24.2, p. 340.

TABLE 17.3	PERCENTILE VALUES FOR MAXIMAL AEROBIC POWER

	Males								
	Age 20–29				Age 30–39				
%	**Balke Treadmill (Time)**	**Max $\dot{V}O_2$ (mL/kg/min)**	**12-min Run (Miles)**	**1.5-Mile Run (Time)**	**Balke Treadmill (Time)**	**Max $\dot{V}O_2$ (mL/kg/min)**	**12-min Run (Miles)**	**1.5-Mile Run (Time)**	
99	32:00	61.2	2.02	8:22	30:00	58.3	1.94	8:49	
95	28:31	56.2	1.88	9:10	27:11	54.3	1.82	9:31	S
90	27:00	54.0	1.81	9:34	26:00	52.5	1.77	9:52	
85	26:00	52.5	1.77	9:52	24:45	50.7	1.72	10:14	
80	25:00	51.1	1.73	10:08	23:30	47.5	1.67	10:38	E
75	23:40	49.2	1.68	10:34	22:30	47.5	1.63	10:59	
70	23:00	48.2	1.65	10:49	22:00	46.8	1.61	11:09	
65	22:00	48.8	1.61	11:09	21:00	45.3	1.57	11:34	
60	21:15	45.7	1.58	11:27	20:20	44.4	1.55	11:49	G
55	21:00	45.3	1.57	11:34	20:00	43.9	1.53	11:58	
50	20:00	43.9	1.53	11:58	19:00	42.4	1:49	12:25	
45	19:26	43.1	1.51	12:11	18:15	41.4	1.46	12:44	
40	18:50	42.2	1.49	12:29	18:00	41.0	1.45	12:53	F
35	18:00	41.0	1.45	12:53	17:00	39.5	1.41	13:25	
30	17:30	40.3	1.43	13:08	16:15	38.5	1.38	13:48	
25	17:00	39.5	1.41	13:25	15:40	37.6	1.36	14:10	
20	16:00	38.1	1.37	13:58	15:00	36.7	1.33	14:33	P
15	15:00	36.7	1.33	14:33	14:00	35.2	1.29	15:14	
10	14:00	35.2	1.29	15:14	13:00	33.8	1.25	15:56	
5	12:00	32.3	1.21	16:46	11:10	31.1	1.18	17:30	
1	8:00	26.6	1.05	20:55	8:00	26.6	1.05	20:55	VP
	n = 2,606				*n* = 13,158				

Total *n* = 15,764

S, superior; E, excellent; G, good; F, fair; P, poor; VP, very poor.

(continued)

is the difference between maximal oxygen consumption ($\dot{V}O_{2max}$) and resting ($\dot{V}O_{2rest}$). To use the $\dot{V}O_2R$ method to determine intensity, the following equations can be used:

$$\text{Target } \dot{V}O_2 \text{ (lower end of range)} = [(0.40) \times (\dot{V}O_{2max} - \dot{V}O_{2rest})] + \dot{V}O_{2rest}$$

$$\text{Target } \dot{V}O_2 \text{ (upper end of range)} = [(0.85) \times (\dot{V}O_{2max} - \dot{V}O_{2rest})] + \dot{V}O_{2rest}$$

$\dot{V}O_{2rest}$ has been estimated to be 3.5 mL · kg^{-1} · min^{-1} (also referred to a one metabolic equivalent or 1 MET) and is used for all individuals. If a Personal Trainer has access to $\dot{V}O_{2max}$ information, then these equations can be used. The percentages used to determine the appropriate $\dot{V}O_2$ range must be made with the client's fitness level and goals in mind. Low-fit clients will need to start on the lower end of the range, whereas more active clients will require intensities toward the upper end of the range to receive the appropriate overload. Normative values for $\dot{V}O_{2max}$ are found in Table 17.3, which allows the Personal Trainer to see the percentile rank for males and females of various ages.

TABLE 17.3	**PERCENTILE VALUES FOR MAXIMAL AEROBIC POWER (Continued)**

	Males								
	Age 40–49				Age 50–59				
%	Balke Treadmill (Time)	Max $\dot{V}O_2$ (mL/kg/min)	12-min Run (Miles)	1.5-Mile Run (Time)	Balke Treadmill (Time)	Max $\dot{V}O_2$ (mL/kg/min)	12-min Run (Miles)	1.5-Mile Run (Time)	
99	29:06	57.0	1.90	9:02	27:15	54.3	1.82	9:31	
95	26:16	52.9	1.79	9:47	24:00	49.7	1.69	10:27	S
90	25:00	51.1	1.73	10:09	22:00	46.8	1.61	11:09	
85	23:14	48.5	1.66	10:44	20:31	44.6	1.55	11:45	
80	22:00	46.8	1.61	11:09	19:35	43.3	1.52	12:08	E
75	21:02	45.4	1.58	11:32	18:32	41.8	1.47	12:37	
70	20:15	44.2	1.54	11:52	18:00	41.0	1.45	12:53	
65	20:00	43.9	1.49	11:58	17:00	39.5	1.41	13:25	
60	19:00	42.4	1.45	12:25	16:10	38.3	1.38	13.53	G
55	18:02	41.0	1.44	12:53	16:00	38.1	1.37	13:58	
50	17:34	40.4	1.41	13:05	15:02	36.7	1.33	14:33	
45	17:00	39.5	1.38	13:25	14:56	36.6	1.33	14:35	
40	16:12	38.4	1.36	13:50	14:00	35.2	1.29	15:14	F
35	15:38	37.6	1.33	14:10	13:05	33.9	1.26	15:53	
30	15:00	36.7	1.13	14:33	12:38	33.2	1.24	16:16	
25	14:20	35.7	1.31	15:00	12:00	32.3	1.21	16:46	
20	13:35	34.6	1.28	15:32	11:10	31.1	1.18	17:30	P
15	12:45	33.4	1.24	16:09	10:15	29.8	1.14	18:22	
10	11:40	31.8	1.20	17:04	9:15	28.4	1.10	19:24	
5	10:00	29.4	1.13	18:39	7:30	25.8	1.03	21:40	
1	7:00	25.1	1.01	22:22	4:20	21.3	0.90	27:08	VP
	$n = 16,534$				$n = 9,102$				

Total $n = 25,636$

S, superior; E, excellent; G, good; F, fair; P, poor; VP, very poor.

(continued)

To determine an appropriate workload, various metabolic equations are available (2). These equations are found in Box 17.2. These equations can estimate the oxygen consumption required by the body during constant, submaximal activity (including walking, jogging/running, stationary cycling, arm cranking, and stepping). In Box 17.3, an extended example shows the application of the various equations to a client's exercise prescription. Underestimating the workload may leave a person below the appropriate target intensity (and the accompanying health benefits). Overestimating commonly results in frustration with exercise and poor adherence. These equations will give initial starting points. Intensity levels may still need to be adjusted on the basis of individual HR responses and perceived levels of exertion.

A simpler method, not requiring extensive calculations, is to take the oxygen consumption values (for the upper and lower end of the target range) and convert them to MET values. This is accomplished by taking the oxygen consumption values and dividing by 3.5 (as 1 MET = 3.5 mL $\cdot$ kg^{-1} $\cdot$ min^{-1}). Tables are available that will help the Personal Trainer determine appropriate workloads. See Tables 17.4 to 17.8 for walking, jogging/running, leg cycle ergometry, arm

| TABLE 17.3 | PERCENTILE VALUES FOR MAXIMAL AEROBIC POWER (*Continued*) |

	Males								
	Age 60–69				Age 70–79				
%	Balke Treadmill (Time)	Max V̇O₂ (mL/kg/ min)	12-min Run (Miles)	1.5-Mile Run (Time)	Balke Treadmill (Time)	Max V̇O₂ (mL/kg/ min)	12-min Run (Miles)	1.5-Mile Run (Time)	
99	25:02	51.1	1.74	10:09	24:00	49.7	1.69	10:27	
95	21:33	46.1	1.60	11:20	19:00	42.4	1.49	12:25	S
90	19:30	43.2	1.51	12:10	17:00	39.5	1.41	13:25	
85	18:00	41.0	1.45	12:53	16:00	38.1	1.37	13:57	
80	17:00	39.5	1.41	13:25	14:34	36.0	1.32	14:52	E
75	16:00	38.1	1.37	13:58	13:25	34.4	1.27	15:38	
70	15:00	36.7	1.33	14:33	12:27	33.0	1.23	16:22	
65	14:30	35.9	1.31	14:55	12:00	32.3	1.21	16:46	
60	13:51	35.0	1.29	15:20	11:00	30.9	1.17	17:37	G
55	13:04	33.9	1.26	15:53	10:30	30.2	1.15	18:05	
50	12:30	33.1	1.23	16:19	10:00	29.4	1.13	18:39	
45	12:00	32.3	1.21	16:46	9:20	28.5	1.11	19:19	
40	11:21	31.4	1.19	17:19	9:00	28.0	1.09	19:43	F
35	10:49	30.6	1.17	17:49	8:21	27.1	1.07	20:28	
30	10:00	29.4	1.13	18:39	7:38	26.0	1.04	21:28	
25	9:29	28.7	1.11	19:10	7:00	25.1	1.01	22:22	
20	8:37	27.4	1.08	20:13	6:00	23.7	0.97	23:55	P
15	7:33	25.9	1.03	21:34	5:00	22.2	0.93	25:49	
10	6:20	24.1	0.99	23:27	4:00	20.8	0.89	27:55	
5	4:55	22.1	0.93	25:58	3:00	19.3	0.85	30:34	
1	2:29	18.6	0.83	31:59	2:00	17.9	0.81	33:30	VP
	n = 2,682				*n* = 467				
Total *n* = 3,149									

S, superior; E, excellent; G, good; F, fair; P, poor; VP, very poor.

(*continued*)

ergometry, and stair stepping (1). Although simpler than the calculations found in Box 17.2, the limitation of using the tables is more restricted to specific workout options. For example, for the walking table, only certain grade and speed options are presented. In Box 17.4, an example is included regarding the use of these tables to determine exercise workload ranges. Other tables (2) are available with more diverse activities (ranging from cleaning the house to hunting to sports and fitness activities).

Anytime a workload is determined using oxygen consumption, the Personal Trainer must realize individual differences in skill and efficiency doing the particular exercise. In addition to using the metabolic calculations or MET tables, a Personal Trainer should monitor the client's response to the exercise (including HR, rating of perceived exertion [RPE], and any other signs or symptoms of overexertion). The Personal Trainer

A Personal Trainer should monitor the client's response to the exercise (including HR, rating of perceived exertion [RPE], and any other signs or symptoms of overexertion).

| TABLE 17.3 | PERCENTILE VALUES FOR MAXIMAL AEROBIC POWER (*Continued*) |

Females

%	Age 20–29 Balke Treadmill (Time)	Max V̇O₂ (mL/kg/ min)	12-min Run (Miles)	1.5-Mile Run (Time)	Age 30–39 Balke Treadmill (Time)	Max V̇O₂ (mL/kg/ min)	12-min Run (Miles)	1.5-Mile Run (Time)	
99	27:43	55.0	1.84	9:23	26:00	52.5	1.77	9:52	
95	24:24	50.2	1.71	10:20	22:06	46.9	1.62	11:08	S
90	22:30	47.5	1.63	10:59	20:34	44.7	1.56	11:43	
85	21:00	45.3	1.57	11:34	19:03	42.5	1.50	12:23	
80	20:04	44.0	1.54	11:56	18:00	41.0	1.45	12:53	E
75	19:42	43.4	1.52	12:07	17:30	40.3	1.43	13:08	
70	18:06	41.1	1.46	12:51	16:30	38.8	1.39	13:41	
65	17:45	40.6	1.44	13:01	16:00	38.1	1.37	13:58	
60	17:00	39.5	1.41	13:25	15:02	36.7	1.33	14:33	G
55	16:00	38.1	1.37	13:58	15:00	36.7	1.33	14:33	
50	15:30	37.4	1.35	14:15	14:00	35.2	1.29	15:14	
45	15:00	36.7	1.33	14:33	13:30	34.5	1.27	15:35	
40	14:11	35.5	1.30	15:05	13:00	33.8	1.25	15:56	F
35	13:36	34.6	1.27	15:32	12:03	32.4	1.21	16:43	
30	13:00	33.8	1.25	15:56	12:00	32.3	1.21	16:46	
25	12:04	32.4	1.22	16:43	11:00	30.9	1.17	17:38	
20	11:30	31.6	1.19	17:11	10:20	29.9	1.15	18:18	P
15	10:42	30.5	1.16	17:53	9:39	28.9	1.12	19:01	
10	10:00	29.4	1.13	18:39	8:36	27.4	1.08	20:13	
5	7:54	26.4	1.05	21:05	7:16	25.5	1.02	21:57	
1	5:14	22.6	0.94	25:17	5:20	22.7	0.94	25:10	VP
	n = 1,350				*n* = 4,394				
Total *n* = 5,744									

S, superior; E, excellent; G, good; F, fair; P, poor; VP, very poor.

(continued)

should assist the client with making adjustments to workload based on the individual's response to the exercise load (1).

Heart Rate. Often, a Personal Trainer will not have access to oxygen consumption information. Heart rate and oxygen consumption have a linear relationship, or in other words, when one increases, the other increases as well. Therefore, in the absence of oxygen consumption information, HR can be used. The ACSM recommends intensity levels for exercise between 64% and 70% (64%/70%) to 94% of maximal HR (2). The following calculation can be used to determine the target HR:

$$\text{Target HR (lower end of range)} = [\text{maximal HR}] \times 0.64$$

$$\text{Target HR (upper end of range)} = [\text{maximal HR}] \times 0.94$$

For example, for a 20-year-old with an estimated maximal HR of 200 (220 − 20 = 200), the range will be 128–188 beats per minute. The resulting target HR range may be so wide that it is not helpful to guide the client's exercise session. The Personal Trainer must therefore consider

| TABLE 17.3 | PERCENTILE VALUES FOR MAXIMAL AEROBIC POWER (*Continued*) | | | | | | | |

Females

%	Age 40–49				Age 50–59				
	Balke Treadmill (Time)	Max $\dot{V}O_2$ (mL/kg/min)	12-min Run (Miles)	1.5-Mile Run (Time)	Balke Treadmill (Time)	Max $\dot{V}O_2$ (mL/kg/min)	12-min Run (Miles)	1.5-Mile Run (Time)	
99	25:00	51.1	1.74	10:09	21:00	45.3	1.57	11:34	
95	20:56	45.2	1.57	11:35	17:16	39.9	1.42	13:16	S
90	19:00	42.4	1.49	12:25	16:00	38.1	1.37	13:58	
85	17:20	40.0	1.43	13:14	15:00	36.7	1.33	14:33	
80	16:34	38.9	1.40	13:38	14:00	35.2	1.29	15:14	E
75	16:00	38.1	1.37	13:58	13:15	34.1	1.26	15:47	
70	15:00	36.7	1.33	14:33	12:23	32.9	1.23	16:26	
65	14:14	35.6	1.30	15:03	12:00	32.3	1.21	16:46	
60	13:56	35.1	1.29	15:17	11:23	31.4	1.19	17:19	G
55	13:02	33.8	1.25	15:56	11:00	30.9	1.17	17:38	
50	12:39	33.3	1.24	16:13	10:30	30.2	1.15	18:05	
45	12:00	32.3	1.21	16:46	10:00	29.4	1.13	18:39	
40	11:30	31.6	1.19	17:11	9:30	28.7	1.11	19:10	F
35	11:00	30.9	1.17	17:38	9:00	28.0	1.09	19:43	
30	10:10	29.7	1.14	18:26	8:30	27.3	1.07	20:17	
25	10:00	29.4	1.13	18:39	8:00	26.6	1.05	20:55	
20	9:00	28.0	1.09	19:43	7:15	25.5	1.02	21:57	P
15	8:07	26.7	1.06	20:49	6:40	24.6	1.00	22:53	
10	7:21	25.6	1.03	21:52	6:00	23.7	0.97	23:55	
5	6:17	24.1	0.98	23:27	4:48	21.9	0.92	26:15	
1	4:00	20.8	0.89	27:55	3:00	19.3	0.85	30:34	VP
	n = 4,834				*n* = 3,103				
Total *n* = 7,937									

S, superior; E, excellent; G, good; F, fair; P, poor; VP, very poor.

(*continued*)

the client's health history as well as his or her goals to narrow the range. For apparently healthy individuals, the range is often narrowed to 70%–85% of maximal HR (1). Therefore, for the 20-year-old, moderately active client, the target HR range will be 140–170 beats per minute. If a client is very deconditioned or unfit, then a lower percentage will be used (e.g., 55%–70%). Selection of the intensity range must be made with the client's health status and fitness goals in mind.

Heart rate reserve can also be used. Heart rate reserve is the difference between maximal HR and resting HR. This method is often referred to as the Karvonen method (1). The formulas used resemble those used with the $\dot{V}O_2R$ method:

$$\text{Target HR (lower end of range)} = [(0.40) \times (HR_{max} - HR_{rest})] + HR_{rest}$$

$$\text{Target HR (upper end of range)} = [(0.85) \times (HR_{max} - HR_{rest})] + HR_{rest}$$

Thus, when using this method for a 20-year-old client who has a resting HR of 75, the range will be 125–181 beats per minute. This range is too wide to be useful and, thus, reflection must be made

TABLE 17.3	PERCENTILE VALUES FOR MAXIMAL AEROBIC POWER (*Continued*)

	Females								
	Age 60–69				Age 70–79				
%	Balke Treadmill (Time)	Max V̇O₂ (mL/kg/ min)	12-min Run (Miles)	1.5-Mile Run (Time)	Balke Treadmill (Time)	Max V̇O₂ (mL/kg/ min)	12-min Run (Miles)	1.5-Mile Run (Time)	
99	19:00	42.4	1.49	12:25	19:00	42.4	1.49	12:25	
95	15:09	36.9	1.34	14:28	15:00	36.7	1.33	14:33	S
90	13:33	34.6	1.27	15:32	12:50	33.5	1.25	16:06	
85	12:28	33.0	1.23	16:22	11:46	32.0	1.20	16:57	
80	12:00	32.3	1.21	16:46	10:30	30.2	1.15	18:05	E
75	11:04	31.0	1.18	17:34	10:00	29.4	1.13	18:39	
70	10:30	30.2	1.15	18:05	9:15	28.4	1.10	19:24	
65	10:00	29.4	1.13	18:39	8:43	27.6	1.08	20:02	
60	9:44	29.1	1.12	18:52	8:00	26.6	1.05	20:54	G
55	9:11	28.3	1.10	19:29	7:37	26.0	1.04	21:45	
50	8:40	27.5	1.08	20:08	7:00	25.1	1.01	22:22	
45	8:15	26.9	1.06	20:38	6:39	24.6	1.00	22:54	
40	8:00	26.6	1.05	20:55	6:05	23.8	0.98	23:47	F
35	7:14	25.4	1.02	22:03	5:28	22.9	0.95	24:54	
30	6:52	24.9	1.01	22:34	5:00	22.2	0.93	25:49	
25	6:21	24.2	0.99	23:20	4:45	21.9	0.92	26:15	
20	6:00	23.7	0.97	23:55	4:16	21.2	0.90	27:17	P
15	5:25	22.8	0.95	25:02	4:00	20.8	0.89	27:55	
10	4:40	21.7	0.92	26:32	3:00	19.3	0.85	30:34	
5	3:30	20.1	0.87	29:06	2:00	17.9	0.81	33:32	
1	2:10	18.1	0.82	33:05	1:00	16.4	0.77	37:26	VP
	n = 1,088				*n* = 209				

Total *n* = 1,297

Reprinted with permission from the Cooper Institute, Dallas, Texas. For more information: www.cooperinstitute.org
S, superior; E, excellent; G, good; F, fair; P, poor; VP, very poor.

on the client's fitness. If the client is moderately active, using a range of 60%–80% may be more appropriate. The HR range program is therefore 150–175 beats per minute. If the client is deconditioned, a range of 40%–50% may be more appropriate.

Rating of Perceived Exertion. Rating of perceived exertion is a guideline to use when setting exercise intensity (2). Two scales are typically used. Table 17.9 lists the 6–20 RPE scale as well as the category-ratio scale that rates exercise intensity on a 0–10 scale (1). RPE can be used to subjectively rate overall feelings of exertion and so can be helpful in guiding exercise intensity (1). The threshold level for cardiorespiratory benefits appears to be between 12 and 16 on the original scale and 4–5 on the ratio scale (2). The verbal descriptors for this range include "somewhat hard" to "hard." When using RPE, the Personal Trainer should keep in mind the variability between individuals (e.g., the RPE value will not necessarily correspond directly with a particular percentage of maximal HR or percentage of HR reserve) and must then make adjustments as needed (1). RPE is helpful

BOX 17.2 Metabolic Equations for Gross $\dot{V}O_2$ in Metric Units

Activity	Resting Component	Sum of These Components Horizontal Component	Vertical Component/ Resistance Component	Limitations
Walking	3.5	$0.1 \times$ speed[a]	$1.8 \times$ speed[a] $\times$ grade[b]	Most accurate for speeds of 1.9–3.7 mph (50–100 m · min^{-1})
Running	3.5	$0.2 \times$ speed[a]	$0.9 \times$ speed[a] $\times$ grade[b]	Most accurate for speeds >5 mph (134 m · min^{-1})
Stepping	3.5	$0.2 \times$ steps per min	$1.33 \times (1.8 \times$ step height[c] $\times$ steps per min)	Most accurate for stepping rates of 12–30 steps per min
Leg cycling	3.5	3.5	$(1.8 \times$ work rate[d]$)/$ body mass[e]	Most accurate for work rates of 300–1200 kg · m · min^{-1} (50–200 W)
Arm cycling	3.5		$(3 \times$ work rate[d]$)/$ body mass[e]	Most accurate for work rates between 150–750 kg · m · min^{-1} (25–125 W)

[a]Speed in m · min^{-1}.
[b]Grade is percent grade expressed in decimal format (e.g., 10% = 0.10).
[c]Step height in m.
Multiply by the following conversion factors:
 lb to kg: 0.454
 in to cm: 2.54
 ft to m: 0.3048
 mi to km: 1.609
 mph to m · min^{-1}: 26.8
 kg · m · min^{-1} to w: 0.164
 W to kg · m · min^{-1}: 6.12
 $\dot{V}O_2$max L · min^{-1} to kcal · min^{-1}: 4.9
 $\dot{V}O_2$max mL · kg^{-1} · min^{-1} to MET: 3.5
[d]Work rate in kilogram meters per minute (kg · m · min^{-1}) is calculated as resistance (kg) $\times$ distance per revolution of flywheel $\times$ pedal frequency per minute.
Note: Distance per revolution is 6 m for Monark leg ergometer, 3 m for the Tunturi and BodyGuard ergometers, and 2.4 m for Monark arm ergometer.
[e]Body mass in kg.
Adapted from American College of Sports Medicine. *ACSM's Guidelines for Exercise Testing and Prescription.* 8th ed. Philadelphia (PA): Lippincott Williams & Wilkins; 2010. p. 158.

for individuals having difficulty determining exercise HR or who are taking medications, which influence HR.

Talk Test. Another very simple way to consider intensity is the "talk test" (7). This simply means that as clients exercise, they should be able to respond to someone. When comfortable speech is not possible (e.g., gasping for breath after every word or two), it may indicate that the intensity is moving above the level typically prescribed. Thus, the goal is to exercise close to the point at which speech first becomes difficult. Although very simple, it appears that the use of the talk test does allow for consistent training intensities.

> *When comfortable speech is not possible (e.g., gasping for breath after every word or two), it may indicate that the intensity is moving above the level typically prescribed.*

EXERCISE SESSION DURATION

Duration and intensity are inversely related. As one increases, the other decreases. ACSM recommends 20–60 minutes of aerobic activity (1). This can be in one exercise session or could be accomplished intermittently (minimum number of minutes per session is 10 if done intermittently).

| BOX **17.3** | **Example for Metabolic Calculations** |

Client (Anne) characteristics:

$$Age = 29 \text{ years}$$
$$Weight = 150 \text{ lb } (68.2 \text{ kg})$$
$$Height = 69 \text{ in } (1.75 \text{ m})$$
$$\dot{V}O_{2max} = 45 \text{ mL} \cdot kg^{-1} \cdot min^{-1} (12.9 \text{ METS})$$

To calculate $\dot{V}O_2R$, use the following formula:

$$\text{Target } \dot{V}O_2 = [(\text{percentage}) \times (\dot{V}O_{2max} - \dot{V}O_{2rest})] + \dot{V}O_{2rest}$$

Because Anne's $\dot{V}O_{2max}$ puts her just above the 80th percentile (Table 17.3), she is considered to be excellent. As a result, her Personal Trainer decides to prescribe a range of 60%–80% $\dot{V}O_2R$. To determine the target $\dot{V}O_2$ range, the calculations for Anne are as follows:

$$\text{Target } \dot{V}O_2 \text{ (lower end)} = [(0.60) \times (45 - 3.5)] + 3.5 = 28.4 \text{ mL} \cdot kg^{-1} \cdot min^{-1} (8.1 \text{ METS})$$

$$\text{Target } \dot{V}O_2 \text{ (upper end)} = [(0.80) \times (45 - 3.5)] + 3.5 = 36.7 \text{ mL} \cdot kg^{-1} \cdot min^{-1} (10.5 \text{ METS})$$

Thus, the workouts will range between 28.4 and 36.7 mL $\cdot kg^{-1} \cdot min^{-1}$ (8.1–10.5 METS). Anne indicates that using her club membership, she enjoys brisk walking and jogging on the treadmill as well as some stationary cycling and bench stepping. She has had trouble determining the right speed and grade resulting in either an insufficient stress or working too hard, exhausting her in a short period of time.

WALKING

Taking the equation for walking from Box 17.2, the Personal Trainer uses walking on the treadmill as the lower end of the intensity range. The Personal Trainer must determine the grade necessary to reach 28.4 mL $\cdot kg^{-1} \cdot min^{-1}$ as Anne has indicated that she feels comfortable walking at around 4.0 miles/hour (mph) (6.4 kph).

The walking equation is as follows:

$$\dot{V}O_2 \text{ (mL} \cdot kg^{-1} \cdot min^{-1}) = (0.1 \times \text{speed}) + (1.8 \times \text{speed} \times \text{grade}) + 3.5 \text{ mL} \cdot kg^{-1} \cdot min^{-1}$$

Therefore, if Anne enjoys walking at 4.0 mph (6.4 kph), the first thing the Personal Trainer must calculate is the speed in m $\cdot min^{-1}$ (as required in the formula). This can be accomplished by multiplying speed in mph by 26.8 (26.8 m $\cdot min^{-1}$ = 1 mph). Therefore, 4.0 mph (6.4 kph) is 107.2 m $\cdot min^{-1}$.

$$28.4 \text{ mL} \cdot kg^{-1} \cdot min^{-1} = (0.1 \times 107.2) + (1.8 \times 107.2 \times \text{grade}) + 3.5 \text{ mL} \cdot kg^{-1} \cdot min^{-1}$$
$$\text{Grade} = 0.07 = 7\%$$

For the lower end of the intensity range, Anne will walk on the treadmill at 4.0 mph (6.4 kph) with a 7% grade.

RUNNING

When working toward the upper end of the intensity range, Anne will be running on the treadmill. She prefers to have little grade and thus the formula for running will be used to determine the speed. The running equation (Box 17.2) is as follows:

$$\dot{V}O_2 \text{ (mL} \cdot kg^{-1} \cdot min^{-1}) = (0.2 \times \text{speed}) + (0.9 \times \text{speed} \times \text{grade}) + 3.5 \text{ mL} \cdot kg^{-1} \cdot min^{-1}$$

Therefore, if Anne wants to run with a 1% grade (note: 1% = 0.01) on the treadmill, the running formula will be used to determine the speed.

$$36.7 \text{ mL} \cdot kg^{-1} \cdot min^{-1} = (0.2 \times \text{speed}) + (0.9 \times \text{speed} \times 0.01) + 3.5 \text{ mL} \cdot kg^{-1} \cdot min^{-1}$$
$$\text{Speed} = 158.9 \text{ m} \cdot min^{-1} = 5.9 \text{ mph } (9.4 \text{ kph})$$

continued >

Box 17.3 Example for Metabolic Calculations (*Continued*)

CYCLING

Anne will be cycling on a Monark cycle ergometer. As with treadmill exercise, her Personal Trainer will determine the workload at the lower and upper ends of her target range (corresponding with 28.4 and 36.7 mL · kg^{-1} · min^{-1}). The formula for cycling from Box 17.2 is as follows:

$$\dot{V}O_2\,(mL \cdot kg^{-1} \cdot min^{-1}) = \frac{1.8 \times \text{work rate in kgm} \cdot min^{-1}}{\text{Body mass}} + 7$$

The Personal Trainer discussed a preferred cycling cadence with Anne and found that she is most comfortable at 70 revolutions per minute. This will be used to determine the resistance level. First the overall work rate is calculated as follows:

$$28.4\,mL \cdot kg^{-1} \cdot min^{-1} = \frac{1.8 \times \text{work rate in kgm} \cdot min^{-1}}{68.2} + 7$$

Thus for the lower end of the range, the work rate is 811 kgm · min^{-1}. To determine the resistance (weight) to place on the flywheel, the following calculation is used:

Work rate (kgm · min^{-1}) = revolutions per minute × length of flywheel in meters × resistance in kilograms

Because Anne desires to pedal at a rate of 70 revolutions per minute on a Monark bike (whose distance per revolution is a constant of 6 meters), the calculation of resistance is:

$$811\,kgm \cdot min^{-1} = 70\,rpm \times 6\,meters \times resistance$$
$$Resistance = 1.9\,kg$$

For the upper end of the target intensity, the work rate is determined using the following formula:

$$36.7\,mL \cdot kg^{-1} \cdot min^{-1} = \frac{1.8 \times \text{work rate in kgm} \cdot min^{-1}}{68.2} + 7$$

Thus the work rate is 1125 kgm · min^{-1} and then, assuming 70 rpm, the resistance at this level would be 3.0 kg.

$$1125\,kgm \cdot min^{-1} = 70\,rpm \times 6\,meters \times resistance$$
$$Resistance = 2.7\,kg$$

STEPPING

Anne owns a 12-in step (12 in = 30.48 cm = 0.3048 meters) and is interested in knowing how quickly she would need to step to be within her target intensity range. A step is defined as a four-part movement (1):

lifting one leg onto a box, fixed bench or step; pushing with this leg to raise the body; placing the other leg on the box; and stepping down with the first and then second leg in a repetitive fashion.

Once again, her Personal Trainer references the formulas in Box 17.2. For stepping, the formula is as follows:

$$\dot{V}O_2\,(mL \cdot kg^{-1} \cdot min^{-1}) = (0.2 \times frequency) + (1.33 \times 1.8 \times height \times frequency) + 3.5$$

For the lower end of Anne's target range, the frequency would be 26 steps per minute:

$$28.4\,mL \cdot kg^{-1} \cdot min^{-1} = (0.2 \times frequency) + (1.33 \times 1.8 \times 0.3048 \times frequency) + 3.5$$

For the upper end of Anne's target range, the frequency would be 36 steps per minute:

$$36.7\,mL \cdot kg^{-1} \cdot min^{-1} = (0.2 \times frequency) + (1.33 \times 1.8 \times 0.3048 \times frequency) + 3.5$$

Anne now has some starting points for her exercise. Initially she can begin toward the lower end of the range. Over time, she will progress toward the higher end of her intensity range. Heart rate and ratings of perceived exertion will be used to fine-tune this prescription.

For Personal Trainers interested in more details on the metabolic equations, please see Chapter 7 in the *ACSM's Guidelines for Exercise Testing and Prescription,* 8th edition (1).

TABLE 17.4	**APPROXIMATE ENERGY REQUIREMENTS IN METS FOR HORIZONTAL AND GRADE WALKING**					
	mph	1.7	2.0	2.5	3.0	3.4	3.75
% Grade	m · min^{-1}	45.6	53.6	67.0	80.4	91.2	100.5
0		2.3	2.5	2.9	3.3	3.6	3.9
2.5		2.9	3.2	3.8	4.3	4.8	5.2
5.0		3.5	3.9	4.6	5.4	5.9	6.5
7.5		4.1	4.6	5.5	6.4	7.1	7.8
10.0		4.6	5.3	6.3	7.4	8.3	9.1
12.5		5.2	6.0	7.2	8.5	9.5	10.4
15.0		5.8	6.6	8.1	9.5	10.6	11.7
17.5		6.4	7.3	8.9	10.5	11.8	12.9
20.0		7.0	8.0	9.8	11.6	13.0	14.2
22.5		7.6	8.7	10.6	12.6	14.2	15.5
25.0		8.2	9.4	11.5	13.6	15.3	16.8

From American College of Sports Medicine. *ACSM's Guidelines for Exercise Testing and Prescription*. 7th ed. Baltimore: Lippincott Williams & Wilkins; 2006. Table D-2.

TABLE 17.5	**APPROXIMATE ENERGY REQUIREMENTS IN METS FOR HORIZONTAL AND GRADE JOGGING/RUNNING**					
	mph	5	6	7	7.5	8	9	10
% Grade	m · min^{-1}	134	161	188	201	214	241	268
0		8.6	10.2	11.7	12.5	13.3	14.8	16.3
2.5		9.5	11.2	12.9	13.8	14.7	16.3	18.0
5.0		10.3	12.3	14.1	15.1	16.1	17.9	19.7
7.5		11.2	13.3	15.3	16.4	17.4	19.4	
10.0		12.0	14.3	16.5	17.7	18.8		
12.5		12.9	15.4	17.7	19.0			
15.0		13.8	16.4	18.9				

From American College of Sports Medicine. *ACSM's Guidelines for Exercise Testing and Prescription*. 7th ed. Baltimore: Lippincott Williams & Wilkins; 2006. Table D-3.

TABLE 17.6	**APPROXIMATE ENERGY REQUIREMENTS IN METS DURING LEG AND CYCLE ERGOMETRY**					
		Power Output (kg · m · min^{-1} and W)					
Body Weight		300	450	600	750	900	1050	1200 (kg · m · min^{-1})
kg	lb	50	75	100	125	150	175	200 (W)
50	110	5.1	6.6	8.2	9.7	11.3	12.8	14.3
60	132	4.6	5.9	7.1	8.4	9.7	11.0	12.3
70	154	4.2	5.3	6.4	7.5	8.6	9.7	10.8
80	176	3.9	4.9	5.9	6.8	7.8	8.8	9.7
90	198	3.7	4.6	5.4	6.3	7.1	8.0	8.9
100	220	3.5	4.3	5.1	5.9	6.6	7.4	8.2

From American College of Sports Medicine. *ACSM's Guidelines for Exercise Testing and Prescription*. 7th ed. Baltimore: Lippincott Williams & Wilkins; 2006. Table D-4.

TABLE 17.7	APPROXIMATE ENERGY REQUIREMENTS IN METS DURING ARM ERGOMETRY					
Body Weight		Power Output (kg · m · min^{-1} and W)					
kg	lb	150	300	450	600	750	900 (kg . m . min^{-1})
		25	50	75	100	125	150 (W)
50	110	3.6	6.1	8.7	11.3	13.9	16.4
60	132	3.1	5.3	7.4	9.6	11.7	13.9
70	154	2.8	4.7	6.5	8.3	10.2	12.0
80	176	2.6	4.2	5.8	7.4	9.0	10.6
90	198	2.4	3.9	5.3	6.7	8.1	9.6
100	220	2.3	3.6	4.9	6.1	7.4	8.7

From American College of Sports Medicine. *ACSM's Guidelines for Exercise Testing and Prescription*. 7th ed. Baltimore: Lippincott Williams & Wilkins; 2006. Table D-5.

Sedentary individuals should start exercising gradually. Short bouts (i.e., 5 minutes) of low-intensity exercise may be used until more extended periods of time can be completed without excessive fatigue. The rate of progression will vary depending on the health status and age of the individual.

Intensity of the exercise is a consideration when determining the duration. For more fit individuals, the intensity level may necessarily be higher than used with a sedentary individual because the threshold for cardiorespiratory benefits will be higher. Risk (1) does increase with higher-intensity exercise (both cardiovascular and orthopedic). For most individuals engaging in exercise to improve health and fitness, a prescription targeting 77%–90% of maximal HR or 60%–80% of HR reserve for 20–30 minutes is sufficient. This time frame does not include warm-up and cool-down, both of which should be done in addition to the time spent at the target exercise program (1).

EXERCISE FREQUENCY

Exercise frequency is the final component in a complete exercise program. For sedentary individuals, incorporating even a couple of days per week can initiate improvements in cardiorespiratory fitness (2). The optimal frequency appears to be 3–5 days per week (1,4). As with intensity, although additional benefits may be achieved above the upper end of the target range, the risk of injuries also

TABLE 17.8	APPROXIMATE ENERGY REQUIREMENTS IN METS DURING STAIR STEPPING					
Step Height		Stepping Rate per Minute					
In	m	20	22	24	26	28	30
4	0.102	3.5	3.8	4.0	4.3	4.5	4.8
6	0.152	4.2	4.6	4.9	5.2	5.5	5.8
8	0.203	4.9	5.3	5.7	6.1	6.5	6.9
10	0.254	5.6	6.1	6.5	7.0	7.5	7.9
12	0.305	6.3	6.8	7.4	7.9	8.4	9.0
14	0.356	7.0	7.6	8.2	8.8	9.4	10.0
16	0.406	7.7	8.4	9.0	9.7	10.4	11.1
18	0.457	8.4	9.1	9.9	10.6	11.4	12.1

From American College of Sports Medicine. *ACSM's Guidelines for Exercise Testing and Prescription*. 7th ed. Baltimore: Lippincott Williams & Wilkins; 2006. Table D-6.

BOX **17.4** **Example for Use of MET Tables**

Client (Joe) characteristics:

$$Age = 40 \text{ years}$$
$$Weight = 175 \text{ lb } (80 \text{ kg})$$
$$Height = 70 \text{ in } (1.78 \text{ m})$$
$$\dot{V}O_{2max} = 45 \text{ mL} \cdot \text{kg}^{-1} \cdot \text{min}^{-1}$$

To calculate $\dot{V}O_2R$, use the following formula:

$$Target \ \dot{V}O_2 = [(\text{percentage}) \times (\dot{V}O_{2max} - \dot{V}O_{2rest})] + \dot{V}O_{2rest}$$

Because Joe's $\dot{V}O_{2max}$ puts him at approximately the 75th percentile (Table 17.3), he is considered to be in the good category. As a result, his Personal Trainer decides to prescribe a range of 60%–75% $\dot{V}O_2R$. To determine the target $\dot{V}O_2$ range, the calculations for Joe are as follows:

$$Target \ \dot{V}O_2 \ (\text{lower end}) = [(0.60) \times (45 - 3.5)] + 3.5 = 28.4 \text{ mL} \cdot \text{kg}^{-1} \cdot \text{min}^{-1} \ (8.1 \text{ METS})$$
$$Target \ \dot{V}O_2 \ (\text{upper end}) = [(0.75) \times (45 - 3.5)] + 3.5 = 34.6 \text{ mL} \cdot \text{kg}^{-1} \cdot \text{min}^{-1} \ (9.9 \ (\text{METS})$$

Thus, the workouts will range between 28.4 and 34.6 mL $\cdot$ kg^{-1} $\cdot$ min^{-1} (8.1 – 9.9 METS). Joe indicates that he wants to use the treadmill as well as a stationary bike.

Joe's Personal Trainer will use Tables 17.4, 17.5, and 17.6. To use these tables, the Personal Trainer must convert the oxygen consumption from units of mL $\cdot$ kg^{-1} $\cdot$ min^{-1} to METs. This is accomplished by dividing the lower and upper ends of the target zone by 3.5 as shown below.

$$28.4 \text{ mL} \cdot \text{kg}^{-1} \cdot \text{min}^{-1}/3.5 = 8.1 \text{ METS}$$
$$34.6 \text{ mL} \cdot \text{kg}^{-1} \cdot \text{min}^{-1}/3.5 = 9.9 \text{ METS}$$

Determination of a walking intensity on the lower end of the range (~8.1 METs) is possible by using Table 17.4. Note that many options are available close to the 8.1-MET target including walking at 1.7 mph (2.7 km/hour) with 25% grade (8.2 MET level) and walking at 2.5 mph (4 km/hour) with a 15% grade (8.1 METs). This would be a rather awkward workload due to the very steep grade. Therefore, the Personal Trainer would discuss with Joe various options. Joe indicated that he likes walking on incline when exercising on the treadmill and thus the Personal Trainer suggests 3.4 mph with a 10% grade.

For the upper end of the workload range (9.9 METs), Joe would rather jog. He prefers to jog on a level treadmill. Using Table 17.5, the Personal Trainer sees that 6 mph (9.6 km/hour) with no grade will be 10.2 METs. Joe will be instructed to monitor his heart rate and RPE as well to make adjustments to these workloads as he becomes accustomed to the exercise.

Joe also requested guidance on determining appropriate settings on a stationary bike. To use Table 17.6 (leg cycle ergometry), the Personal Trainer must know Joe's body weight. Body weight is 175 lb (80 kg). Going across the row for 80 kg in Table 17.6, the workloads approximating 8.1 METs and 9.9 METs are slightly over 900 kgm $\cdot$ min^{-1} (150 W) and 1200 kgm $\cdot$ min^{-1} (200 W). These settings will provide Joe with guidance on what workloads to begin his exercise.

increases. Admittedly, individuals focused on competition or performance will likely train six or more days per week. Different goals will require different exercise programs and thus involve different associated risks. ACSM suggests that 3 days per week is sufficient to improve maximal oxygen consumption when exercising at 77%–90% of maximal HR or 60%–80% of HR reserve (1). If weight loss is a goal, then exercise frequency may need to be more frequent (3). Similarly, if the exercise intensity is held at the lower end of the target range, then the frequency can be increased (1). In some situations, for deconditioned individuals, multiple short daily exercise sessions may be more appropriate (1).

TABLE 17.9	CATEGORY AND CATEGORY-RATIO SCALES FOR RATINGS OF PERCEIVED EXERTION (CATEGORY SCALE) AND FOR SENSATIONS, EXPERIENCES AND FEELINGS, INCLUDING PAIN (CATEGORY-RATIO SCALE)	
Category Scale	**Category-Ratio Scale**	**Descriptor**
6 No exertion at all	0 Nothing at all	
7 Extremely light	0.3	
8	0.5 Extremely weak	Just noticeable
9 Very light	0.7	
10	1 Very weak	
11 Light	1.5	
12	2 Weak	Light
13 Somewhat hard	2.5	
14	3 Moderate	
15 Hard (heavy)	4	
16	5 Strong	Heavy
17 Very hard	6	
18	7 Very strong	
19 Extremely hard	8	
20 Maximal exertion	9	
	10 Extremely strong	"Maximal"
	11	
	⸮	
	• Absolute maximum	Highest possible

Copyright Gunnar Borg. Reproduced with permission. For correct use of the Borg scales, it is necessary to follow the administration and instructions given in Borg G. *Borg's Perceived Exertion and Pain Scales*. Champaign (IL): Human Kinetics; 1998.

CALORIES EXPENDED: A SUMMARY OF THE ENDURANCE PHASE

Selection of mode, intensity, duration, and frequency determines the calories expended during the activity. This caloric expenditure can be used to provide an overall summary of the workout. ACSM recommends expending 150–400 calories in physical activity each day (1). Previously sedentary individuals will begin on the lower end of the range and progress upward. Expenditures of approximately 1,000 calories per week are associated with decreases in the risk of all-cause mortality (1). For weight loss, overweight and obese adults should strive toward expending 2,000 calories per week or more (3).

> *Selection of mode, intensity, duration, and frequency determines the calories expended during the activity.*

Some shortcomings of caloric expenditure estimates include coordination and skill influences. An experienced swimmer, for example, will expend less energy to swim the same pace as someone with inefficient stroke patterns. Even though at a similar pace, the calories expended by the inexperienced swimmer will be much higher than those expended by the experienced athlete. Thus, interindividual differences limit the precision of this estimation and are related to classifications of exercises discussed previously in this chapter. Realizing the limitations, the Personal Trainer may use the following equation to approximate the number of calories expended per minute of a given activity (1):

$$(\text{METs} \times 3.5 \times \text{body weight in kilograms})/200 = \text{calories per minute}$$

The attractive aspect of using this approach is the inclusion of both time and the intensity of the prescribed exercise mode. For example, if a client runs on the treadmill at 0% grade (level) and 7 miles/hour (mph) (11.2 km/hour) for 45 minutes, the Personal Trainer can "summarize" the workout by using the formula for calories per minute. Using Table 17.5, the MET level for 7 mph (11.2 km/hour) and 0% grade is 11.7 METS. If the client weighs 150 lb (68.2 kg), then the number of calories expended for the total workout can be determined as follows:

$$(11.7 \times 3.5 \times 68.2)/200 = 14 \text{ calories per minute}$$

$$14 \text{ calories per minute} \times 45 \text{ minutes} = 630 \text{ calories for the workout}$$

Tracking the calories expended can be helpful because the time, intensity, and mode of exercise are all factors in the outcome. Also, for clients focusing on weight loss, it is very helpful to be able to calculate the number of calories expended in a given activity.

WEEKLY SUMMARY FOR THE ENDURANCE PHASE

Use of MET levels can also be used to provide a weekly summary. In the updated recommendations for adults from ACSM and the American Heart Association, a minimum goal is 450–750 $\text{MET} \cdot \text{min}^{-1} \cdot \text{week}^{-1}$ (5). For example, if a person walks 30 minutes on 5 days of the week:

$$3 \text{ mph (4.83 kph) is equal to 3.3 METS}$$

$$30 \text{ minutes at this intensity} = 3.3 \text{ METS} \times 30 \text{ minutes} = 99 \text{ MET} \cdot \text{min}^{-1}$$

$$\text{For the week (5 days of activity)} = 99 \times 5 = 495 \text{ MET} \cdot \text{min}^{-1} \text{ for the week}$$

For someone exercising at a higher intensity, 5 mph (8.05 kph) jogging for 20 minutes 3 days per week:

$$5 \text{ mph (8.05 kph) is equal to 8.6 METS}$$

$$20 \text{ minutes at this intensity} = 8.6 \times 20 = 172 \text{ MET} \cdot \text{min}^{-1}$$

$$\text{For the week (3 days of activity)} = 172 \times 3 = 516 \text{ MET} \cdot \text{min}^{-1} \text{ for the week}$$

This method is also useful when individuals combine various activities of different intensity levels. If a client enjoyed walking and jogging, then a total could also be achieved. For example, 2 days per week walking 3 mph (4.83 kph) for 30 minutes and 2 days per week jogging 5 mph (8.05 kph) would result in a total of 542 $\text{MET} \cdot \text{min}^{-1}$ for the week, determined as follows:

$$30 \text{ minutes at 3 mph (4.83 kph) (3.3 METS)} = 3.3 \text{ METS} \times 30 \text{ minutes} = 99 \text{ MET} \cdot \text{min}^{-1}$$

$$\text{For the week (2 days of activity)} = 99 \times 2 = 198 \text{ MET} \cdot \text{min}^{-1} \text{ for the week}$$

PLUS

$$20 \text{ minutes at 5 mph (8.6 METS)} = 8.6 \times 20 = 172 \text{ MET} \cdot \text{min}^{-1}$$

$$\text{For the week (2 days of activity)} = 172 \times 2 = 344 \text{ MET} \cdot \text{min}^{-1} \text{ for the week}$$

Some MET values are shown in Tables 17.4 through 17.8 for select activities. For a more extensive list, please see the Compendium of Physical Activities (2) or http://prevention.sph.sc.edu/tools/compendium.htm. Note that the MET values in various tables may differ slightly as these are approximations.

Cool-Down

The cool-down is a transition from the higher intensity of the endurance phase back toward resting levels. The cool-down allows HR, blood pressure, and respiration rate to shift downward and back toward resting levels. By allowing a gradual progression toward resting rather than abruptly stopping exercise, the client will also avoid postexercise hypotension (low blood pressure) and resulting dizziness (due to lack of blood flow back to the heart and brain because of blood pooling in the legs). A gradual decrease in intensity also helps dissipate body heat, promotes lactate removal (metabolic end-product that the body can actually break down for fuel during low levels of activity rather than being inactive), and attenuates the rise in catecholamines (hormones released that increase HR and blood pressure), which often follows exercise (1).

> *The cool-down allows HR, blood pressure, and respiration rate to shift downward and back toward resting levels.*

The cool-down period is one of gradual recovery from the endurance phase of the workout. As with the warm-up, approximately 10 minutes of activities of diminished intensity is appropriate (1). For higher-intensity exercise, a longer cool-down may be warranted. For example, to return to the client who uses brisk walking as an exercise mode for the endurance phase, an appropriate cool-down would include slow walking for 5 minutes followed by 5 minutes of total body stretches.

SAMPLE CARDIOVASCULAR TRAINING PROGRAMS

In the following pages, examples of various cardiorespiratory endurance programs are presented. For each, an overall scheme of training progression is shown for an apparently healthy client. Use of the terms to describe the program state—beginner, intermediate, and established—is somewhat subjective. For some individuals, the initial beginner stage may present too much of a challenge. If so, starting out with 5- to 10-minute bouts of exercise as tolerated may be more appropriate. The focus is not on starting aggressively or achieving target goals quickly, but rather to gradually increase the overall workload to promote adherence. Progression should be individualized on the basis of health status, age, individual goals, and current functional capacity (1).

For each of the stages, a range rather than a single number is included for frequency, intensity, and duration. The role of a Personal Trainer is to assist the client with the appropriate balance based on individual responses. Frequency of exercise progresses gradually over the 6-month period outlined from 3 days per week up to a target of 3–5 days per week. Intensity increases from relatively low to a target of 70%–85% HR reserve. By slowly increasing the intensity, the client is able to adapt to the higher levels of exercise without becoming discouraged or experiencing retrogression (i.e., a reversal of gains due to excessive overload). The duration of the exercise session also increases in small steps to allow for appropriate adaptations.

Fitness Gains for Beginners

Tables 17.10 through 17.12 include examples of training programs for various types of activities for a person who has not been previously active. Table 17.10 provides a sample workout schedule for a walking program. Recall that walking is a Group A activity due to the relative ease in maintaining a constant intensity. Table 17.11 provides a sample workout schedule for a swimming program. Swimming is an example of a Group C activity due to the skill level required to maintain a constant intensity for a sufficient period of time. Table 17.12 is a mixture of activities, which may be available at a health club. Note the sequence in time, intensity, and frequency as well a progression

TABLE 17.10	SAMPLE WALKING PROGRAM			
Fitness Level	**Time Point**	**Warm-Up**	**Workout**	**Cool-Down**
Beginner	First week	Slow easy walking pace and gentle body stretches for 5 min	Walk at a pace that gives a fairly light level of exertion (RPE 11-12) for 10–15 min (3 d/wk)	Slow easy walking pace for 5 min
	Later weeks	Slow easy walking pace and gentle body stretches for 10 min	Walk at a pace that gives a moderate level of exertion (RPE 12-13) for 20–25 min (3-4 d/wk)	Slow easy walking pace for 10 min
Intermediate	Initial weeks	Slow easy walking pace and gentle body stretches for 10 min	Walk at a pace that feels somewhat hard (RPE 13-14) for 20–25 min (3-4 d/wk)	Easy walking pace for 10 min
	Middle weeks	Slow easy walking pace and gentle body stretches for 10 min	Walk at a pace that feels somewhat hard to hard (RPE 13-15) for 25–30 min (3-5 d/wk)	Easy walking pace for 10 min
	Later weeks	Slow easy walking pace and gentle body stretches for 10 min	Walk at a pace that feels hard (RPE 15-16) for 30–35 min (3-5 d/wk)	Easy walking pace for 10 min
Established	Continue	Slow easy walking pace and gentle body stretches for 10 min	Walk at a pace that feels hard (15-16) for 30–40 min (3-5 d/wk)	Easy walking pace for 10 min

Reprinted with permission from Bushman B, Young JC. *Action Plan for Menopause*. Champaign (IL): Human Kinetics; 2005. p. 142.

in the different types of activities. Including new modes of exercise can provide much-appreciated variety but should be introduced gradually so that appropriate adjustments can be made (i.e., appropriate overload).

Fitness Gains and Weight Loss

Clients who have not been active and are striving to achieve a healthier body weight often consult Personal Trainers. The ACSM Position Stand, "Appropriate Intervention Strategies for Weight Loss and Prevention of Weight Regain for Adults" (3) indicates that to assist in weight loss, increasing activity levels to 45–60 minutes per day may be required for overweight adults. In Box 17.5, an example is given for a male who is sedentary and overweight.

IMPLEMENTATION OF CARDIOVASCULAR TRAINING PROGRAMS

Implementation of effective cardiovascular endurance training programs requires the Personal Trainer to have knowledge of the current scientific basis of exercise. This chapter has reviewed in detail the ACSM guidelines regarding intensity, frequency, and duration. These guidelines provide a framework rather than a rigid checklist. The Personal Trainer must evaluate each client individually. This includes an understanding of health status and cardiovascular risks (see Chapter 13). Individual fitness assessments (see Chapter 14) provide baseline information, which is used to determine an appropriate initial level of exercise. Creating the exercise program is like a master chef. Unlike a novice,

> *Implementation of effective cardiovascular endurance training programs requires the Personal Trainer to have knowledge of the current scientific basis of exercise.*

TABLE 17.11	**SAMPLE SWIMMING PROGRAM**			
Fitness Level	**Time Point**	**Warm-Up**	**Workout**	**Cool-Down**
Beginner	First week	Gentle shoulder and arm stretches, easy swimming pace for 5 min (change strokes as needed)	Use kickboard and swim laps (alternating strokes and type of kicking) at a fairly light level of exertion (RPE 11-12) for 10–15 min (3 d/wk)	Easy swim pace (use favorite stroke) for 5 min, stretch calf and shoulder muscles
	Later weeks	Shoulder and arm stretches, easy pace swim and kick (change strokes and kicks as needed) for 10 min	Use kickboard, pull buoy, and swim laps (alternating strokes and type of kicking) at a moderate level of exertion (RPE 12-13) for 20–25 min (3–4 d/wk)	Easy swim pace (use 2 favorite strokes) for 10 min, stretch calf and shoulder muscles Total distance: approximately 500 yd (depends on skill level)
Intermediate	Initial weeks	Shoulder and arm stretches, easy pace swim and kick (change strokes and kicks as needed) for 10 min	Use kickboard, pull buoy, and swim laps (alternating strokes and type of kicking) at a pace that feels somewhat hard (RPE 13-14) for 20–25 min (3–4 d/wk)	Easy swim and pull for 10 min, stretch calf and shoulder muscles
	Middle weeks	Shoulder and arm stretches, easy pace swim and kick (change strokes and kicks as needed) for 10 min	Use kickboard, pull buoy, and swim laps (alternating strokes and type of kicking), keeping RI at :15-:20, at a pace that feels somewhat hard to hard (RPE 13-15) for 25–30 min (3–5 d/wk)	Easy swim and pull for 10 min, stretch calf and shoulder muscles
	Later weeks	Shoulder and arm stretches, easy pace swim and kick (change strokes and kicks as needed) for 10 min	Use kickboard, pull buoy, and swim laps (alternating strokes and type of kicking), keeping RI at :10-:15, at a pace that feels hard (RPE 15-16) for 30–35 min (3–5 d/wk)	Easy swim and pull for 10 min, stretch calf and shoulder muscles Total distance: 900–1350 yd (depends on skill level)
Established	Continue	Shoulder and arm stretches, easy pace swim and kick (change strokes and kicks as needed) for 10 min	Swim, kick, pull, keeping RI at :10-:15, at a pace that feels hard (RPE 15-16) for 30–40 min; use repeated sets, ascending, descending, or Fartlek swims (3–5 d/wk)	Easy swim and pull for 10 min, stretch calf and shoulder muscles Total distance: 1500–2000 yd (depends on skill level)

Reprinted with permission from Bushman B, Young JC. *Action Plan for Menopause.* Champaign (IL): Human Kinetics; 2005. p. 144.

Note: For the workout, those with more advanced swimming skill can alternate strokes (freestyle, backstroke, breaststroke) and add repeated sets of swims, pulls, and kicks. For example, intermediate-skill swimmers: swim 2 × 50, 2 × 100 with RI of :15-:20; established swimmers: swim 4 × 100 with :10-:15 RI, kick 4 × 75 with :10-:15 RI, pull 6 × 50 with :10-:15 RI.

TABLE 17.12	SAMPLE CROSS-TRAINING PROGRAM AT A HEALTH CLUB			
Fitness Level	**Time Point**	**Warm-Up**	**Workout**	**Cool-Down**
Beginner	Early weeks	Slow easy walking pace and gentle body stretches for 5 min	Pick one activity each day at RPE 11-12 (fairly light level of exertion) for 10–15 min (3–4 d/wk): • Walking on the treadmill • Stationary bike	Slow easy walking pace for 5 min
	Later weeks	Slow easy walking pace and gentle body stretches for 10 min	Pick one activity each day at RPE 12-13 (moderate level of exertion) for 20–25 min (3–4 d/wk): • Brisk walking on the treadmill • Stationary bike • Stair stepper	Slow easy walking pace for 10 min
Intermediate	Early weeks	Slow easy walking pace and gentle body stretches for 10 min	Pick one activity each day at RPE 13-14 (somewhat hard level of exertion) for 20–25 min (3–4 d/wk): • Brisk walking or jogging on the treadmill • Stationary bike • Stair stepper • Elliptical trainer • Nordic ski machine	Easy walking pace for 10 min
	Middle weeks	Slow easy walking pace and gentle body stretches for 10 min	Pick one activity each day at RPE 13-15 (somewhat hard to hard level of exertion) for 25–30 min (3–5 d/wk): • Brisk walking or jogging on the treadmill • Stationary bike • Stair stepper • Elliptical trainer • Nordic ski machine • Floor or step aerobics class	Easy walking pace for 10 min
	Later weeks	Slow easy walking pace and gentle body stretches for 10 min	Pick one activity each day at RPE 15-16 (hard level of exertion) for 30–35 min (3–5 d/wk): • Brisk walking or jogging on the treadmill • Stationary bike • Elliptical trainer • Stair stepper • Nordic ski machine • Floor or step aerobics class • Spinning class	Easy walking pace for 10 min
Established	Continue	Slow easy walking pace and gentle body stretches for 10 min	Pick an exercise that provides you with an intensity that feels hard (15-16) for 30–40 min (3–5 d/wk)	Easy walking pace for 10 min

Reprinted with permission from Bushman B, Young JC. *Action Plan for Menopause*. Champaign (IL): Human Kinetics; 2005. p. 145–146.

BOX **17.5** **Example for Obese Client**

Client (Bob) characteristics:

$$\text{Age} = 35 \text{ years}$$
$$\text{Weight} = 210 \text{ lb } (95.5 \text{ kg})$$
$$\text{Height} = 71 \text{ in } (1.80 \text{ m})$$

Bob has led an inactive lifestyle and desk/office job and desires to start an exercise program to assist him with his weight-loss goals. He is consulting a dietician regarding better food choices and realizes the importance of exercise in helping him lose the weight and in maintaining the weight loss. Bob's Personal Trainer will develop a comprehensive program, including cardiorespiratory endurance training, resistance training, and flexibility. Listed below is the starting point for Bob's cardiorespiratory training program.

The Personal Trainer has reviewed Bob's health history and finds that, other than his weight (which for his height results in a body mass index of 29.5), which places him in the overweight classification and his sedentary lifestyle, he has no other risk factors for coronary artery disease. With this in mind, his ACSM risk stratification is "moderate risk" (see Table 13.1 and Figure 13.5) so beginning a moderate-intensity program is appropriate.

Using a cardiorespiratory fitness assessment (see examples in Chapter 14), the Personal Trainer estimates Bob's $\dot{V}O_{2max}$ to be 39 mL $\cdot$ kg^{-1} $\cdot$ min^{-1} ("poor" category according to Table 17.3). Bob's target range ($\dot{V}O_2R$ method) will be lower than previous examples in this chapter because of his lower fitness level. The Personal Trainer decides to start with 45%–60% $\dot{V}O_2R$. This is calculated as follows:

$$\text{Target } \dot{V}O_2 \text{ (lower end)} = [(0.45) \times (39 - 3.5)] + 3.5 = 19.5 \text{ mL} \cdot \text{kg}^{-1} \cdot \text{min}^{-1} \text{ (5.6 METS)}$$

$$\text{Target } \dot{V}O_2 \text{ (upper end)} = [(0.60) \times (39 - 3.5)] + 3.5 = 24.8 \text{ mL} \cdot \text{kg}^{-1} \cdot \text{min}^{-1} \text{ (7.1 METS)}$$

Getting an idea of a starting speed for treadmill walking can be done by consulting Table 17.4. To use this table, oxygen consumption values in mL $\cdot$ kg^{-1} $\cdot$ min^{-1} must be converted to METs (divide each by 3.5). This results in a range of 5.6–7.1 METs. Going to Table 17.4, the Personal Trainer selects 3.0 miles/hour (mph) (4.8 km/hour) with a 5% grade as a starting point for the endurance phase of the exercise session.

To adjust the workout based on Bob's responses, the Personal Trainer has determined a heart rate range (using HR reserve method). HR_{max} will be estimated from Bob's age (220 − age = 220 − 35 = 185). Bob's HR_{rest} is 70. To determine the lower end of the heart rate range, the following has been calculated:

$$\text{Target HR (lower end of range)} = [(0.45) \times (HR_{max} - HR_{rest})] + HR_{rest}$$

$$\text{Target HR (lower end of range)} = [(0.45) \times (185 - 70)] + 70 = 122$$

To determine the upper end of the heart rate range, the following has been calculated:

$$\text{Target HR (upper end of range)} = [(0.60) \times (HR_{max} - HR_{rest})] + HR_{rest}$$

$$\text{Target HR (upper end of range)} = [(0.60 \times (185 - 70)] + 70 = 139$$

Bob's Personal Trainer will use this information to make adjustments to Bob's exercise prescription.

After an initial warm-up, Bob begins walking on the treadmill at 3 mph (4.8 km/hour) with a 5% grade. Using a heart rate monitor to assist with tracking intensity, the Personal Trainer notes that Bob's heart rate is stabilizing at around 132 beats per minute. Noting that this is toward the upper end of the target heart rate range (122–139 beats per minute), the Personal Trainer lowers the grade to 3% and finds that Bob's heart rate responds by lowering to 126 beats per minute. The use of heart rate along with the predetermined workload allows for a well-controlled exercise prescription. Subjectively, Bob can also use the rating of perceived exertion and talk test.

Initially Bob will walk only for 10 minutes. Establishing a baseline level of fitness and a pattern of activity is the goal for new exercisers. Bob's Personal Trainer will make small weekly adjustments to continue to provide an appropriate overload. Using Table 15.5 can be very helpful in providing appropriate exercise program progression.

A long-term goal for Bob to promote sustained weight loss will be to incorporate 200–300 minutes of physical activity each week (3) into his lifestyle. A regular exercise program, in addition to positive nutritional changes, is the key to Bob's weight-loss goals as well as his ability to keep the weight off.

who would be tied to a recipe, the master chef is able to take knowledge of various ingredients to create individualized, appealing dishes. In a similar manner, a qualified Personal Trainer does not try to fit all clients into a single mode (i.e., recipe approach) but rather has a solid understanding of the ingredients (i.e., mode, frequency, intensity, and duration) and is able to customize the combination of those ingredients for the benefit of the client.

SUMMARY

When considering the balance of intensity, duration, and frequency, the Personal Trainer must take into account the goals of the client (e.g., general fitness, weight loss, competition), life situations (e.g., work schedule, availability of exercise time), and client preferences. Cardiorespiratory endurance training is an essential part of a client's exercise program. Other important components include resistance and flexibility training, which are detailed in Chapters 16 and 18. A cardiorespiratory endurance training session includes three basic components: warm-up, endurance phase, and cool-down. A cardiorespiratory endurance program includes consideration of intensity, duration, and frequency. The Personal Trainer must determine the appropriate balance of these three factors based on the client's current health status and fitness goals.

REFERENCES

1. American College of Sports Medicine. *ACSM's Guidelines for Exercise Testing and Prescription.* 8th ed. Philadelphia: Lippincott Williams & Wilkins; 2010.
2. American College of Sports Medicine. *ACSM's Resource Manual for Guidelines for Exercise Testing and Prescription.* 6th ed. Philadelphia: Lippincott Williams & Wilkins; 2010.
3. American College of Sports Medicine. Position stand: appropriate intervention strategies for weight loss and prevention of weight regain for adults. *Med Sci Sports Exerc.* 2001;33:2145–56.
4. American College of Sports Medicine. Position stand: the recommended quantity and quality of exercise for developing and maintaining cardiorespiratory and muscular fitness, and flexibility in health adults. *Med Sci Sports Exerc.* 1998;30:975–91.
5. Haskell WL, Lee IM, Pate RR, et al. Physical activity and public health: Updated recommendations for adults from the American College of Sports Medicine and the American Heart Association. *Med Sci Sports Exerc.* 2007;39(8):1423–34.
6. Nelson ME, Rejeski WJ, Blair SN, et al. Physical activity and public health in older adults: Recommendations from the American College of Sports Medicine and the American Heart Association. *Med Sci Sports Exerc.* 2007;39(8):1435–45.
7. Persinger R, Foster C, Gibson M, et al. Consistency of the talk test for exercise prescription. *Med Sci Sports Exerc.* 2004;36:1632–6.
8. U.S. Department of Health and Human Services. [Internet] 2008 physical activity guidelines for Americans. ODPHP Publication No. U0036, 2008 [cited 2008 Nov 12]. Available from www.health.gov/paguidelines

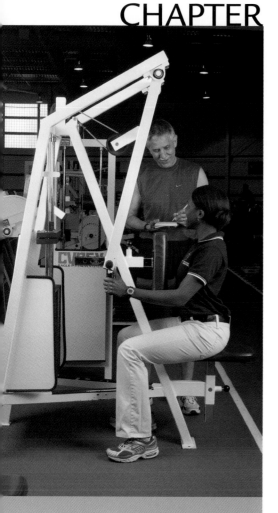

CHAPTER

18

Guidelines for Designing Flexibility Programs

OBJECTIVES

- Introduce flexibility as a health-related dimension of fitness
- Present three basic types of stretching (static, dynamic, proprioceptive neuromuscular facilitation)
- Discuss concepts and current controversy surrounding stretching
- Outline factors that influence flexibility and the response to training
- Suggest safe and effective stretches to perform
- Provide sample flexibility programs

Flexibility refers to the degree to which a joint moves throughout a normal, pain-free range of motion (ROM). As most physical activities and sports consist of numerous multijoint movements, it is essential that musculoskeletal function not be compromised by inadequate flexibility. Stretching is the method used most commonly to increase joint ROM. In its current Position Stand on exercises to develop and maintain fitness and flexibility in adults, the American College of Sports Medicine recommended the inclusion of general stretching exercises emphasizing the major skeletal muscle groups at least 2–3 days a week (3). Like body composition, cardiorespiratory fitness, or muscular strength, flexibility is classified as a health-related dimension of fitness (13). This means that flexibility contributes to an overall improved quality of life in athletes and the general public alike.

The purpose of this chapter is to present flexibility as an essential ingredient of health-related fitness and to provide Personal Trainers with a basic understanding of how to properly incorporate flexibility training into the exercise programs of healthy individuals.

DETERMINANTS OF FLEXIBILITY

Hamill and Knutzen (28) suggest that several factors determine flexibility. These factors include joint structure, health of soft tissue around the joint, length of antagonist muscles, and temperature of the tissues being stretched in addition to the viscoelastic ("rubber band–like") properties of the tissues surrounding the joint. Not surprisingly then, flexibility is largely determined by how well these factors facilitate movement. To better understand the importance of these factors, study Figure 18.1 carefully. Figure 18.1 depicts an anterior view (*left panel*) and cross-sectional view (*right panel*) of a typical joint—the human knee.

Notice that the knee is padded with fat and is secured into place by ligaments. These tissues influence knee ROM both at the joint itself and elsewhere in the lower extremity. There are several examples of this influence to consider. For example, tightness of the ligaments as illustrated in Figure 18.1 or excessive fat surrounding the thigh could inhibit knee ROM during flexion. In fact, one belief about bodybuilders is that they are "muscle bound" and possess a more limited joint ROM as a result of the additional bulk. This is true to a certain extent because thick skeletal muscles can certainly limit ROM. Although flexibility is the theme of this chapter, it is important to understand that it is only one component of health-related fitness. If the training demands of an athlete or the natural (healthy) body composition of a client predispose them toward muscle bulk rather than flexibility, a more limited joint ROM may be tolerable.

Because muscles bring about bone movement, the reader can also see from Figure 18.1 that contraction of the quadriceps femoris will produce leg extension if the knee is bent at the start of the movement. However, a tight quadriceps femoris (perhaps as a result of soreness or poor conditioning) can restrict leg extension and limit flexibility. Notice too from Figure 18.1 that the joint is restricted by the very architecture of the bones themselves. Leg extension is limited by what are termed "bony blocks," which consist of nothing more than the ends of the femur and tibia resisting hyperextension during full leg extension brought about by the quadriceps femoris. Of course,

> *It is also important to understand that injury, disease, and poor soft tissue integrity can also contribute to hypermobility or a condition in which individuals have excessive ROM in a joint.*

it is also important to understand that injury, disease, and poor soft tissue integrity can also contribute to hypermobility or a condition in which individuals have excessive ROM in a joint. The possibility of hypermobility can also be imagined when studying Figure 18.1.

The point of this brief anatomical review was to establish that joints have inherent structural properties that determine full ROM. Not surprisingly, these properties differ by joint and among individuals and often explain joint ROM differences expressed during testing and physical activity. Some of these factors can be controlled, whereas others cannot. Although the anatomical structure

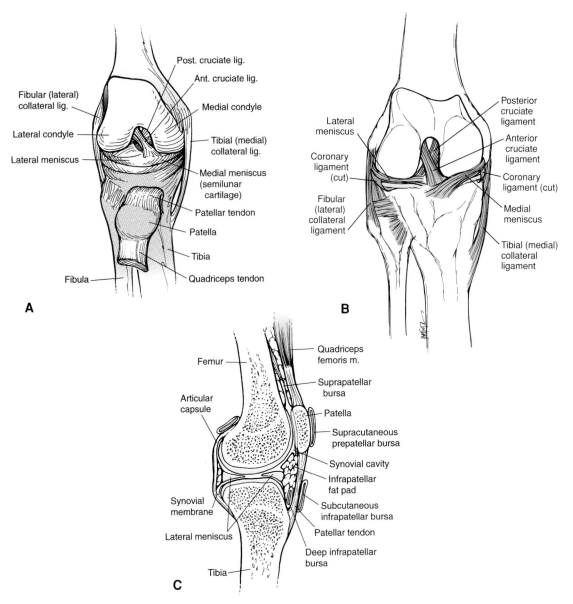

Ligament	Insertion	Action
Anterior cruciate	Anterior intercondylar area of tibia to medial surface of lateral condyle	Prevents anterior tibial displacement; resists extension, internal rotation, flexion
Arcuate	Lateral condyle of femur to head of fibula	Reinforces back of capsule
Coronary	Meniscus to tibia	Holds menisci to tibia
Medial collateral	Medial epicondyle of femur to medial condyle of tibia and medial meniscus	Resists valgus forces; taunt in extension; resists internal, external rotation
Lateral collateral	Lateral epicondyle of femur to head of fibula	Resists varus forces; taut in extension
Patellar	Inferior patela to tibial tuberosity	Transfers force from quariceps to tibia
Posterior cruciate	Posterior spine of tibia to inner condyle of femur	Resists posterior tibial movement; resists flexion and rotation
Posterior oblique	Expansion of semimembranosus muscle	Supports posterior, medial capsule
Transverse	Medial meniscus to lateral meniscus in front	Connects menisci to each other

FIGURE 18.1. Typical joint anatomy. (Reprinted with permission from Hamill J, Knutzen KM. *Biomechanical Basis of Human Movement.* 3rd ed. Philadelphia: Lippincott Williams & Wilkins; 2009. p. 212.)
A = anterior; B = posterior; C = lateral

of the joint clearly influences ROM, there are other influences. Commonly, these influences include age, gender, and physical activity history.

Age

As we grow older, the ability to move through a full ROM becomes compromised with an overall loss of flexibility of approximately 25%–30% by age 70 (7,16,23,27). The decreases in flexibility that one may experience will depend on the joint itself. Brown and Miller (9) determined a 30% loss in hamstring flexibility from the age of 20–29 to 70+ years, whereas Germain and Blair (23) found a 15% loss in shoulder flexion from the age of 20–30 to 70+ years.

Loss of ROM within a joint may have several causes. With age, changes occur in the framework of the connective tissue collagen fibers as demonstrated by increased rigidity of the tissue (4). This increased rigidity is attributed to tighter cross-linkage within and between collagen fibers, which makes the joint more resistant to bending (36,57). There is also a reduction of elastin as well as a deterioration of the cartilage, ligaments, tendons, synovial fluid, and muscles with age that may decrease joint ROM (1,10,47). Physiological changes are not the only suspect in the age-related loss of flexibility. Decreased physical activity appears to accelerate the age-related loss of physical activity (10,41).

Gender

Numerous studies suggest that females are more flexible than males owing to a different pattern of skeletal architecture and connective-tissue morphology and certain hormonal differences (8,20,22,58). The differences in ROM between genders may result from differences in joint and bone structures (2). For example, females typically have broader and shallower hips than males, which creates the possibility of a greater ROM in the pelvic region (2). Gelabert (22) also suggested that females generally have a greater range of extension in the elbow because of a shorter upper curve of the olecranon process of the elbow than males. Females may also have greater potential for flexibility in trunk flexion after puberty because of a comparatively lower center of gravity and shorter leg length (12).

Physical Activity History

An individual's history of physical activity has an impact on his or her joint ROM. Studies have shown that an individual who is physically active is also more likely to have a greater ROM than a sedentary individual (14,30,32). Cornu et al. (14) demonstrated that volleyball players exhibited greater flexibility in wrist extension than sedentary individuals. In another sport-related study, Jaeger et al. (30) found that elite field hockey players had significantly greater hip ROM than sedentary individuals. Studies have not been limited to sport activity, though. In a study by Voorrips et al. (53) that examined different habitual physical activity of older women, it was found that the more active older women had significantly greater flexibility in the hip and spine than moderately active and sedentary older women.

BENEFITS AND RISKS OF FLEXIBILITY TRAINING

As with other forms of physical training, flexibility training is believed to present clients with certain benefits and risks. These benefits and risks are frequently categorized from the personal experiences of coaches, clinicians, and exercise leaders. It is important for Personal Trainers to understand, though, that while such perspectives have their place in the apprenticeship of the fitness professional, the only sound forms of training come from those rooted in an understanding of human anatomy and physiology, biomechanics, and the unique physical and psychological qualities of

> *The existing science of flexibility training often presents fitness professionals with more questions than answers regarding the benefits and risks of stretching.*

the client. Unfortunately, the existing science of flexibility training often presents fitness professionals with more questions than answers regarding the benefits and risks of stretching. The following two sections will provide you with a short review of what are commonly held to be the benefits and risks associated with flexibility training.

Benefits

IMPROVED ROM IN SELECTED JOINTS

Flexibility training has been shown to improve an individual's joint ROM (35,40,53). In a long-term study on the effects of exercise on shoulder and hip ROM by Misner et al. (40), it was found that the flexibility program used produced significant increases in shoulder extension (5.7%), shoulder transverse extension (10.4%), hip flexion (13.3%), and hip rotation (6.3%). A minor improvement (5.5%) was also observed in shoulder flexion. Improvements in flexibility could be seen in a relatively short time period. Kerrigan et al. (32) recorded improved ROM values in both static and dynamic hip extension when participants followed the program twice daily for 10 weeks. Kukkanen et al. (35) also found improvements in spinal ROM and greater hamstring flexibility after subjects followed a 3-month program.

IMPROVED PERFORMANCE FOR ACTIVITIES OF DAILY LIVING

The extent to which individuals can live independently in the community depends on their ability to perform basic daily tasks such as self-care and essential household chores. Individuals 65 years and older, living independently or in nursing home facilities, are especially good candidates for training programs that help improve overall physical functionality. These individuals allocate most of their activity time to the performance of tasks that are formally termed "activities of daily living" (ADLs). As they become older, executions of ADLs are often reported to be extremely difficult, if not impossible (40). The ability to perform ADLs has been highly correlated with joint mobility (51). In other words, ADLs are easier to perform when an individual possesses an acceptable ROM within the joint. It has also been found that flexibility training can improve ADL functioning (24,26). Klein et al. (33) found that flexibility training improved the execution of certain ADLs within an older adult population.

Risks

JOINT HYPERMOBILITY

Hypermobility syndrome is known as "congenital laxity" of ligaments and joints. This condition is characterized by extreme ROM accompanied by mild- to moderate-intensity pain (18). Although it is suggested that certain athletes (e.g., gymnasts) and individuals may possess extraordinary joint ROM, there is insufficient scientific evidence to link hypermobility to flexibility training.

DECREASED STRENGTH

There is some evidence to suggest that stretching may contribute to decreased muscular strength. In a recent study, Nelson et al. (45) found reduced muscle strength and endurance performance after short-term static stretching in physical education college students. Fowles et al. (19) found similar results after prolonged stretching of the ankle plantarflexors. This voluntary strength deficit lasted for up to an hour after stretching. In addition, Kokkonen et al. (34) demonstrated that stretching prior to the execution of a one repetition maximum decreased the performance of the lift. Although these studies suggest that strength may be compromised following a short-term stretching session, studies need to be conducted to determine the long-term effects of stretching on strength and should not be discouraged for this reason alone.

INEFFECTIVENESS OF FLEXIBILITY TRAINING

In their 2004 review of the literature, Thacker et al. (50) were unable to conclude whether or not stretching before or after exercise contributed to injury prevention among competitive or recreational athletes. This was an important finding from the literature because flexibility training is often promoted as a means of reducing injury risk. Witvrouw et al. (56) also reviewed the literature regarding injury prevention and flexibility. They concluded that the type of sport activity in which an individual participates is critical when determining the value of flexibility training to reduce injury. The more explosive the skills involved in an activity, the more likely stretching may be needed to decrease injury.

Interestingly, the duration of increased flexibility after stretching may not be as long as Personal Trainers may think. In two of the more recently conducted studies, DePino et al. (15) recruited 30 male subjects and found that hamstring static stretch–induced knee ROM gains likely lasted no longer than approximately 3 minutes. These authors further suggest that athletes who statically stretch and then wait longer than 3 minutes before activity can expect to lose ROM gained as a result of the preceding bout of stretching. Spernoga et al. (49) also recruited 30 male subjects, used proprioceptive neuromuscular facilitation (PNF) techniques, and found increased hamstring flexibility that lasted only 6 minutes after the stretching protocol ended. The mechanism, however, and the overall impact are unclear and should not deter Personal Trainers from encouraging stretching exercises to clients.

EVALUATING FLEXIBILITY

Assessment of clients' ROM is an essential component of developing their exercise programs. Goniometry assessment provides the fitness professional with several important pieces of information. These include the following:

> *Assessment of clients' ROM is an essential component of developing their exercise programs.*

- ➤ Immediate ROM feedback
- ➤ Identification of muscular imbalances
- ➤ Current ROM prior to the start of the exercise program
- ➤ Insight into the client's learning preferences and a baseline measurement from which plans can be made for future exercise goals

Please refer to Chapter 14 for a more comprehensive look at evaluating flexibility of a client.

THREE TYPES OF STRETCHING

Several methods exist to improve flexibility and increase joint ROM, and nearly all of them involve some form of stretching. Stretches can be performed by the client (active stretching) or by the Personal Trainer (passive stretching). Although passive stretching can be very helpful for improving flexibility, it is most safely performed by a Personal Trainer with adequate knowledge and experience to prevent injury to the client. There are generally three types of stretching that can be performed using active or passive techniques to improve flexibility. These include static, dynamic, and PNF.

> *There are generally three types of stretching that can be performed using active or passive techniques to improve flexibility. These include static, dynamic, and PNF.*

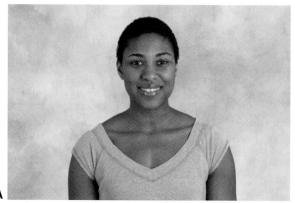

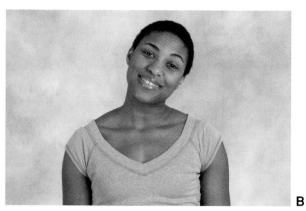

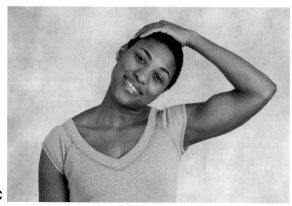

FIGURE 18.2. Progression of a static stretch. **A.** 1. Facing forward, tilt head to the left, moving only in the sagittal plane. 2. Hold and then return to the starting position. **B.** 3. Repeat with the other side. 4. A good cue for this exercise is "right ear to right shoulder." **C.** 1. Reach with one arm in opposite direction from head tilt. 2. With or without a partner, pull from top of head toward the direction of stretch, applying gentle pressure only.

Static

Static stretching is undoubtedly the method used most commonly to improve flexibility. Static stretching can be performed actively and passively and consists of slow movements into position and holding the position for a few seconds at peak tension. For example, to actively stretch the sternocleidomastoid (neck) muscles, the client would perform a lateral flexion of the neck as depicted in Figure 18.2. This position would be held at peak tension for 10–30 seconds before returning the head upright. Static stretches can be modified too, as depicted in Figure 18.2, so that the client can better hold at peak tension or truly achieve peak tension via self-assistance and support. Furthermore, lateral flexion of the neck also serves as a good example of how static stretches can be passive stretches. Through careful movements, the Personal Trainer could also guide the client's head into position and hold at peak tension for a designated period.

Despite the popularity of static stretching, little agreement has been reached among experts with respect to how long the static stretch should be held at peak tension. In its 1998 Position Stand on exercises to develop and maintain cardiorespiratory and muscular fitness and flexibility in adults, the American College of Sports Medicine suggested a hold range of 10–30 seconds (3). Data from Nelson and Bandy (43) supports the ACSM Position Stand that static stretches of 30 seconds, 3 days a week, for 6 weeks, significantly improved hamstring flexibility in high school–aged males compared with unstretched controls. Most of the newer published studies that have found flexibility improvements with static stretching have also used 30-second hold times.

Dynamic

Dynamic stretching is a form of stretching that incorporates movement along with muscle tension development. Dynamic stretches should be performed only as active stretches. In the broadest sense, dynamic stretches are built into every mode of exercise and physical activity. Jeffreys (31) has

---

| BOX **18.1** | **Ballistic Stretching—Understanding the Controversy** |

Some flexibility experts fail to distinguish dynamic stretching from another form of movement termed **ballistic** stretching. Unfortunately, these oversights have resulted in a great deal of confusion by fitness professionals, so much so that trainees and students are often discouraged from performing dynamic stretches. As stated earlier in this chapter, whether the movement is a soccer ball kick or a tennis serve, physical movements impose dynamic stretches on the soft tissues that bring about these movements. What ballistic stretching most often refers to is the short ROM bouncing action that produces jerky movements in an attempt to move into position and hold at peak muscle tension. For example, a client seated upright on the floor could extend his or her arms in an effort to reach the toes. By moving slowly into that position and holding for a few seconds at peak tension, the client would be performing an active static stretch. If the client reached toward the toes, however, and tried tapping them repeatedly with short, successive, bouncing flexions at the hip, he or she would be performing a ballistic stretch. Not unlike dynamic stretching, these movements can also be quite common during sport participation.

Considering the confusion, novice trainers might question the utility or safety of ballistic stretching. The claim is most often made that ballistic stretching is unsafe or at least ineffective for improving flexibility possibly because ballistic stretching imposes too rapid of a stretch on muscles that may be in the process of contracting during each successive "bounce" movement. Smith et al. (48) found that similar bouts of static and ballistic stretching brought on significant increases in delayed-onset muscle soreness in 20 male subjects unaccustomed to such exercise. However, these researchers also concluded that the static stretching actually induced significantly more delayed-onset muscle soreness than did ballistic stretching. More recently, Nelson and Kokkonen (44) concluded that acute ballistic muscle stretching inhibited maximal strength performance, but Unick et al. (52) found no statistically significant difference in vertical jump performance as a result of static or ballistic stretching among actively trained women.

No attempt is being made here to settle the controversy surrounding ballistic stretching. Novice trainers should recognize that both dynamic and ballistic movements are normal components of sport activity and may have legitimate roles in the training and rehabilitation of athletes (44).

characterized dynamic stretching as being very similar to a sport- or function-specific warm-up. It is difficult to depict examples of dynamic stretching on paper. Consider the movements of a boxer in the ring prior to a fight. Jabs he makes with the upper extremities and quick turns of the torso all serve as good examples of dynamic stretch. TaeBo® movements and stereotypical medicine ball exercises provide further examples of dynamic stretching. Ideally, dynamic stretches incorporate movements that are specific to sport movements of interest, but excellent dynamic stretches can also be developed on the basis of the flexibility needs of the medically cleared population at large (Box 18.1).

Proprioceptive Neuromuscular Facilitation

Proprioceptive neuromuscular facilitation involves both active and passive techniques designed to improve joint ROM. This form of stretching requires an experienced Personal Trainer and a cooperative client, but several muscle groups can be trained when PNF techniques are properly used. PNF stretching is commonly believed to elicit a relaxation response from the neuromuscular system. This response can occur in the prime mover (agonist), synergist, and antagonist muscles across a particular joint. With a stretch-induced reduction in muscle tone, joint ROM increases during subsequent stretches and eventually during physical activity.

In a recently published review, however, Chalmers (11) refutes this rationale and points to studies that suggest that PNF improves ROM mainly because of changes in the ability to tolerate stretching and/or changes in the viscoelastic properties of the stretched muscle. The basis for ROM change continues to be studied, and PNF techniques have long been shown to increase joint ROM. PNF stretching should be performed only by competent and trained practitioners as overstretching is possible if the technique is not fully understood.

RATIONALE FOR FLEXIBILITY TRAINING

Despite the importance of full, pain-free joint ROM for sport and physical activity, the justification for certain flexibility training techniques is controversial. Moreover, little scientific evidence exists to support or discontinue even the most common stretching habits designed for injury prevention among competitive or recreational athletes (50). Not surprisingly, the novice Personal Trainer is bound to be confused with respect to the inclusion or omission of flexibility exercises in the overall conditioning of clients.

One approach to this problem involves conducting a thorough fitness assessment of the client to determine the extent to which inflexibility limits sport and/or general physical performance. Should ROM deficiencies be evident in the client, the basic stretching techniques described in this chapter are those most often used to improve flexibility. It is reasonable to employ these suggested techniques and continue to monitor the flexibility needs of the client. While at least one early study (37) found significant improvements in flexibility with all three methods, Personal Trainers are encouraged to select an approach that best suits the needs, limitations, and abilities of the client while continuing to monitor joint ROM and its ultimate impact on sport and physical activity performance.

GENERAL GUIDELINES TO CONSIDER WHEN DESIGNING A FLEXIBILITY TRAINING PROGRAM

There are some preliminary training guidelines unique to the design of flexibility programs. These involve warm-up, breathing, and posture.

Warm-Up

Although stretches can be performed at the start, in the middle, and/or at the finish of the workout, it is common to precede stretching with a brief, aerobic exercise warm-up. Wenos and Konin (54) have even found that active warm-up reduces the resistance to stretch. It has been established that increasing the temperature of a muscle increases the elastic properties or the ability to stretch (21,25,46,57). Warm muscle tissue responds less stiffly than cold muscle tissue. Little evidence suggests that the exercise warm-up should be altered to accommodate flexibility training exclusively. Typical warm-up exercises include stationary cycling, treadmill running, and rowing machine work.

Breathing

Proper breathing techniques are often helpful in relaxing the client and allowing movement into position more comfortably. Flexibility training is no time to perform a Valsalva maneuver (air expiration against a closed glottis). Use this time in the program design to allow the client to participate in a relaxing form of exercise, which may help reduce stress levels and voluntary muscle tension. In general, exercisers should exhale slowly as they move toward the end point of a stretch, and inhale as they return to the starting position.

Posture

In the design of a flexibility training program, Personal Trainers should understand the proper positioning of the stretch to target the appropriate muscle group. Focus on maintaining proper body alignment during the execution of the exercises. Posture is discussed extensively in Chapter 14. For example, consider the stretch depicted by Figure 18.21. Posture can be greatly improved by using the hand *not* grasping the ankle to grab a pillar, railing, or the back of a chair to maintain balance. Emphasis should be made to avoid pressing the elevated foot to the gluteals (i.e., hyperflexion at the knee) or leaning into the stretch for additional force development. Some reminders for correct postural alignment are listed below:

➤ Maintain neutral position of the spine (characterized by having a slight inward curve at the cervical and lumbar spines and a slight outward curve of the thoracic spine)
➤ Shoulders should remain back and away from the ears
➤ Hips should be in a neutral and level position. See Figures 18.23 and 18.29 for examples of proper hip placement

Precautions for Individuals with Health Concerns

> *Considering the three types of stretching presented in this chapter, there is little reason to avoid flexibility training in the apparently healthy individual.*

Considering the three types of stretching presented in this chapter, there is little reason to avoid flexibility training in the apparently healthy individual. However, there are several conditions that may present challenges to the novice trainer when designing flexibility training programs. Four of these conditions are arthritis, muscular imbalance, osteoporosis, and hip fracture/replacement, and they are most commonly seen in older exercisers and can be anticipated on the basis of the client's recently completed health history questionnaire.

Arthritis

According to the U.S. National Center for Chronic Disease Prevention and Health Promotion (42), 46 million Americans suffer from arthritis or other joint pain and inflammation. Arthritis is believed to limit physical activity in nearly 19 million adult Americans. Arthritis is defined as an inflammation of a joint resulting in damage to the joint structure. There are more than 100 different types of arthritis, with the two most common types being osteoarthritis and rheumatoid arthritis (55). Osteoarthritis is a chronic degenerative condition that develops over time and results in abnormal wear and tear of cartilage covering the ends of the bones. Rheumatoid arthritis is classified as an autoimmune disease in which the body attacks and destroys the joint surface. In either case, individuals with arthritis tend to limit movement because of pain and stiffness, which may result in an increased loss of flexibility and joint motion. Fortunately, flexibility and joint range can be improved in an individual with arthritis through training (38).

According to the American College of Sports Medicine (55), exercise programming for the individual with arthritis includes the following:

➤ Perform flexibility exercise one to two times daily, using pain-free ROM as an index of intensity
➤ In a single exercise session, progress from flexibility exercises for the affected joints to neuromuscular muscle function exercises (strength and endurance) to aerobic activities.
  • Avoid exercise during arthritic flare-ups
➤ Avoidance of vigorous, highly repetitive exercises
➤ Morning exercises for rheumatoid arthritis clients if the client reports significant morning stiffness (although some patients may benefit from the increased circulation from the exercise).

According to the American College of Sports Medicine (55), exercise programming should recognize that if the client experiences greater joint pain following a training session, the session may have been too intense for the joints and may need to be modified. To avoid overworking individuals who have taken anti-inflammatory medications (e.g., aspirin, ibuprofen, and naproxen sodium), pay close attention to their effort during exercise because these drugs can temporarily lessen musculoskeletal pain.

Muscular Imbalance

Many clients possess muscular imbalances of the body, which may create postural alignment issues and injury. Repetitive movements, poor posture, and weak or tight muscles can cause these muscular imbalances but they are also seen in athletes too. Consider the baseball or tennis athlete who trains and plays with distinct joint dominance. When the body experiences an imbalance in muscular forces on opposite sides of a joint, ROM may be affected (2). The obvious goal to correct the muscular imbalance would be to strengthen the weak muscle and stretch the shorter muscle if ROM is compromised.

Osteoporosis

Osteoporosis (brittle bone disease) and osteopenia (low bone density) affects both males and females. As the bones lose density, they are more prone to fractures. The most common sites for bone loss include the spine, hips, and wrists. ROM guidelines for these populations include the following:

➤ Avoiding repetitive exercises that involve excessive or heavily loaded spinal flexion or twisting
➤ Suggesting exercises to help improve posture and spinal alignment

Hip Fracture/Replacement

For individuals who have recently had a hip fracture or hip replacement, it is recommended to avoid flexibility exercises that involve excessive:

➤ Internal rotation of the hip (turning the foot inward)
➤ Hip adduction (crossing the legs beyond the midline)
➤ Hip flexion (thigh more than parallel to floor)

FLEXIBILITY PROGRAM DEVELOPMENT

> *Flexibility programs follow the parameters of the FIDM acronym (Frequency, Intensity, Duration, and Mode).*

Developing a flexibility training program is easy to do for a wide range of clients. Flexibility programs follow the parameters of the FIDM acronym (*F*requency, *I*ntensity, *D*uration, and *M*ode). As discussed earlier, however, there is considerable controversy about nearly every constituent of the flexibility training program. What follows are the FIDM recommendations condensed from the American College of Sports Medicine's current Position Stand on exercises to develop and maintain fitness and flexibility in adults (3). These parameters can be used by Personal Trainers to structure flexibility training programs. Unless otherwise indicated, the guidelines apply to all three of the stretching techniques presented in Figures 18.3 through 18.31. As the Personal Trainer skill improves, adaptations to these parameters can be made.

Frequency

It is currently recommended that stretches be performed at least 2–3 days a week, including two to four stretch repetitions per muscle group. Bandy et al. (6) found no increase in hamstring flexibility in 93 female and male subjects when the frequency of stretching was increased from one to three times per day. Little research exists to refute the practice of stretching daily whether followed by other physical activity or not.

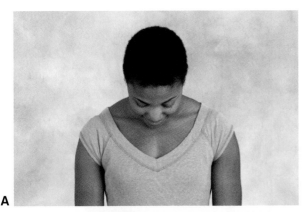

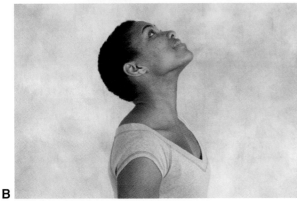

FIGURE 18.3. Forward flexion and extension. **A.** 1. Facing forward, move head forward to tuck chin into chest, hold. 2. Move slowly from this flexion position to extension. **B.** 3. Extension should involve looking up to ceiling until a 45° angle is reached, hold. 4. Avoid dropping head back onto the upper back.

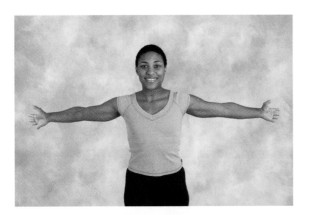

FIGURE 18.4. Chest stretch. 1. Shoulders should be relaxed, not elevated. 2. Move extended arms to the back. 3. Arms should be kept at or a little below shoulder height. 4. A good cue for this stretch is "open arms wide."

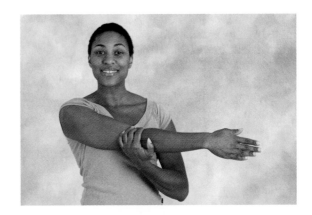

FIGURE 18.5. Arms across the chest. 1. Facing forward, extend the right arm and draw across the chest. 2. Arm should be as straight as possible, with gentle tension developed on the right shoulder. 3. Grasp right elbow with the left hand. 4. Apply gentle pressure with the left hand to increase tension on the right shoulder. 5. Repeat with the other arm/other side.

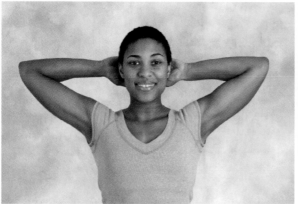

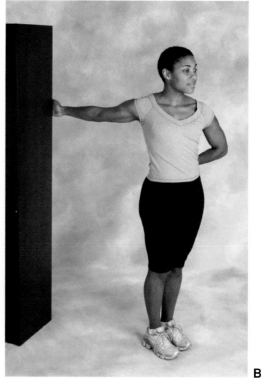

A

B

FIGURE 18.6. Chest stretch (progression). **A.** 1. Place the palms of the hand on the back of the head and bring elbow to the back. **B.** 2. Place extended arms against an open doorway and lean forward, feeling gentle tension develop across the chest.

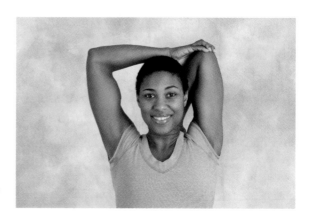

FIGURE 18.7. Elbow behind the head. 1. Facing forward, bring right arm up, bend from the elbow, and drop the hand behind the head. 2. Try to reach left shoulder with right hand. 3. Repeat with other arm/other side. Bring right hand to left shoulder and gently pull left elbow rightward to increase tension on left arm (triceps brachii).

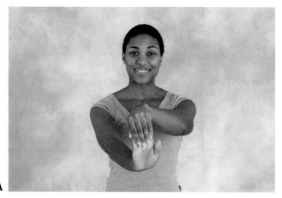

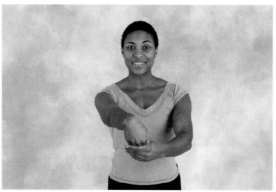

A

B

FIGURE 18.8. Palm up/palm down. **A.** 1. This exercise can be performed while standing or seated. 2. Extend right arm perpendicular to the body. 3. Extend wrist so the palm faces away from the body. 4. Gently pull right hand (fingertips) toward body until tension develops in the forearm flexors. 5. Repeat with other arm/other side. **B.** 1. This exercise can be performed while standing or seated. 2. Extend right arm perpendicular to the body. 3. Flex wrist so the palm faces the body. 4. Gently pull right hand with left hand until tension develops in the forearm extension.

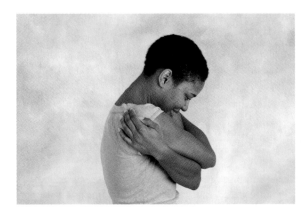

FIGURE 18.9. Arm hug. 1. Cross the arms around the body, elbows pointing forward. 2. Let the upper body round.

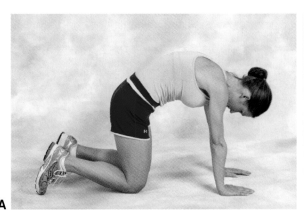

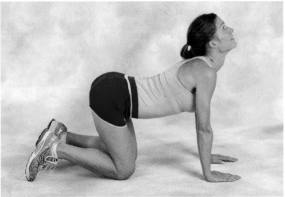

A

B

FIGURE 18.10. Kneeling cat. **A.** 1. Kneel in quadruped position. 2. Draw in abdominals and contract the gluteals. **B.** 3. Round throughout the entire spine.

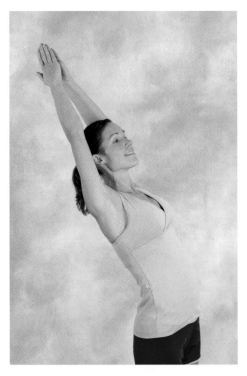

FIGURE 18.11. Pillar/overhead reach. 1. Facing forward, stand erect and extend arms above head, keeping shoulders in neutral position. 2. Interlock fingers and use the palms to press upward. 3. Stretch can also involve the trunk muscles (torso) by moving in frontal plane to one side of the body and back. 4. Hold when tension is developed in the torso on the side opposite reach.

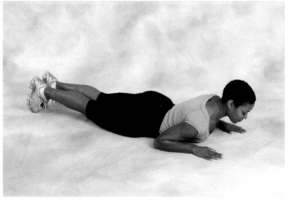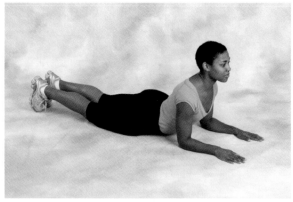

A   B

FIGURE 18.12. Modified cobra. **A.** 1. Lie prone on the floor with the head resting on the forearms and the legs extended. 2. Place the elbows directly under the shoulders with the hands facing forward. **B.** 3. Press into the forearms and raise the upper body, keeping the hips on the floor.

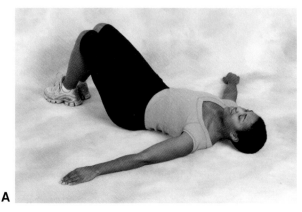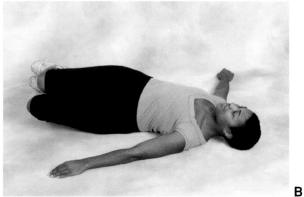

A   B

FIGURE 18.13. Supine rotational stretch. **A.** 1. Lie face up on the floor. 2. Bend knees to that the feet are flat on the floor. 3. Extend arms across the floor to stabilize upper body with movement. **B.** 4. Slowly move both legs with the knees bent to the right side of the body. 5. Maintain upper back against the floor and the abdomen oriented toward the ceiling. 6. Repeat by moving the legs to the left side.

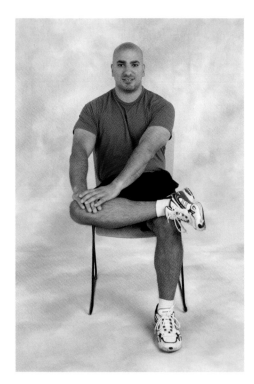

FIGURE 18.14. Seated hip rotator stretch level I. 1. Sit upright on a sturdy, nonmovable chair. 2. Cross right ankle onto bent left knee. 3. Gently press down on right knee until tension develops in the outer portion of the right thigh. 4. Repeat with the opposite side.

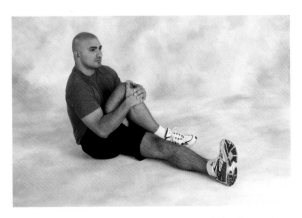

FIGURE 18.15. Seated hip rotator stretch level II. 1. Sit upright on the floor, with left leg extended and right knee bent. 2. Place the right foot over the left leg. 3. Hug the knee toward the chest. 4. Repeat on other side.

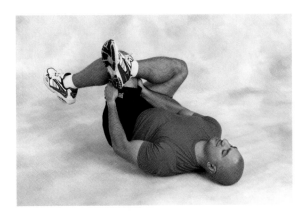

FIGURE 18.16. Supine hip rotator stretch (progression from seated). 2. Lie face up on floor with knees bent so feet are flat on the floor. 2. Cross right ankle onto bent left knee. 3. Lift left foot off the floor. 4. Wrap hands around the left leg and draw into the body. 5. Focus on opening up the right knee until tension develops in the outer portion of the right thigh. 6. Repeat on the opposite side.

Intensity

Moving into position of mild discomfort before holding a stretch is the current recommendation on static flexibility training intensity. Obviously, this subjective feeling of discomfort will vary from client to client. Fitness professionals will be interested to learn that individual effort can be standardized in the laboratory using maximal voluntary isometric contractions. Feland and Marin (17) found that a submaximal form of PNF produced comparable gains in hamstring flexibility to those produced by maximal voluntary isometric contractions in 72 male subjects aged 18–27 years. These authors concluded that PNF stretching using submaximal contractions might reduce injury risk associated with PNF stretching. Because most Personal Trainers will not have access to isokinetic equipment, it is recommended that fitness professionals employ a Borg Rating of Perceived Exertion scale and suggest that clients position themselves for (static) stretching at an intensity that corresponds to a 13–15 range.

Duration

Two points are at issue with respect to the parameter of duration. First, current recommendations involve stretching hold times of 10–30 seconds for active static stretches and the same for PNF techniques when preceded by a 6-second active contraction. There seems to be little additional flexibility benefit to static stretch hold times that exceed 30 seconds (5).

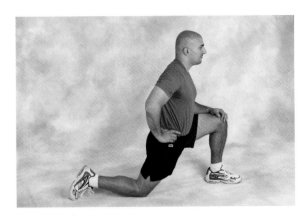

FIGURE 18.17. Kneeling hip flexors stretch. 1. Kneel on both knees with upper body lifted. 2. Plant the right foot on the floor until you reach a 90° angle with both the front and back legs. 3. Shift the weight forward while keeping the upper body lifted.

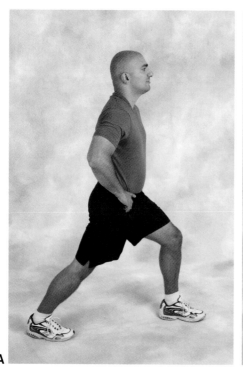
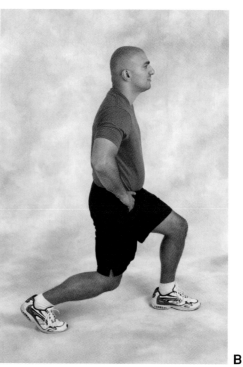

A   B

FIGURE 18.18. Standing hip flexor stretch. **A**. 1. Stand erect and keep hands on the hips. 2. Step forward with left foot into a lunge position; right heel may be elevated to facilitate this movement. **B**. 3. Shift the hips forward. 4. Maintain this position, feeling tension develop in hips, quadriceps, and buttocks. 5. Repeat with the opposite side.

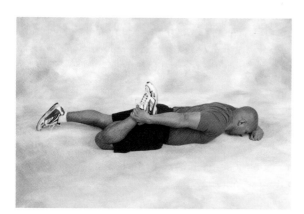

FIGURE 18.19. Prone quadriceps stretch. 1. Lie prone on the floor with legs extended. 2. Draw right heel back toward the gluteals.

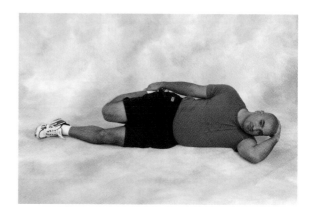

FIGURE 18.20. Side-lying quadriceps stretch (progression). 1. Lie on floor with left side of the body; the trunk should be perpendicular to the floor. 2. Bend right knee, keeping knees and hips stacked. 3. Reach with the right hand across the front of the right foot. 4. Gently pull thigh back slightly using the right arm. 5. Allow the left arm to stabilize the torso by pressing against the floor. 6. Repeat with the left thigh by positioning the body with the right side against the floor.

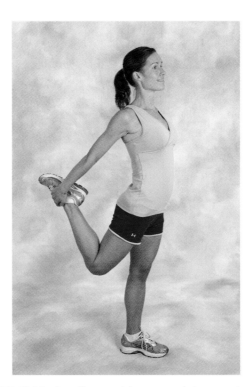

FIGURE 18.21. Standing quadriceps stretch (progression).
1. While in a standing position (a chair may be used to hold onto for support), bend the right knee toward the gluteals.
2. Grasp the right ankle with the right hand. 3. Gently pull thigh back slightly using the right arm.

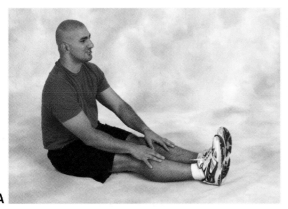

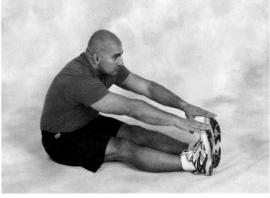

A   B

FIGURE 18.22. Seated hamstring stretch. **A.** 1. Sit upright on the floor with both legs extended and hands resting on the quadriceps. **B.** 2. Slowly walk the hands forward toward the feet, keeping the chest lifted.

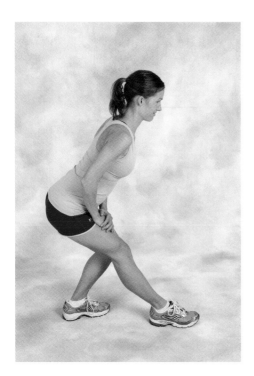

FIGURE 18.23. Standing hamstring stretch (progression). 1. Standing upright, bring the right foot slightly ahead of the left foot. 2. Slowly draw the hips back while slightly bending the left knee and extending the right knee. 3. Bring the toes of the right foot off the floor and toward the body. 4. Hold and then return to the starting position. 5. Repeat with the opposite leg.

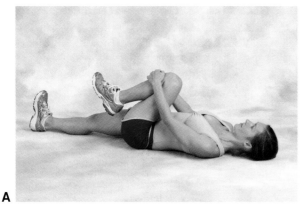
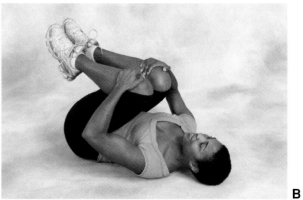

A

B

FIGURE 18.24. Supine knees to chest. 1. Lie supine on the floor. 2. Hug the knees to the chest. Can be done with one leg **(A)** or two legs **(B)**.

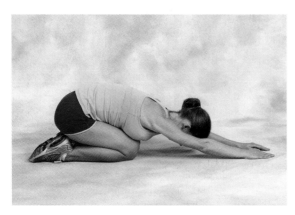
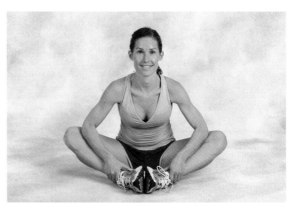

FIGURE 18.25. Child's pose. 1. Kneel in a quadruped position. 2. Sit back onto heels with arms extended.

FIGURE 18.26. Butterfly stretch. 1. Sit upright on the floor with the soles of the feet together. 2. Draw the knees to the floor. 3. Lean forward from the hips.

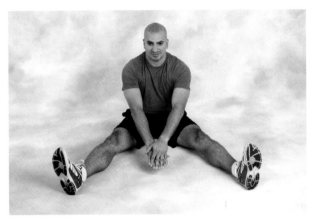

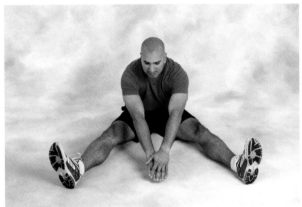

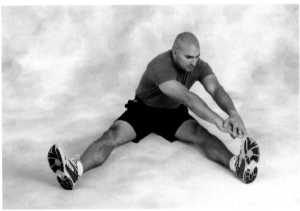

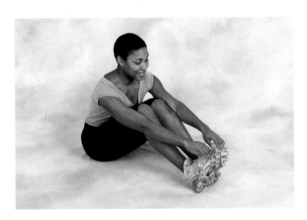

FIGURE 18.27. Straddle. 1. Sit upright on floor with both legs extended together. 2. Slowly spread legs apart so that feet are as far from each other as possible. 3. Gently reach toward center or alternate reach from right to left.

FIGURE 18.28. Seated calf stretch. 1. Sit upright with both legs extended. 2. Turn the toes toward the ceiling. 3. Draw the tops of the toes toward the upper body.

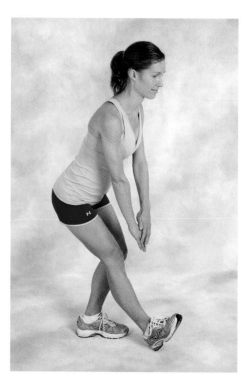

FIGURE 18.29. Standing calf stretch. Place your body weight on the left leg with your right leg forward, heel on the ground. 2. Grasp banister or handrail for support if necessary. Bring the toes of the right foot toward the body as you sit back slightly onto the left leg. 3. Feel the stretch develop in the right calf. 4. Slowly return to the starting position and repeat with the opposite side.

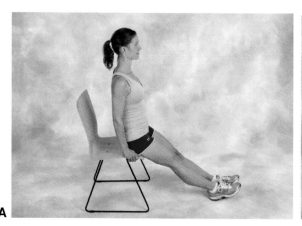
A

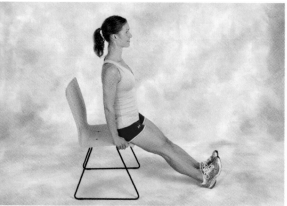
B

FIGURE 18.30. Dynamic foot ROM. 1. Sit upright on a chair with both legs extended together. **A.** 2. Point toes away from the body. **B.** 3. Move toes toward the body.

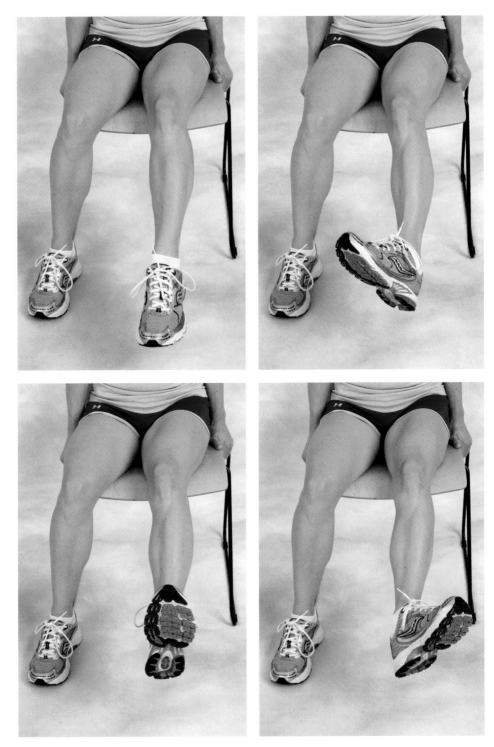

FIGURE 18.31. Dynamic foot ROM. Sit on a chair and rotate feet clockwise and counterclockwise.

Mode

It is recommended that a general stretching routine be used to best improve flexibility. This means that stretches should involve the major muscle and tendon groups of the body. Some of the more commonly performed static stretches are presented in the previous pages. For an example of how these parameters can be incorporated into a flexibility training program, see Box 18.2. Because PNF techniques require advanced skill and experience, Personal Trainers are encouraged to continue their education and readings on this subject and practice employing these stretches when ready. For more information about PNF techniques, readers are referred to Houglum (29).

BOX **18.2** **Sample Training Program**

By incorporating the FIDM (*Frequency, Intensity, Duration,* and *Mode*) parameters discussed in this chapter, even the novice trainer can structure a basic flexibility training program for a wide range of trainees. Here is a sample training program that uses the stretches presented in this chapter.

Client: 40-year-old female, medically cleared to begin consistent exercise program

Height = 168 cm (5′ 6″), weight = 68 kg (150 lb)

No history of orthopedic problems, mild chronic back pain

Objectives: Improve flexibility as measured by goniometry
Session: 15-minute warm-up using a NordicTrack CX 1055 elliptical trainer
(average heart rate: 108 bpm)

Body Region	Exercise	Comments
Neck	Lateral flexion	Begin as an active stretch, move head slowly to prevent dizziness
Shoulders	Arms across chest	Avoid bending the elbow as the arm is brought across the chest
Chest	Chest stretch	Maintain relaxed shoulders
Arms	Elbow extension	
Back	Kneeling cat	Discontinue stretch if it produces immediate back pain
Torso	Modified cobra	Discontinue stretch if it produces immediate back pain
Hips	Seated hip rotator, level I	Progress to level II exercise when level I can be performed for 30 seconds without pain
Thigh (anterior)	Prone quadriceps	
Thigh (posterior)	Seated hamstring	Maintain upright posture and natural spinal curves
Calves	Standing calf step	

Trainer's Notes: Be sure to follow the FIDM guidelines for flexibility training suggested in this chapter, keeping in mind that they can certainly be adapted to the progress and individual needs of the client. If one or more of the recommended parameters do not seem to be effective, adapt as needed.

This program can and should be modified as the client progresses to greater low back ROM. Goniometer remeasures can be made every 4–6 weeks to assess the influence of the training program over time and as a result of the training session. By following the chart of stretches listed in this chapter, this client will be able to progress from these basic stretches to more complex ones. The order of exercises performed during a session is not important.

SUMMARY

The purpose of this chapter was to present flexibility as an essential ingredient of health-related fitness and to provide Personal Trainers with a basic understanding of how to properly incorporate flexibility training into the exercise programs of healthy individuals. Although the science of flexibility training is often conflicting, Personal Trainers should use this aspect of flexibility training as motivation for staying abreast of the scientific literature as it develops. Moreover, Personal Trainers should make use of their good judgment and entire education in the exercise sciences to design training programs that suit the specific needs of their clients.

REFERENCES

1. Adrian MJ. Flexibility in the aging adult. In: Smith EL, Serfass RC, editors. *Exercise and Aging: The Scientific Basis*. Hillside (NJ): Enslow Publishers; 1981. p. 45–57.
2. Alter MJ. *Science of Flexibility*. 3rd ed. Champaign (IL): Human Kinetics; 2004.
3. American College of Sports Medicine. Position stand: the recommended quantity and quality of exercise for developing and maintaining cardiorespiratory and muscular fitness, and flexibility in healthy adults. *Med Sci Sports Exerc*. 1998;30:975–91.
4. Bailey AJ. Ageing of the collagen of the musculoskeletal system. *Int J Sports Med*. 1989;10:S86–90.
5. Bandy WD, Irion JM. The effect of time on static stretch on the flexibility of the hamstring muscles. *Phys Ther*. 1994;74(9):845–52.
6. Bandy WD, Irion JM, Briggler M. The effect of time and frequency of static stretching on flexibility of the hamstring muscles. *Phys Ther*. 1997;77(10):1090–6.
7. Bassey EJ, Morgan K, Dallosso HM, Ebrahim SBJ. Flexibility of the shoulder joint measured as range of abduction in a large representative sample of men and women over 65 years of age. *Eur J Appl Phys*. 1989;58:353–60.
8. Bell R, Hoshizaki T. Relationships of age and sex with joint range of motion of seventeen joint actions in humans. *Can J Appl Sports Sci*. 1981;6:202–6.
9. Brown DA, Miller WC. Normative data for strength and flexibility of women throughout their life. *Eur J Appl Phys*. 1998;78: 77–82.
10. Buckwalter JA. Maintaining and restoring mobility in middle and old age: the importance of the soft tissues. *Instr Course Lect*. 1997;46:459–69.
11. Chalmers G. Re-examination of the possible role of Golgi tendon organ and muscle spindle reflexes in proprioceptive neuromuscular facilitation muscle stretching. *Sports Biomech*. 2004;3(1):159–83.
12. Corbin CB. *A Textbook of Motor Development*. 2nd ed. Dubuque (IA): Brown; 1980.
13. Corbin CB, Welk GJ, Corbin WR, Welk KA. *Fundamental Concepts of Fitness and Wellness*. 2nd ed. Boston: McGraw-Hill; 2006:1–302.
14. Cornu C, Maisetti O, Ledoux I. Muscle elastic properties during wrist flexion and extension in healthy sedentary subjects and volley-ball players. *Int J Sports Med*. 2003;24(4):277–84.
15. DePino GM, Webright WG, Arnold BL. Duration of maintained hamstring flexibility after cessation of an acute static stretching protocol. *J Athl Train*. 2000;35(1):56–9.
16. Einkauf DK, Gondes ML, Jensen MJ. Changes in spinal mobility with increasing age in women. *Phys Ther*. 1987;67:370–5.
17. Feland JB, Marin HN. Effect of submaximal contraction intensity in contract-relax proprioceptive neuromuscular facilitation stretching. *Br J Sports Med*. 2004;38(4):E18.
18. Finsterbush A, Pogrund H. The hypermobility syndrome: musculoskeletal complaints in 100 consecutive cases of generalized joint hypermobility. *Clin Orthop*. 1982;168:124–7.
19. Fowles JR, Sale DG, MacDougall JD. Reduced strength after passive stretch of the human plantarflexors. *J Appl Physiol*. 2000;89(3):1179–88.
20. Gabbard C, Tandy R. Body composition and flexibility among prepubescent males and females. *J Hum Move Stud*. 1988;14(4): 153–9.
21. Garrett WE, Best TM. Anatomy, physiology, and mechanics of skeletal muscle. In: Buckwalter JA, Einhorn TA, Simon SR, editors. *Orthopaedic Basic Science Biology and Biomechanics of the Musculoskeletal System*. 2nd ed. American Academy of Orthopaedic Surgeons; 2000:684–716.
22. Gelabert RR. *Gelabert's Anatomy for the Dancer*. New York: Danad; 1966.
23. Germain NW, Blair SN. Variability in shoulder flexion with age, activity and sex. *Am Correct Ther J*. 1983;37:156–60.
24. Gersten JW, Ager C, Anderson K, Cenkovich F. Relation of muscle strength and range of motion to activities of daily living. *Arch Phys Med Rehabil*. 1970;3:137–42.
25. Gillette T, Holland GJ. Relationship of body core temperature and warm-up to hamstring range of motion. *J Orthop Sports Phys Ther*. 1991;13(3):126–31.
26. Guralnik JM, Simonsick EM. Physical disability in older Americans. *J Gerontol*. 1993;48:3–10.
27. Hageman PA, Blanke DJ. Comparison of gait in young women and elderly women. *Phys Ther*. 1986;66:1382–7.
28. Hamill J, Knutzen KM. *Biomechanical Basis of Human Movement*. 3rd ed. Philadelphia: Lippincott Williams & Wilkins; 2009. p. 121–4.

29. Houglum PA. *Therapeutic Exercise for Musculoskeletal Injuries*. 2nd ed. Champaign (IL): Human Kinetics; 2005.

30. Jaeger M, Friewald J, Englehardt M, Lange-Berlin V. Differences in hamstring muscle stretching of elite field hockey players and normal subjects. *Sortverletz Sportschaden*. 2003;17(2):65–70.

31. Jeffreys I. Warm-up and stretching (Chapter 13). In: Baechle TR, Earle RW, editors. *Essentials of Strength Training and Conditioning*. 3rd ed. Champaign (IL): Human Kinetics; 2008. p. 296–324.

32. Kerrigan DC, Xenopoulos-Oddsson A, Sullivan MJ, et al. Effect of hip flexor-stretching program on gait in the elderly. *Arch Phys Med Rehabil*. 2003;84(1):1–6.

33. Klein DA, Stone WJ, Phillips WT, et al. PNF training and physical function in assisted-living older adults. *J Aging Phys Activity*. 2002;10:476–88.

34. Kokkonen J, Nelson AG, Cornwell A. Acute muscle stretching inhibits maximal strength performance. *Res Q Exerc Sport*. 1998;69(4):411–5.

35. Kukkanen T, Malkia E. Effects of a three-month therapeutic exercise programme on flexibility in subjects with low back pain. *Physiother Res Int*. 2000;5(1):46–61.

36. LaBella FS, Paul G. Structure of collagen from human tendon as influenced by age and sex. *J Gerontol*. 1965;20:54–9.

37. Lucas RC, Koslow R. Comparative study of static, dynamic, and proprioceptive neuromuscular facilitation stretching techniques on flexibility. *Percept Mot Skills*. 1984;58(2):615–8.

38. MacDonald CW, Whitman JM, Cleland JA, Smith M, Hoeksma HL. Clinical outcomes following manual physical therapy and exercise for hip osteoarthritis: a case series. *J Orthop Sports Phys Ther*. 2006;36(8):573.

39. Mahieu NN, McNair P, De Muynck M, et al. Effect of static and ballistic stretching on the muscle-tendon tissue properties. *Med Sci Sports Exerc*. 2007;39(3):494–501.

40. Misner JE, Massey BH, Bemben M, et al. Long-term effects of exercise on the range of motion of aging women. *J Orthop Sports Phys Ther*. 1992;16(1):37–42.

41. Munns K. Effects of exercise on the range of joint motion in elderly subjects. In: Smith EL, Serfass RC, editors. *Exercise and Aging: The Scientific Basis*. Hillside (NJ): Enslow Publishers; 1981. p. 167–178.

42. National Center for Chronic Disease Prevention and Health Promotion [Internet]. Atlanta (GA): Centers for Disease Control and Prevention [cited 2008 Sept 22]. Available from http://www.cdc.gov/arthritis

43. Nelson RT, Bandy WD. Eccentric training and static stretching improve hamstring flexibility of high school males. *J Athl Train*. 2004;39(3):254–8.

44. Nelson AG, Kokkonen J. Acute ballistic muscle stretching inhibits maximal strength performance. *Res Q Exerc Sport*. 2001;72(4):415–9.

45. Nelson AG, Kokkonen J, Arnall DA. Acute muscle stretching inhibits muscle strength endurance performance. *J Strength Cond Res*. 2005;19(2):338–43.

46. Sapega AA, Quedenfeld TC, Moyer RA, Butler RA. Biophysical factors in range-of-motion exercise. *Phys Sports Med*. 1981;9(12):57–65.

47. Shepard RJ. *Physical Activity and Aging*. Chicago: Yearbook Medical Publishers; 1978. p. 45–48.

48. Smith LL, Brunetz MH, Chenier TC, et al. The effects of static and ballistic stretching on delayed onset muscle soreness and creatine kinase. *Res Q Exerc Sport*. 1993;64(1):103–7.

49. Spernoga SG, Uhl TL, Arnold BL, Gansneder BM. Duration of maintained hamstring flexibility after a one-time, modified hold-relax stretching protocol. *J Athl Train*. 2001;36(1):44–8.

50. Thacker SB, Gilchrist J, Stroup DF, Kimsey CD Jr. The impact of stretching on sports injury risk: a systematic review of the literature. *Med Sci Sports Exerc*. 2004;36(3):371–8.

51. Thompson CJ, Osness WH. Effects of an 8-week multimodal exercise program on strength, flexibility, and golf performance in 55 to 79-year-old men. *J Aging Phys Activity*. 2004;12(2):144–56.

52. Unick J, Kieffer HS, Cheesman W, Feeney A. The acute effects of static and ballistic stretching on vertical jump performance in trained women. *J Strength Cond Res*. 2005;19(1):206–12.

53. Voorrips LE, Lemmink KAPM, Van Heuvelen MJG, et al. The physical condition of elderly women differing in habitual physical activity. *Med Sci Sports Exerc*. 1993;25(10):1152–7.

54. Wenos DL, Konin JG. Controlled warm-up intensity enhances hip range of motion. *J Strength Cond Res*. 2004;18(3):529–33.

55. Whaley MH, Brubaker PH, Otto RM. *ACSM's Guidelines for Exercise Testing and Prescription*. 7th ed. Philadelphia (PA): Lippincott Williams & Wilkins; 2006.

56. Witvrouw E, Mahieu N, Danneels L, McNair P. Stretching and injury prevention. *Sports Med*. 2004;34:443–9.

57. Wright V, Johns RJ. Observations on the measurement of joint stiffness. *Arch Rheum*. 1960;3:328–40.

58. Youdas JW, Krause DA, Hollman JH, et al. The influence of gender and age on hamstring muscle length in healthy adults. *J Orthop Sports Phys Ther*. 205;35(4):246–52.

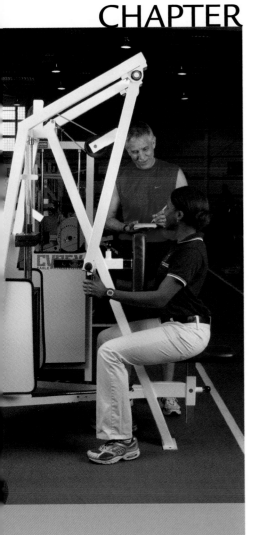

19

Sequencing the Personal Training Program

OBJECTIVES

- Provide the Personal Trainer with a "how-to" guide for the first training session as well as for subsequent sessions and program variables
- Review basic customer service skills as they are applied in a fitness facility and during a personal training session
- Educate the Personal Trainer on communication skills and client–trainer relationships
- Provide the Personal Trainer with comprehensive criteria for an optimal personal training session
- Review the four phases of the personal training session: preparation, transition, workout, and review
- Provide the Personal Trainer with the purpose and template for developing useful training notes for proper documentation and effective program management

Personal training is a challenging job. Many clients have no idea where to start with their exercise program. Others take what they have read in the latest bodybuilding magazine and launch into an exercise program that may be inappropriate for their needs. Others are simply unmotivated, which makes it difficult to get them to exercise effectively and consistently, regardless of their level of knowledge and understanding.

Many clients arrive for their session with their body and minds prepared for anything but a good workout. The Personal Trainer's job is to make every minute of each session effective. This is achieved through a preplanned series of exercises designed to meet the individual's training goals and learning objectives for that particular session. The Personal Trainer must also maximize the trainee's physical performance within any orthopedic and/or physiological limitations or barriers.

> **The Personal Trainer's job is to make every minute of each session effective.**

The celebrity, the corporate executive, the model, the professional athlete, and the housewife each need and deserve the best possible training session. Results that come from productive work make each session worthwhile. The achievement of goals will encourage the client to want to continue working with the Personal Trainer or, at the very least, motivate the client to continue to exercise for a lifetime. It is the Personal Trainer's job as a professional to create this situation for each and every client. Personal Trainers must take pride in their job and train clients productively, with safety as a primary concern. Doing so ensures that both Personal Trainers and clients alike will experience their desired results.

The purpose of this chapter is to take the theoretical framework presented in the earlier chapters of this book, or the science of personal training, and demonstrate the art of personal training—how it may be applied at the "point of service"—which is the personal training session. By doing so, the Personal Trainer will be able to combine these training principles and modalities into an effective training session. This chapter also provides a framework for a Personal Trainer's job responsibilities, record-keeping procedures, and a step-by-step approach to delivering a personal training session.

This chapter specifically addresses the needs and typical activities of the Personal Trainer working in a membership fitness facility. It takes into account the barriers and situations that are common in such a work environment. The specific tenets and recommendations with regards to professionalism, customer service, and the step-by-step approach to the personal training session remain consistent regardless of the Personal Trainer's work environment.

OPTIMAL CLIENT CARE AND CUSTOMER SERVICE

It is important, first and foremost, that regardless of the training venue, the highest degree of client care is essential for every Personal Trainer. It does not matter if the Personal Trainer is an employee at a fitness center or a sole proprietor running his or her own business. Safe and effective customer service is the primary responsibility of every Personal Trainer.

> **Personal Trainers should keep in mind that every person they come in contact with throughout their work day, who is not on staff, is considered a "customer."**

There are some customer service skills that will go a long way to provide this optimal care and certainly enhance service delivery for every Personal Trainer. Personal Trainers should keep in mind that every person they come in contact with throughout their work day, who is not on staff, is considered a "customer." This includes all training clients, facility members, and guests (prospective clients). Table 19.1 presents basic customer service skills that every Personal Trainer should strive to perfect.

TABLE 19.1	BASIC CUSTOMER SERVICE SKILLS FOR THE PERSONAL TRAINER
Skill	**Description**
10-foot/5-foot rule	When a customer comes within 10 feet of a Personal Trainer, the Personal Trainer will stop what he/she is doing and make eye contact. When a customer comes within 5 feet, the Personal Trainer will speak to him or her.
Speaking first and last—and clearly	The Personal Trainer will initiate conversation with customers and will also have the last word with them. Greeting them with hello, etc., and ending with "have a nice day," "thank you for coming in," "my pleasure," etc. The Personal Trainer will also speak clearly and distinctly.
Posture	The Personal Trainer will assume a professional posture. Hands at side or behind back, stand upright and alert, look interested in the client, good body language (no slouching, hands in pocket, folded arms, etc.).
Smile/pleasant expression AND eye contact when greeting client	The Personal Trainer will greet the customer with eye contact and a smile or other pleasant expression.
Use the customer's name	The Personal Trainer will use the customer's name as often as possible.
Wear the name tag	The Personal Trainer will be neatly dressed in a clean and untattered uniform complete with a nametag (whenever appropriate).
Staff behavior is NOT hectic or chaotic	The Personal Trainer will behave in a controlled and orderly fashion.
Staff acknowledges customers in public places	The Personal Trainer speaks, nods, or otherwise acknowledges customers in public places.
The Personal Trainer speaks in a respectful tone to customers AND staff	The Personal Trainer will speak to customers in a respectful tone. The Personal Trainer will also speak to staff in a respectful manner. No derogatory slurs and no religious, ethnic, or sexual jokes, comments, or epithets will be made.
The Personal Trainer does not engage in distracting personal chatter or horseplay	The Personal Trainer will act in a professional manner around all customers. He or she will be alert to the customers' needs and proactive in his/her response.
The Personal Trainer does not eat, drink, or chew gum in public areas	
The "Barney Principle"	"Please" and "thank you" are the magic words. Using common manners (staff members not competing with customers for equipment). Choosing words that *positively* impact the customer. ("my pleasure" vs. "no problem").

EFFECTIVE PROFESSIONAL DAILY HABITS

Client Safety

The safety of the client is of primary concern. The Personal Trainer should understand the short- and long-term physiological changes that will result from the training. The confidence that the client is placing in the Personal Trainer makes it imperative that the Personal Trainer know the client's physical limitations as ascertained from the health history and a fitness evaluation. The Personal Trainer should also be sensitive to any daily fluctuations in the client's physical status. Any medical limitation affected by exercise should be referred to the client's physician for evaluation and treatment. The Personal Trainer should apply all phases of the exercise program with safety in mind. Form, speed of movement, weight selection, and monitoring of training intensities are all examples of safety consciousness.

Planning Each Workout

The Personal Trainer should map out specific goals and objectives in conjunction with the recommendations specified by current ACSM guidelines (1). Training programs should be planned accordingly, taking into account all structural and metabolic limitations when planning long- and short-term goals. Progressions should be planned so that each session can be as productive as possible. Clients should be challenged to their physical potential through a planned routine that is safe. Checking with clients daily or before each session on their physical/emotional readiness to exercise is crucial. This will assist the Personal Trainer in deciding on an optimal motivational approach. The Personal Trainer should be sensitive to the clients' needs and either talk to clients frequently, if they respond to that type of encouragement, or back off and keep vocal encouragement to a minimum if it is their preference.

Proper Charting

Proper charting is a "must-have"—not only from a customer service perspective but also from an ethical and liability standpoint. Documenting all activities and events will help the Personal Trainer provide the optimal service while limiting exposure risk. Each session should follow long- and short-term goals and objectives as agreed on at the initial fitness evaluation and interview (see Chapter 7). The Personal Trainer should record workout specifics such as appropriate weights/reps/sets, physiological data such as training HR/rating of perceived exertion (RPE)/BP responses or changes, signs and/or symptoms that may have occurred during a session, and, in certain cases, any special routines that will assist another staff member who might train that client next. The purpose of the notes are to:

> Keep track of exercise programs so they can be subsequently evaluated for effectiveness based on the results of posttesting
> Make the client's routine somewhat consistent regardless of the instructor
> Reinforce long-/short-term objectives
> Keep track of the trainee's progression in relation to changes in the applied program intensities

Professional Conduct in the Training Facility

The Personal Trainer must pay attention to the clients, whether he or she is working directly with them or not. It is understood that a Personal Trainer who is training a client is focused on that client alone. He or she should talk to that client only, give the client positive encouragement, and spot when necessary. A Personal Trainer who is not currently working with a client should talk to the trainees who are stretching or warming up/cooling down. Personal Trainers can take a HR, ask clients about their diets, and show them that they care. Proper body language is also an extremely important concept. For example, a Personal Trainer should not sit on a piece of equipment while the client is on another piece of equipment or lean up against the wall while the client is on the treadmill. Aside from the safety factor, if the client perceives that the Personal Trainer is disinterested and not caring, the quality of the workout will be compromised. These little things will differentiate the professional Personal Trainer from others (Fig. 19.1).

A Personal Trainer should not sit on a piece of equipment while the client is on another piece of equipment or lean up against the wall while the client is on the treadmill.

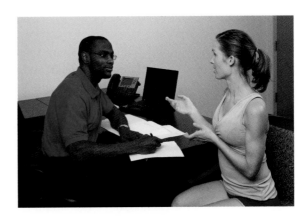

FIGURE 19.1. Proper body language is critical to the success of the Personal Trainer.

Facility Cleanliness

During nontraining time, check the facility to make sure that all is in order, the weights are put back, and the facility looks presentable. Personal Trainers should make periodic checks of the changing rooms and locker room facilities. They should try to go out of their way, depending on the facility, to make sure that the clients know where everything is, familiarize them with the phone system, show them where the emergency alarm is, and above all make sure that the room is clean.

Proper Exercise Protocols

Any major changes in the client's program as outlined from the client's fitness evaluation should be indicated in the client's fitness program chart. A Personal Trainer should be sure to update the fitness program chart as soon as any change in medical or structural condition presents itself. Take the appropriate steps, speak to the client regarding those conditions that affect the program, and ask the client's permission to contact his or her physician if warranted. The more closely the Personal Trainer monitors the client's day-to-day or week-to-week variations, the more effective, safe, and valid the exercise programs will be.

Daily Personal Trainer Improvement

A Personal Trainer should set short- and long-term career goals and make a concerted effort to reach those goals. Reading related literature, attending clinics, sharing information with other Personal Trainers, and observing other Personal Trainers with attention to detail will enhance the educational and vocational abilities of the Personal Trainer. Networking with other trainers and allied exercise and healthcare professionals, such as dieticians, allows Personal Trainers to refer if and when necessary and helps promote the profession from within.

PERSONAL TRAINING SESSION CRITERIA

Although Personal Trainers are found in a variety of work environments, there are common work performance criteria that will set apart the professional trainer from others. The comprehensive list below outlines some of the these important work habits that should be continuously practiced and perfected.

There are common work performance criteria that will set apart the professional trainer from others.

Greeting

The Personal Trainer's appearance must be neat and professional. Personal Trainers who are not required to wear a uniform might consider developing their own to create a consistently professional image. Like effective branding does for any product on the shelf, a consistently professional appearance will speak volumes about a Personal Trainer. First impressions are important, and it is up to the Personal Trainer to portray a professional appearance that will produce the desired impression for every client and prospective client.

The Personal Trainer should greet the client in an appropriate manner. A friendly, professional greeting with a handshake and a smile goes a long way to setting the tone and opening the door to building rapport with the client. Inappropriate language (i.e., demeaning comments; racial, ethnic, or sexist epithets; or "locker-room talk") has no place in a personal training session. Personal conversation should be kept to a minimum. A Personal Trainer should focus completely on the client's needs from the moment he or she greets the client through the farewell at the end of the session.

The Personal Trainer should always greet the client and start the session on time. Starting a session late tells the client that the Personal Trainer does not value the client's time. It clearly relates an uncaring feeling to the client and displays the epitome of unprofessionalism. Like any service provider, the Personal Trainer must always exhibit good client rapport. The client must trust the Personal Trainer's guidance, skills, and knowledge to benefit from the symbiotic client–trainer relationship.

Warm-Up Phase

The Personal Trainer must select an appropriate warm-up modality that:

➤ Is relevant to any structural or metabolic limitations
➤ Is relevant to goals and structure of workout
➤ Includes:
  • A minimum of 3–5 minutes in length
  • Appropriate intensity (i.e., at low end of training zone)
  • Monitoring of HR and/or RPE

Progression

A Personal Trainer must follow an appropriate exercise progression throughout the personal training session. Workouts should be constructed and proceed on the basis of the following general guidelines:

➤ Dynamic warm-up (as detailed above)
➤ Cardiovascular aerobic or anaerobic interval work when indicated (occurs within workout content after appropriate warm-up and includes appropriate cool-down)
➤ Flexibility component after appropriate warm-up (when indicated)
➤ Strength/muscular endurance component
➤ Core strengthening
➤ Condition-specific exercises (e.g., orthopedic protocols, pregnancy protocol) should occur at a logical point within the workout (pelvic tilt or floor work exercises should be introduced within the workout without making the client move back and forth from standing/seating to a reclining position several times).

Continuity

The "flow" of the personal training session should proceed in a continuous, uninterrupted manner (i.e., the Personal Trainer should not be charting the workout while the client waits to proceed to the next exercise). Make efficient use of floor space and choice of exercise modality when the training floor is crowded. It is up to the Personal Trainer to be creative and make alternative choices of exercises in an expedient manner.

Cool-Down Phase

The Personal Trainer should build in a gradual decrease in exercise intensity at the end of any cardiovascular exercise bout for the purpose of an effective cool-down. It should be a minimum of 2–5 minutes in length (cool-downs are client and situation specific in almost all cases), depending on the exercise intensity, duration, time exercising, and client-specific conditions (i.e., less-fit clients should be allowed a longer cool-down period to allow HR and BP to decrease). Exercise HR and/or RPE should be monitored. Additionally, a cool-down should occur after any hard bout of exercise or at any point within the workout, prior to final flexibility and abdominal, or core, work.

Flexibility

The Personal Trainer should follow appropriate flexibility training guidelines. Flexibility training with a client should be done only after an adequate warm-up. The type of flexibility training program depends on the client's needs and orthopedic history. Clients who have specific range-of-motion concerns should have more attention given to flexibility prior to any strength training or weight work, as well. The Personal Trainer, regardless of methodology, should follow ACSM guidelines (1) and hold static stretches for a minimum of 10–30 seconds. Proprioceptive neuromuscular facilitation stretches can be held for 6–10 seconds. However, it is vitally important to teach clients to listen to the needs of their body where stretching is concerned. Stretching exercises should include stretching of the major muscle groups as well as any specific areas of concern highlighted within the fitness assessment. Any muscle groups that may be sore from the previous workout and muscle groups worked at a high intensity during the workout should be given special consideration.

Monitoring Metabolic and Perceived Exertion

> *The Personal Trainer should monitor HR or RPE throughout various stages of the entire workout.*

The Personal Trainer should monitor HR or RPE throughout various stages of the entire workout, including the following:

- Warm-up phase
- Cardiovascular phase
- During weight/resistance training
- Postworkout
- During any interval work

Rating of perceived exertion is used for any clients taking medication that affects HR (e.g., β-blockers) during aerobic exercises and may be used during all modes of exercise for everyone. HR and RPE should be monitored throughout the workout. All perceptual signs and responses are observed in conjunction with HR and RPE, and exercise is monitored accordingly. This is especially important for clients who have a tendency to work hard and underestimate their RPE. Clients should be monitored for ataxia (unsteadiness of gait) or other physical signs of fatigue or stress (1).

Exercise Selection

The Personal Trainer must take several factors into account when selecting appropriate exercise progressions. These factors include the following:

- Client's goals
- Client's advisor program

➤ Client's skill level
➤ Structural or conditional specifics
➤ Considerations on the particular training day (e.g., client is tired, sore, has been ill, hasn't trained regularly, hasn't trained in over 1 month)
➤ Availability of equipment and other activities occurring within the fitness center

Spotting: Hands-On Interaction

The Personal Trainer should provide appropriate spotting during all aspects of the exercise session. This includes the following:

➤ *Cardiovascular work:* The Personal Trainer should be in a position to monitor the client's HR and RPE and give any assistance that is necessary
➤ *Resistance training machines:* Ranges of motion, feedback on speed of movement, verbal cues, and hands-on feedback during any machine weight work
➤ *Free weights:* Appropriate spotting occurs at all times with all clients (the Personal Trainer should be in a position to assist clients with the weights if they are not able to maintain good form or are unable to complete the activity)
➤ *Core work:* The Personal Trainer should assist the client and/or correct form, breathing, etc.
➤ *Stretching:* The Personal Trainer should direct appropriate stretching progression at the end of the session, within the context of the workout and based on the client need
➤ *Balancing equipment:* The Personal Trainer should be properly positioned to prevent the client from falling or provide adequate support for the client during balance training drills

The hands-on interaction that occurs during the workout should be based on the client, the exercises used, the appropriate feedback needed, and the overall program. Determine whether teaching cues and safety precautions are proper and appropriate for each client.

Equipment Use/Replacement

The Personal Trainer should use a variety of equipment during the workout. Any equipment used during the workout must be returned to a neat, orderly condition during the course of the workout to maintain safety and not interfere with any other workouts that are occurring within the same time frame. The variety and progression depend on several factors, including the following:

The Personal Trainer should use a variety of equipment during the workout.

➤ The client's individual goals
➤ Structural or metabolic barriers and needs
➤ The previous exercise session
➤ Gym floor traffic

Charting

The Personal Trainer must document all pertinent information in the client's fitness program chart. The client's chart for the day should include specific information regarding the following:

➤ The day's objectives
➤ Client's subjective comments
➤ Observations made by the Personal Trainer (as relevant)
➤ A clear, and neat, write-up of the workout performed
➤ Any new exercises or new machines used and how the client felt and performed the exercises

➤ Any particular changes in the client's fitness level as noted on a specific machine (e.g., "Client ran 0.3 miles farther than usual today" or "Client wasn't able to complete usual distance on bike due to hard workout previously")
➤ Recommendations for changes/updates in fitness program
➤ Recommendation for a reassessment
➤ Recommendations for the next exercise session

Adherence to Fitness Program Specifics

The Personal Trainer should adhere to the specific fitness program recommendations as based on the initial or follow-up fitness evaluations and interviews. Adhere to and expand on these recommendations within each workout. Such fitness program specifics include the following:

➤ Specific work or exercises for a structural and metabolic condition as recommended by a physician (e.g., perform exercises as specifically recommended for the client's shoulder impingement syndrome)
➤ Exercises used within a workout based on the client's overall structural or metabolic specifics (e.g., low back stabilization exercises included for the client who is on a low back protocol)
➤ Exercises or workout design based on short- and long-term goals (e.g., weight loss, workout includes CV and circuit work)

Attentiveness

Attentiveness begins the moment the client walks onto the exercise floor and finishes with the Personal Trainer saying goodbye to the client (including plans for the next session/workout and when it will occur, i.e., scheduling the client's next workout). Attention to every detail within the workout is important. Pertinent details include the following:

> **Attention to every detail within the workout is important.**

➤ Monitoring signs and symptoms
➤ Providing water and a towel, if appropriate
➤ Modification of exercises based on the client's ability to perform them correctly
➤ Exercise occurring within the desired target training zone and appropriate modifications as needed during the course of the session
➤ Ensuring proper breathing and form during all exercises
➤ Adherence to fitness program-specific recommendations

Innovation and Problem-Solving Skills

The Personal Trainer must have the ability to improvise and modify any aspect of the client's workout based on the following:

➤ Other activities occurring within the fitness center
➤ Availability of equipment within the fitness center
➤ Specific injuries and/or limitations
➤ Exercise prescription and training recommendations for a particular sporting event
➤ Previous exercise sessions
➤ Client attitude, level of motivation, or stage of readiness

Table 19.2 serves as a checklist for Personal Trainer managers to use when evaluating other trainers' skills and execution of a personal training session (2).

TABLE 19.2	**PERSONAL TRAINING SESSION EVALUATION CRITERIA/CHECKLIST**

I. Greeting

☐ Personal Trainer's appearance is neat and professional
☐ Appropriate greeting and reception
☐ Picks up client on time
☐ Displays good client rapport

II. Warm-up phase

Appropriate CV equipment utilized:
☐ Relevant to any structural or metabolic limitations
☐ Relevant to workout and program goals

Includes:
☐ A minimum of 3–5 minutes in length
☐ Appropriate intensity (i.e., at low end of training zone)
☐ Monitors and documents intensity responses (HR, RPE)

III. Exercise selection

Exercise selection takes into account:
☐ Client's goals (long-term and short-term)
☐ Overall training program
☐ Client's skill and fitness levels
☐ Any structural or metabolic conditions
☐ Any day-to-day considerations (i.e., client is tired, sore, had recent illness, inconsistent attendance, hasn't trained in over 1 month)
☐ Availability of equipment and other activities occurring within fitness center (See Innovation and problem-solving skills in section V below)
☐ A logical rationale for exercises (order, progression, continuity, etc.) or equipment and within accepted standards of care
☐ Previous exercise sessions

IV. Spotting, hands-on interaction, and attentiveness

Spotting occurs during all aspects of the exercise session:
☐ CV work: Personal Trainer is positioned to monitor the client's training HR/RPE, provide assistance
☐ Properly monitoring the range of motion on resistance training exercises, feedback on speed of movement, verbal cues, and hands-on feedback during exercises
☐ Free weights: Appropriate spotting occurs **at all times** with all clients. Personal Trainer is in a position to assist the clients with the weights if they are not able to maintain good form or are unable to complete the activity
☐ Abdominals: Personal Trainer models correct form, assists the client with form, breathing etc.
☐ Stretching: Hands-on stretching occurs at the end of the session and within the context of the workout as needed
☐ Balancing exercises: proper positioning to prevent client from falling
☐ Teaching cues are safe, accurate, and appropriate for the client

* The hands-on interaction should be based upon the client, the exercises utilized, the appropriate feedback needed and their overall program.

V. Innovation and problem-solving skills

Ability to improvise and modify any aspect of client's workout based upon:
☐ Other activities occurring within the fitness center
☐ Availability of equipment within the fitness center
☐ Specific injuries, limitations, or complaints of pain/discomfort
☐ Exercise prescription and training requests for a particular sporting event
☐ Previous exercise sessions

VI. Monitors metabolic and structural considerations

HR, RPE, and/or BP are monitored throughout various stages of the entire workout:
☐ Warm-up phase
☐ CV phase
☐ Resistance phase
☐ For hypertensive clients, BP is to be monitored before, during, and after a CV bout, interval, or resistance training phase.
☐ Trainer should ask for constant feedback of joint pain, fatigue, etc., from client.

* RPE is utilized for any **hypertensive clients** on medication that affects heart rate. Heart rate and RPE are to be monitored throughout workout with **pregnant clients.** Perceptual signs/signals (like ataxia (unsteadiness of gait), or other physical signs of fatigue) should be monitored in conjunction with HR, BP, and RPE, and exercise is modified accordingly. This is especially important in clients who have a tendency to work hard and underestimate their RPE.

(continued)

TABLE 19.2	PERSONAL TRAINING SESSION EVALUATION CRITERIA/CHECKLIST (*Continued*)

VII. Cool-down phase

☐ A slow decrease in exercise intensity occurs at the end of any CV bout, any hard bout of exercise, or at any point within the workout, prior to final flexibility and abdominal work.

☐ 2′–5′ in length; dependent upon the exercise intensity, time exercising, and client-specific conditions (e.g., provide hypertensive client and less-fit clients a longer cool-down period to allow for HR and BP to return toward pre-exercise levels without blood pooling or orthostatic hypotensive responses).

☐ Vital and perceptual signs are monitored

VIII. Flexibility work

☐ Occurs after an adequate physical preparation

☐ Depending upon the individual, at a minimum, at the end of the workout.

☐ Static stretches held for 10–30 seconds, proprioceptive neuromuscular facilitation stretches can be held for 6–7 seconds.

☐ Includes stretching the major muscle groups, any specific areas highlighted within the fitness assessment, or muscle groups emphasized during the workout.

IX. Charting/program update

The client's session should include specific information regarding:

☐ The day's objectives

☐ Client's subjective comments

☐ Relevant observations made by Personal Trainer

An update of the workout program after completion, taking into consideration:

☐ New exercises/machines utilized, how the client felt and performed the exercises

☐ Any particular changes in the client's fitness level as noted on a specific machine (e.g., "ran 0.3 m farther than usual today"; "wasn't able to complete usual distance due to hard workout")

☐ Recommendations for reassessment, suggested exercises for next workout session, etc.

☐ Any pain or discomfort that occurred during the session

☐ Any notes for next workout.

EDUCATION AND MOTIVATION

Exercise the body in a logical progression. Preplanning of the workout with consideration to muscular and systematic functions (e.g., aerobic, anaerobic power, sprint, postural problems) will make the entire session more efficient for the client. If time and machine availability make this preparation impractical, the general workout objective should be formulated and adhered to carefully. Remember to consider both the muscular and cardiorespiratory systems in every workout.

The Personal Trainer should emphasize the muscle groups and systematic functions that are specific to the trainee's individual goals and objectives. Even though many clients are in a "general conditioning" mode, each individual has a specific area of concern to which the Personal Trainer can gear the exercise routines to make them more meaningful. Some clients, for example, want to "tone up" their hips and buttocks. Explain the effectiveness of squatting exercises in relation to this individual goal. The Personal Trainer should talk to each client about how the tailored routine he or she has designed relates to the client's training objectives. Sport-specific emphasis can be obtained by exercising the muscles specific to performing the activity (e.g., exercising the quadriceps muscles for skiing, improving flexibility for golf). When prudent, appropriate orthopedic protocols should be implemented and explained as to how they will be integrated into the client's program to improve or prevent further injury.

The Personal Trainer should take proper notes for each workout. The short-term goal for each session should be included in this procedure. Specific objectives can be listed in order of priority. Specific exercises with weights/reps/sets, and HR/RPE responses when appropriate, can also be included in the notes. Any incidental aches and pains must be recorded. Any Personal Trainer should be able to train every client with the help of the workout notes.

> ***Any Personal Trainer should be able to train every client with the help of the workout notes.***

The Personal Trainer should emphasize correct form in all training sessions. The safety of an exercise is based in the form of execution, not the amount of weight or the number of reps. The Personal Trainer must make sure to exercise each targeted muscle group through a proper range of motion. Emphasize specific targeted muscles and coach the trainee not to contract extraneous muscles. This applies especially to the lower back, the neck/shoulder area, and the forearms. Ensure that the muscles lift and support the weight. The client should not support heavy weight with the moving joint(s) "locked out" (e.g., overhead press, bench press, and leg press). The Personal Trainer should teach and reinforce proper breathing techniques. The client should never hold his or her breath during any contraction. This increases intrathoracic (inside the chest) pressure and as a result increases blood pressure, which may or may not be dangerous for the specific client but is certainly unnecessary. The client should exhale when performing a concentric contraction and inhale during the eccentric phase.

The Personal Trainer should include the proper proportion of supervised aerobic exercise in each workout. The Personal Trainer should know the appropriate training HR range and record RPE when applicable. These measurements of intensity should be used to guide the progression of the applied workloads. Some aerobic components can be prescribed before or after the actual supervised session. This will depend on the client's overall physical condition, daily schedule, and specific training goals and objectives. The Personal Trainer should make sure that clients understand how to operate the prescribed aerobic modality and that they can either take their own HR or gauge RPE effectively, before they exercise without supervision. It is important to ask clients what additional activities they are performing outside of the facility. This will assist the Personal Trainer in the design of their training sessions. The Personal Trainer should teach each client the physiological basis of the RPE scale and explain how this will assist in monitoring exercise intensity and how it will make the sessions more efficient.

Personal Trainers must make each workout as interesting and as varied as possible. They must motivate the clients in every way they can. This variation is effective both psychologically and physiologically. Attention span is increased when topics of focus are divided into small diverse blocks relative to a client's physiological, structural, and motivational status. Mixing up the routine in this manner will help the client concentrate on the workout and its quality.

It is easy to train a client who is motivated and interested in the session. The Personal Trainer's job is to ensure that interest so that the effectiveness of each workout will be maximized. This can be achieved by incorporating static stretching in the session after a high-intensity strength set or mixing in aerobic or anaerobic intervals at specific points in the routine. The Personal Trainer should keep the client moving, minimize unnecessary conversation, and be alert to all of the overt signs of workout intensity. Personal Trainers must be creative in all of their sessions. This makes the Personal Trainer's job a lot more interesting and enjoyable.

> *The Personal Trainer should keep the client moving, minimize unnecessary conversation, and be alert to all of the overt signs of workout intensity.*

THE PHASES OF A PERSONAL TRAINING SESSION

Many dynamics are involved in a personal training session. Although sessions may vary on the basis of the different clients' goals and abilities, the Personal Trainer should always have a systematic approach to the personal training session. These sequential systems are not limited to the actual training session itself. Many of the systems that may be implemented will happen before and after the actual training session itself. These systems may be broken down into four phases: preparation phase, transitional phase, the workout, and the review.

Preparation Phase

Prior to a client's arrival, the Personal Trainer's objective should be to obtain as much information about him or her as possible. This information can be gathered while the client is on the phone scheduling the first session and should include such questions as the following:

➤ How did you hear about us?
➤ Are you currently exercising?
➤ What are your goals?
➤ Are there any medical conditions that a Personal Trainer should be aware of?

At the end of the conversation, the Personal Trainer should avoid commitment remorse from the client by telling the client what to expect on the first day. Here is a sample phone conversation that the Personal Trainer could use when trying to obtain information from a prospective client:

Michael: Thank you for calling the Fitness Center. How may I be of service?
Julie: Yes. I am calling to schedule my first personal training session.

Michael: Great, Julie, before I schedule that with you, I would like to ask you some questions so I can prepare a program that is specific to you. Is that okay?
Julie: Sure.

Michael: What are some of your goals?
Julie: I would like to lose some weight and tone my arms.

Michael: Are you currently exercising?
Julie: Yes. I walk and do free weights twice a week.

Michael: Wow! That's great. What are you hoping to get from this program that you are not receiving from your current program?
Julie: Well, I have been doing the same thing for over a year and I am not seeing any results.

Michael: That is quite normal, don't worry. Is there any medical condition that I should be aware of?
Julie: No.

Michael: Okay Julie, when you arrive, we are going to ask you to fill out some informational paperwork prior to your session, so try to arrive about 10 minutes early. After you finish, we are going to do a light warm-up before beginning the actual session. Once you complete the warm-up, I am going to take you through the workout that I will have designed for you, so wear comfortable clothes. Sound good?
Julie: Yes. Thank you.

It is important to take notes during this conversation for two reasons. First, it will help the Personal Trainer develop a program that is conducive to the client's needs. Moreover, when the client arrives, the Personal Trainer can reiterate this information to the client, which shows interest and builds credibility. The first impression is the most important stage of developing a Personal Trainer–client relationship. A well-prepared Personal Trainer has a much greater chance of client retention.

On the day of the client's scheduled appointment, the Personal Trainer should be present and ready to begin well before the new client's workout time. The client's folder with the information that was obtained on the phone should be retrieved, as well as the program that the Personal Trainer prepared prior to the client's arrival. The Personal Trainer should review the exercise prescription and notes taken from the phone conversation. All pertinent forms should be on the Personal Trainer's clipboard and prepared for the session.

When the new client arrives, the Personal Trainer should be introduced with a smile, shake the client's hand, and make eye contact. The client should be invited to a waiting area or office to fill out any forms that the facility may require, such as an information sheet, medical questionnaire, or Physical Activity Readiness Questionnaire. Once the client finishes filling out the forms, the Personal Trainer is going to want to take a minute to review the forms with the client, looking for anything that may assist in the training process or that may have been overlooked during the initial conversation (Fig. 19.2). Personal Trainers may occasionally need to contact the client's physicians if medical conditions are present requiring medical clearance. This should be done prior to any exercise program participation.

When the new client arrives, the Personal Trainer should be introduced with a smile, shake the client's hand, and make eye contact.

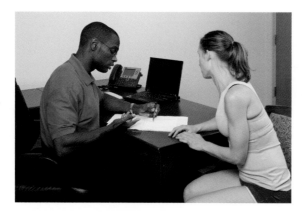

FIGURE 19.2. Personal Trainer reviewing pre-evaluation forms with a client.

It is at this point that the Personal Trainer is going to begin the transition from filling out the forms to the actual workout, also known as the transitional phase. Here is a review of the components of the preparation phase:

1. Ask permission to obtain as much information as possible before meeting the new client.
2. Inform the client about what he or she can expect during the session, to prevent commitment remorse.
3. Take notes of the conversation to aid in program development and building rapport.
4. Develop a program on the basis of the client's goals.
5. Arrive 15 minutes prior to the session to review the client's folder.
6. Introduce yourself and ask the client to fill out proper forms.
7. Review the forms with your client and begin warm-up.

Transitional Phase

Once the Personal Trainer and the client have reviewed the proper paperwork, it is time to begin the client's warm-up. Select a cardiovascular machine that is going to correspond to the client's ability. Begin slowly and after 30 seconds, ask whether the client is comfortable. Once the client is comfortable, it is time to go over exactly what he or she will be doing during the workout. Some of the key points that the Personal Trainer should convey to the client are the muscle groups that will be working, how the client will be feeling, and teaching the client to use a modified RPE scale from 1 to 10 (Fig. 19.3). A sample explanation might go something like the following:

> *Michael: Julie, typically our clients come in and train three times per week. Therefore, we will be working your entire body every time you come in. Based on your primary goal of weight loss, we are going to be moving fairly quickly from exercise to*

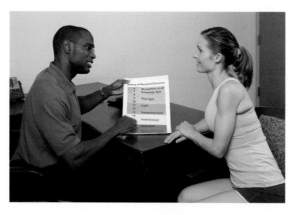

FIGURE 19.3. Personal Trainer explaining the use of the rating of perceived exertion chart to a client.

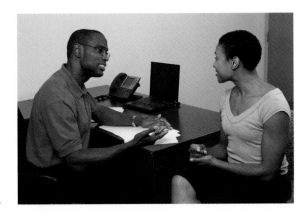

FIGURE 19.4. Personal Trainer briefing a client.

exercise with very little rest, with higher repetitions and lower weights. You are going to be out of breath and sweating. That's okay. It's very normal. After each exercise I am going to be asking you how you feel on a scale from 1 to 10, 10 being the hardest thing you have ever done in your life and 1 being the easiest. This is what I am going to use to judge if you can keep the same pace or if we need to modify the intensity in any way. So just shout out "Mike, that was a 3" or "Mike, that was a 7" so I know what is your perceived exertion is. If you have any questions at all, please feel free to ask.

During that brief conversation (Fig. 19.4), the Personal Trainer:

1. Told what muscles will be working
2. Restated the primary goal to enforce personal attention
3. Explained how the client would be feeling
4. Used a modified RPE
5. Told the client to please feel free to ask any questions

A simple conversation can bring a level of comfort between the Personal Trainer and the client. Once the Personal Trainer describes what is about to happen, he or she should make sure to set up the first exercise for the client and prepare the area where the training session will occur. Finally, check the client's HR to get a baseline reading for the workout. Once a baseline measurement has been established, it is time to begin the actual workout. Here is a review of the stages of the transitional phase:

1. Set up the client on a piece of cardiovascular equipment that corresponds to his or her ability.
2. After the client is set up, go over what will happen during the workout, to further develop a sense of comfort for the client. Remember to reiterate primary goals to enforce personal attention.
3. Set up the first exercise or several exercises that will be performed with the client as well as the area where the Personal Trainer will be working if necessary.
4. Take the client's HR to determine a baseline.

The Workout

Communication with the client is going to be extremely important throughout the workout. A Personal Trainer who is training someone for the first time cannot assume that the client knows the proper form of an exercise or where the Personal Trainer will be placing his or her hands to spot them effectively. Before each exercise the Personal Trainer must explain the following details: proper form, proper breathing, and where the Personal Trainer will be touching the client to be able to spot them. All of these factors are imperative for the client's comfort and your liability. Two things that should not be incorporated in this dialogue are the amount of weight being used and the number of repetitions. If the Personal Trainer tells the client he or she is going to perform 15 repetitions and the Personal Trainer happens to overestimate the amount of weight the client can handle and he or

> *A Personal Trainer who is training someone for the first time cannot assume that the client knows the proper form of an exercise or where the Personal Trainer will be placing his or her hands, to spot them effectively.*

she can perform only 10 repetitions, the client will now have a sense of failure and a "this is too hard" attitude. A sample explanation might go as follows:

> *Michael: Julie, the first exercise we are going to perform is the dumbbell chest press. You are going to be lying on the bench with your hands up in the air. I am going to hand you the dumbbells and then stand behind you and spot you from your wrist. I want you to take a big deep breath in through your nose on the way down, bending your elbows and bringing your hands just above your chest. Then you are going to exhale as you push the dumbbells straight up in the air. Throughout the exercise, I want you to try and keep five points of contact: your head, shoulders, lower back, glutes, and feet. Do you have any questions?*

Once again, from the simple dialogue the Personal Trainer was able to describe the proper form of the exercise, the proper breathing technique, and how the client would be spotted. Upon completion of the exercise, the client should be asked how he or she feels on a scale from 1 to 10 and then the Personal Trainer should establish a pace based on the client's first sets.

Throughout the workout, maintain constant involvement and enthusiasm. Keeping the client motivated is one of the main goals of the workout. The other key factor is time management. The Personal Trainer always wants to stay ahead of the client, having all of the weights and exercises prepared in advance. Breaks will be limited, on the basis of the client's goals and ability. If after three exercises a client informs the Personal Trainer that he or she is at an RPE of 9 out of 10, slow down the workout by explaining the theories behind the designed workout. This will considerably slow down the pace of the workout, while the client does not get a sense of failure. Monitor the client's HR to determine the necessary length of the breaks.

With about 15 minutes remaining in the session, tell what exercises are remaining, so the client can mentally prepare for the finish (Fig. 19.5). With approximately 10 minutes remaining, it is time to cool down and stretch. After competing the stretching, it is time to move into the review phase. Here is a review of the stages of the workout:

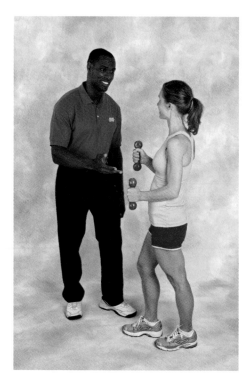

FIGURE 19.5. Personal Trainer communicating effectively with a client upon the completion of an exercise.

1. Before beginning each exercise, explain to the client the proper form, proper breathing, and where you will be touching the client to spot them.
2. After each exercise, ask the client how he or she feels on a scale from 1 to 10
3. Establish a pace based on the client's ability.
4. Converse during breaks if the workout needs to slow down or increase in intensity.
5. With 15 minutes left in the workout, tell the client what exercises are remaining so he or she mentally prepares for the finish.
6. With 10 minutes remaining, cool down and stretch.

The Review

Upon completion, thank the client for a good workout. Once the client is gone, the Personal Trainer must restore the training area to its proper form, racking the weights and wiping down all equipment. It is then time to record all of the information that has just been obtained throughout the workout. On the client's chart, record the client's RPE for each exercise, whether the client had any difficulty throughout any of the exercises, and any modifications that have been made for the next workout. Finally, place the folder back in the storage facility and prepare for the next client. Once again, the stages of the review phase include the following:

1. Thanking the client for a good workout.
2. Restoring the training room to proper form.
3. Recording information from the client's workout, including RPE and any modifications for the next workout.
4. Placing the client's folder back in the storage facility.

TRAINING NOTES

Training notes are the Personal Trainer's equivalent to medical charts. They contain valuable pieces of information that are vital to the proper treatment of each client. Although recording information and transferring data from sheet to sheet can be tedious, it is extremely important to the success of any applied training regimen. Analysis of the chart will enable the Personal Trainer to structure workouts for maximum results. The objectives for the notes are as follows:

> *Training notes are the Personal Trainer's equivalent to medical charts.*

- ➤ To keep track of the exercise program so that its effectiveness can be evaluated through the reevaluation procedure
- ➤ To ensure that the client's program is consistent regardless of the instructor
- ➤ To reinforce long- and short-term objectives
- ➤ To keep track of the trainee's progression in relation to changes in workout intensity

All notes should be thorough and concise. Note only relevant information and be sure to sign your name to each session. The following types of information are a sample of what might be included in a client's training notes:

1. *Subjective (SUB)*: Describes how the client feels on the day of a particular workout. It serves as a barometer for the Personal Trainer in structuring the physiological and psychological climate of the workout.
2. *Observation (OBS)*: Notes any signs of tissue trauma (e.g., edema, extreme redness), ecchymosis (black and blue), or joint dysfunction (i.e., limping or impaired ROM). If any of these signs exist, it might be recommended to ask the client to see his or her physician.
3. *Objectives (OBJ)*: Describes specific objectives for that session. It should be based on the long- and short-term goals with consideration of daily SUB and OBS.

4. *Workout (WO)*: Notes the major components of that session (i.e., modes, exercises, sets, reps, weights, workloads, HR/RPE responses).

5. Comments are noted at the end of each session. This section may include plans for the next workout (e.g., pain associated with a specific movement) or any other relevant comments.

6. Personal Trainer's signature

SUMMARY

It is obvious that, like any other "technical" job task, personal training has very specific protocols that should be followed to optimize the level of service delivered to the client. In addition to following accepted standard guidelines with regard to exercise, the Personal Trainer must also strive to deliver the highest level of customer service and accurately and completely document every aspect of the client's program and individual session.

REFERENCES

1. American College of Sports Medicine. *Guidelines for Exercise Testing and Prescription.* 8th ed. Baltimore: Lippincott Williams & Wilkins; 2010.

2. Plus One Training Department. *Exercise Specialist Training Manual.* 6th ed. New York: Plus One; 2004.

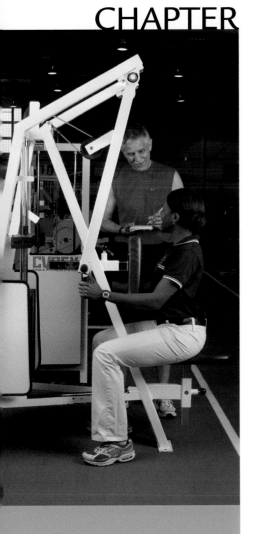

20

Special Populations

OBJECTIVES

- Provide a description of special populations that makes them unique when compared with individuals who do not have disease
- Learn how to create programs for older adults who may have comorbidities
- Develop a knowledge of cardiovascular disease
- Learn how to develop programs for women who are pregnant from the first trimester to the last trimester
- Learn the distinction between Type 1 and Type 2 diabetes
- Review the categories of obesity and how Personal Trainers develop lifestyle modification programs for them
- Provide the Personal Trainer with the correct tools to develop programs for clients who have been diagnosed with hypertension

I
n 2005, less than half (49.1%) of U.S. adults met the Centers for Disease Control and Prevention (CDC)/ACSM physical activity recommendation with 23.7% reporting no leisure-time activity (2). Physical inactivity is associated with at least numerous unhealthy conditions, including obesity, hypertension, gestational and Type 2 diabetes, and atherosclerotic cardiovascular disease (CVD), and contributes annually to 250,000 premature deaths (14). Older Americans are currently both the least physically active and the most rapidly growing of any age group. Over the next several decades, millions of baby boomers will continue to turn 65 years of age (49). These factors make it increasingly likely that the Personal Trainer will be interacting with clientele other than apparently healthy adults. This chapter discusses the special considerations and scope of practice of exercise program design for the following subpopulations: older adults, cardiac disease, pregnancy, diabetes mellitus, obesity, and hypertension.

PROGRAMMING FOR OLDER ADULTS

Older adults can be defined as men and women 65 years and older and adults aged 50–64 years with clinically significant chronic conditions and/or functional limitations that impact movement ability, fitness, or physical activity (49). Despite these age ranges, the Personal Trainer should not assume that chronological age is equivalent to physiological or functional age. Individuals of similar ages can differ remarkably in functional capacity, which in turn will affect how they respond to exercise. Although it is inevitable that physiological function will decline with age, the rate and magnitude of change are dependent on a complex mixture of genetics, individual health, presence of disease/injury, and exercise history. Safe and effective exercise programming for older adults requires that Personal Trainers have knowledge of the effects of aging on physiological function at rest and throughout the exercise intensity spectrum. A list of key physiological aspects of aging is presented in Table 20.1.

> *Individuals of similar ages can differ remarkably in functional capacity, which in turn will affect how they respond to exercise.*

Lastly, an awareness of the physiological aspects of aging will assist the Personal Trainer in establishing realistic program goals for clientele. Previously sedentary, older adults initiating an exercise program can expect improvements in numerous health benefits. However, because of the natural decline in function associated with aging, the Personal Trainer should interpret maintenance of function as a successful outcome. For example, research suggests an average 1% decrease in cardiorespiratory fitness per year (26). A Personal Trainer who works with a client for 3 years and observes no change in his or her cardiorespiratory fitness level over that time has designed and implemented an effective program. Why? The inevitable decline in physiological function, in this case cardiorespiratory fitness, has been delayed. Personal Trainers should design programs for older adults with three primary goals in mind:

1. Prevent or retard the progression of chronic diseases (and possibly aid in "reversing" as in normalizing blood glucose)
2. Maintain or enhance cardiorespiratory fitness levels (i.e., functional capacity)
3. Prevent functional limitations and disabilities

Because of the likelihood of clinically significant or underlying chronic disease in older adults, it is imperative that Personal Trainers always complete a thorough preparticipation health screening and risk stratification (as detailed in Chapter 13) before beginning an exercise program with this population. The next section will describe design considerations for cardiorespiratory fitness, muscular strength, flexibility, and balance.

Aerobic Activity for Older Adults

Cardiorespiratory fitness is arguably the most important goal of an exercise program for older adults as low cardiorespiratory fitness may contribute to premature mortality in middle-aged and

TABLE 20.1	PHYSIOLOGICAL ASPECTS OF AGING	
System	**Parameter**	**Change**
Cardiovascular	Maximal heart rate and stroke volume	↓
	Maximal cardiac output	↓
	Resting and exercise blood pressure	↑
	Maximal oxygen consumption	↓
Environmental	Cold tolerance (heat production/blood redistribution)	↓
	Heat tolerance (sweat capacity/blood redistribution)	↓
Musculoskeletal	Lean body mass	↓
	Fat mass	↑
	Muscle strength	↓
	Bone mineral density	↓
	Flexibility	↓
Metabolic	Glucose tolerance	↓
	Insulin sensitivity	↓
Other	Balance	↓
	Reaction time	↑*

*Reaction time increases with age (i.e., it will take longer to accomplish a task).

older adults (35). The literature suggests a 15% reduction in mortality for a 10% improvement in cardiorespiratory fitness (11,29). Moreover, decreased cardiorespiratory fitness contributes to a reduction in physiological functional capacity and eventually can result in loss of independence (26,38). Personal Trainers should design programs for older adults with the intention of fulfilling the population-wide recommendation of moderate-intensity aerobic activity for a minimum of 30 minutes on 5 days each week (or 150 minutes) or vigorous-intensity aerobic activity for a minimum of 25 minutes on 3 days each week (or 75 minutes) or an equivalent combination of both (49). When not feasible for older adults to fulfill these guidelines due to debilitating chronic conditions, it is imperative that Personal Trainers encourage these individuals to be as physically active as their condition permits (2). It is imperative that older adult clientele be counseled to avoid physical inactivity. The general cardiorespiratory training principles of exercise prescription detailed in Chapter 18 apply to older adults, although depending on the disease and functional status of the individual, modifications to the program may be warranted (Table 20.2).

Muscle Strengthening Activity for Older Adults

Aging is associated with a reduction in muscle mass, which in turn contributes to decreased muscle strength and a decline in functional capacity. Undeterred, the process can ultimately result in balance impairments, mobility problems, and lack of independence for the older adult (53). Furthermore, decreased muscle mass plays a role in the development of glucose intolerance and Type 2 diabetes. For these reasons, the Personal Trainer should recognize the importance of implementing a resistance training program for older adult clientele to attenuate the loss of muscle mass. The general resistance training principles of exercise prescription detailed in Chapter 16 with several considerations that account for function and possible disease status also apply to older adults (Table 20.3).

Flexibility Activity for Older Adults

Flexibility is an essential component of fitness and decreases with age and physical inactivity. Poor flexibility, coupled with decreased musculoskeletal strength, has been associated with a diminished ability to perform activities of daily living (2). Consequently, the beneficial effect of static stretching

TABLE 20.2	AEROBIC EXERCISE PROGRAM MODIFICATIONS FOR OLDER ADULTS
Program Component	**Program Modification**
Exercise mode	Walking is an excellent mode of exercise for many older adults Modality should not impose excessive orthopedic stress Aquatic, stationary cycle, and recumbent stepper exercise may be preferable for clients with a diminished ability to tolerate weight-bearing exercise Modality should be accessible, convenient, and enjoyable to promote adherence A group setting may provide social reinforcement to adherence
Exercise intensity	To minimize complications and promote long-term compliance, intensity for inactive older adults should start low and progress according to client preference and tolerance. Initiating a program at less than 40% HRR or VO_2R is not unusual Many adults have clinically diagnosed conditions or likely have underlying chronic diseases; thus, a conservative approach to increasing intensity may be required Exercise need not be vigorous and continuous to be beneficial; a daily accumulation of 30 minutes of moderate-intensity physical activity can provide health benefits Measured peak heart rate is preferable to age-predicted peak heart rate because of the variability in peak heart rate in clients $>$ 65 yrs and their greater risk for underlying CAD Activities performed at a given MET level represent greater relative intensities in older adults than in younger clients because of the decrease in peak METs with age (Table 20.1) Older adults are likely to be taking medications that can influence heart rate
Exercise session duration	To prevent injury, ensure safety, and promote adherence, older adults should increase exercise duration prior to intensity Duration need not be continuous to produce benefits. Clients who have difficulty sustaining exercise for 30 min or who prefer shorter bouts of exercise can be advised to exercise for 10-min bouts throughout the day
Exercise frequency	Moderate-intensity exercise should be performed most days of the week Vigorous-intensity exercise bouts should be alternated with rest of moderate-intensity exercise days

From American College of Sports Medicine. *ACSM's Guidelines for Exercise Testing and Prescription.* 8th ed. Baltimore: Lippincott Williams & Wilkins; 2010.

TABLE 20.3	RESISTANCE TRAINING GUIDELINES FOR OLDER ADULTS
Program Component	**Program Modification**
Exercise mode	Perform 8–10 exercises using the major muscle groups Dynamic muscle strengthening activities include machine and free weights, weight-bearing calisthenics, resistance bands, and similar resistance exercises that use major muscle groups
Exercise intensity	Perform each lift or movement with a resistance that allows for 10–15 repetitions per exercise Level of effort for muscle-strengthening activities should be moderate to high. On a 10-point scale, where no movement =0, and maximal effort =10, moderate-intensity effort =5 or 6, and high-intensity effort =7 or 8
Exercise session duration	Complete 1 set of each exercise Allow adequate rest between exercises to prevent carry-over fatigue
Exercise frequency	Resistance training should be performed on two or more nonconsecutive days per week

Adapted from American College of Sports Medicine. *ACSM's Guidelines for Exercise Testing and Prescription.* 8th ed. Baltimore: Lippincott Williams & Wilkins; 2009; and Nelson ME, Rejeski WJ, Blair SN, et al. Physical activity and public health in older adults: recommendation for adults from the American College of Sports Medicine and the American Heart Association. *Med Sci Sports Exerc.* 2007;39:1435–45.

on the achievement and maintenance of flexibility should not be overlooked. The guidelines for designing flexibility programs that are detailed in Chapter 18 apply to older adults.

The last 10 years have seen much scientific inquiry on the topic of stretching and performance/risk of injury. Collectively, present research findings suggest that there are no ergogenic benefits, and potentially detrimental effects (decreased muscle strength and endurance, impaired balance, and diminished reaction time), to the incorporation of static stretching exercises into the warm-up routine (57). These findings are consistent among different populations and research designs, including untrained and trained individuals, recreational and competitive athletes, males and females, and with or without an aerobic warm-up (57). The Personal Trainer should be mindful of this evidence when designing programs for older adult clientele and consider sequencing the workout so that flexibility follows the aerobic and resistance training components.

Balance Exercise for Older Adults

Fall incidence rates currently pose a serious health problem for older adults. In persons 65 years and older, it has been estimated that 35%–45% of otherwise healthy, community-dwelling adults fall at least once a year (7). Decreased balance is attributable to an age-related decline in multiple physiological systems that contribute to decreased muscle flexibility and strength, reduced central processing of sensory information, and slowed motor responses (7). In addition to an increased risk of falls, diminished balance and mobility may limit activities of daily living or participation in leisure-time activities. Accordingly, Personal Trainers must include balance exercises in older adults' exercise programs. Although research has yet to identify the optimal frequency, duration, and type of balance exercises, it has been recommended that balance training be performed 3 days per week for 10–15 minutes each session. Balance training can be integrated into various phases of the exercise session, including warm-up, main component, or cool-down. Sample balance exercises and training progression (from simple to complex) are presented in Table 20.4 and are shown in Figures 20.1, 20.2, and 20.3.

> *Personal Trainers must include balance exercises in older adults' exercise programs.*

TABLE 20.4	**BALANCE EXERCISES AND TRAINING PROGRESSION FOR OLDER ADULTS**
Position	**Balance Exercise**
Sitting	Sit upright and complete progressions listed below Perform leg activities (heel, toe, or single-leg raises, marching)
Standing	"Clock"—balance on one leg (45° or 90° angle), Personal Trainer calls out time, client moves nonsupport leg to time called (i.e., 5 o'clock, 9 o'clock), alternate legs Perform leg activities (heel, toe, or single-leg raises—45° or 90° angle, marching) "Spelling"—balance on one leg, Personal Trainer asks the client to spell word working with nonsupport leg (i.e., client's name, day of week, favorite food), alternate legs
In motion	Heel-to-toe walking along 15-ft line on floor (first with and then without partner) "Excursion"—alternating legs, lunge over a space separated by two lines of tape. Progress to hopping or jumping (using single-leg or double-leg) back and forth across the space Dribble basketball around cones that require the client to change direction multiple times
Training progression	Arm progressions: use surface for support, hands on thigh, hands folded across chest Surface progressions: chair, balance discs, foam pad, physioball Visual progressions: open eyes, sun glasses or dim room lighting, closed eyes Tasking progressions: single tasking, multitasking (i.e., balance exercise + pass/catch ball)

Number of repetitions per exercise and rest intervals will be dependent on client conditioning and functional status.

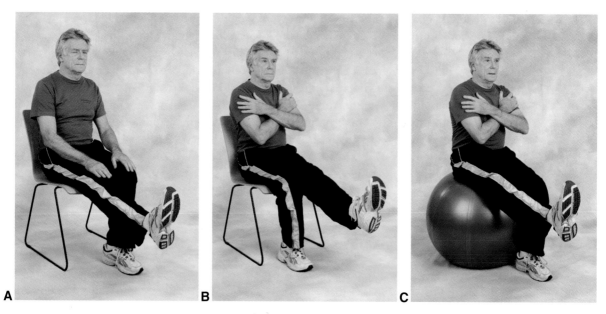

FIGURE 20.1. Sample progression of sitting balance exercises: **(A)** closed eyes; **(B)** arms crossed; and **(C)** physioball.

PROGRAMMING FOR CLIENTS WITH CVD

According to the American Heart Association, more than 79 million Americans have one or more types of CVD (55). Although the prevalence of CVD-related deaths has declined since the 1980s, it remains the leading cause of death in the United States (55). In 2004, CVD claimed 870,000 lives, and over half were attributed to coronary artery disease (CAD) (55). Patterns of nutrient intake and physical inactivity underlie the global epidemic of chronic diseases, including obesity, hypertension, dyslipidemia, and Type 2 diabetes, which all serve as risk factors that contribute to the process of

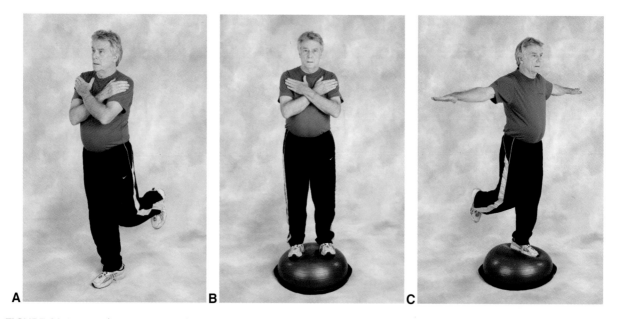

FIGURE 20.2. Sample progression of standing balance exercise, with arms crossed on floor **(A)** and with arms crossed **(B)** and open **(C)** on balance training equipment.

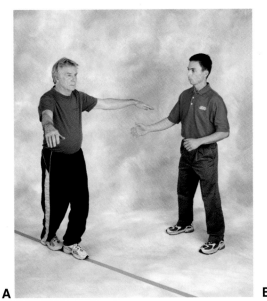
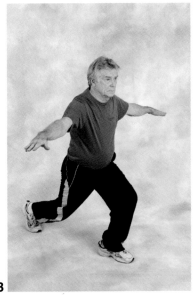
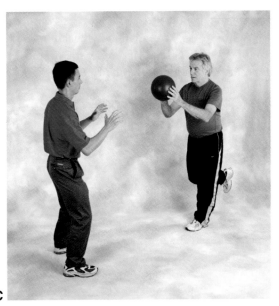

FIGURE 20.3. Sample progression of in-motion balance exercises: **(A)** heel-to-toe; **(B)** excursion; and **(C)** multitasking.

> *The Personal Trainer should recognize that primary prevention of atherosclerotic risk factors is preferable; individuals who are able to reach the age of 50 years with no risk factors have markedly higher survival rates than those with any combination of risk factors.*

CAD. Importantly, the Personal Trainer should recognize that primary prevention of atherosclerotic risk factors is preferable; individuals who are able to reach the age of 50 years with no risk factors have markedly higher survival rates than those with any combination of risk factors. Even those individuals who have one risk factor at middle age are at a much higher risk for CVD and CAD (47). Alternatively, exercise programs can be designed for individuals with known CAD that can stabilize and even reverse the process of atherosclerosis.

Programming Goals

Positive risk factor modification is the primary goal of an aerobic exercise program for clients with heart disease. Scientific research has demonstrated that there is a dose–response relationship between exercise and multiple health outcomes, including risk of CAD and all-cause mortality, obesity, dyslipidemia, Type 2 diabetes, and perhaps most importantly cardiorespiratory fitness (72). It has been suggested that cardiorespiratory fitness is the ultimate marker for health outcomes and risk stratification. Studies have consistently demonstrated an inverse relationship between $\dot{V}O_{2max}$ values and risk of CVD (10,11). Moreover, it has been shown that risk for CVD and all-cause mortality in men and women is highest for individuals with low levels of cardiorespiratory fitness compared with other traditional risk factors such as hypertension, dyslipidemia, and obesity (12). Each 1-MET increase ($3.5 \text{ mL} \cdot \text{kg}^{-1} \cdot \text{min}^{-1}$) in cardiorespiratory fitness can reduce the risk of CVD and all-cause mortality by 8%–17%.

Based on the dose–response relationship between exercise and health outcomes, both the ACSM and U.S. Surgeon General have noted that the health benefits of a program are closely associated with total weekly energy expenditure (2,68). The ACSM has recommended a target energy expenditure of $150-400 \text{ kcal} \cdot \text{day}^{-1}$. The lower end of this range corresponds to $1,000 \text{ kcal} \cdot \text{week}^{-1}$, whereas the upper end is equivalent to approximately $3,000 \text{ kcal} \cdot \text{week}^{-1}$. Additionally, recent studies have shown that exercise programs with energy expenditure recommendations (14 and 23 $\text{kcal} \cdot \text{kg}^{-1} \cdot \text{week}^{-1}$) based on individual differences in body mass lead to significant improvements in cardiorespiratory fitness and other important risk factors for CAD, including dyslipidemia, body composition, and insulin sensitivity (31,41,46,60). Accordingly, the Personal Trainer should individually design the parameters of the aerobic exercise prescription (frequency, intensity, time, and type—the FITT principle) to fulfill total weekly energy expenditure levels that have been shown to elicit positive adaptations to CAD risk factors. Achievement of this objective will positively modify the process of atherosclerosis and subsequently reduce the likelihood of future cardiac events (66).

Aerobic Activity for Cardiac Disease

Exercise training is relatively safe for the majority of clients with CVD provided that appropriate assessment and screening is performed before beginning the program. The likelihood of an adverse event, although not entirely preventable, can be markedly reduced with baseline assessments, risk stratification, patient education, and client adherence to established exercise recommendations (2). Critically, all CVD clients should have physician clearance and consent to participate in an exercise program. Additionally, it is recommended that the Personal Trainer stratify the cardiac client according to the risk stratification model presented in Table 20.5. Clients stratified as Class B will be appropriate clients to begin an exercise program in your facility. In contrast, Class C and D risk–stratified clientele require medical supervision and should not begin an exercise program in your facility and can be referred to an existing clinically supervised program.

Once it has been established that it is reasonably safe for the cardiac client to begin, the specific details of an exercise program can be formulated. The next step is to establish a baseline measure of cardiorespiratory fitness. This is critical as one of your goals is to improve cardiorespiratory fitness and, without a baseline value, it will be impossible to evaluate the successfulness of your program. Most of the cardiorespiratory assessments described in Chapter 14 can be provided to cardiac clients after proper screening and clinical evaluations including a recent clinical exercise test. Additionally, appropriate exercise intensity is dependent on the baseline cardiorespiratory fitness level. The Personal Trainer must recognize the critical importance of exercise intensity to the exercise prescription model, particularly for this population. Failure to meet minimal threshold values may result in lack of a training effect, while exceeding appropriate intensities can lead to overtraining and negatively impact adherence to an exercise program (37). Furthermore, excessively high exercise intensity

TABLE 20.5 AMERICAN HEART ASSOCIATION RISK STRATIFICATION CRITERIA

Risk classification for exercise training (Class A):
Apparently healthy individuals

This classification includes the following:
1. Children, adolescents, men aged <45 years, and women aged <55 years who have no symptoms or known presence of heart disease or major coronary risk factors.
2. Men ≥45 years and women ≥55 years who have no symptoms or known presence of heart disease and with <2 major cardiovascular risk factors.
3. Men ≥45 years and women ≥55 years who have no symptoms or known presence of heart disease and with ≥2 major cardiovascular risk factors.

Activity guidelines: No restrictions other than basic guidelines
Supervision required: None[a]
ECG and blood pressure monitoring: Not required

Risk classification for exercise training (Class B):
Presence of known, stable cardiovascular disease with low risk for complications with vigorous exercise, but slightly greater than for apparently healthy individuals

This classification includes individuals with any of the following diagnoses:
1. CAD (MI, CABG, PTCA, angina pectoris, abnormal exercise test, and abnormal coronary angiograms); those whose conditions are stable and who have the clinical characteristics outlined below
2. Valvular heart disease, excluding severe valvular stenosis or regurgitation with the clinical characteristics as outlined below
3. Congenital heart disease; risk stratification for patients with congenital heart disease should be guided by the 27th Bethesda Conference recommendations.
4. Cardiomyopathy: ejection fraction ≤30%; includes stable patients with heart failure with clinical characteristics as outlined below but not hypertrophic cardiomyopathy or recent myocarditis
5. Exercise test abnormalities that do not meet any of the high-risk criteria outlined in Class C below

Clinical characteristics (must include all of the following):
1. New York Heart Association Class 1 or 2
2. Exercise capacity ≤6 METs
3. No evidence of congestive heart failure
4. No evidence of myocardial ischemia or angina at rest or on the exercise test ≤6 METs
5. Appropriate rise in systolic blood pressure during exercise
6. Absence of sustained or nonsustained ventricular tachycardia at rest or with exercise
7. Ability to satisfactorily self-monitor intensity of activity

Activity guidelines: Activity should be individualized, with exercise prescription provided by qualified individuals and approved by primary healthcare provider.
Supervision required: Medical supervision during initial prescription session is beneficial.
Supervision by appropriate trained nonmedical personnel for other exercise sessions should occur until the individual understands how to monitor his or her activity. Medical personnel should be trained and certified in Advanced Cardiac Life Support. Nonmedical personnel should be trained and certified in Basic Life Support (which includes cardiopulmonary resuscitation).
ECG and blood pressure monitoring: Useful during the early prescription phase of training, usually 6–12 sessions.

Risk classification for exercise training (Class C):
Those at moderate-to-high risk for cardiac complications during exercise and/or unable to self-regulate activity or to understand recommended activity level

This classification includes individuals with any of the following diagnoses:
1. CAD with the clinical characteristics outlined below.
2. Valvular heart disease, excluding severe valvular stenosis or regurgitation with the clinical characteristics as outlined below.
3. Congenital heart disease; risk stratification for patients with congenital heart disease should be guided by the 27th Bethesda Conference recommendations.

(*continued*)

TABLE 20.5	AMERICAN HEART ASSOCIATION RISK STRATIFICATION CRITERIA (*Continued*)

4. Cardiomyopathy: ejection fraction ≤30%; includes stable patients with heart failure with clinical characteristics as outlined below but not hypertrophic cardiomyopathy or recent myocarditis.
5. Complex ventricular arrhythmias not well controlled.

Clinical characteristics (any of the following):
1. New York Heart Association Class 3 or 4.
2. Exercise test results
   Exercise capacity <6 METs
   Angina or ischemic ST depression at a workload <6 METs
   Fall in systolic blood pressure below resting levels during exercise
   Nonsustained ventricular tachycardia with exercise
3. Previous episode of primary cardiac arrest (i.e., cardiac arrest that did not occur in the presence of an acute myocardial infarction or during a cardiac procedure).
4. A medical problem that the physician believes may be life-threatening

Activity guidelines: Activity should be individualized with exercise prescription provided by qualified individuals and approved by primary healthcare provider
Supervision: Medical supervision during all exercise sessions until safety is established.
ECG and blood pressure monitoring: Continuous during exercise sessions until safety is established, usually ≥12 sessions.

Risk classification for exercise training (Class D):
Unstable disease with activity restriction[b]

This classification includes individuals with any of the following:
1. Unstable ischemia.
2. Severe and symptomatic valvular stenosis or regurgitation.
3. Congenital heart disease; criteria for risk that would prohibit exercise conditioning in patients with congenital heart disease should be guided by the 27th Bethesda Conference recommendations.
4. Heart failure that is not compensated.
5. Uncontrolled arrhythmias.
6. Other medical conditions that could be aggravated by exercise.

Activity guidelines: No activity is recommended for conditioning purposes.
Attention should be directed to treating the patient and restoring the patient to Class C or better. Daily activities must be prescribed on the basis of individual assessment by the patient's personal physician.

Modified from Fletcher GF, Balady GJ, Amsterdam EA, et al. Exercise standards for testing and training. A statement for health care professionals from the American Heart Association. *Circulation.* 2001;104:1694–1740.
[a]It is suggested that persons classified as Class A-2 and particularly Class A-3 undergo a medical examination and possibly a medically supervised exercise test before engaging in vigorous exercise.
[b]Exercise for conditioning purposes is not recommended.

for a cardiac client may elicit abnormal clinical symptoms. For most previously sedentary cardiac clients, the threshold intensity for improving cardiorespiratory fitness approximates 45% of HRR or $\dot{V}O_2R$ (63). Other exercise intensity considerations are presented in Table 20.6.

Lastly, despite the prevailing notion that higher-intensity exercise in individuals with cardiac disease carries an added risk, some researchers have concluded that vigorous physical activity appears to be more cardioprotective than moderate-intensity physical activity. The Personal Trainer should initially design an exercise program (Table 20.7) aimed at fulfilling the threshold exercise intensity and total energy expenditure requirements (1,000 kcal $\cdot$ week^{-1} or 14 kcal $\cdot$ kg^{-1} $\cdot$ week^{-1}) necessary to modify the risk factors that mediate the process of atherosclerosis. Progression of total weekly energy expenditure should be the next goal of the aerobic exercise program. Ultimately, provided there are no contraindications, the Personal Trainer can incorporate vigorous exercise intensity into the program.

TABLE 20.6	**EXERCISE INTENSITY CONSIDERATIONS FOR CLIENTS WITH CARDIAC DISEASE**

Program Modification

Deconditioned and low-functional capacity clients may need to start at low intensities (20%–30% HRR or $\dot{V}O_2R$)
Target exercise intensity should fall 10–15 beats per minute below a heart rate that has previously elicited abnormal clinical symptoms (i.e., chest pain or other angina symptoms)

β-Blockers and other heart rate–lowering medications will decrease the accuracy of exercise intensity prescription methods based on an age-predicted maximal heart rate

Rating of Perceived Exertion (RPE) levels of 11 (*fairly light*) to 13 (*somewhat hard*) typically correspond to the target heart rate for cardiac clients first initiating an exercise program. RPE can be progressed (14–16) after several months of training when conditioning has improved and no complications are present

From American College of Sports Medicine. *ACSM's Guidelines for Exercise Testing and Prescription.* 8th ed. Baltimore: Lippincott Williams & Wilkins; 2010.

Resistance Training Exercise Prescription for Cardiac Disease

Personal Trainers should incorporate resistance training into the exercise programs of low-risk (Class B) clients with cardiac disease with two primary goals (53) in mind:

1. to maintain and improve muscular strength levels for performing activities of daily living and
2. to reduce the cardiac demands (e.g., lower heart rate and blood pressure) associated with completing these tasks.

TABLE 20.7	**EXAMPLE OF EXERCISE PROGRAM DESIGN FOR CLIENTS WITH CARDIAC DISEASE**

Client (Anni) characteristics:

$$\text{Age} = 66 \text{ years}$$
$$\text{Weight} = 132 \text{ lb (60 kg)}$$
$$\dot{V}O_{2max} = 31.4 \text{ mL} \cdot \text{kg}^{-1} \cdot \text{min}^{-1}$$

To calculate $\dot{V}O_2R$, use the following formula:

$$\text{Target } \dot{V}O_2 = [(\text{percentage}) \times (\dot{V}O_{2max} - \dot{V}O_{2rest})] + \dot{V}O_{2rest}$$

Because Anni's $\dot{V}O_{2max}$ puts her in the 70th percentile (Table 17.3), she is considered to be above average. Accordingly, her Personal Trainer establishes her exercise intensity at 45% $\dot{V}O_2R$. To determine the target $\dot{V}O_2$, the calculations for Anni are as follows:

$$\text{Target } \dot{V}O_2 = [(0.45) \times (31.4 - 3.5)] + 3.5 = 16.1 \text{ mL} \cdot \text{kg}^{-1} \cdot \text{min}^{-1} \text{ (4.6 METs)}$$

Anni had her left knee replaced 2 years ago and reports discomfort when performing weight-bearing activities. Furthermore, balance impairment is a concern as Anni reports three previous falls in the last 6 months, including one on the treadmill. Consequently, Anni's Personal Trainer determines cycle ergometry will be a safe exercise modality. Using Table 17.6, Anni's Personal Trainer determines that 50 W is the appropriate workload that corresponds with Anni's target $\dot{V}O_2$.

The Personal Trainer can estimate the number of calories expended per minute at the 50-W cycle ergometer workload with the following equation:

$$(4.6 \times 3.5 \times 60)/200 = 4.8 \text{ kcal} \cdot \text{min}^{-1}$$

The Personal Trainer can now determine the minutes per week at the target workload required for Anni to meet the minimal energy expenditure recommendation of 14 kcal $\cdot$ kg^{-1} $\cdot$ wk^{-1} that research has suggested to be effective at reducing the risk factors for CAD.

$$[(14 \text{ kcal} \cdot \text{kg}^{-1} \cdot \text{wk}^{-1} \times 60 \text{ kg}) = 1000 \text{ kcal} \cdot \text{wk}^{-1}] \div 5 \text{ kcal} \cdot \text{min}^{-1} = 175 \text{ kcal} \cdot \text{wk}^{-1}$$

Accumulating 175 min $\cdot$ wk^{-1} at an intensity of 50 W on the cycle ergometer or the metabolic equivalent will ensure that Anni is achieving the ACSM weekly energy expenditure goal that has been shown to positively modify the risk factors that contribute to the process of CAD. This could be accomplished by exercising at the target intensity 5 d/wk for 35 min $\cdot$ d^{-1} or any other combination of frequency and duration that totals 175 min $\cdot$ wk^{-1}.

TABLE 20.8	RESISTANCE TRAINING GUIDELINES FOR CLIENTS WITH CARDIAC DISEASE
Program Component	**Program Modification**
Exercise mode	Perform 8–10 exercises using the major muscle groups Dynamic muscle strengthening exercises include machine and free weights, weight-bearing calisthenics, resistance bands, and similar resistance exercises that use major muscle groups Isometric exercise is not recommended for clients with cardiovascular disease
Exercise intensity	Begin program with a low weight for each exercise 10–15 repetitions per exercise to "moderate" fatigue, which approximately corresponds to a Rating of Perceived Exertion range of 11–13 (*light* to *somewhat hard*) on the Borg scale The rate-pressure product (heart rate × systolic blood pressure) should not be greater than that prescribed during aerobic exercise
Exercise session duration	Complete 1 set of each exercise Allow adequate rest between exercises to prevent carry-over fatigue
Exercise frequency	Resistance training should be performed on two nonconsecutive days per week

Adapted from American College of Sports Medicine. *ACSM's Guidelines for Exercise Testing and Prescription.* 8th ed. Baltimore: Lippincott Williams & Wilkins; 2010; and Pollock ML, Franklin BA, Balady GJ, et al. Resistance exercise in individuals with and without cardiovascular disease: benefits, rationale, safety, and prescription: An advisory from the Committee on Exercise, Rehabilitation, and Prevention, Council on Clinical Cardiology, American Heart Association; Position paper endorsed by the American College of Sports Medicine. *Circulation.* 2000;101:828-33.

The Personal Trainer should request clients to receive physician or cardiologist approval before integrating resistance training into the exercise routine. Importantly, clients should inquire with their medical team about any limitations the Personal Trainer should be aware of when designing the re-sistance-training program (e.g., clients should avoid resistance training within 3 months of CABG surgery). Clients with heart disease will require careful monitoring for proper technique and breathing patterns. Straining, tight gripping of weight handles/bars, and the Valsalva maneuver are all activities that should be avoided. Progression of resistance training should be gradual ($\sim$2–5 lb · week^{-1} [1–2.3 kg] for upper body and 5–10 lb · week^{-1} [2.3–4.5 kg] for lower body) and, similar to the older adult; maintenance may be the more realistic objective.

> *Clients should inquire with their medical team about any limitations the Personal Trainer should be aware of when designing the resistance-training program (e.g., clients should avoid resistance training within 3 months of CABG surgery).*

Lastly, because of the potential disproportionate increase in blood pressure during resistance train-ing (relative to aerobic exercise) and the subsequent increased metabolic oxygen demand imposed on the myocardium, any number of repetitions to fatigue (1- or 10-repetition maximum [1RM or 10RM]) is discouraged. General resistance training guidelines for clients with cardiac diseases are presented in Table 20.8.

PROGRAMMING FOR PREGNANCY AND POSTPARTUM

Pregnancy is associated with multiple anatomical and physiological changes. Originally, prevailing opinion was that physical activity should be discouraged during this period of the lifespan because of the supposed increased maternal and fetal risk of untoward events (1). However, current research suggests that unless a specific obstetric or medical condition is present, the likelihood of adverse events or complications following acute exercise or chronic training in the mother and fetus is minimal (9). The Personal Trainer should recognize that, similar to other populations, physical activity throughout

> *The Personal Trainer should recognize that, similar to other populations, physical activity throughout pregnancy and the postpartum period confers numerous benefits and should be encouraged.*

TABLE 20.9	ABSOLUTE AND RELATIVE CONTRAINDICATIONS TO EXERCISE DURING PREGNANCY
Absolute Contraindications	**Relative Contraindications**
Hemodynamically significant heart disease	Severe anemia
Restrictive lung disease	Unevaluated maternal cardiac dysrhythmia
Incompetent cervix/cerclage	Chronic bronchitis
Multiple gestation at risk for premature labor	Poorly controlled Type 1 diabetes
Persistent second- or third-trimester bleeding	Extreme morbid obesity
Placenta previa after 26 wks of gestation	Extreme underweight (BMI < 12)
Premature labor during current pregnancy	History of extremely sedentary lifestyle
Ruptured membranes	Intrauterine growth restriction in current pregnancy
Preeclampsia/pregnancy-induced hypertension	Poorly controlled hypertension
	Orthopedic limitations
	Poorly controlled seizure disorder
	Poorly controlled hyperthyroidism
	Heavy smoker

From American College of Sports Medicine. *ACSM's Guidelines for Exercise Testing and Prescription*. 8th ed. Baltimore: Lippincott Williams & Wilkins; 2010.

pregnancy and the postpartum period confers numerous benefits and should be encouraged. Collectively, the Personal Trainer, client, and obstetric healthcare provider can establish the following exercise program goals: avoid excessive weight gain, reduce the risk of gestational diabetes, lower the incidence of low back pain, and prevent excessive decreases in cardiorespiratory and muscular fitness (9).

Screening and Risk Stratification

Prior to participation in an exercise program, women with or without a previously sedentary lifestyle should be evaluated by their obstetric provider to determine whether exercise is contraindicated (Table 20.9). Personal Trainers are encouraged to administer the Physical Activity Readiness Medical Examination for Pregnancy (PARmed-X for Pregnancy) questionnaire (available at http://www.csep.ca) to prospective clients to determine the appropriateness of participation in a fitness routine. The PARmed-X includes a tear-away medical clearance form to be signed by the obstetric provider verifying the safety of exercise, along with recommendations for cardiorespiratory and resistance training activities. Personal Trainers should be knowledgeable of, and able to educate clients on, the potential signs that would warrant the termination of exercise (Table 20.10).

TABLE 20.10	WARNING SIGNS TO TERMINATE EXERCISE DURING PREGNANCY	
Sign or Symptom		**Sign or Symptom**
Vaginal bleeding		Muscle weakness
Dyspnea prior to exertion		Calf pain or swelling
Dizziness		Preterm labor
Headache		Decreased fetal movement
Chest pain		Amniotic fluid leakage

From American College of Sports Medicine. *ACSM's Guidelines for Exercise Testing and Prescription*. 8th ed. Baltimore: Lippincott Williams & Wilkins; 2010.

General Exercise Considerations for Pregnancy and Postpartum

Fatigue, nausea, and vomiting may limit exercise, especially during the first trimester. Importantly, the Personal Trainer should recognize the increased nutritional requirements of pregnant clientele. After the 13th week, pregnancy requires approximately an additional 300 kcal · day^{-1} to fulfill the increased metabolic demands of pregnancy (2). The caloric requirement will be higher depending on the energy expenditure of the exercise program. Personal Trainers are encouraged to utilize the metabolic calculations presented in Chapter 16 to estimate the total energy expenditure of the client's exercise program in order to recommend appropriate dietary modifications to clients.

Pregnant women will have diminished thermoregulatory control throughout pregnancy and consequently the Personal Trainer should encourage clients to maintain adequate hydration. Additionally, pregnant women should be encouraged to wear appropriate clothing that will facilitate heat dissipation and avoid exercise in hot, humid conditions (1). Choose environmentally controlled indoor settings in these situations.

The physiological changes associated with pregnancy persist for 4–6 weeks postpartum; however, women typically can gradually return to exercise provided the delivery was uncomplicated. Women who are nursing may elect to feed their babies prior to exercise to alleviate the discomfort of engorged breasts and to reduce the likelihood of feeding problems due to acidity in the breast milk (1). Lastly, the Personal Trainer should remind clients that pregnancy is not a time to expect large improvements in fitness and ultimately, throughout the gestational period, it is normal for numerous fitness parameters to decline (9).

Aerobic Exercise Prescription for Pregnancy

The general cardiorespiratory training principles of exercise prescription detailed in Chapter 18 apply to pregnant and postpartum women, although the profound anatomical and physiological changes will require the Personal Trainer to make a number of special adaptations to the training program (Table 20.11). The consensus statement for regular physical activity from the U.S. Surgeon General (30-min of moderate-intensity physical activity on most, preferably all, days of the week) is an appropriate target aerobic exercise program for most women during uncomplicated pregnancies. Recreational and competitive athletes may train safely at higher intensities and volumes throughout pregnancy with the understanding that they are undergoing closer obstetric supervision (9).

Resistance Training and Flexibility Prescription for Pregnancy

The general resistance and flexibility training principles of exercise prescription detailed in Chapters 16 and 18, with several adjustments that account for morphological and physiological changes, apply to pregnant and postpartum women. After the first trimester, resistance and flexibility training exercises in the supine position should be avoided because of the potential obstruction of venous return and subsequent risk of orthostatic hypotension (2). Isometric or heavy resistance training may elicit a pressor response (sudden increase in heart rate and blood pressure) and is not recommended (9). Joint range of motion will be enhanced during pregnancy because of increased circulating levels of relaxin and therefore the potential exists for ligament and joint capsule damage with an overly aggressive flexibility program (9). Consequently, Personal Trainers are encouraged to focus on maintaining normal joint range of motion with slow, static stretching throughout pregnancy.

PROGRAMMING FOR CLIENTS WITH DIABETES

Diabetes mellitus is a metabolic disorder that is associated with a variety of diseases (cardiovascular, renal, eye, musculoskeletal, nervous, urinary, etc.) stemming from abnormal pancreatic insulin production and/or diminished peripheral action of insulin. Looking at current data, it is clear that

TABLE 20.11	**AEROBIC EXERCISE PROGRAM MODIFICATIONS FOR PREGNANT WOMEN**
Program Component	**Program Modification**
Exercise mode	Walking and cycling may be easier to monitor for exercise intensity Activities that increase the risk of falls (e.g., skiing and skating), abdominal trauma (e.g., basketball and softball), and excessive joint stress (e.g., jogging and tennis) should be avoided and generally are not recommended Activities at elevations greater than 6,000 ft and scuba diving are contraindicated
Exercise intensity	Target heart rate (e.g., %HR$_{max}$ or %HRR) should not be employed as a method to monitor exercise intensity due to the variability in maternal resting and maximal heart rate throughout pregnancy. Likewise, target VO$_2$ (e.g., %VO$_2$R) is not a valid tool to monitor intensity due to the progressive decrease in cardiorespiratory fitness over the course of the pregnancy Rating of Perceived Exertion values of 11–13 (light to somewhat hard) on the 6–20 scale can be used to accurately and safely monitor exercise intensity The talk test may also be used to monitor appropriate exercise intensity. Pregnant women should exercise at an intensity that permits conversation. Intensity should be decreased when conversation is not possible.
Exercise session duration	Accumulating 30 minutes of exercise in 15-min intermittent bouts may attenuate energy balance and thermoregulatory concerns.
Exercise frequency	Moderate-intensity exercise should be regular rather than sporadic in nature. Exercise should be performed at least 3 days, preferably 5–7 d/wk.

Adapted from American College of Obstetricians and Gynecologists. Exercise during pregnancy and the postpartum period. ACOG Committee Opinion No. 267. *Obstet Gynecol*. 2002;99:171–73; and Artal R, O'Toole M. Guidelines of the American College of Obstetricians and Gynecologists for exercise during pregnancy and the postpartum period. *Br J Sports Med*. 2003;37:6–12; and American College of Sports Medicine. *ACSM's Guidelines for Exercise Testing and Prescription*. 8th ed. Baltimore: Lippincott Williams & Wilkins; 2010.

diabetes continues to be a significant problem in the United States. To date, 23.6 million Americans (7.8% of the U.S. population) have diabetes. Of that total, 17.9 million are diagnosed cases with 1.6 million new cases for people 20 years and older reported in 2007 (21).

The development of diseases of the heart, vascular system (e.g., stroke and hypertension), kidneys, eyes, and nervous system is positively associated with diabetes. Diabetes was the seventh leading cause of death in 2006 and contributed to 233,619 deaths in 2005 (21). The cause of death in diabetic individuals stems from complications of the diseases associated with diabetes, with heart disease being the most prominent cause.

Two distinct categories are used to classify individuals with diabetes: Type 1 and Type 2. Type 1 diabetes is the least common form in adults (usually striking children and younger adults) and comprises approximately 5%–10% of all diagnosed cases of diabetes. This leaves 90%–95% of all diagnosed adults in the category of Type 2 diabetes. In general, the incidence and development of Type 2 diabetes are associated with the sedentary lifestyle and the obesity epidemic in this country and rightfully so; however, exercise professionals must also consider diabetes as a disease of aging. According to 2007 CDC statistics, 23.8% of individuals 60 years

> *Personal Trainers should turn their attention to the prevention of diabetes not only in the obese but also in the older adult population as well as in children.*

and older have diabetes with 536,000 new cases reported and the prevalence increases across the lifespan (21,32). Therefore, Personal Trainers should turn their attention to the prevention of diabetes not only in the obese but also in the older adult population as well as in children.

Because the growth of diabetes in the U.S. population suggests no slowing trend, enhancing the ability to implement diabetes management and prevention programs should be a major focus as we look to the future. The demand for competent Personal Trainers to provide appropriate guidance and supervision to individuals with diabetes will continue to increase in the health and medical fitness settings. Therefore, health and fitness professionals must be prepared to meet this challenge.

Pathophysiology of Type 1 and Type 2 Diabetes

Normally, insulin is released by the pancreas in response to a rise in blood glucose following the intake and digestion of food. In Type 1 diabetes, pancreatic β-cells that produce insulin are destroyed by an autoimmune disorder, creating an absolute insulin deficiency (no insulin production) in the body. In Type 2 diabetes, insulin is produced but is ineffective at controlling blood glucose, thereby introducing an insulin resistance in body tissues. The pancreas must increase insulin production to overcome this resistance, causing an excess of blood insulin in these individuals. Hyperinsulinemia (elevated blood insulin concentration) over time can contribute to a host of problems such as hypertension, hypercholesterolemia, excessive blood clotting, atherosclerosis, and kidney stones to name a few (21,43). In general, a normal resting blood glucose level is less than $100 \text{ mg} \cdot \text{dL}^{-1}$ of blood, whereas diabetes can be diagnosed when fasting blood glucose is $126 \text{ mg} \cdot \text{dL}^{-1}$ or greater on two or more occasions.

The cause of diabetes differs slightly between both types. Family history and/or a genetic predisposition to developing the disease may be common to both Type 1 and Type 2 diabetes (8). Factors related to Type 1 are environmental causes or viral infections that trigger the autoimmune response. Increasing age, race, and obesity are more related to the development of Type 2 diabetes. Whatever the underlying cause, the main goal in the management of diabetes is adequately controlling blood glucose levels (2). Exercise, among other treatment strategies, can be used effectively to achieve this goal.

Programming Goals

Exercise training fits into the management of diabetes by addressing various health and subclinical factors. The main exercise programming goals for individuals with diabetes are to (2,4,15,16,33,42,58,61,70):

1. improve insulin sensitivity and blood glucose control and decrease insulin requirements,
2. improve blood lipid profiles,
3. reduce blood pressure,
4. improve muscular strength and endurance through enhancing skeletal muscle mass,
5. improve flexibility and joint range of motion,
6. reduce body weight (particularly reduce intra-abdominal fat), and
7. assist with decreasing the risk of diabetic complications.

Consistency in a daily routine is a major pillar in diabetes care. This regularity refers to when meals are eaten and the amount/type of food, when medications are taken, and frequency, intensity, and time (duration and time of day) of physical activity. Personal Trainers, when working with clients with diabetes, should maintain regular contact with the client's physician or other healthcare provider when designing or making changes to the exercise program. This will enable a more consistent and appropriate treatment plan for the client/patient.

Aerobic Training for Clients with Diabetes

The majority of research regarding exercise training and diabetes has been done in the area of aerobic exercise. Thus, aerobic programming is much more understood and the guidelines more clear than for resistance training. Interestingly, the positive effects of aerobic exercise on glucose metabolism and insulin sensitivity in clients with diabetes are rather acute, meaning that the changes that do occur are lost within a few days following the cessation of training (4). For Personal Trainers, this again speaks to the previous discussion of providing a consistent training regimen for clients with diabetes. If these clients are to realize the benefits of aerobic exercise, the program must involve frequent exercise activities with total adherence on a day-to-day basis (66). Regular exercise in clients with diabetes assists in controlling blood glucose, enhancing insulin sensitivity, decreasing and managing body weight, improving lipid profiles and decreasing blood pressure, increasing cardiovascular fitness and exercise capacity, and managing some diabetic complications such as coronary heart disease or peripheral vascular disease (2,4,15,16,19,32,39,43,52).

FREQUENCY

ACSM recommends a basic target range of 3–4 days per week to achieve minimal benefits from exercise (2). Greater frequencies of physical activity have been shown to be effective in improving glucose tolerance and insulin sensitivity with minimal exercise-induced complications (27). Personal Trainers should consider progressing clients to 5 days per week, or perhaps daily, provided that there is an appropriate mix of intensity and duration. Clients who are obese or are taking insulin may benefit most by a daily schedule as it allows for greater consistency and an opportunity for increasing caloric expenditure for weight management purposes (4).

INTENSITY

ACSM recommends a range of 50%–80% of $\dot{V}O_2$ or HR reserve for clients with diabetes (2). This range has been well substantiated in research (4,15,16). With such a large range, Personal Trainers can exercise some flexibility in what intensity they choose to start clients at providing plenty of room for progression when warranted. For clients who are overweight, sedentary, and/or less familiar with exercise, an appropriate starting point would be 50% of $\dot{V}O_2$ or HR reserve or slightly lower depending on the client's initial fitness level and tolerance to exercise. The decision to progress the client through the intensity range should be made while keeping their ability to tolerate exercise, age, and individual goals in mind. In general, frequency and duration goals should be met before a significant progression in intensity is made (2).

As an adjunct method, Personal Trainers are encouraged to use the Rating of Perceived Exertion (RPE) scale when determining intensity as some clients with a long history of diabetes may incur a condition that can affect the heart rate (and blood pressure) response to exercise (2). An RPE range of 11–15 (on the 6–20 scale) falls in line with the prescribed $\dot{V}O_2$ and HR reserve values with adjustments made on the basis of the percent values.

TIME

ACSM recommends a range of 20–60 minutes for clients with diabetes (2). Once again, the Personal Trainer is given a great amount of room to adjust and progress within this large range. Recent research provides a worthy minimal goal of 150 min $\cdot$ week^{-1} to elicit positive changes in glucose tolerance and insulin sensitivity and potential changes in body weight (15,16,27). This amount may seem high for the client who is overweight, deconditioned, or older. However, exercise may not need to be continuous to provide a benefit; therefore, Personal Trainers should consider using multiple bouts of exercise throughout the day (>10 minutes) to achieve the overall initial exercise time goal (40). Target the client's exercise time progression to 30 minutes of continuous activity to achieve his or her caloric expenditure goals in the program. Because intensity will be relatively low, frequency and duration will be the most important factors determining caloric expenditure. If weight loss is a goal, and for many clients it will be, ACSM recommends 2,000 kcals $\cdot$ week^{-1} or more and daily exercise to achieve this goal.

TYPE

Guidelines for choosing a mode of exercise are similar to those for an apparently health adult. In general, the exercise modality should be chosen by clients as something that they will enjoy using to assist in their adherence to the program. Walking is the most common form of exercise for clients with diabetes (4). However, there are some considerations to be made for clients with diabetes. For those clients who are obese or experience diabetic complications (peripheral neuropathy is one), Personal Trainers should minimize high-impact, weight-bearing activities or those that require a greater amount of balance and coordination (2). Therefore, alternating weight-bearing activities with non–weight-bearing activities such as cycling, upper body ergometry, swimming, may enhance the safety and appropriateness of the exercise program.

Resistance Training for Clients with Diabetes

A resistance training program is essential for clients with diabetes to assist in managing their disease and associated complications as well as maintaining their physiological function through improving strength and endurance. Some believe that the increased risk of diabetes with increasing age is partly due to loss of muscle mass that negatively impacts the ability to remain recreationally active, perform activities of daily living, and maintain independence (32). Other benefits include improving skeletal muscle quality, improving glycemic control and insulin sensitivity, decreasing glycosylated hemoglobin (HbA_{1C}) levels, decreasing intra-abdominal fat, and improving the overall metabolic profile in clients with diabetes (4,15,17,20,30,33,42,52,67). Below is a summary of the programmatic variables for resistance training clients with diabetes.

RESISTANCE

For clients with both Type 1 and Type 2 diabetes, a 1-RM test can be done to determine maximal strength provided that diabetes is well-controlled and no complications are present (especially diabetic retinopathy). In general, most clients will tolerate a resistance of 30%–50% of 1-RM; however, others recommend a range of 40%–60% of 1-RM as being safe and effective at improving strength and endurance (2,42). Progress resistance slowly based on the clients' tolerance to the resistance. If they can perform their exercise easily at the upper ranges of their repetition range and they are experiencing no adverse effects, it would then be appropriate to progress within the program. Other authors have demonstrated greater effects on muscle strength and lean body mass and adequate feasibility of performing high-intensity resistance training (75%–85% 1-RM), but the Personal Trainer must weigh the benefits of such training with the risks of higher-intensity exercise in clients with diabetes (30).

SETS AND REPETITIONS

An appropriate starting point for clients with diabetes is 1–2 sets per exercise (2,33). Repetitions can be set similarly to what an apparently healthy individual would follow in a resistance program. Use the client's individual goals (e.g., general strength vs. endurance) and their ability to tolerate exercise as the guide in choosing the repetition range. Begin the program with a 10–15 repetition range and use 15–20 repetitions as a progression goal if appropriate (2,33). Rest periods between sets can be set at 30 seconds to a minute in length when using these repetition ranges.

FREQUENCY

The recommended minimal frequency for clients with diabetes is 2 days per week to see benefits from the program (2,33). In addition, ACSM also recommends at least 48 hours between sessions to allow for full recovery from each resistance training workout. Although past research has also shown the effectiveness of a higher volume of resistance training performed at a moderate intensity (40%–50% 1-RM). Ishii and colleagues (42) trained subjects with Type 2 diabetes at a frequency of 5 days · week^{-1} and demonstrated a 48% increase in insulin sensitivity following the training program.

Again, these findings underscore the importance of a consistent, possibly daily, activity regimen for clients with diabetes. The maintenance of chronic training changes in these clients may be influenced most by a consistent training program, which should be the overall goal (4,65). However, the Personal Trainer must consider that most clients with diabetes will be sedentary, overweight, and potentially inexperienced with exercise; thus, increasing the frequency of an exercise program must be introduced slowly.

EXERCISES

Number, type, and order of exercises can be prescribed in a similar manner to nondiabetic clients. Therefore, clients should perform one exercise per body part up to a total of 8–10 exercises working from large to small muscle groups. Research has demonstrated the effectiveness of circuit training for managing and preventing diabetes (32,33,48). Thus, Personal Trainers should seriously consider adding a circuit training regimen to the training program to enhance both muscle strength and endurance.

Combining Strength and Endurance Training for Clients with Diabetes

After considering the previous two sections on resistance and aerobic training programs, it may be most beneficial for Personal Trainers to prescribe a program for their clients that combine both aspects of training. In his review, Eriksson (32) comments that the best training program for individuals with Type 2 diabetes should be targeted to improve cardiorespiratory fitness, muscular strength, and muscular endurance. This can be gained by following a combination program or a circuit-type resistance training. From an adherence viewpoint, combining modes of exercise within the program may help achieve the overall, main goal of the client's program to consistently participate in long-term exercise.

> *Combining modes of exercise within the program may help achieve the overall, main goal of the client's program to consistently participate in long-term exercise.*

Other authors have documented the success of such combination programs for clients with diabetes. Sigal and colleagues (58) showed greater positive effects of a moderate-intensity aerobic and resistance training program on HbA$_{1C}$ values in clients with Type 2 diabetes compared with resistance or aerobic exercise alone. Maiorana and others (48) demonstrated that circuit training is an effective method for improving cardiovascular endurance, increasing muscle mass and decreasing body fat, improving strength, and decreasing both fasting blood glucose and HbA$_{1C}$ following training in individuals with Type 2 diabetes. Finally, Tokmakidis and others (67) elicited improvements in glucose control (decreased HbA$_{1C}$), insulin sensitivity, muscular strength, and aerobic endurance in as little as 4 weeks of combined aerobic and resistance training in women with Type 2 diabetes. The overall intensity of this program was moderate with resistance loads set at 60% 1-RM and aerobic intensities of 60%–70% HR$_{max}$ progressing to higher intensities of 70%–80% HR$_{max}$.

Other Considerations for Clients with Diabetes

The main programmatic considerations for Personal Trainers involve minimizing the risks involved with exercising individuals with diabetes. A list of preexercise contraindications is presented in Table 20.12. In cases where the individual has complications of diabetes such as diabetic retinopathy, peripheral neuropathy, or nephropathy, consult the client's physician before beginning the exercise program. These clients may need referral to a medically supervised environment if the condition limits overall exercise tolerance or if they have signs and/or symptoms of CVD. If the clients have been cleared to exercise, it is prudent for the Personal Trainer to be aware of very specific exercise considerations for each of these conditions (Tables 20.13 and 20.14).

It is also important to attempt to minimize the risk of your client developing hypoglycemia (blood glucose < 80 mg $\cdot$ dL^{-1}) during or after exercise as this is the most common problem with

TABLE 20.12	**EXERCISE CONTRAINDICATIONS FOR CLIENTS WITH DIABETES**
Any complications involving diabetic retinopathy
High resting blood glucose – uncontrolled hyperglycemia (>250–300 mg $\cdot$ dL^{-1})
Exercising during time of peak medication activity
Changes (increase or decrease) in blood pressure with exertion
Resting blood glucose of <100 mg $\cdot$ dL^{-1} prior to exercise

From American College of Sports Medicine. *ACSM's Guidelines for Exercise Testing and Prescription.* 8th ed. Baltimore: Lippincott Williams & Wilkins; 2010.

exercise (2). Remember that exercise has an insulin-like effect on circulating blood glucose, even in the absence of blood insulin, and this effect can be enhanced if special precautions are not taken. Therefore, Personal Trainers should use the following strategies (2) with their clients to avoid this problem:

1. avoid exercising during the time when the medication is working at its peak,
2. eating 1–2 hours before exercise,
3. eating a snack immediately before exercise (and possibly during the exercise if duration is prolonged),
4. checking blood glucose before exercise (eat if blood glucose <100 mg $\cdot$ dL^{-1}),
5. exercising with a partner for safety reasons, and
6. know the warning signs of hypoglycemia (and hyperglycemia) (refer to Table 20.14 for a list of signs and symptoms).

Regarding diet strategies, clients should consult with their dietitians or physicians on what foods are appropriate to eat before, during, and after exercise. In addition, clients with diabetes should also avoid exercising late at night if possible as this may produce low blood glucose during sleep (nocturnal hypoglycemia) and inadvertently cause a potentially life-threatening situation. Thus, if late night exercise cannot be avoided, the clients should eat following exercise according to their physicians' or dieticians' guidelines.

Lastly, Personal Trainers should provide their clients with a list of general exercise guidelines that are specific to the proper management of diabetes. Warm-up and cool-down (5–10 minutes each) are particularly important in this population to avoid exercise-induced cardiovascular complications. Proper footwear is also very important for clients with diabetes, especially for those with or at risk for peripheral neuropathy and peripheral vascular disease. Because many of these clients may also be obese and hypertensive, maintaining adequate hydration and avoiding hot/humid environments to

TABLE 20.13	**COMPLICATIONS ASSOCIATED WITH DIABETES AND RELATED EXERCISE PRECAUTIONS**
Complications	**Exercise Precautions**
Retinopathy (eyes)	Avoid excessive blood pressures during exercise (>170 mmHg)
Peripheral Neuropathy (nerve and vascular)	Avoid exacerbating lower-extremity ulcerations, if present Avoid exercise that requires greater balance or coordination challenges Be cautious of greater muscle weakness Consider non–weight-bearing activities (cycle, swimming, upper body ergometry, etc.)
Nephropathy (kidney)	Reduced endurance capacity/increased fatigability, avoid prolonged exercise duration/high intensity with poor tolerance

From American College of Sports Medicine. *ACSM's Guidelines for Exercise Testing and Prescription.* 8th ed. Baltimore: Lippincott Williams & Wilkins; 2010.

TABLE 20.14	SELECTED SIGNS AND SYMPTOMS OF HYPERGLYCEMIA AND HYPOGLYCEMIA	
Hyperglycemia (>300 mg $\cdot$ dL^{-1})	**Hypoglycemia (<80 mg $\cdot$ dL^{-1} or rapid drop in glucose)**	
Dry skin	Dizziness and headache	
Hunger	Weakness and fatigue	
Nausea/vomiting	Shaking	
Blurred vision	Tachycardia (fast heart rate)	
Frequent urination	Irritable	
Extreme thirst	Confusion	
Drowsiness	Sweating	
Acetone breath ("fruity breath")	Slurred speech	
	Anxious	
	Hunger	

From American College of Sports Medicine. *ACSM's Guidelines for Exercise Testing and Prescription.* 8th ed. Baltimore: Lippincott Williams & Wilkins; 2010.

assist with appropriate thermoregulation and blood pressure responses to exercise will also allow the client to tolerate exercise better. Also, consider using lighter workloads for individuals with diabetic complications (retinopathy is a big one), as blood pressure will not increase or spike as much as it does with higher loads.

PROGRAMMING FOR OBESE CLIENTS

Obesity is defined as having a very high amount of body fat in relation to overall lean body mass or having a BMI ≥ 30 kg $\cdot$ m^{-2} (23). Looking back over the previous 20 years, data demonstrate a dramatic increase in obesity in the United States. Recent 2007 data show that only one state's population (Colorado) had a prevalence of obesity less than 20%. Thirty states were equal to or greater than 25% and three of these (Alabama, Mississippi, and Tennessee) had a prevalence equal to or greater than 30% (24). According to the National Health and Nutrition Examination Survey, more than one third (72 million) of U.S. adults in 2005–2006 were con-

> *According to the National Health and Nutrition Examination Survey, more than one third (72 million) of U.S. adults in 2005–2006 were considered as being obese with the highest prevalence (~40%) occurring in men and women aged 40–59 years (50).*

sidered as being obese with the highest prevalence (~40%) occurring in men and women aged 40–59 years (50). These trends are startling, although there may be a bit of good news. While still very high, the prevalence of obesity in the United States has not significantly increased since 2003–2004 (50).

The obesity problem facing medical, health, and fitness professionals in the United States is very complex. Obesity is associated with the development of diabetes mellitus, CVD, hypertension, and certain types of cancers, and increases the risk of disability and all-cause mortality (44,50,74). Thus, obesity impacts the healthcare delivery system through its relationships with several diseases and conditions. It is thought that obesity is the end result of a number of factors including increased caloric consumption (overconsumption), decreased levels of physical activity, genetics, cultural, environmental (home, school, work, and community life), and disease (69). Therefore, Personal Trainers should be prepared to interact and consult with a variety of professionals such as dietitians, health nurses, physicians, public health professionals, and others.

Programming Goals

Personal Trainers can make their greatest impact with obese clients by providing sound exercise programs that focus on weight management and promoting adherence to an active lifestyle that matches closely with appropriate dietary strategies. This is a challenge because it is common for overweight or obese individuals to have many deeply rooted negative behaviors and barriers to activity that must be addressed before they can truly adhere to a program. Personal Trainers are encouraged to obtain further experience in motivational counseling, goal-setting strategies, and determining readiness for change before planning to work with obese clients. Some general exercise program goals for these individuals are as follows (2,5,13,18,51,54,59,74):

1. weight loss or management through maximizing caloric expenditure,
2. maintain or increase lean body mass to maintain resting metabolic rate,
3. improve metabolic profile,
4. lower the risk of comorbidities (e.g., hypertension, diabetes, orthopedic problems),
5. lower mortality risk, and
6. promote appetite control and improve mood state.

Aerobic Training for Obese Clients

From a weight management viewpoint, physical activity in the form of exercise is the most significant predictor of long-term success (2). In terms of successful weight loss, diet with caloric restriction is the most important predictor. However, regular aerobic exercise should be used in concert with a low-calorie, low-fat, and high-fiber diet plan thereby helping provide a negative caloric balance to achieve weight loss through maximizing energy expenditure (2). Below is the optimal exercise prescription for obese clients.

FREQUENCY

ACSM recommends a training frequency of 5–7 days per week to maximize energy expenditure in obese clients (2). Other studies have shown the effectiveness of a high-frequency exercise program on fat loss provided that the intensity is set appropriately (18,51,59).

INTENSITY

Because of the potential of orthopedic injuries, ACSM recommends an initial intensity range of 40%–60% $\dot{V}O_2$ or HRR (2). This low-to-moderate intensity range places more emphasis initially on frequency and time (together these variables create a significant exercise volume) to determine energy expenditure during exercise. Later progression into higher ranges of intensities may not be appropriate for some obese clients and should be individualized on the basis of the client's goals and history. Past research supports moderate-intensity exercise as an effective method for supporting weight loss and successful weight management (5,54,59).

TIME

ACSM recommends an exercise duration of 45–60 minutes per session (2,5). This amount of exercise is consistent with past research and previous guidelines for weight loss and weight management strategies (5,18,28,56,59). However, some clients may be too severely deconditioned or have conditions that limit their ability to exercise for this long. In these cases, prescribing multiple bouts of exercise ($\geq$10 min · session^{-1}) may be best to begin with and gradually shift to more continuous exercise later on in the program (2,5,40).

In summary, successful weight control may be likely when obese clients are exercising 45–60 minutes per session (200–300 min · week^{-1}), expending at least 300 kcals per session, and a total of 2,000 kcals or more per week (2,5). In terms of caloric expenditure relative to body weight,

Personal Trainers should follow recommendations of 4 kcal $\cdot$ kg^{-1} $\cdot$ session^{-1} or 23 kcal $\cdot$ kg^{-1} $\cdot$ week^{-1} for clients who wish to lose fat and maintain weight loss (59).

TYPE

The primary mode of exercise should involve large muscle groups and be aerobic in nature to provide the greatest caloric expenditure during exercise (2).

Resistance Training for Obese Clients

Resistance training programs are commonly treated as an adjunct to a regular, aerobic exercise program and should not be used in lieu of an aerobic program. The benefits of resistance training for clients who are obese are similar to the apparently healthy adult; thus, following the resistance training guidelines that are recommended for apparently healthy adults is appropriate for obese clients.

The greatest benefit a resistance training program can provide might be in the maintenance of lean body mass in clients following a calorically restricted diet (18). In addition, resting metabolic rate will be preserved along with lean body mass that could help support the successful maintenance of long-term weight loss. However, as was shown in this study, the volume of training may have to be high. In another study, the combination of moderate-intensity resistance (3 days $\cdot$ week^{-1}) and aerobic exercise (3 days $\cdot$ week^{-1}) was more successful at decreasing subcutaneous and visceral fat compared with aerobic (6 days $\cdot$ week^{-1}) exercise alone (51). Subsequently, lean body mass was more preserved in the combined group than in the aerobic-only group. These two studies provide excellent evidence to encourage Personal Trainers to include a resistance training program as a component of the total exercise program.

Other Considerations for Obese Clients

Personal Trainers should keep a few considerations in mind when working with obese clients. First, because of general fitness issues and greater amounts and the makeup of adipose tissue, obese clients do not regulate their body temperature as effectively as leaner clients (2).

Therefore, Personal Trainers should educate their clients on proper exercise clothing, hydration, environmental issues (hot/humid environments), and signs of heat exhaustion/stroke. Second, obese clients are at greater risk of experiencing orthopedic injuries because of greater stress on joints due to their overall weight (2). Personal Trainers should keep this in mind during program design, in particular with the intensity portion. Considerations should also be made to include non–weight-bearing modalities when appropriate to minimize orthopedic stress. Also, Personal Trainers should be prepared to modify the exercise program on the basis of the presence of other conditions (diabetes, CAD, hypertension, etc.) that may require an adjustment from the prescription given above for obese clients. Lastly, because of size limitations, certain exercise modalities may not be able to accommodate an obese client; thus, Personal Trainers may need to be more creative in their exercise planning and utilize equipment that can accommodate their particular clients (2). Table 20.15 includes some additional recommendations to follow for weight loss programs.

> *Personal Trainers should be prepared to modify the exercise program on the basis of the presence of other conditions (diabetes, CAD, hypertension, etc.) that may require an adjustment from the prescription given above for obese clients.*

PROGRAMMING FOR CLIENTS WITH HYPERTENSION

With more than 73 million adults (1 in 3) with hypertension, it remains the most prevalent form of CVD in the United States (55). It is often called the "silent killer" because of the lack of noticeable signs or symptoms of the disease, which is until serious problems develop. Currently, the

TABLE 20.15	ADDITIONAL RECOMMENDATIONS FOR WEIGHT LOSS PROGRAMS
Gradual weight loss of 1 kg/wk or less	
Daily, negative caloric balance should not exceed 500-1000 kcals	
Goal for long-term weight loss of at least 5%-10% of total weight	
Employ behavioral modification strategies to enhance adherence	
Dietary intake should not be <1200 kcals per day	
Balanced diet with fat intake <30% of total calories consumed	

From American College of Sports Medicine. *ACSM's Guidelines for Exercise Testing and Prescription.* 8th ed. Baltimore: Lippincott Williams & Wilkins; 2010.

> *It is often called the "silent killer" because of the lack of noticeable signs or symptoms of the disease, which is until serious problems develop.*

definition of hypertension remains as an elevated arterial blood pressure of greater than or equal to 140/90 mm Hg.

Hypertension is the major contributor to the risk of stroke and is also related to the development of CAD (leading to myocardial infarction), heart failure, kidney disease, peripheral vascular disease, and blindness (2,22). The Seventh Report of the Joint National Committee (JNC7) on Prevention, Detection, Evaluation, and Treatment of High Blood Pressure indicated that above a pressure of 115/75 mm Hg, CVD risk doubles for each increment of 20/10 mm Hg and those who have "normal" blood pressure at 55 years of age will have a 90% risk of developing hypertension over the remainder of their life (25,71). Thus, the prevalence of hypertension greatly increases with age. The JNC7 report also offered a new classification termed "prehypertension" to describe blood pressures between 120–139 and 80–89 mm Hg (a range that was previously considered "upper normal") that emphasized the need for early management of moderately elevated levels of blood pressure and prevent the conversion of prehypertension to hypertension. Personal Trainers can make a positive impact on their clients who have hypertension or prehypertension through appropriate exercise programming as part of a comprehensive lifestyle management strategy (diet, stress reduction, smoking cessation, lower alcohol consumption, etc.) or medication regimen.

Programming Goals

General programming goals in the management of hypertension are as follows (6,25):

1. lower systolic and diastolic blood pressures at rest and during exercise,
2. lower the risk of mortality from CVD (myocardial infarction, stroke, heart failure, etc.),
3. lower the risk of other comorbidities (kidney disease, eye problems, diabetes, etc.), and
4. incorporate opportunities for clients to pursue other lifestyle changes (stress management, diet, smoking cessation, weight management, etc.).

Aerobic Training for Clients with Hypertension

Just as was seen with obese clients, aerobic exercise is the cornerstone activity in the total program for clients with hypertension. On average, clients may experience a decline of approximately 3–4 mm Hg for systolic blood pressure and approximately 2–3 mm Hg decline for diastolic blood pressure from aerobic exercise training with greater changes (~1 mm Hg or more) seen in those with diagnosed hypertension (34,73). Taken alone, these changes may not seem very significant; however, when coupled with other treatment strategies (diet, medication, etc.), the effect will be much more appreciable. It is also important to note that several studies have shown that higher cardiorespiratory fitness provides a cardioprotective effect of lower mortality risk from all causes and CVD in individuals with hypertension (62). Thus, improving overall fitness in clients with hypertension may be a worthy goal to pursue independent of the direct effects exercise may have on lowering blood pressure. Below are recommendations for aerobic exercise programs targeted at eliciting positive changes in blood pressure.

FREQUENCY

ACSM recommends exercise for clients with hypertension on most, if not all, days of the week. Personal Trainers should encourage their clients to participate in daily, regular exercise as the subacute response of blood pressure following a bout of aerobic exercise is to remain below levels measured prior to exercise (6). This translates into more controlled and consistent blood pressure levels from day to day, which is ideal for clients with hypertension. In their review of past research studies, Whelton and colleagues (73) found a greater decrease in blood pressure as exercise frequency increased (>150 min · week^{-1}).

INTENSITY

ACSM recommends moderate-intensity exercise, 40%–70% of $\dot{V}O_2$ or HR reserve, as the primary intensity prescription for individuals with hypertension (2,6). In the reviews by Fagard (34) and also Whelton and others (73), low- to moderate-intensity levels were more effective at reducing blood pressure than higher-intensity level. For Personal Trainers, this is particularly important information to apply for hypertensive clients who are deconditioned or older or have conditions that can affect their risk of experiencing cardiovascular complications during exercise (diabetes, CAD, etc.).

Rating of Perceived Exertion may need to be used to help determine intensity instead of HR in the presence of certain medications that can affect the client's HR response during exercise (β-blockers are the main culprit). An RPE range of 11–14 is appropriate for these clients to achieve low- to moderate-intensity exercise.

TIME

ACSM recommends an exercise time of 30–60 minutes of continuous or accumulated exercise per session. There appears to be little difference in chronic blood pressure changes between 30 and 60 minutes of exercise training; therefore, Personal Trainers should choose the exercise time goal based on individual client goals and personal history (6,34,73). A caloric expenditure goal of 2,000 kcals or more per week should be considered if weight loss is indicated to help treat persons with hypertension.

TYPE

Clients with hypertension should primarily engage in aerobic endurance activities that involve large muscle groups and are rhythmic in nature. Avoid activities that emphasize isometric muscle contractions or elicit large pressor responses in your clients.

Resistance Training for Clients with Hypertension

Resistance training should not be prescribed as the primary form of activity for clients with hypertension (2). Although studies have demonstrated a favorable blood pressure response to resistance training, the overall effect is not as great as the response to aerobic exercise training (45). Specific resistance training recommendations for these clients are similar to those used for apparently healthy adults. As an adjunct to this general recommendation, Personal Trainers should focus on designing resistance programs that incorporate a higher number of repetitions (~15) per exercise and balancing this with low to moderate resistance (40%–60% 1-RM). The primary reason for this is to prevent large increases in blood pressure during resistance training. In addition, teaching clients proper exercise technique, proper breathing, and avoiding larger amounts of isometric work during resistance training will also help minimize these blood pressure responses.

Other Considerations for Clients with Hypertension

The primary focus of these considerations is safety during and after exercise. As stated previously, hypertension is often associated with a variety of conditions that may require special attention and specific precautions during exercise. In these cases, the general exercise prescription may need to be modified to address these issues (6).

> *Hypertension is often associated with a variety of conditions that may require special attention and specific precautions during exercise.*

The majority of clients with hypertension will most likely be taking some form of antihypertensive medication. The greatest risk these medications pose is in eliciting an abnormal drop in blood pressure (hypotension) following exercise. Therefore, engaging in gradual and prolonged cool-down activities will be important in minimizing the risk for excessive postexercise hypotension. The cool-down should never be omitted for sake of time. Antihypertensive medications are very diverse in their overall action and number. Thus, Personal Trainers are encouraged to familiarize themselves regarding the types, names, actions, and what the exercise responses are to these medications before working with hypertensive clients. The 8th edition *ACSM Guidelines for Exercise Testing and Prescription* (2) is an excellent text to use as a starting point for this information.

Lastly, Personal Trainers working with this population are encouraged to gain skill or enhance existing skills in blood pressure monitoring. Accurate measurement of blood pressure before, during, and after exercise will enhance the safety and appropriateness of the client's program. Precautions dictate that exercise be avoided if resting blood pressure exceeds 200/110 mm Hg, and exercise terminated if blood pressure exceeds 220/105 mm Hg or the client experiences a 10 mm Hg or more drop in blood pressure during exercise (2).

SUMMARY

This chapter explored the special considerations of exercise program design for older adults, obesity, hypertension, diabetes mellitus, cardiac disease, and pregnancy. Below are important questions, among many others, that were addressed in this section:

- What is the weekly volume of exercise necessary for stabilizing the process of CAD?
- Is moderate- or vigorous-intensity exercise best for improving cardiorespiratory fitness?
- What are the important health outcomes for older adults and for clients with diabetes or hypertension?
- What are the most critical safety concerns when working with pregnant or obese clients?

Personal Trainers are ultimately responsible for designing safe and effective programs that make a positive difference in the lives of their clients, regardless of their overall condition. To answer such questions, Personal Trainers are encouraged to use evidence-based practice to guide their selection and use of a specific intervention in a given situation. Evidence-based practice is the integration of best research **evidence** with professional **expertise** and **client values**. Personal Trainers should consider all three dimensions when formulating daily decisions with clientele and developing the exercise program. The rationale for basing decisions on sound evidence is clear—programs supported by research lead to an informed action plan that minimizes risk and optimizes effectiveness. Therefore, Personal Trainers should develop themselves as proficient consumers of scientific research to best apply evidence-based principles and practices with their clients.

REFERENCES

1. American College of Obstetricians and Gynecologists. Exercise during pregnancy and the postpartum period. ACOG Committee Opinion No. 267. *Obstet Gynecol.* 2002;99:171–73.

2. American College of Sports Medicine. *ACSM's Guidelines for Exercise Testing and Prescription.* 8th ed. Baltimore: Lippincott Williams & Wilkins; 2010.

3. American College of Sports Medicine. Position stand: the recommended quantity and quality of exercise for developing and maintaining cardiorespiratory and muscular fitness and flexibility in healthy adults. *Med Sci Sports Exerc.* 1998;30:975–91.

4. American College of Sports Medicine. Position stand: exercise and Type 2 diabetes. *Med Sci Sports Exerc.* 2000;32:1345–60.

5. American College of Sports Medicine. Position stand: appropriate intervention strategies for weight loss and prevention of weight regain for adults. *Med Sci Sports Exerc.* 2001;33:2145–56.

6. American College of Sports Medicine. Position stand: exercise and hypertension. *Med Sci Sports Exerc.* 2004;36:533–53.

7. American Geriatrics Society, British Geriatrics Society, and American Academy of Orthopedic Surgeon Panel on Falls Prevention. Guideline for the prevention of falls. *JAGS.* 2001;49:664–72.

8. Annis AM, Caulder MS, Cook ML, Duquette D. Family history, diabetes, and other demographic and risk factors among participants of the National Health and Nutrition Examination Survey 1999–2002. *Prev Chronic Dis.* 2005;2:1–12.

9. Artal R, O'Toole M. Guidelines of the American College of Obstetricians and Gynecologists for exercise during pregnancy and the postpartum period. *Br J Sports Med.* 2003;37:6–12.

10. Blair SN, Kohl HW III, Paffenbarger RS, Clark DG, Cooper KH, Gibbons LW. Physical fitness and all-cause mortality: a prospective study of healthy men and women. *JAMA.* 1989;262:2395–401.

11. Blair SN, Kohl HW III, Barlow CE, Paffenbarger RS Jr, Gibbons LW, Macera CA. Changes in physical fitness and all-cause mortality. *JAMA.* 1995;273:1093–8.

12. Blair SN, Kampert JB, Kohl HW III, et al. Influences of cardiorespiratory fitness and other precursors on cardiovascular disease and all-cause mortality in men and women. *JAMA.* 1996;276:205–10.

13. Blissmer B, Riebel D, Dye G, Ruggerio L, Greene G, Caldwell M. Health-related quality of life following a clinical weight loss intervention among overweight and obese adults: intervention and 24 month follow-up effects. *Health Qual Life Outcomes.* 2006;4:43.

14. Booth FW, Gordon SE, Carlson CJ, Hamilton MT. Waging war on modern chronic diseases: primary prevention through exercise biology. *J Appl Physiol.* 2000;88:774–87.

15. Boulé NG, Haddad E, Kenny GP, Wells GA, Sigal RJ. Effects of exercise on glycemic control and body mass in Type 2 diabetes mellitus: a meta-analysis of controlled clinical trials. *JAMA.* 2001;286:1218–27.

16. Boulé NG, Weisnagel SJ, Lakka TA, et al. Effects of exercise training on glucose homeostasis: the HERITAGE Family Study. *Diabetes Care.* 2005;28:108–14.

17. Brooks N, Layne JE, Gordon PL, Roubenoff R, Nelson ME, Castaneda-Sceppa C. Strength training improves muscle quality and insulin sensitivity in Hispanic older adults with Type 2 diabetes. *Int J Med Sci.* 2006;4:19–27.

18. Bryner R, Ullrich I, Sauers J, et al. Effects of resistance vs. aerobic training combined with an 800 calorie liquid diet on lean body mass and resting metabolic rate. *J Am Coll Nutr.* 1999;18:115–21.

19. Burnet DL, Elliott LD, Quinn MT, Plaut AJ, Schwartz MA, Chin MH. Preventing diabetes in the clinical setting. *J Gen Intern Med.* 2006;21:84–93.

20. Castaneda C, Layne J, Munoz-Orians L, et al. A randomized controlled trial of resistance exercise training to improve glycemic control in older adults with Type 2 diabetes. *Diabetes Care.* 2002;25:2335–41.

21. Centers for Disease Control and Prevention. *National Diabetes Fact Sheet: General Information and National Estimates on Diabetes in the United States, 2007.* Atlanta (GA): U.S. Department of Health and Human Services, Centers for Disease Control and Prevention; 2008.

22. Centers for Disease Control and Prevention. What is high blood pressure? Atlanta (GA): Centers for Disease Control and Prevention Web site [Internet]; [cited 2008 Aug 12]. Available from http://www.cdc.gov/bloodpressure/about.htm

23. Centers for Disease Control and Prevention. Defining obesity and overweight. Atlanta (GA): Centers for Disease Control and Prevention Web site [Internet]; [cited 2008 Aug 10]. Available from http://www.cdc.gov/nccdphp/dnpa/obesity/defining.htm

24. Centers for Disease Control and Prevention. U.S. obesity trends 1985–2007. Atlanta (GA): Centers for Disease Control and Prevention Web site [Internet]; [cited 2008 Aug 10]. Available from http://www.cdc.gov/nccdphp/dnpa/obesity/trend/maps/index.htm

25. Chobanian A, Bakris G, Black H, et al. Seventh Report of the Joint National Committee on Prevention, Detection Evaluation, and Treatment of High Blood Pressure. *Hypertension.* 2003;42:1206–52.

26. Dempsey J, Seals D. Aging, exercise, and cardiopulmonary function. In: Lamb DR, Gisolfi CV, Nadel E, editors. *Exercise in Older Adults.* Carmel (IL): Cooper Publishing Group; 1995. p. 237–304.

27. Diabetes Prevention Program Research Group. Reduction in the incidence of Type 2 diabetes with lifestyle intervention or metformin. *N Engl J Med.* 2002;346:393–403.

28. *Dietary Reference Intakes for Energy, Carbohydrate, Fiber, Fat, Fatty Acids, Cholesterol, Protein, and Amino Acids (Macronutrients).* Washington (DC): National Academies Press; 2005.

29. Dunn AL, Marcus BH, Kamper JB, et al. Comparison of lifestyle and structured interventions to increase physical activity and cardiorespiratory fitness: a randomized trial. *JAMA.* 1999;281:327–34.

30. Dunstan D, Daly R, Owen N, et al. High-intensity resistance training improves glycemic control in older patients with Type 2 diabetes. *Diabetes Care.* 2002;25:1729–36.

31. Duscha BD, Slentz CA, Johnson JL, et al. Effects of exercise training amount and intensity on peak oxygen consumption in middle-age men and women at risk for cardiovascular disease. *Chest.* 2005;128:2788–93.

32. Eriksson J. Exercise and the treatment of Type 2 diabetes mellitus. An update. *Sports Med.* 1999;27:381–91.

33. Eriksson J, Taimela S, Eriksson K, Parviainen S, Peltonen J, Kujala U. Resistance training in the treatment of non-insulin dependent diabetes mellitus. *Int J Sports Med.* 1997;18:242–6.

34. Fagard R. Exercise characteristics and the blood pressure response to dynamic physical training. *Med Sci Sports Exerc.* 2001;33:S484–92.

35. Fitzgerald MD, Tanaka H, Tran ZV, Seals DR. Age-related declines in maximal aerobic capacity in regularly exercising vs. sedentary women: a meta-analysis. *J Appl Physiol.* 1997;83:160–5.

36. Fletcher GF, Balady GJ, Amsterdam EA, et al. Exercise standards for testing and training. A statement for health care professionals from the American Heart Association. *Circulation.* 2001;104:1694–740.

37. Franklin BA: Fitness: the ultimate marker for risk stratification and health outcomes? *Prev Cardiol.* 2007;10:42–6.

38. Hagberg JM. Physical activity, fitness, health, and aging. In: Bouchard C, Shephard RJ, Stephens T, editors. *Physical Activity, Fitness, and Health.* Champaign (IL): Human Kinetics; 1994. p. 993–1006.

39. Harris S, Petrella R, Leadbetter W. Lifestyle interventions for Type 2 diabetes: relevance for clinical practice. *Can Fam Physician.* 2003;49:1618–25.

40. Haskell WL, Lee I-M, Pate RR, et al. Physical activity and public health: updated recommendation for adults from the American College of Sports Medicine and the American Heart Association. *Med Sci Sports Exerc.* 2007;39:1423–34.

41. Houmard JA, Tanner CJ, Slentz CA, Duscha BD, McCartney JS, Kraus WE. Effect of the volume and intensity of exercise training on insulin sensitivity. *J Appl Physiol.* 2004;96:101–6.

42. Ishii T, Yamakita T, Sato T, Tanaka S, Fujii S. Resistance training improves insulin sensitivity in NIDDM subjects without altering maximal oxygen uptake. *Diabetes Care.* 1998; 21:1353–5.

43. Iqbal N. The burden of Type 2 diabetes: strategies to prevent or delay onset. *Vasc Health Risk Manag.* 2007;3:511–20.

44. Kahn B, Flier J. Obesity and insulin resistance. *J Clin Invest.* 2000;106:473–81.

45. Kelley G, Kelley K. Progressive resistance exercise and resting blood pressure: a meta-analysis of randomized controlled trials. *Hypertension.* 2000;35:838–43.

46. Kraus WE, Houmard JA, Duscha BD, et al. Effects of the amount and intensity of exercise on plasma lipoproteins. *N Engl J Med.* 2002;347:1483–92.

47. Lloyd-Jones DM, Dyer AR, Wang R, Daviglus ML, Greenland P. Risk factor burden in middle age and lifetime risks for cardiovascular and non-cardiovascular death (Chicago Heart Association Detection Project in Industry). *Am J Cardiol.* 2007;99:535–40.

48. Maiorana A, O'Driscoll G, Goodman C, Taylor R, Green D. Combined aerobic and resistance exercise improves glycemic control and fitness in Type 2 diabetes. *Diabetes Res Clin Pract.* 2002;56:115–23.

49. Nelson ME, Rejeski WJ, Blair SN, et al. Physical activity and public health in older adults: recommendation for adults from the American College of Sports Medicine and the American Heart Association. *Med Sci Sports Exerc.* 2007;39:1435–45.

50. Ogden CL, Carroll MD, McDowell MA, Flegal KM. *Obesity Among Adults in the United States— No Change since 2003–2004.* NCHS data brief no 1. Hyattsville (MD): National Center for Health Statistics; 2007.

51. Park S, Park J, Kwon Y, Kim H, Yoon M, Park H. The effect of combined aerobic and resistance exercise training on abdominal fat in obese middle-aged women. *J Physiol Anthropol.* 2003;22:129–35.

52. Peirce N. Diabetes and exercise. *Br J Sports Med.* 1999;33:161–73.

53. Pollock ML, Franklin BA, Balady GJ, et al. Resistance exercise in individuals with and without cardiovascular disease: benefits, rationale, safety, and prescription: An advisory from the Committee on Exercise, Rehabilitation, and Prevention, Council on Clinical Cardiology, American Heart Association; Position paper endorsed by the American College of Sports Medicine. *Circulation.* 2000;101:828–33.

54. Racette S, Weiss E, Hickner R, Holloszy J. Modest weight loss improves insulin action in obese African Americans. *Metabolism.* 2005;54:960–65.

55. Rosamond W, Flegal K, Furie K, et al. American Heart Association Statistics Committee and Stroke Statistics Subcommittee. Heart disease and stroke statistics—2008 update: a report from the American Heart Association Statistics Committee and Stroke Statistics Subcommittee. *Circulation.* 2008;117:e25–146.

56. Saris WH, Blair SN, van Baak MA, et al. How much physical activity is enough to prevent unhealthy weight gain? Outcome of the IASO 1st Stock Conference and consensus statement. *Obes Rev.* 2003;4:101–14.

57. Shrier I. Does stretching improve performance? A systematic and critical review of the literature. *Clin J Sport Med.* 2004;14: 267–73.

58. Sigal R, Kenny G, Boulé N, et al. Effects of aerobic training, resistance training or both on glycemic control in Type 2 diabetes. *Ann Intern Med.* 2007;147:357–69.

59. Slentz C, Aiken L, Houmard J, et al. Inactivity, exercise, and visceral fat. STRRIDE: a randomized, controlled study of exercise intensity and amount. *J Appl Physiol.* 2005;99:1613–18.

60. Slentz CA, Duscha BD, Johnson JL, et al. Effects of the amount of exercise on body weight, body composition, and measures of central obesity: STRRIDE—a randomized controlled study. *Arch Intern Med.* 2004;164:31–9.

61. Soukup J, Maynard TS, Kovaleski JE. Resistance training guidelines for individuals with diabetes mellitus. *Diabetic Educ.* 1994;20:129–37.

62. Sui X, LaMonte M, Blair S. Cardiorespiratory fitness and risk of nonfatal cardiovascular disease in women and men with hypertension. *Am J Hypertens.* 2007;20:608–15.

63. Swain DP, Franklin BA. Is there a threshold intensity for aerobic training in cardiac patients. *Med Sci Sports Exerc.* 2002;34: 1071–5.

64. Swain BP, Franklin BA. Comparison of cardioprotective benefits of vigorous versus moderate intensity aerobic exercise. *Am J Cardiol.* 2006;97:141–7.

65. Taylor JD. The impact of a supervised strength and aerobic training program on muscular strength and aerobic capacity in individuals with Type 2 diabetes. *J Strength Cond Res.* 2007;21:824–30.

66. Thompson PD, Buchner D, Pina IL, et al. Exercise and physical activity in the prevention and treatment of atherosclerotic cardiovascular disease: a statement from the Council on Clinical Cardiology (Subcommittee on Exercise, Rehabilitation, and Prevention) and the Council on Nutrition, Physical Activity, and Metabolism (Subcommittee on Physical Activity). *Circulation.* 2003;107;3109–16.

67. Tokmakidis SP, Zois CE, Volaklis KA, Kotsa K, Touvra AM. The effects of a combined strength and aerobic exercise program on glucose control and insulin action in women with Type 2 diabetes. *Eur J Appl Physiol.* 2004;92:437–42.

68. U.S. Department of Health and Human Services. *Physical Activity and Health: A Report of the Surgeon General.* Atlanta (GA): U.S. Department of Health and Human Services, Centers for Disease Control and Prevention, National Center for Chronic Disease and Health Promotion; 1996.

69. U.S. Department of Health and Human Services. *The Surgeon General's Call to Action to Prevent and Decrease Overweight and Obesity.* Atlanta (GA): U.S. Department of Health and Human Services, Office of the Surgeon General; 2001. Available from http://www.surgeongeneral.gov/topics/obesity/

70. Valitutto M. Common crossroads in diabetes management. *Osteo Med Prim Care.* 2008;2:4.

71. Vasan R, Beiser A, Seshadri S, et al. Residual lifetime risk for developing hypertension in middle-aged women and men: The Framingham Heart Study. *JAMA.* 2002;287:1003–10.

72. Warburton DER, Nicol CW, Bredin SSD. Health benefits of physical activity: the evidence. *CMAJ.* 2006;174:801–9.

73. Whelton S, Chin A, Xin X, He J. Effect of aerobic exercise on blood pressure: a meta-analysis of randomized, controlled trials. *Ann Intern Med.* 2002;136:493–503.

74. Wilborn C, Beckham J, Campbell B, et al. Obesity: prevalence, theories, medical consequences, management, and research directions. *J Int Soc Sports Nutr.* 2005;2:4–31.

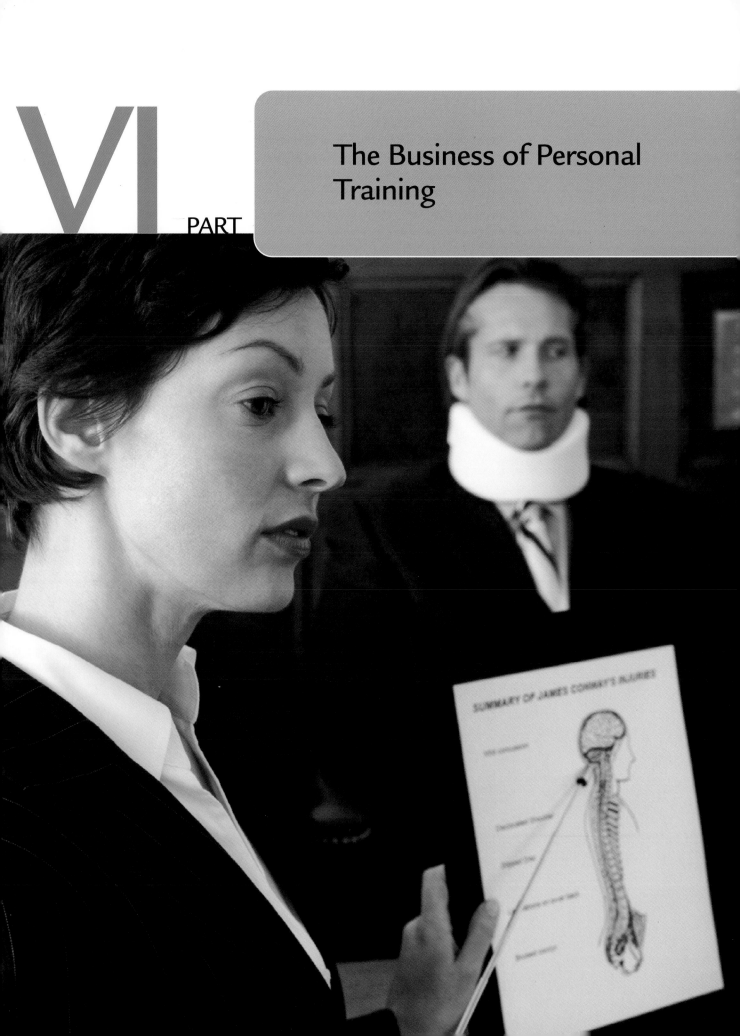

VI PART

The Business of Personal Training

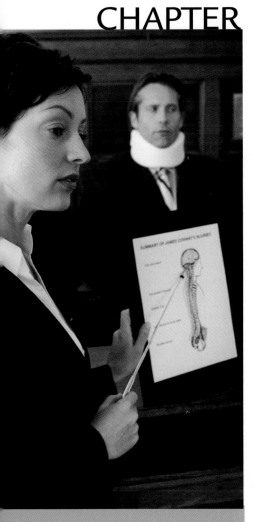

21

Business Basics and Planning

OBJECTIVES

- Learn how to sell and market training services to potential clients
- Learn how to price training sessions
- Learn how to maintain professional standards that will protect a business reputation

A Personal Trainer may be very knowledgeable and skilled in exercise science principles and their application in a personal training session, but an understanding of the business of personal training is equally important for his or her success. Whether working as an entrepreneur, a fitness center employee, or an independent contractor, a Personal Trainer needs business expertise in how to sell and market training services to potential clients, how to price training sessions, and how to maintain professional standards that will protect a business reputation. For success as a self-employed Personal Trainer, business planning, business models, and budgeting are also needed before a business can be started. Finally, business success will also depend on finding a work–life balance, as personal training can involve long days with many training sessions and interaction with many different people.

> *For success as a self-employed Personal Trainer, business planning, business models, and budgeting are also needed before a business can be started.*

THE PERSONAL TRAINER'S POSITION

A Personal Trainer can work in several different, yet distinct settings. Some of the more common venues or "job classifications" include the solo Personal Trainer, the employee or independent contractor, and the manager or personal training business owner. The independent Personal Trainer is commonly known as a Personal Trainer who is independent of another business entity. The Personal Trainer of this type typically markets to potential clients and schedules and delivers training sessions in the client's home, outside, or in the gym. The employee or independent contractor is typically hired or contracted by a business owner to provide training services for the business's clients. The Personal Trainer/manager/owner typically supervises the business operations and staff management of a personal training business. Whether the Personal Trainer is a sole proprietor or an employee, success will be based on how well he or she can sell the training services. The "Sales" section in this chapter provides a comprehensive approach to selling personal training services. Although the emphases on specific job tasks might differ from one setting to another, the goal is ultimately the same: to follow sound business practices and develop a profitable enterprise by delivering the optimal level of service to the end user, the training client.

There are various compensation models for personal training programs in the fitness center setting. Some facilities compensate Personal Trainers a percentage of the revenue generated by the services they deliver, otherwise known as commission-based compensation. Other facilities hire Personal Trainers as hourly or salaried employees with designated work shifts and pay them an additional commission for "fee for service" sessions delivered to the members. Individual salaries or commission rates for Personal Trainers typically vary on the basis of education, certification, experience, seniority, job performance, and volume of revenue produced. Regardless of the compensation model, it is important that all program costs be considered during the business planning phase. General and administrative costs for marketing, administrative support, meetings, uniforms, payroll taxes, liability insurance, and continuing education can dramatically affect the profitability of the personal training program (2).

BUSINESS SUCCESS

> *Long-term viability relies greatly upon the ability of the Personal Trainer to establish and maintain repeat business.*

Success in the personal training business is very much dependent on the same factors affecting other service-based industries. Consequently, long-term viability relies greatly upon the ability of the Personal Trainer to establish and maintain repeat business.

Managing a Personal Training Department

If working in a health club, corporate fitness facility, or a nonprofit recreation center, a Personal Trainer may be employed to manage the personal training department, while still maintaining a schedule of training clients. This added responsibility requires good organizational skills and time management. Skills in interviewing, hiring, employee training, service pricing, marketing, sales, and policy-setting are needed by the personal training manager.

Hiring Personal Trainers

The following are important steps to follow when hiring a Personal Trainer:

1. Résumé should be reviewed carefully for educational background, current certifications, recent training experience with a variety of clientele, and innovative training programs.
2. Applicants should be asked to bring copies of current fitness and CPR-AED/First Aid certifications to the interview appointment. This may prevent an undesired realization after hiring that the Personal Trainer's certifications have expired.
3. The Personal Trainer/manager should create a list of questions to ask all personal training applicants. The questions should be practical, including scenarios that require the Personal Trainer to discuss training program options for hypothetical clients.
4. The Personal Trainer's availability and scheduling preference for appointments should be clearly assessed and agreed to at the time of the interview and prior to a job offer. If the department needs an evening Personal Trainer and the interviewee is already training elsewhere in the evening, the Personal Trainer/manager needs to know that information to effectively plan for staffing needs.
5. A practical or "hands-on" component should be a part of the interview process. The Personal Trainer should demonstrate exercises and spotting techniques on the fitness floor. Someone should be designated to be a hypothetical client. The Personal Trainer/manager should observe and assess how the Personal Trainer interacts with this person.
6. A practical component consisting of fitness assessments should also be a part of the interview process. Utilizing a designated hypothetical client, the Personal Trainer should explain and demonstrate commonly used fitness assessments, such as resting blood pressure and heart rate, strength and flexibility measures, body composition, and cardiovascular endurance testing. The Personal Trainer should also be able to compare the results with norms and provide the results to the hypothetical client.

Setting Training Standards

The personal training manager is ultimately responsible for the safety and customer satisfaction of every personal training client. Therefore, it is necessary to set standards for delivering personal training services in a manner that is consistent with industry standards for safety and that will ensure that excellent customer service is consistently delivered. Here are some guidelines for setting the department's service standards:

1. Personal Trainers must give their undivided attention to their clients (1). This means that Personal Trainers must watch clients at all times and spot exercises with appropriate techniques. Policy parameters should be specific. Talking on cell phones, talking with other Personal Trainers or other members, and watching TV monitors are examples of unacceptable behaviors that would not meet training standards. In addition, a Personal Trainer who spends much of the training session talking about his or her personal affairs will have difficulty focusing fully on the client's workout and exercise technique (1).
2. The Personal Trainer must begin training sessions on time and end training sessions on time, and respect the training client's time and schedule.
3. There should be a dress standard for the department's Personal Trainers. If possible, Personal Trainers should wear a shirt with a facility logo and the words "Personal Trainer." The shirt, along with

established standards for pants and shoes, will ensure a professional look for the personal training department, while also providing advertising to other members.

4. The Personal Trainer should keep written documentation of every client's workout as well as any measurements, tests, and performance tracking for that client (1). The personal training department manager should provide a standardized "training card" for Personal Trainers to use. There should be a designated training file in which the training cards are kept that is accessible to both the training client and other Personal Trainers. If a client wants to work out without the Personal Trainer or another Personal Trainer needs to cover a training session because of illness or vacation, the training cards are readily available.

5. A client confidentiality policy should be maintained. Personal Trainers should be reminded that they should never discuss any client's personal information with others. Personal Trainers must respect their clients' privacy and be trustworthy (1).

6. Honesty and scope of practice standards should be emphasized. If a Personal Trainer does not know the answer to a client's health- or fitness-related questions, the Personal Trainer needs to admit that he or she does not have that information. The Personal Trainer can volunteer to research the topic and provide an answer at the next training session. If the client is asking for medical advice or a diagnosis, the Personal Trainer must not overstep his or her scope of practice but should explain that the client needs to consult a physician for that information (1). Ideally, the Personal Trainer should establish a network of allied healthcare professionals through which referrals can be made to physicians, physical therapists, dieticians, and other experts.

> *It is necessary to set standards for delivering personal training services in a manner that is consistent with industry standards for safety and that will ensure that excellent customer service is consistently delivered.*

7. Personal Trainers must maintain personal training certifications, CPR certification, and liability insurance, if it is not provided by the fitness facility. Records of certification and professional liability insurance should be kept in employee files (2).

TRAINING AND EMPOWERING PERSONAL TRAINERS

Personal Trainers should be encouraged to continuously read and learn, staying current on the latest industry standards and changing trends. The Personal Trainer/manager can subscribe to trade journals and publications and make them available to his Personal Trainers. Budget permitting, some Personal Trainer/managers can provide an annual educational stipend for each Personal Trainer that will subsidize his or her participation in continuing education to maintain personal training certification. Others provide CEC-approved in-house educational sessions to make it convenient and cost-effective for Personal Trainers to attend and earn credit for continuing education or recertification. Others hold weekly staff meetings with Personal Trainers and even have them take turns providing continuing education with handouts and discussion.

Managers should empower Personal Trainers by encouraging them to share training program ideas in meetings, help plan and implement new training program approaches such as small-group training or sport-specific training, and share ideas for how to increase clientele and sales. Personal Trainers should be included in discussions about pricing of training sessions and their compensation rates. They should be treated as professionals, and their creative ideas and opinions should be valued. They should feel like an integral part of the training team.

FITNESS MANAGEMENT

A Personal Trainer may also be placed in charge of a fitness department in a health club, corporate fitness facility, or nonprofit recreation center. Other Personal Trainers may also be part of this department. In addition to overseeing the personal training sales and delivery, the fitness department manager may also be responsible for fitness equipment purchases, emergency drills, maintenance and repairs, special fitness programming events, and, in some cases, the group fitness program. Even with all of these responsibilities, the fitness manager may still be expected to retain personal training clients for additional department revenue and to supplement his or her income in addition to that received managing the fitness department. A checklist along with some practical guidelines may include the following:

> *The fitness department manager may also be responsible for fitness equipment purchases, emergency drills, maintenance and repairs, special fitness programming events, and, in some cases, the group fitness program.*

1. Setting a schedule for available times for training and for management responsibilities
2. Using a time-management system to stay organized
3. Training exercise specialists and Personal Trainers to follow routine procedures (such as turning in time cards) that will simplify the workload
4. Explaining tasks to other fitness staff and then delegating these tasks to those who will get them done correctly and on time (e.g., assign the planning of monthly emergency drills/procedure reviews to a fitness staff member and have this person plan and execute the drills and reviews with all fitness staff, including Personal Trainers)
5. Taking time to lead by example for both members and fitness staff by leading a healthy lifestyle of regular exercise and practicing good nutritional habits

STARTING A BUSINESS

> *There are five basic business models from which to choose for a personal training business: sole proprietorship, independent contractor, partnership, corporation, and S corporation.*

Before starting a personal training business, it is important to evaluate an appropriate business model from which to operate. There are five basic business models from which to choose for a personal training business: sole proprietorship, independent contractor, partnership, corporation, and S corporation.

Sole Proprietorship

In a sole proprietorship, one person owns the business. As the simplest, least-expensive business model, often the only requirement before starting operations is a license from the state and/or local city where the business will be located. Personal income tax is paid on any business earnings. Two drawbacks to this model can be capital expenses for business startup/expansion and personal liability for any incurred debt (4). In the eyes of the law and the Internal Revenue Service, the business and the individual are one and the same. Another point to consider as a sole proprietor is the lack of assistance with day-to-day operations during your absence.

Independent Contractor

An independent contractor provides certain services for other individuals or businesses. Many Personal Trainers are independent contractors who provide personal training services to health clubs; the client pays the club for the services and the club pays the Personal Trainer. Personal Trainers who are independent contractors often work at multiple locations, set their own schedules, are paid by the session, and often have some control over training session format and fees. However, the percentage of the training fees that the individual contractor receives is often determined by the health club management (4). An independent contractor is similar to a sole proprietorship except the Personal Trainer actually operates his or her own business within the health club. The primary advantage of this arrangement is the Personal Trainer's access to health club members and equipment.

Partnership

A business partnership is formed by two or more people, either with an informal agreement or with a formal written contract filed with local or state government. Partnerships are loosely governed by state and federal regulations and are subject to personal income tax based on each partner's ownership share. Forming a partnership allows pooled financial resources and talents, but ownership transfer among partners may be difficult, and each partner can be held liable if another partner fails to meet business-related obligations (4).

Corporation

A corporation is a formal business entity subject to laws, regulations, and the demands of stockholders. Governed by a charter and bylaws, a corporation is a legal entity completely separate from its owners and managers and is taxed as such. The corporate profits paid as dividends are also taxed for each shareholder. Investors, whose personal risk for financial liability is limited, are often part of a corporation's startup and growth. Corporation ownership can be more easily transferred than ownership in a sole proprietorship or partnership (4).

S Corporation

The S corporation (or subchapter S corporation), a popular alternative for small businesses, combines the advantages of the sole proprietorship, partnership, and corporation. The benefits include the following:

➤ Limited risk and exposure of personal assets
➤ No double taxation on both salary and business income
➤ Freedom for each partner to distribute dividends (4)

ADMINISTRATION

To establish and administer a business, the Personal Trainer should first develop a business plan. The business plan includes a demographic and competitor analysis, establishing a budget, developing management policies, marketing, sales, and pricing.

The first step involved in creating a solid business plan is a comprehensive demographic analysis. One must acquire data about the population located in the area one plans to conduct business in. Depending on the scope of the Personal Training operation, this might include anyone living in a 2- to 10-mile radius from a specified location. During this phase of the plan, one should examine the total number of people, number of households, household income, number of families, and a variety of other population characteristics. These demographic markers will provide the business operator with the preliminary information necessary to determine whether there's a chance his or her business can be successful in the chosen marketplace.

The first step involved in creating a solid business plan is a comprehensive demographic analysis.

Once the demographic analysis has been conducted, the business operator should thoroughly evaluate the competition inside the market area. Virtually all fitness centers offer personal training, so these entities will represent the greatest competitive threat to your business viability. Other potential competitors might include gender-specific clubs, group training studios, and hospital-based wellness programs. The strength or weakness of the competition will help you determine the percentage of market share you can reasonably expect to cultivate with your entity.

Establishing a Budget

A market analysis will provide valuable information useful in developing an annual operating budget. It provides the baseline data to build the budget from the ground up. Personal training businesses typically begin with determining sales goals. The sales goals are set by determining the projected number of training sessions over the course of a week, month, and year multiplied by the average rate per session. These totals will help determine expenses over each period of time, because direct expenses correlate with sessions delivered multiplied by the cost per session. To establish a budget, the Personal Trainer should consider the following:

1. Estimate business expenses (exclusive of salary) needed to operate annually, including the following:
   a. Gas/vehicle maintenance
   b. Income tax
   c. Liability insurance
   d. Telephone
   e. Uniforms
   f. Professional memberships/certifications
   g. Conferences and training
   h. Business supplies (computer, office supplies, postage, printing, etc.)
   i. Fitness equipment
   j. Client gifts/awards
   k. Accountant fees
2. Determine a realistic number of training hours annually that fit into a realistic schedule (factor in vacation days, personal days for medical checkups and family emergencies, sick days, etc.)
3. Determine a charge per training session to achieve a gross annual income that will cover business expenses and personal expenses and will allow some funds to be put aside for savings and/or investments (5). Consider the average price point for personal training services in your region and specifically what the competition is charging.

Management and Policies

To manage a business effectively, the Personal Trainer must work from a business plan, which should include the creation of a business vision, mission statement, business values, a brief description of the business services (Box 21.1), the choice of a business model, and the listing of operational policies (6) such as the following:

> Billing (Will clients prepay for each session or will you bill them monthly?)
> Cancellation policy (How many hours will you need without charging the client?)
> Late arrival policy (Will you charge for the entire session anyway?)
> Vacation policy (What will this be for both the Personal Trainer and the client?)
> Payment methods (Will the client pay by cash, check, or credit card?)
> "Insufficient funds" check policy (Will there be a penalty and if so, what?)

Marketing

The personal training market includes different groups of people with varying needs. A market niche represents a client group with similar needs and goals. Personal Trainers often choose to focus their marketing efforts on one or several of these groups. For example, a Personal Trainer could select the niche market based on the following:

A market niche represents a client group with similar needs and goals.

| BOX **21.1** | **Sample Mission Statement** |

THE PERSONAL TRAINING ACADEMY

Our Vision
✓ To grow profitably by delighting customers and achieving undisputed leadership in the field of personal training.

Our Mission
✓ To create value for shareowners through our marketplace leadership in personal training and fitness programming that helps all of our clients achieve their goals.

Our Values
✓ **Integrity,** honesty, and the highest ethical standards
✓ **Mutual respect** and trust in our working relationships
✓ **Innovation** and encouragement to challenge the status quo
✓ **Communication** that is open, consistent, and two-way
✓ **Teamwork** and meeting our commitments to one another
✓ **Continuous improvement,** development, and learning in all we do
✓ **Diversity** of people, cultures, and ideas
✓ **Performance** with recognition for results

Service Description
✓ The Personal Training Academy provides personal training clients with the best possible physical and psychological advantage by improving their focus, discipline, and self-confidence. This is achieved through the most advanced state-of-the-art personal training techniques available, thus enhancing the client's ability to compete and achieve success both in fitness and in life.

➤ Client type (e.g., gender, age, fitness level)
➤ Training needs (e.g., sport-specific training, prenatal fitness, group training)
➤ Training location (e.g., in-home training, health club training, sport location training)

Personal Trainers should ask the following questions when selecting their market niches:

➤ What is the potential for income with this market?
➤ Is this market readily accessible in my geographical area?
➤ Does this market fit well with my training skills and interest?
➤ Can I highlight my knowledge, services, certifications, and skills in such a way to reach this market as my clientele?

One of the best ways to market personal training services is to ask for referrals from satisfied clients. Personal Trainers sometimes are hesitant to do this, but if the Personal Trainer truly believes that a client has benefited greatly from the training, then other potential clients may want to also receive these same benefits. Other ways of marketing personal training include volunteering to speak at community events and organizations and networking with other business professionals in the community. Advertising in the phone book, the newspaper, and by direct mail can be costly and may not provide a good return on the investment at first. Establishing a Web site and profiling the training style and qualifications are other good approaches for marketing a business and staying competitive in the personal training business.

Personal training businesses use a variety of strategies to attract clients. Among the more popular strategies are:

1. Client referral (the most focused strategy)
   a. The focus is on generating prospects and clients.
   b. The process involves existing clients providing the names of potential new clients.
   c. Clients are provided with referral cards to hand in the names of prospects.
   d. Incentives are typically given to clients for providing referrals.
   e. It is usually an ongoing strategy.
2. Lead boxes (provides a very low rate of return)
   a. This strategy primarily serves as a source for leads (names).
   b. The boxes are placed in business locations that tend to serve customer bases that are demographically similar to the targeted audiences.
   c. Businesses are given awards for allowing the lead boxes to be placed in their locales.
3. Advertising (most expensive and lowest rate of return on investment)
   a. In general, this strategy is designed to build brand recognition in the marketplace, enhance the image of the organization, create leads, or occasionally generate prospects.
   b. This technique is a shotgun approach to reaching clients (vs. more targeted methods).
   c. Cable television, radio, newspapers, billboards, and external or internal signage are examples of this method.
   d. The most effective type of advertising for generating leads or prospects provides a "Call to Action" and typically creates urgency by establishing a deadline.
   e. It is important to know the marketing target niche before the advertising medium is selected.
4. Alliances with Homeowner Associations (HOAs) and realtors
   a. This strategy is a good source for qualified leads and even prospects (HOAs and realtors whose customers match the organization's target market should be engaged in the process).
   b. HOAs and realtors can provide the names of new people in the area.
   c. A strategy involves providing the HOAs or realtors with a certificate or letter to give to customers that offers some complimentary service (i.e., training session or preactivity screening and goals analysis).
5. Direct mail (the return rate for this technique is usually 1%–3% for mailed pieces and 7%–15% for e-mails)
   a. This strategy is primarily a technique for creating leads or turning leads into prospects.
   b. This method is a more focused technique than advertising.
   c. Direct mail lists from agencies should be used (very targeted lists—such as ZIP codes or even specific delivery routes—can be obtained to best match the desired market area and demographics of the target audience).
   d. The piece that is mailed is typically simple, with an attention-grabbing call to action and normally incorporates an incentive to create urgency and generate an action response.
6. Community involvement (ideal for service and relationship-driven businesses like personal training)
   a. This strategy focuses on creating relationships to uncover prospects.
   b. The technique involves creating a specific image within the community and becoming a recognized professional in the community.
   c. An example of this approach is to become active in community organizations, such as the local chambers of commerce, the Rotary Club, church groups, and other civic organizations.
   d. Another option is hosting community events in the training facility or sponsoring community events at other locations.
   e. Volunteer as a speaker for community organizations and special events. Offer your services to provide simple screenings while advertising your services.
   f. Join small business groups and pair up with others and exchange services. For example, you can provide personal training to another small business owner in exchange for marketing services.

7. Reputation management
   a. This strategy is used to enhance the public image of the organization.
   b. Over time, this approach can be a great source for prospects.
   c. The technique involves developing a press kit on the Personal Trainer or the business as a whole (e.g., a background, fact sheet).
   d. This strategy requires establishing positive relationships with the local media.
   e. The approach requires regularly issuing press releases of human interest involving the club and following up with the media.
8. Promotional materials
   a. This strategy is normally used to help convert leads to prospects or prospects to members.
   b. The materials are designed to create a positive image of the business and to help educate consumers on personal training in general, the business, and its Personal Trainers.
   c. Web sites, print brochures, and video brochures are examples of this technique.
   d. These materials are normally given to leads and more often to prospects.
9. Strategic alliances
   a. This strategy is designed to create partnerships between businesses and organizations with similar target audiences.
   b. This technique is good at bringing in leads and prospects.
   c. The approach involves cross-marketing between the businesses (e.g., a Personal Trainer might partner with a home fitness equipment retailer offering equipment purchasers a complimentary "orientation to the purchased equipment," with the objective of converting them into personal training clients; the retailer has a "value-added service"—the Personal Trainer—which might be an inducement for the customer to purchase the equipment).
   d. The customers of each business become potential customers for the other partner (an alliance group) (2).

Sales

Too often, Personal Trainers focus their "sales" efforts on creating signs, flyers, and brochures, hoping that clients will flock to them for training. The mistake often made is that such efforts are "low-percentage" marketing activities that offer a low return on the investment of time, money, and effort. In addition, these activities do not close the sale for the Personal Trainer; they only weed out potential prospects for the Personal Trainer's services. The Personal Trainer is depending on the client to respond to the marketing piece. The key to sales success is for the Personal Trainer to use available resources, proactively cultivate warm-market "suspects" to convert them into prospects, and finally ask the prospect for the sale.

> *The key to sales success is for the Personal Trainer to use available resources, proactively cultivate warm-market "suspects" to convert them into prospects, and finally ask the prospect for the sale.*

Before going into the sales process, "sale" must first be defined. A sale is simply an agreement—a quid pro quo—between the Personal Trainer, the client, and at times the facility where the training sessions will take place. A sale is not an imposition on the client. All too often, a Personal Trainer is "apologetic" when asking for the sale. In actuality, every sale is a "win–win" situation, because all participants position themselves to get what they want. Clients are securing the direction, expertise, or motivation they desire, and the Personal Trainer is contracting his or her professional services. The ingredient needed to fulfill the sale is commitment. The client must commit to what was agreed to at the point of sale (i.e., showing up prepared for the training session at the scheduled time), and the Personal Trainer must commit to

TABLE 21.1	BENEFITS OF PERSONAL TRAINING
Client achieves results more quickly	
Reduces the risk of injury to the client	
Increases the client's motivational levels	
Provides more focused workouts for the client	
Utilizes the client's time more efficiently	

deliver on the service "promise" to the client (i.e., delivering a safe, individualized, goal-oriented workout).

In the gym or fitness center environment, the Personal Trainer's primary source of business is the membership base. This captive audience is the Personal Trainer's main resource for "prospects." It is important for the Personal Trainer to be established as an expert and to build rapport with the members, creating a warm market for the Personal Trainer to target, market to, and ultimately, to ask for the sale.

Before approaching members on the exercise floor, Personal Trainers should have a clear understanding of what their objective is and what value they bring to the potential client. It is important to be empathetic and see things through the eyes of the member. Why should the member consider personal training? What is in it for the member? The Personal Trainer should know what the benefits of personal training are to the client (Table 21.1).

The Personal Trainer needs to be aware of the prospect's questions and concerns. What are the prospect's perceptions? Will personal training help get the participant more fit? Will it help the participant look better? Will it help the participant be healthier? These are all valuable benefits and perceived outcomes for the participant, but ultimately, even a prospect who perceives these outcomes as real still might not make the commitment to purchase training sessions. Why? It is because it is all about the prospect's emotions. The Personal Trainer must consider how the prospect feels about his or her goals and how he or she will feel when they are fulfilled.

Effective sales generation is simply a step-by-step process outlined on the following pages (and in Table 21.2), which could be used for a facility-based Personal Trainer.

TABLE 21.2	THE FITNESS FACILITY-BASED PERSONAL TRAINER'S SALES CHECKLIST
Be proactive. Approach prospects and always remember to smile—*be positive and upbeat, no matter how bad a day you are having*	
Top priority is to build rapport—to develop a relationship of mutual trust and confidence	
Sell *benefits* of personal training but key into *how they'll feel* when achieving those benefits	
Be empathetic—see their world as if it was your own	
Be genuine—exude sincerity	
Be warm—treat prospects with respect	

It's a win–win!
    Clients take control of their goals by using an expert's assistance
    Personal Trainers practice their profession, increase their earning potential, and add valuable experience, which enhances their value to the employer or facility and the fitness industry in general.
    The facility enhances the service delivered to clients by providing one-on-one management of the member
    You must *ask* for the sale!—*It is a numbers game. The more prospects you ask, the more sales you'll make.*	

STEP 1: MAKING CONTACT

Getting a foot in the door. A personal Trainer needs to proactively approach a facility member or client exercising on the gym floor. The Personal Trainer should greet the member with a smile and offer his or her expertise on the basis of his or her observations of the member.

Sample "openings" may include the following:

➤ "Hi! May I help you with your exercise program?"
➤ "Hey Mark, let me show you a more effective way to do this exercise"
➤ "Hello Linda, I noticed you're really focusing on your lower body. Can I show you a great new combination of exercises for your hips and thighs?"

STEP 2: BUILDING RAPPORT

"Trust me?" *Yes!!!* Personal Trainers must build rapport and trust so that prospects believe in them and their ability in helping the clients achieve established goals. A Personal Trainer builds trust by taking a personal interest in the prospect, making mental notes of the prospect's likes, dislikes, or personal information that the prospect may share with the Personal Trainer.

Sample rapport-building "blurbs" include the following:

➤ "Hi John, it's good to see you're back on track after the holidays."
➤ "Hello Marie, how was your business trip?"
➤ "Hi Jessica, did your daughter decide between colleges?"

STEP 3: ASSESSING NEED

The Personal Trainer needs to "shut up and listen!!!" The best salespersons are seldom the best talkers—they're usually the best listeners. The Personal Trainer should key into "What's in it for the prospect?" and focus on not just "what" the prospect wants but also learn *why* the prospect wants it. Ask simple open-ended questions that encourage the prospect to share information.

STEP 4: THE TEASE

This is how Personal Trainers continue to build trust and demonstrate and build their value. The simplest way is to assist a prospect with an exercise or make program suggestions. A Personal Trainer can spot the prospect as he or she is progressing through a workout and suggest a "better way." The Personal Trainer can also demonstrate a new exercise or literally "train" the client for 5 or 10 minutes, just giving the prospect a "taste" of what it is like to work with him or her. This sampling of the Personal Trainer's prowess is the "tease" that should keep the prospect wanting more.

STEP 5: PRESENTING A WINNING PROPOSITION

Asking for the sale. The Personal Trainer must present a winning solution to the prospect's need before asking for the sale. This "frames" the pitch so that the prospect responds affirmatively when asked for the sale.

➤ "With your high school reunion coming up, it's a great time to specialize your exercise program, don't you think?"
➤ "If I can show you how I can help you reach your goal, would that interest you?"

STEP 6: "THE CLOSE"

The Personal Trainer should give the prospect "either/or" choices, never "yes" or "no." A sample "yes-or-no" proposal may include something like "Marie, would you like to set up a training appointment?"

A sample "either/or" proposal might be "Marie, you're usually here in the morning, I'm available to help you any two mornings per week at 6 AM or 7 AM. Which works best for you?" Giving the prospect a choice between two "yeses" increases the likelihood that the Personal Trainer will close the sale.

STEP 7: THE FALL-BACK

Opening the backdoor—"the tickler file." Every prospect that says "no" becomes a "future prospect." The Personal Trainer should maintain a database of contact and personal information (e.g., likes, dislikes, occupation) of these prospects for further rapport building, always looking for the opportunity to once again ask for the sale. The Personal Trainer should continue to deliver a service (e.g., assistance on the training floor) and communicate through every available vehicle (in person, phone, e-mail, etc.) increasing his or her value as a Personal Trainer. Photocopying clips of fitness articles that prospects might be interested in and providing them to clients, e-mailing a Web-based link to a pertinent Web site, and even a press release with the Personal Trainer's own "success story" are all examples of how to effectively "drip" on prospects to build a Personal Trainer's value. Personal Trainers in a fitness center setting should also do whatever they can to keep the prospect coming in to work out, even if the prospect continues to train on his or her own. Doing so helps maintain the Personal Trainer's "warm market" so that the prospect remains a prospect and is also a source of referrals to the Personal Trainer.

STEP 8: KEEP IN MIND

It's a "numbers game." An insurance company study conducted several years back showed that even the worst approach to selling can be successful if the salesperson simply goes through the numbers and "keeps asking." With this in mind, understand that a prospect is always a potential customer, so practice cautious persistence.

Pricing

Once the framework for the personal training business is complete, specific pricing and budgets can be established. Typical direct expenses include salaries, payroll taxes, and benefits. Operational expenses include marketing expenses, program materials, and facility use charges. Pricing is typically established through consideration of a number of factors. It is essential to consider the general business objectives (e.g., profit, overall client retention, the projected number of clients, and average number of sessions per client per unit of time) before establishing pricing. To conduct programs within established budgetary guidelines, revenues and expenses should be reviewed regularly (2).

Ultimately, what a Personal Trainer charges for training services depends on market forces. Completing a market analysis will help determine perceived value in the marketplace and thus price point. Some key elements of a market analysis include the following:

➤ Demographic study: How many potential clients are there in the geographical area?
➤ Competitive analysis: What are other Personal Trainers charging for their services?
➤ Consumer survey: What is the prospective client's perceived value?
➤ Demand projections: How large is the market?
➤ Financial considerations: Based on budgetary projections, what is the required revenue per unit sale? What volume is required to meet budget?
➤ Focus group information: What are the perceived needs of the prospect base?
➤ Consider the four E's when considering what to charge clients (3).
  • Education
    • Bachelor's or Master's degree in exercise science/physiology; level of certification (e.g., ACSM, ACE, NSCA, NASM)
  • Experience
    • Years working as a certified personal trainer
    • Types of training (sports specific, special medical populations)

- Environment/location
  - Where you are physically (facility) and geographically (city, state)
  - Business or studio location (owner/operator)
- Expenses
  - Equipment, clothing, gas (traveling trainers), personal liability insurance, advertising/marketing materials, certification/membership fees, rent/electricity/insurance

> *Completing a market analysis will help determine perceived value in the marketplace and thus price point.*

- The components under each of the four E's are not exhaustive, nor are they intended to be. As the personal training industry continues to grow, so will the needs of certified personal trainers and their businesses.

Business Planning

Budgets are necessary to forecast financial expectations and goals, provide accountability, track progress of actual results versus projected results, and allow justification and scrutiny. Completing an accurate, reliable, and analyzable budget without a computer is not easy. Simple software programs like QuickBooks or MYOB (Manage Your Own Business) are available and recommended, even for the solo Personal Trainer; they will help organize business finances and make tax reporting easier (2).

> *Although there are many resources available for the Personal Trainer/manager/owner, it remains prudent to enlist the guidance of a legal and accounting professional.*

Although there are many resources available for the Personal Trainer/manager/owner, it remains prudent to enlist the guidance of a legal and accounting professional. The Internal Revenue Service Web site is a great resource for obtaining specific tax forms and information. It is accessible at http://www.irs.gov/.

PROFESSIONAL STANDARDS

A Code of Ethics for ACSM Certified and Registered Professionals has been established, which helps guide the ethical practice of Personal Trainers. This code (see Chapter 1) helps bring the profession of personal training in line with other professions and healthcare disciplines.

SUMMARY

It is no longer true that the best "technical Personal Trainer" is the most successful. Whether the Personal Trainer is "going solo" or is a manager of a large personal training department within a fitness center, today's Personal Trainers need to be proficient in both exercise science and business management. Only by combining these varied skills can they ensure their success and that of their clients.

REFERENCES

1. American College of Sports Medicine. *ACSM's Resources for the Personal Trainer*. 2nd ed. Baltimore: Lippincott Williams & Wilkins; 2005.
2. American College of Sports Medicine. *ACSM's Resource Manual for Guidelines for Exercise Testing and Prescription*. 6th ed. Baltimore: Wolters Kluwer/Lippincott Williams & Wilkins; 2009.
3. Churilla JR. Starting a personal training business. *ACSM's Certified News*. 2008;18(2):1–7.
4. Holland T. Ten important personal training guidelines. *Am Fitness*. 2001;19(1):42.
5. Miller W. One-on-one: choosing a market niche. *Strength Cond*. 1994;16(4):68–9.
6. Schreiber K. One-on-one: setting up a budget for a personal training business. *Strength Cond*. 1994;16(5):64–5.

CHAPTER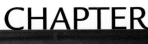

22

Legal Issues and Responsibilities

OBJECTIVES

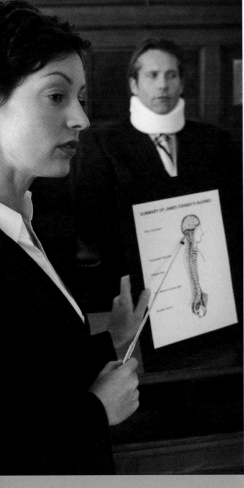

* Understand the primary areas of potential liability
* Understand the role of industry standards and guidelines
* Learn practical strategies to manage risk

Personal Trainer must understand legal issues and responsibilities before assuming the task of training any person. Regardless of Personal Trainers' business model, whether associated with a personal training department or running their own business, Personal Trainers need to know what areas of potential liability affect their practice, what industry standards and guidelines direct these areas, and what measures they can take to manage risk effectively. All physical activity involves risk of injury; accidents can and will happen. To maintain professionalism and to protect the longevity of a personal training career, a Personal Trainer needs to proactively anticipate these areas of risk and to manage them with common sense. This knowledge of, and commitment to, safety and injury prevention not only minimizes the likelihood of professional liability but also improves quality of service and may save lives.

> *All physical activity involves risk of injury; accidents can and will happen.*

This chapter discusses liability specifically related to working with clients and does not expand into broader issues such as type of business organization, copyright, or trademark issues that are more appropriately covered in other chapters and books devoted specifically to business practices. Local rules and regulations, definitions of standards of care, and the acceptability of waivers of liability vary from state to state, county to county, and even city to city. This chapter is not intended to be legal advice and should not be considered a substitute for legal counsel on specific liability issues pertaining to individual situations.

POTENTIAL AREAS OF PROFESSIONAL LIABILITY

Legal considerations affect many aspects of the personal training experience. Areas of potential exposure to liability include the physical setting where program activities occur; the equipment used; the nature and quality of training techniques, advice, and services rendered; the degree of emergency preparedness and responsiveness; and the method of keeping and protecting records. Although legal principles affect the training environment, as a practical matter most cases today are settled out of court and therefore never actually create case law. To help Personal Trainers understand the practical ramifications, this chapter is organized according to the most common types of incidents likely to occur during day-to-day business. The application of legal concepts such as negligence to particular circumstances is then examined, and the role of professional standards, guidelines, position statements, and recommendations from professional organizations is considered. Personal training is a business/invitee relationship. In these types of relationships, the ante for invitee responsibilities is raised

> *Personal training is a business/invitee relationship. In these types of relationships, the ante for invitee responsibilities is raised.*

Safe Premises

Although most Personal Trainers focus on educating themselves on the latest training techniques and aspects of program design, in reality, Personal Trainers are vulnerable to professional liability for incidents that result from conditions of the physical setting where program activities occur. In general (11), any business owner who allows people to enter upon land or into a building is required to provide a reasonably safe environment under theories of tort law (Box 22.1). The area of tort law that regulates these issues is termed "premises liability." The ACSM (4) has identified six fundamental standards to which facilities must adhere (Box 22.2). Because a Personal Trainer may offer services in a variety of locations, including a health/fitness facility, the outdoors, or in a client's home, the Personal Trainer should take basic precautions to help ensure that every training setting is reasonably safe.

> *The Personal Trainer should take basic precautions to help ensure that every training setting is reasonably safe.*

BOX **22.1**	**Key Terms**

Contract law: Body of law that regulates the rights and obligations of parties that enter into a contract. A contract is an agreement between two or more parties that creates an obligation to do, or not to do, something that creates a legal relationship. If the agreement is broken, the parties have the right to pursue legal remedies. A contract can be written or verbal. The important elements of a contract include an offer and an acceptance, also referred to as a "meeting of the minds" and the exchange of something of value.

Duty of care: Refers to the level of responsibility that one has to protect another from harm. In general, the legal standard is reasonable care under the circumstances, which is based on an examination of factual details.

Informed consent: A process that entails conveying complete understanding to a client or patient about his or her option to choose to participate in a procedure, test, service, or program.

Negligence: A failure to conform one's conduct to a generally accepted standard or duty.

Release or waiver: An agreement by a client before beginning participation, to give up, relinquish, or waive the participant's rights to legal remedy (damages) in the event of injury, even when such injury arises as a result of provider negligence.

Risk management: A process whereby a service or program is delivered in a manner to fully conform to the most relevant standards of practice and that uses operational strategies to ensure day-to-day fulfillment, ensure optimum achievement of desired client outcomes, and minimize risk of harm to clients.

Tort law: Body of law that regulates civil wrongdoing.

*Adapted from Herbert DL, Herbert WG, Herbert TG. *Legal Aspects of Preventive, Rehabilitative and Recreational Exercise Programs.* 4th ed. Canton (OH): PRC Publishing; 2002; Koeberle BE. *Legal Aspects of Personal Fitness Training.* 2nd ed. Canton (OH): PRC Publishing; 1994; American College of Sports Medicine. *ACSM's Resource Manual for Guidelines for Exercise Testing and Prescription.* 6th ed. Baltimore: Wolters Kluwer/Lippincott Williams & Wilkins; 2010; Cotten DJ, Cotten MB. *Legal Aspects of Waivers in Sport, Recreation and Fitness Activities.* Canton (OH): PRC Publishing; 1997.

SLIP AND FALL

The number one claim against fitness facilities and professionals is for injuries related to falls on the training premises, according to many insurance providers (6). Courts have consistently held that clients are entitled to "reasonably safe" conditions. Personal Trainers can foster reasonably safe conditions by a regular practice of inspection for, and correction and warning of, any hazards in the workout and access areas to the workout location (12). For example, if items are on the floor that may cause a fall, the trainer should clear these away before beginning the session. If floor surfaces

BOX **22.2**	**ACSM Standards of Care for Health and Fitness Facilities**

1. A facility must be able to respond in a timely manner to any reasonably foreseeable emergency event that threatens the health and safety of facility users. Toward this end, a facility must have an appropriate emergency plan that can be executed by qualified personnel in a timely manner.
2. A facility must offer each adult member a preactivity screening that is appropriate to the physical activities to be performed by the member.
3. Each person who has supervisory responsibility for a physical activity program or area at a facility must have demonstrable professional competence in that physical activity program or area.
4. A facility must post appropriate signage alerting users to the risks involved in their use of those areas of a facility that present potential increased risk(s).
5. A facility that offers youth services or programs must provide appropriate supervision.
6. A facility must conform to all relevant laws, regulations, and published standards.

Adapted and modified from American College of Sports Medicine. *ACSM's Health/Fitness Facility Standards and Guidelines.* 3rd ed. Champaign (IL): Human Kinetics; 2007.

are wet and incapable of correction before the session occurs, the session should be either moved or rescheduled. If safety conditions require, it is always better to be conservative and reschedule rather than to continue training in the presence of known dangers. Personal Trainers who work in aquatics facilities need to be particularly vigilant about deck conditions and pool access areas, as wet surfaces increase the likelihood of a slip-and-fall incident.

In addition to routinely inspecting locations before and during training sessions, Personal Trainers should follow a procedure of proper equipment storage when equipment is not in use (6). Regardless of the training setting, encourage designating specific storage places for equipment so items are not left where people can trip over them. Different types of equipment require different types of storage. Make sure to use storage practices that not only store equipment effectively out of people's way but also protect it from being used for inappropriate purposes. For example, many types of personal training equipment are attractive to young children and may be best stored in locked cabinets if children potentially have access.

Objects that are part of the facility environment but that are not necessarily fitness equipment can also pose risks. In one case, a client brought suit against a health club after he sustained injuries resulting from a fall that occurred as the client was reaching to adjust a television that was positioned on an overhead rack. The Personal Trainer's assessment of the fitness facility environment should include all areas and objects. Many legal tests for liability will revolve around the concept of what potential injuries are reasonably foreseeable. An example of a foreseeable risk would be if a skier hits a bump on a ski slope and breaks a leg. The skier could have anticipated that the accident could be a reasonable foreseeable risk of skiing.

Personal Trainers should also educate clients about appropriate clothing and footwear to prevent injury and to enhance training. Clothing should be comfortable, breathable, and allow movement. In particular, Personal Trainers need to check footwear and should not allow clients to train with inadequate shoes. Factors such as poor fit, excess wear, and unsuitability to the activity all increase the risk of injury. Recognition of foot and leg care issues is especially important if the Personal Trainer works with clients who have diabetes, venous insufficiency, or other medical conditions that may impact the lower extremities. An awareness of these issues will permit the Personal Trainer to make physician referrals when appropriate. Personal Trainers who work with people who are new to exercise may want to create a client handout that outlines appropriate exercise apparel and other exercise safety issues. If the Personal Trainer trains clients in a setting in which protection is necessary, such as a helmet for cycling or pads for inline skating, the Personal Trainer should make sure that the client wears protective equipment (12).

Equipment Use

According to insurance providers, the second leading reason for claims against Personal Trainers is injury resulting from the use of equipment (12). These cases are based on legal theories from tort law that a Personal Trainer's duty or standard of care (Box 22.1) is to exercise reasonable care that the client does not suffer injury. A Personal Trainer who fails to take reasonable precautions, which is determined on the basis of an evaluation of facts surrounding an incident, could be deemed to be negligent and therefore liable or responsible. Professional organizations such as the ACSM and NSCA also offer industry guidelines relating to matters of facility and equipment setup, inspection, maintenance, repair, and signage. Although these standards and guidelines do not have the force of law, they can be introduced as evidence via expert testimony of the Personal Trainer's duty or standard of care. Keep in mind that the law does not envision that accidents never happen; laws and industry standards and guidelines exist to encourage proactive safe behavior to avoid preventable accidents.

> *The law does not envision that accidents never happen; laws and industry standards and guidelines exist to encourage proactive safe behavior to avoid preventable accidents.*

As a practical matter, when it comes to using equipment safely, the question then becomes what steps Personal Trainers can take to prevent foreseeable accidents. Personal Trainers should always use safe, reliable, and appropriate equipment and use equipment for its intended purposes according to manufacturer guidelines (1). Whenever a Personal Trainer directs a client to use equipment, the Personal Trainer should provide proper instructions and supervision. In addition, policies and procedures for routine safety inspections, maintenance, and repair should be in place and observed systematically. Personal Trainers or facility managers should keep written records to demonstrate compliance with these policies and procedures. The importance of thorough documentation cannot be overemphasized. All of these steps are likely to minimize the risk of an accident. And, if an accident occurs and everything has been done to prevent it, then it is likely to be considered the type of accident that could not have been prevented by taking reasonable precautions.

Many clients will ask Personal Trainers to recommend equipment. It is important for the Personal Trainer to work only with reliable fitness equipment dealers when recommending equipment to clients. Personal Trainers who do not have a reliable vendor with whom to work should not recommend one piece of equipment over another. The topic of product liability is complex and outside the scope of this chapter. However, the Personal Trainer should be warned that equipment product managers are now pursuing clubs and Personal Trainers for improper installation and maintenance in cases that they lose under product liability.

FREE WEIGHTS

For a concrete example of potential liability for client injury from equipment use, consider this common scenario that involves an experienced Personal Trainer supervising an apparently healthy client who is performing a squat or similar exercise with free weights. The Personal Trainer encourages the client to use a heavier weight and perform more repetitions even though the client complains of fatigue. The client suffers a debilitating back injury and sues the Personal Trainer and fitness facility.

Under theories of negligence, the Personal Trainer owes this client a duty to exercise reasonable care to prevent injury. Reasonable steps that a Personal Trainer can take to avoid this type of incident include fostering open communications with the client to encourage feedback and listening when the client communicates that he or she is reaching fatigue. Personal Trainers should know how to spot signs of fatigue and be conservative when implementing program progressions. Injuries are not uncommonly sustained by clients who are new to exercise. In one instance (*Lumpkin v. Fitness Together I, Inc., et al.*, Jefferson County Circuit Court Case Number CV-2005-6512, Jefferson County, Alabama), a client filed suit alleging that he was pushed too aggressively by a Personal Trainer to continue squats after the client reported severe muscle fatigue and pain with accompanying physical symptoms of trembling and an inability to stand. The client subsequently developed rhabdomyolysis requiring hospitalization. Although such an outcome is not always predictable, strong lines of communication increase the likelihood that the attuned Personal Trainer will recognize and can appropriately respond to feedback provided by the client.

Another step that a Personal Trainer could take is to keep detailed records of numbers of repetitions, sets, and weight loads on specific training days. In this manner, a client can follow a reasonable plan of progression that minimizes injury risk. Before implementing progression in a program, Personal Trainers can discuss the client's feeling of readiness to increase intensity and further evaluate whether the timing is appropriate for such a change. If specific records are maintained, the Personal Trainer is also in a position to evaluate whether or not a client's response to a particular exercise session is abnormal and requires referral to a physician (3).

WEIGHT MACHINES

Even though machines carry a reduced risk of injury because the client's body is more stable and movement is more restricted than with free weights, injuries still occur. Most injuries happen when a client is encouraged to handle a weight that is too heavy; a weight plate slips and falls because a pin was not properly inserted; or a cable breaks. Weight plates have fallen and crushed ankles and feet or hit people in the head. Clients suffer physical injuries and sue the Personal Trainer, fitness facility, and equipment manufacturer.

Here again, a Personal Trainer can exercise reasonable care to ensure that the client does not suffer this type of injury through a consistent practice of regular inspections and correction of any known hazards such as worn or faultily maintained equipment; through keeping records of what weight the client has been able to lift, the number of repetitions, and sets; and through following a conservative plan to increase intensity in close communication with the client. When working with weight training equipment, the Personal Trainer can develop a procedure of instruction and supervision for each exercise that includes an equipment and body scan to check for proper equipment setup and body alignment. Creating this type of instructional technique so that an inspection becomes a routine part of each and every exercise can go a long way toward preventing accidents.

Factors that courts have looked at in equipment-related cases include whether or not the equipment has been maintained appropriately and used for its intended purpose per specific manufacturer guidelines. In particular, courts examined whether or not parts had been replaced in a timely manner and whether or not facility owners had ensured that routine inspections and maintenance were conducted and documented (6). Regardless of the setting, a Personal Trainer should be proactive in learning about equipment safety inspections, maintenance, and record-keeping policies as well as the procedures for reporting the need for repairs. Before putting a client on any piece of equipment, the Personal Trainer should have firsthand knowledge of its readiness for use.

> **Before putting a client on any piece of equipment, the Personal Trainer should have firsthand knowledge of its readiness for use.**

Keep in mind that courts also examine appropriateness of use. In one case (*Nelson v. Sheraton Operating Corp.*, 87 Wash. App. 1038, Not Reported in P.2d, 1997 WL 524034; Wash. App. Div. 1, 1997), hotel management had placed equipment in a hotel gym that was intended for private home use. The court found the hotel liable for injuries suffered by the client. A training facility should provide commercial equipment; manufacturers do not design home equipment to withstand the wear and tear of frequent use by multiple users. A Personal Trainer who owns or manages a training studio should use professional equipment.

CARDIOVASCULAR MACHINES

Treadmills are currently among the most popular form of exercise equipment in fitness facilities; however, it is imperative that their familiarity not lead the Personal Trainer to assume that clients will be familiar with their use. Numerous cases feature instances in which a client loses control and falls from a treadmill. These cases often involve middle-aged or older adult clients who are unfamiliar with the machine's workings and unable to keep up with the movement speed. In once instance (*Corrigan v. Musclemakers, Inc.*, 258 A.D.2d 861, 686 N.Y.S.2d 143; N.Y.A.D.; 3 Dept 1999), a 49-year-old client who had never patronized a gym and who had never been on a treadmill was placed on one by a Personal Trainer. The Personal Trainer provided no instruction on the use of the machine, including no instruction on how to adjust the speed, stop the belt, or operate the controls. The client was thrown from the machine and suffered a broken ankle. Subsequently, a lawsuit concerning the injury was filed. This case is consistent with others that show that the consequences from falls include back, neck, shoulder, and other joint injuries, broken bones, and even death. Clients (or their survivors) sue the Personal Trainer, fitness facility, and equipment manufacturer (6).

> **Personal Trainers must remain alert to the special risks presented and take proactive steps to manage and minimize these risks.**

Of course, these examples should not discourage a Personal Trainer from using equipment to condition clients. Equipment is an essential part of creating effective training programs. These incidents simply underscore that whenever equipment is being used,

Personal Trainers must remain alert to the special risks presented and take proactive steps to manage and minimize these risks. And Personal Trainers should maintain detailed records to document the steps that have been taken (12).

Scope of Practice

Another important area of potential liability for the Personal Trainer pertains to scope of practice. As fitness professionals work more closely together with healthcare providers to deliver a continuum of care to individuals, it is important to define respective roles. According to the American College of Sports Medicine's Code of Ethics for Certified and Registered Professionals, "[Personal Trainers] practice within the scope of their knowledge, skills, and abilities. [Personal Trainers] will not provide services that are limited by state law to provision by another healthcare professional only" (2). This is particularly true of Personal Trainers with advanced academic degrees or training and when working with clients who may have special exercise considerations. Both criminal and civil actions are possible for practicing medicine or some other allied healthcare profession without a license. An injunction against a Personal Trainer's practice is possible. An elevated standard of care is required because malpractice is certainly a viable concern.

The contemporary delivery of healthcare services itself is in a state of flux because of high costs and attempts to reduce costs by expanding the roles of paraprofessionals in the medical context. As a result, states vary widely on what constitutes the practice of medicine and what is appropriate behavior for a nurse, physician assistant, or other paraprofessional. According to fitness law experts David L. and William G. Herbert, many states have defined the practice of medicine broadly so that persons engaged in exercise testing and prescription activities could, under some circumstances, fall within the range of such statutes (5).

> *Personal Trainers who operate their own businesses would be wise to seek the advice of local legal counsel and to take other steps to manage risk effectively, such as maintaining certifications, obtaining releases and waivers or consents as applicable, carrying liability insurance, and keeping detailed written records.*

Personal Trainers, therefore, need to become familiar with the relevant guidelines for scope of practice that are established at their affiliated organizations and institutions. Personal Trainers who operate their own businesses would be wise to seek the advice of local legal counsel and to take other steps to manage risk effectively, such as maintaining certifications, obtaining releases and waivers or consents as applicable, carrying liability insurance, and keeping detailed written records.

SUPPLEMENTS

Claims related to violations of scope of practice occur most frequently in the area of supplements. A high-profile case brought against a Personal Trainer and a large fitness chain (*Capati v. Crunch Fitness Intern, Inc.*, 295 A.D.2d 181, 743 N.Y.S.2d 474; N.Y.A.D. 1 Dept 2002) involved a scenario in which a Personal Trainer sold supplements, including one that contained ephedra, to a client. The client, who had hypertension, died. Survivors filed a suit. In another example, a Personal Trainer sold steroids to a client, who later suffered adverse consequences and filed a claim against the Personal Trainer (6).

In another incident, a personal training company combined supplement sales with its fitness packages to increase revenue. The company eventually had a client who was allergic to an ingredient in the supplement. The problem was compounded when the client assumed that if she took more than the recommended dosage, she would see more results. She ended up in the hospital, and even though she had been a loyal client for some time, she sued the Personal Trainer and the business. The case was settled out of court, and the Personal Trainer lost his business. The problem was not that the Personal Trainer had sold the client the products, but that he had given her a written plan specifying what to eat and when to take the supplements. The fact that the client overdid it did not matter (6).

According to insurers, the problem with supplements is worsened by the fact that most supplement manufacturers do not carry any insurance coverage. Therefore, the people selling the supplements do not have any products liability coverage. Furthermore, most of the insurance policies for fitness professionals do not include protection for products liability.

In today's market, no one, even professional registered dietitians, can be certain about the ingredients in many supplements because they are not subject to government regulation. In addition, one can never be certain regarding who may have severe allergic reactions, including the risk of death, to any particular ingredient. To proactively protect client safety and to minimize the risk of professional liability, Personal Trainers should avoid selling supplements.

MEDICAL OR DIETARY ADVICE

No cases have yet been litigated to conclusion that involved a client suing a Personal Trainer for faulty medical or dietary advice, except in the case of supplements. However, remember that healthcare is a highly regulated area. The consequences of stepping over the line into the protected area of a licensed healthcare practitioner—such as a medical doctor, physical therapist, registered dietitian, or chiropractor—vary by state. You are exposed to potential liability for acting outside the scope of practice if your "advice" could be interpreted as the unauthorized practice of medicine (or some other licensed profession) and if this advice results in a client injury. The Personal Trainer should develop a comprehensive network of allied professionals and actively refer clients who request or require specialized services to the appropriate healthcare provider (5).

Sexual Harassment

Sexual harassment claims represent the third area of potential exposure to liability that is seeing growth in the number of claims against Personal Trainers according to insurance providers (6). Because the personal training relationship can seem "intimate," it lends itself to creating more opportunity for abusive conduct on the part of the Personal Trainer or for a misinterpretation of actions on the part of the client. Numerous cases involve a male Personal Trainer and a female client. The female client believes that inappropriate touching has occurred and that she has been violated. Or, a personal relationship develops between the Personal Trainer and the client who then raises questions about the legitimacy of the business services rendered. The client believes that undue influence was used to create an exploitive situation.

Sexual harassment is difficult to prove and often rests on credibility. Personal Trainers, therefore, should be vigilant and act professionally at all times. One strategy to protect against a claim of inappropriate touching is to always ask a client for permission to use tactile spotting and to avoid it unless absolutely necessary. Some Personal Trainers do not touch clients directly, but spot them through the use of another prop, such as a ball. Also, avoid situations behind closed doors where no one else is present. For example, if skinfold body composition assessments are offered, conduct the procedure in a room with other Personal Trainers, perhaps behind a folding screen, or have another Personal Trainer or staff member present. If a personal relationship develops with a client, discontinue the professional relationship and refer the client to another Personal Trainer.

> *One strategy to protect against a claim of inappropriate touching is to always ask a client for permission to use tactile spotting and to avoid it unless absolutely necessary.*

Proper Qualifications

Although no specific case on the books has held that Personal Trainers have a higher standard of care based on their specific training in individual assessment, program design, and supervision, clients have filed claims after injuring themselves, based on the fact that a Personal Trainer did not have the qualifications represented in a facility's advertising literature. These claims were based on a theory of breach of contract because the facility failed to provide Personal Trainers with the level of qualification that it had promised (5). The facility, through its literature, imposed a higher standard as to the level of qualification by marketing these qualifications.

> *Clients have filed claims after injuring themselves, based on the fact that a Personal Trainer did not have the qualifications represented in a facility's advertising literature.*

The best evidence that a Personal Trainer can show that his or her training services meet professional standards is to maintain certification and to conduct business according to the knowledge, skills, and abilities that are expected as minimum competencies by the certifying organization. The ACSM certified Personal Trainer^{SM} is defined as a fitness professional involved in developing and implementing an individualized approach to exercise leadership in healthy populations and/or those individuals with medical clearance to exercise. This certified professional is deemed to be proficient in writing appropriate exercise recommendations, leading and demonstrating safe and effective methods of exercise, and motivating individuals to begin and continue their healthy behaviors (3).

The issue of a Personal Trainer's responsibility for advising appropriate levels of training intensity is even more critical as more people with special needs seek to work with Personal Trainers. Personal Trainers who advertise their services to targeted clientele such as older adults or people with arthritis, claiming that they are trained to serve these niche markets, need to be sure that they are sufficiently prepared to serve these clients' needs. Evidence of sufficient preparation would include additional education, training, and experience in working with people with particular needs. Personal Trainers should therefore keep written records of all certifications, continuing education, and work-related experience.

An important precaution to help ensure that a Personal Trainer delivers services that are appropriate to the client is preactivity screening to assess health and medical history. In addition, the Personal Trainer needs to be able to properly interpret health risks and determine when a medical clearance is necessary. After all these precautionary steps are taken, the Personal Trainer needs to be able to conduct a safe fitness evaluation to determine the recommended level of training that will be safe and effective to meet the particular client's needs and goals (3). All of these measures should be kept in written records to document the steps taken by the Personal Trainer to create a specific exercise program (3).

The risk of exposure to liability for a Personal Trainer may be even greater when training services are delivered in a medical setting. In a 2003 Indiana case (*Community Hospital v. Avant*, 790 N.E.2d 585; Ind. App. 2003), a court held that even though a Personal Trainer was employed by a hospital and the fitness facility was owned by the hospital, the Personal Trainer was not a healthcare provider. The case, therefore, did not qualify as a medical malpractice case. The significance of this case, however, is that the client did try to sue both the fitness club and the hospital on the basis of injuries sustained while engaged in the personal train-

> *The risk of exposure to liability for a Personal Trainer may be even greater when training services are delivered in a medical setting.*

ing program, and the court did examine the fact that the training occurred in a setting with a close connection to a hospital. Another court might have found that this type of training did need to meet the standards of healthcare practitioners (6,11).

Emergency Response

As yet no specific case has involved a claim against a Personal Trainer for wrongful death in a situation in which a client has had a heart attack or other medical emergency and died while under the supervision of a Personal Trainer. However, as most Personal Trainer certifications require that Personal Trainers have CPR training (and some require first aid training and automated external defibrillator [AED] training), it is possible that a claim could be filed against a Personal Trainer who failed to provide an emergency response if that failure led to a death that could have otherwise been avoided. In addition, numerous states have enacted legislation mandating that health/fitness facilities have at least one AED on the premises (10).

> *It is possible that a claim could be filed against a Personal Trainer who failed to provide an emergency response if that failure led to a death that could have otherwise been avoided.*

The ACSM and the American Heart Association (AHA) published a joint position stand in 1998 with recommendations for health/fitness facilities regarding the screening of clients for the presence of cardiovascular disease, appropriate staffing, emergency policies, equipment, and procedures relative to the client base of a given facility (8). In 2002, the ACSM and the AHA published a joint position stand to supplement the 1998 recommendations regarding the purchase and use of AEDs in health/fitness facilities (7) and supported in 2007 by the ACSM (4). These organizations agree that a comprehensive written emergency plan is essential to promote safe and effective physical activity.

The AHA, the ACSM, and the International Health, Racquet and Sportsclub Association recommend that all fitness facilities have written emergency policies and procedures, including the use of automated defibrillators, which are reviewed and practiced regularly. Staff who have responsibility for working directly with program participants and provide instruction and leadership in specific modes of exercise must be trained in CPR. These staff should know and practice regularly the facility's emergency plan and be able to readily handle emergencies. In addition, these organizations require health/fitness facilities to use AEDs (4,13).

As evidence of professional competency, Personal Trainers should keep CPR, first aid, and AED certifications current. Personal Trainers should proactively familiarize themselves with any affiliated organization's emergency plan and be ready to implement the plan's procedures in case of emergency. For Personal Trainers who operate a business, creating an emergency plan should be a top priority. Personal Trainers who provide training services outdoors or in a client's home should also have written emergency policies and procedures.

In addition to having an emergency plan, Personal Trainers should also document any accident or incident immediately, using an Incident Report Form (Box 22.3). The Personal Trainer should include only the facts surrounding the incident and not any opinions regarding what may or may not have caused the incident. In addition, the names and contact information of witnesses should be included. And, the person who experienced the incident should sign the form. Insurers will provide incident reporting forms, and the Personal Trainer should always carry one to every training session (1,4).

Client Confidentiality

The failure to protect client confidentiality is another emerging area of potential liability for a Personal Trainer. This is rooted in the concept of preventing potential harm to a client's reputation. The Personal Trainer must keep detailed written records from the first client prescreening to notes documenting each training session. These records are critical evidence that can document that the Personal Trainer exercised reasonable care in performing his or her professional duties. At the same time, the Personal Trainer must exercise care to protect this information. The ACSM's guidelines for the fitness testing, health promotion, and wellness area state that "A facility should ensure that its fitness testing, health promotion, and wellness has a system that provides for and protects the complete confidentiality of all user records and meetings. User records should be released only with an individual's signed authorization" (4). Before a Personal Trainer discloses any personal information, even for marketing purposes, such as a client testimonial or "before and after" photos, the Personal Trainer should get and store a signed release form. A law passed by the U.S. Congress requires healthcare professionals to have strict policies regarding the safety and security of private records (the Health Insurance Portability & Accountability Act [HIPAA] of 1996, Public Law 104-191, which amends the Internal Revenue Service Code of 1986, also known as the Kennedy-

BOX **22.3** **Incident Report**

INCIDENT REPORT
TO BE COMPLETED BY INSTRUCTOR

Date: _____

Location/Address of Accident or Incident: _____

Name of Instructor Completing the Form: _____

Date of Accident or Incident: _____

Approximate Time of Accident or Incident: _____ : _____ am pm

Name of Injured Person: _____ Age: _____ Sex: _____

Injured Person's Address _____

City: _____ State: _____ Zip Code: _____

Home Phone #: (   ) _____ Work Phone #: (   ) _____ Cell Phone #: (   ) _____

How long has this person been under your instruction: _____
_____

Describe the accident/incident: _____
_____
_____

Describe possible injury (sprained ankle, etc.): _____
_____
_____

Describe type of equipment involved: _____
_____

List any type of treatment performed by you or by a doctor (include doctor, hospital name): _____
_____
_____

Were there any witnesses to the incident: yes _____   no _____

If yes, please have each witness write a brief statement about what happened.

YOUR SIGNATURE: _____

Adapted from Jeff Frick, Fitness and Wellness Insurance Agency, 380 Stevens Avenue, Suite 206, Solana Beach, CA 92075.

> *The Personal Trainer must keep detailed written records from the first client prescreening to notes documenting each training session.*

Kassebaum Act) and recently came into effect on April 14, 2003. Although it is still unclear whether HIPAA extends to Personal Trainers, it is wise to become familiar with this law and how it may affect the release of any personal information to a third party. It is clear that when a Personal Trainer works under the auspices of a "covered healthcare provider" as defined by HIPAA (e.g., a hospital, physician office), this law will govern the release of client information.

RISK MANAGEMENT STRATEGIES

Personal Trainers should manage risk exposure with a multilayered approach that incorporates a number of important strategies. As the first line of defense, Personal Trainers should create written policies, procedures, and forms that meet industry standards and guidelines and maintain detailed written records that document compliance with these policies. This strategy minimizes the likelihood that the Personal Trainer would fail to demonstrate that he or she exercised reasonable care under the circumstances. In other words, the Personal Trainer should make every effort not to be negligent.

The second strategy involves using a release, waiver, or informed consent, depending on which legal document is recognized under the laws of the place where the Personal Trainer conducts business (9). The purpose of these documents is either (a) to demonstrate that the Personal Trainer fully informed the client of all of the potential risks of physical activity and the client decided to undertake the activity and waive the Personal Trainer's responsibility or (b) to demonstrate that the client knowingly waived his or her right to file a claim against the Personal Trainer even if the Personal Trainer is negligent. Courts have consistently held that in order for a release to operate as an effective

> *As the first line of defense, Personal Trainers should create written policies, procedures, and forms that meet industry standards and guidelines and maintain detailed written records that document compliance with these policies.*

bar to liability, the release should be clear and unambiguous and should refer specifically to the negligence of the party seeking the release. The Personal Trainer should keep these records indefinitely and in a safe place. Consent forms are not infinity contracts so provisions should also be made for an annual signing of these important documents. Each state has its own statutes of limitations on waivers and consent forms. The Personal Trainer is advised to check with legal authorities within their jurisdiction.

A third strategy is to carry professional liability insurance (5,12). This transfers the risk to the insurer. In that instance, even if the Personal Trainer is negligent, the insurance company assumes responsibility for resolving any claims. Most insurers of Personal Trainers provide coverage for certified professionals. A fourth strategy is to incorporate the business to protect personal assets from any potential claims. A fifth strategy is to cultivate strong relationships with your clients and colleagues. Clients are much less likely to sue if they perceive a Personal Trainer as caring, responsible, and responsive to their needs. And, the final strategy is to consult local legal counsel to ensure that your business practices meet the requirements of your specific location (6).

Written Policies, Procedures, and Forms

> *Personal Trainers should conduct their business according to written policies, procedures, and forms that ensure that their business practices conform to the standards set by professional organizations.*

Personal Trainers should conduct their business according to written policies, procedures, and forms that ensure that their business practices conform to the standards set by professional organizations (1,3–6,11,12). In addition to policies discussed in the business practices chapter, every Personal Trainer should also have risk management policies that include a written emergency plan and a preactivity screening procedure. The most important forms for a Personal Trainer include the following:

1. Preactivity screening form such as a PAR-Q
2. Health History Questionnaire
3. Physician's Statement and Medical Clearance
4. Fitness Assessment or Evaluation Form
5. Client Progress Notes
6. Incident Reports

As important as having these forms is using these forms. The Personal Trainer should complete all portions of the forms. A form that is only partially completed is often the source of more questions than answers and may imply that the Personal Trainer was not thorough in their use. When utilizing these forms, blank spaces are unacceptable.

In the event that a Personal Trainer is encouraging a client to train independently on equipment in a particular fitness facility, an equipment orientation form for the client to sign to indicate that he or she has received instruction on the proper setup and use of weight training equipment would be useful to document equipment instruction.

Informed Consent, Release, or Waiver

In numerous states, courts are holding up waivers more and more as valid means of protection against litigation. In 2001, a California case (*Bendek v. PLC Santa Monica, LLC*, 104 Cal.App.4th 1351, 129 Cal.Rptr. 197; Cal.App.2 Dist 2002) was dismissed after a court held that the waiver form signed by a facility member when she joined protected the facility and its owners from liability when the member filed a lawsuit claiming that she slipped and injured herself. This case is consistent with other California cases (6). Depending on where a Personal Trainer lives, he or she may need to have a document entitled one of the following:

➤ Express assumption of the risk
➤ Informed consent
➤ Release or waiver of liability

An Assumption of the Risk or Informed Consent document (Box 22.4) essentially explains the risks of participating in physical activity to a prospective client. The client then agrees that he or she knowingly understands these risks, appreciates these risks, and voluntarily assumes responsibility for taking these risks. These documents help strengthen the assumption of risk defense for the personal trainer when inherent injuries occur, but do not provide protection for negligence.

A Waiver or Release of Liability (Box 22.5) document states that the client knowingly waives or releases the Personal Trainer from liability for any acts of negligence on the part of the Personal Trainer (4). In other words, the prospective client waives his or her right to sue the Personal Trainer, even if the Personal Trainer is negligent (13). A Personal Trainer needs to consult with an attorney in his or her location to determine which type of document is the standard practice for his or her state. For additional forms, please refer to *ACSM's Health/Fitness Facility Standards and Guideline* (3rd ed.) (4).

Professional Liability Insurance

In today's litigious environment, for the most protection, a Personal Trainer should carry professional liability insurance ($2 million per occurrence is the recommended amount), even when working in a business as an employee, where the Personal Trainer may be covered under the business owner's policy. The reason for this is that it is not unusual for a single claim to result in a million dollar judgment. Purchasing the best protection enables the Personal Trainer to practice responsibly and feel confident that his or her business will not be destroyed by one mishap. ACSM Certified Personal Trainers can purchase professional liability insurance through the ACSM.

Professional liability insurance provides a broad spectrum of protection from claims such as those arising from negligence, breach of contract, or even sexual harassment, and it can provide coverage for both injuries to a person or to property. Insurance professionals are expert at handling claims and will take care of all of the details, enabling the Personal Trainer to continue to operate his or her business (6). This includes, when necessary, providing the defense to a lawsuit. Frequently, this duty to defend is as valuable to the insured as is the duty to indemnify.

> *Professional liability insurance provides a broad spectrum of protection from claims such as those arising from negligence, breach of contract, or even sexual harassment, and it can provide coverage for both injuries to a person or to property.*

| BOX 22.4 | **Sample of Informed Consent Form for a Symptom-Limited Exercise Test** |

Informed Consent for an Exercise Test

1. Purpose and Explanation of the Test

You will perform an exercise test on a cycle ergometer or a motor-driven treadmill. The exercise intensity will begin at a low level and will be advanced in stages, depending on your fitness level. We may stop the test at any time because of signs of fatigue or changes in your heart rate, electrocardiogram, or blood pressure, or symptoms you may experience. It is important for you to realize that you may stop when you wish because of feelings of fatigue or any other discomfort.

2. Attendant Risks and Discomforts

There exists the possibility of certain changes occurring during the test. These include abnormal blood pressure, fainting, irregular, fast or slow heart rhythm, and in rare instances, heart attack, stroke, or death. Every effort will be made to minimize these risks by evaluation of preliminary information relating to your health and fitness and by careful observations during testing. Emergency equipment and trained personnel are available to deal with unusual situations that may arise.

3. Responsibilities of the Participant

Information you possess about your health status or previous experiences of heart-related symptoms (e.g., shortness of breath with low-level activity, pain, pressure, tightness, heaviness in the chest, neck, jaw, back, and/or arms) with physical effort may affect the safety of your exercise test. Your prompt reporting of these and any other unusual feelings with effort during the exercise test itself is very important. You are responsible for fully disclosing your medical history as well as symptoms that may occur during the test. You are also expected to report all medications (including nonprescription) taken recently and, in particular, those taken today, to the testing staff.

4. Benefits to Be Expected

The results obtained from the exercise test may assist in diagnosing your illness, in evaluating the effect of your medications, or in evaluating what type of physical activities you might do with low risk.

5. Inquiries

Any questions about the procedures used in the exercise test or the results of your test are encouraged. If you have any concerns or questions, please ask us for further explanations.

6. Use of Medical Records

The information that is obtained during exercise testing will be treated as privileged and confidential as described in the Health Insurance Portability and Accountability Act of 1996. It is not to be released or revealed to any person except your referring physician without your written consent. However, the information obtained may be used for statistical analysis or scientific purposes with your right to privacy retained.

7. Freedom of Consent

I hereby consent to voluntarily engage in an exercise test to determine my exercise capacity and state of cardiovascular health. My permission to perform this exercise test is given voluntarily. I understand that I am free to stop the test at any point if I so desire.

I have read this form, and I understand the test procedures that I will perform and the attendant risks and discomforts. Knowing these risks and discomforts, and having had an opportunity to ask questions that have been answered to my satisfaction, I consent to participate in this test.

_____   _____
        Date   Signature of patient

_____   _____
        Date   Signature of witness

_____   _____
        Date   Signature of physician or authorized delegate

Reprinted with permission from American College of Sports Medicine. *ACSM's Guidelines for Exercise Testing and Prescription.* 8th ed. Baltimore: Wolters Kluwer/ Lippincott Williams & Wilkins; 2010.

BOX **22.5**   **Agreement and Release of Liability Form**

I, _____, the undersigned, wish to participate in a fitness evaluation which consists of a submaximal cardiovascular assessment (bike or treadmill), body fat analysis by skinfold, strength and flexibility assessments, muscular endurance assessment and individualized exercise program at the Fitness Center in Atlanta, Georgia, which is to be conducted on this _____ day of _____, 20____. The evaluation will be conducted under the direction of a Personal Trainer. I understand and acknowledge that participation in the fitness evaluation activities involves an inherent risk of physical injury and I assume all such risks. I understand that I will participate in all fitness exercises in said fitness evaluation. I assume all risks of damage or injury, including death, that may be sustained by me while particpating in the fitness evaluation test.

For and in consideration of The Fitness Center allowing me to take the fitness evaluation, I hereby release and covenant not to sue The Fitness Center, the officers, agents, members and employees of each, from any and from all claims or actions, including those of negligence, which might arise as a result of any personal injury, including death, or property damage which I might suffer as a result of my participation in the fitness evaluation on the date set forth above.

By signing this document, I hereby acknowledge that I am at least 18 years of age and have read the above carefully before signing, and agree with all of its provisions this _____ day of _____, 20____.

_____   _____

Signature of Participant   Witness

NOTE: This form is presented for information purposes only and should be not considered legal advice or used as such. The use of this form in specific situations requires substantive legal judgments and a licensed attorney should be consulted before using the form.

SUMMARY

The personal training industry is in a rapid state of growth and redefinition as more healthcare providers acknowledge the need for exercise training as part of a program of preventive healthcare. In addition, the wellness trend is fueling more and more individuals to assume responsibility for their personal health and to consult with experts such as Personal Trainers to provide training services that enhance the quality of their daily lives. Personal Trainers have great opportunities to work in a variety of settings and make a powerful difference in the lives of clients.

More professional opportunities, however, increase expectations of responsible professional conduct. More professional responsibility means more potential exposure to liability for failing to act responsibly. Today's Personal Trainer must understand these potential areas of risk exposure and the legal issues and industry standards and guidelines that surround these issues to deliver services confidently and to proactively manage risk. This professionalism in all aspects of doing business not only increases the personal and professional rewards of life as a Personal Trainer but also ensures lasting business success amid the growing complexity of our modern legal environment. Ultimately, the purpose of liability is to protect individuals. The most successful Personal Trainers will always keep in mind that the core of personal training is ultimately personal: to protect the best interests of the client at all times and in all ways. To this end, the ACSM has developed a Code of Ethics for ACSM Certified and Registered Professionals (see Chapter 1) that will help establish the Personal Trainer profession.

REFERENCES

1. American College of Sports Medicine. *ACSM's Certification Review*. 2nd ed. Baltimore: Lippincott Williams & Wilkins; 2006.

2. American College of Sports Medicine Code of Ethics for ACSM Certified and Registered Professionals [Internet]. Indianapolis (IN): American College of Sports Medicine; [cited 2008 Aug 8]. Available from http://www.acsm.org/AM/Template.cfm?Section=CCRB_Candidate_Handbook2&Template = /CM/ContentDisplay.cfm&ContentID=3363

3. American College of Sports Medicine. *ACSM's Guidelines for Exercise Testing and Prescription*. 8th ed. Baltimore: Lippincott Williams & Wilkins; 2010.

4. American College of Sports Medicine. *ACSM's Health/Fitness Facility Standards and Guidelines*. 3rd ed. Champaign (IL): Human Kinetics; 2007.

5. American College of Sports Medicine. *ACSM's Resource Manual for Guidelines for Exercise Testing and Prescription*. 6th ed. Baltimore: Lippincott Williams & Wilkins; 2010.

6. Archer S. Reward carries risk: a liability update. *IDEA Personal Trainer*. 2004;15(4):30–4.

7. Balady GJ, Chaitman B, Foster C, et al. Automated external defibrillators in health/fitness facilities: supplement to the AHA/ACSM recommendations for cardiovascular screening, staffing and emergency policies at health/fitness facilities. *Circulation*. 2002;105(9):1147–50.

8. Balady GJ, Chaitman B, Driscoll D, et al. Recommendations for cardiovascular screening, staffing and emergency policies at health/fitness facilities. *Circulation*. 1998;97(22):2283–93.

9. Cotten DJ, Cotten MB. *Legal Aspects of Waivers in Sport, Recreation and Fitness Activities*. Canton (OH): PRC Publishing; 1997.

10. Connaughton JO, Spangler JO, Zhang J. An analysis of automated external defibrillator implementation and related risk management practices in health/fitness clubs. *J Legal Aspects Sport*. 2007;17(1):101–26.

11. Herbert DL, Herbert WG. *Legal Aspects of Preventive, Rehabilitative and Recreational Exercise Programs*. 4th ed. Canton (OH): PRC Publishing; 2002.

12. Koeberle BE. *Legal Aspects of Personal Fitness Training*. 2nd ed. Canton (OH): PRC Publishing; 1994.

13. McInnis K, Herbert W, Herbert D, Herbert J, Ribisl P, Franklin B. Low compliance with national standards for cardiovascular emergency preparedness at health clubs. *Chest* 2001;120(1):283–8.

This appendix details information about American College of Sports Medicine (ACSM) Certification and Registry Programs and gives a complete listing of the current knowledge, skills, and abilities (KSAs) that compose the foundations of these certification and registry examinations. The mission of the ACSM Committee on Certification and Registry Boards is to develop and provide high-quality, accessible, and affordable credentials and continuing education programs for health and exercise professionals who are responsible for preventive and rehabilitative programs that influence the health and well-being of all individuals.

ACSM CERTIFICATIONS AND THE PUBLIC

The first of the ACSM clinical certifications was initiated more than 30 years ago in conjunction with publication of the first edition of *Guidelines for Exercise Testing and Prescription*. That era was marked by rapid development of exercise programs for patients with stable coronary artery disease (CAD). ACSM sought a means to disseminate accurate information on this healthcare initiative through expression of consensus from its members in basic science, clinical practice, and education. Thus, these early clinical certifications were viewed as an aid to the establishment of safe and scientifically based exercise services within the framework of cardiac rehabilitation.

Over the past 30 years, exercise has gained widespread favor as an important component in programs of rehabilitative care or health maintenance for an expanding list of chronic diseases and disabling conditions. The growth of public interest in the role of exercise in health promotion has been equally impressive. In addition, federal government policy makers have revisited questions of medical efficacy and financing for exercise services in rehabilitative care of selected patients. Over the past several years, recommendations from the U.S. Public Health Service and the U.S. Surgeon General have acknowledged the central role for regular physical activity in the prevention of disease and promotion of health.

The development of the health/fitness certifications in the 1980s reflected ACSM's intent to increase the availability of qualified professionals to provide scientifically sound advice and supervision regarding appropriate physical activities for health maintenance in the apparently healthy adult population. Since 1975, more than 35,000 certificates have been awarded. With this consistent growth, ACSM has taken steps to ensure that its competency-based certifications will continue to be regarded as the premier program in the exercise field.

The ACSM Committee on Certification and Registry Boards (CCRB) Publications Sub-Committee publishes *ACSM's Certified News*, a periodical addressing professional practice issues; its target audience is those who are certified. The CCRB Continuing Professional Education Sub-Committee has oversight of the continuing education requirements for maintenance of certification and auditing renewal candidates. Continuing education credits can be accrued through ACSM-sponsored educational programs, such as ACSM workshops (ACSM Certified Personal Trainer^{SM}, ACSM Certified Health Fitness Specialist, ACSM Certified Clinical Exercise Specialist, ACSM Registered Clinical Exercise Physiologist$^{®}$), regional chapter and annual meetings, and other educational programs approved by the ACSM Professional Education Committee. These enhancements are intended to support the continued professional growth of those who have made a commitment to service in this rapidly growing health and fitness field.

In 2004, ACSM was a founding member of the multiorganizational Committee on Accreditation for the Exercise Sciences (CoAES) and assisted with the development of standards and guidelines for educational programs seeking accreditation under the auspices of the Commission on Accreditation of Allied Health Education Programs (CAAHEP). Additional information on outcomes-based, programmatic accreditation can be obtained by visiting www.caahep.org, and specific information regarding the standards and guidelines can be obtained by visiting www.coaes.org. Because the standards and guidelines refer to the KSAs that follow, reference to specific KSAs as they relate to given sets of standards and guidelines will be noted when appropriate.

ACSM also acknowledges the expectation from successful candidates that the public will be informed of the high standards, values, and professionalism implicit in meeting these certification requirements. The college has formally organized its volunteer committee structure and national office staff to give added emphasis to informing the public, professionals, and government agencies about issues of critical importance to ACSM. Informing these constituencies about the meaning and value of ACSM certification is one important priority that will be given attention in this initiative.

ACSM CERTIFICATION PROGRAMS

The ACSM Certified Personal Trainer[SM] is a fitness professional involved in developing and implementing an individualized approach to exercise leadership in healthy populations and/or those individuals with medical clearance to exercise. Using a variety of teaching techniques, the CPT is proficient in leading and demonstrating safe and effective methods of exercise by applying the fundamental principles of exercise science. The CPT is familiar with forms of exercise used to improve, maintain, and/or optimize health-related components of physical fitness and performance. The CPT is proficient in writing appropriate exercise recommendations, leading and demonstrating safe and effective methods of exercise, and motivating individuals to begin and to continue with their healthy behaviors.

The ACSM Certified Health Fitness Specialist (HFS) is a degreed health and fitness professional qualified for career pursuits in the university, corporate, commercial, hospital, and community settings. The HFS has knowledge and skills in management, administration, training, and in supervising entry-level personnel. The HFS is skilled in conducting risk stratification, conducting physical fitness assessments and interpreting results, constructing appropriate exercise prescriptions, and motivating apparently healthy individuals and individuals with medically controlled diseases to adopt and maintain healthy lifestyle behaviors.

The ACSM Certified Clinical Exercise Specialist (CES) is a healthcare professional certified by ACSM to deliver a variety of exercise assessment, training, rehabilitation, risk-factor identification, and lifestyle management services to individuals with or at risk for cardiovascular, pulmonary, and metabolic disease(s). These services are typically delivered in cardiovascular/pulmonary rehabilitation programs, physicians' offices, or medical fitness centers. The ACSM Certified Clinical Exercise Specialist is also competent to provide exercise-related consulting for research, public health, and other clinical and nonclinical services and programs.

The ACSM Registered Clinical Exercise Physiologist® (RCEP) is an allied health professional who works in the application of physical activity and behavioral interventions for those clinical conditions for which they have been shown to provide therapeutic and/or functional benefit. Persons for whom RCEP services are appropriate may include, but are not limited to, those individuals with cardiovascular, pulmonary, metabolic, orthopedic, musculoskeletal, neuromuscular, neoplastic, immunologic, or hematologic disease. The RCEP provides primary and secondary prevention strategies designed to improve fitness and health in populations ranging from children to older adults. The RCEP performs exercise screening, exercise and fitness testing, exercise prescription, exercise and physical activity counseling, exercise supervision, exercise and health education/promotion, and measurement and evaluation of exercise and physical activity related outcome measures. The RCEP works individually or as part of an interdisciplinary team in a clinical, community, or public health setting. The practice and supervision of the RCEP is guided by published professional guidelines, standards, and applicable state and federal regulations.

ACSM also develops specialty certifications to enhance the breadth of knowledge for individuals working in a health, fitness, or clinical setting. For information on KSAs, eligibility, and scope of practice for ACSM specialty certifications, visit www.acsm.org/certification or call 1-800-486-5643.

HOW TO OBTAIN INFORMATION AND APPLICATION MATERIALS

The certification programs of ACSM are subject to continuous review and revision. Content development is entrusted to a diverse committee of professional volunteers with expertise in exercise science, medicine, and program management. Expertise in design and procedures for competency assessment is also represented on this committee. The administration of certification exams is conducted through Pearson VUE authorized testing centers. Inquiries regarding exam registration can be made to Pearson VUE at 1-888-883-2276 or online at www.pearsonvue.com/acsm.

For general certification questions, contact the ACSM Certification Resource Center:

1-800-486-5643
Web site: www.acsm.org/certification
E-mail: certification@acsm.org

KNOWLEDGE, SKILLS, AND ABILITIES (KSAs) UNDERLINING ACSM CERTIFICATIONS

Minimal competencies for each certification level are outlined below. Certification examinations are constructed based on these KSAs. For the ACSM Certified Health Fitness Specialist and the ACSM Certified Clinical Exercise Specialist credentials, two companion ACSM publications, *ACSM's Resource Manual for Guidelines for Exercise Testing and Prescription,* sixth edition, and *ACSM's Certification Review Book,* third edition, may also be used to gain further insight pertaining to the topics identified here. For the ACSM Certified Personal Trainer[SM], candidates should refer to *ACSM's Resources for the Personal Trainer,* current edition, and *ACSM's Certification Review Book,* third edition. For the ACSM Registered Clinical Exercise Physiologist[®], candidates should refer to ACSM's *Resources for Clinical Exercise Physiology,* current edition, and *ACSM's Resource Manual for Guidelines for Exercise Testing and Prescription,* sixth edition. However, neither the *ACSM's Guidelines for Exercise Testing and Prescription* nor any of the above-mentioned resource manuals provides all of the information upon which the ACSM Certification examinations are based. Each may prove to be beneficial as a review of specific topics and as a general outline of many of the integral concepts to be mastered by those seeking certification.

APPENDIX FIGURE 1

Level	Requirements	Recommended Competencies
ACSM Certified Personal Trainer^{SM}	• 18 years of age or older • High school diploma or equivalent (GED) • Possess current adult CPR certification that has a practical skills examination component (such as the American Heart Association or the American Red Cross)	• Demonstrate competence in the KSAs required of the ACSM Certified Personal Trainer™ as listed in the current edition of the *ACSM's Guidelines for Exercise Testing and Prescription* • Adequate knowledge of and skill in risk-factor and health-status identification, fitness appraisal, and exercise prescription • Demonstrate ability to incorporate suitable and innovative activities that will improve an individual's functional capacity • Demonstrate the ability to effectively educate and/or communicate with individuals regarding lifestyle modification
ACSM Certified Health Fitness Specialist	• Associate's degree or a bachelor's degree in a health-related field from a regionally accredited college or university (one is eligible to sit for the exam if the candidate is in the last term of their degree program); AND • Possess current adult CPR certification that has a practical skills examination component (such as the American Heart Association or the American Red Cross)	• Demonstrate competence in the KSAs required of the ACSM Certified Health Fitness Specialist In as listed in the current edition of the *ACSM's Guidelines for Exercise Testing and Prescription* • Work-related experience within the health and fitness field • Adequate knowledge of, and skill in, risk-factor and health-status identification, fitness appraisal, and exercise prescription • Demonstrate ability to incorporate suitable and innovative activities that will improve an individual's functional capacity • Demonstrate the ability to effectively educate and/or counsel individuals regarding lifestyle modification • Knowledge of exercise science including kinesiology, functional anatomy, exercise physiology, nutrition, program administration, psychology, and injury prevention
ACSM Certified Clinical Exercise Specialist	• Bachelor's degree in an allied health field from a regionally accredited college of university (one is eligible to sit for the exam if the candidate is in the last term of their degree program); AND • Minimum of 600 hours of observational and active patient/client care in a clinical exercise program (e.g., cardiac/pulmonary rehabilitation programs; exercise testing; exercise prescription; electrocardiography; patient education and counseling; disease management of cardiac, pulmonary, and metabolic diseases; and emergency management); AND • Current certification as a basic life support provider or CPR for the professional rescuer (available through the American Heart Association or the American Red Cross)	• Demonstrate competence in the KSAs required of the ACSM Certified Clinical Exercise Specialist and Certified Health Fitness Specialist, as listed in the current edition of *ACSM's Guidelines for Exercise Testing and Prescription* • Ability to demonstrate extensive knowledge of functional anatomy, exercise physiology, pathophysiology, electrocardiography, human behavior/psychology, gerontology, graded exercise testing for healthy and diseased populations, exercise supervision/leadership, patient counseling, and emergency procedures related to exercise testing and training situations

(continued)

APPENDIX FIGURE 1	(Continued)	
Level	**Requirements**	**Recommended Competencies**
ACSM Registered Clinical Exercise Physiologist®	• Master's degree in exercise science, exercise physiology, or kinesiology from a regionally accredited college or university • Current certification as a basic life support provider or CPR for the professional rescuer (available through the American Heart Association or the American Red Cross) • Minimum of 600 clinical hours or alternatives as described in the current issue of ACSM's *Certification Resource Guide* (hours may be completed as part of a formal degree program) • Recommendation of hours in clinical practice areas: cardiovascular—200; pulmonary—100 ; metabolic—120; orthopedic/musculoskeletal—100; neuromuscular—40; immunologic/hematologic—40	• Demonstrate competence in the KSAs required of the ACSM Registered Clinical Exercise Physiologist®, ACSM Certified Clinical Excercise Specialist, ACSM Certified Health Fitness Specialist, and ACSM Certified Personal Trainer^{SM} as listed in the current edition of *ACSM's Guidelines for Exercise Testing and Prescription*

Classification/Numbering System for Knowledge, Skills, and Abilities (KSAs)

All the KSAs for a given certification/credential are listed in their entirety across a given practice area and/or content matter area for each level of certification. Within each certification's/credential's KSA set, the numbering of individual KSAs uses a three-part number as follows:

- First number: denotes practice area (1.x.x)
- Second number: denotes content area (x.1.x)
- Third number: denotes the sequential number of each KSA (x.x.1) within each content area. If there is a break in numeric sequence, it indicates that a KSA was deleted in response to the recent job-task analysis from the prior version of the KSAs. From this edition forward, new KSAs will acquire a new KSA number.

The practice areas (the first number) are numbered as follows:

1.x.x	General population/core
2.x.x	Cardiovascular
3.x.x	Pulmonary
4.x.x	Metabolic
5.x.x	Orthopedic/musculoskeletal
6.x.x	Neuromuscular
7.x.x	Neoplastic, immunologic, and hematologic

The content matter areas (the second number) are numbered as follows:

x.1.x	Exercise physiology and related exercise science
x.2.x	Pathophysiology and risk factors
x.3.x	Health appraisal, fitness, and clinical exercise testing
x.4.x	Electrocardiography and diagnostic techniques
x.5.x	Patient management and medications
x.6.x	Medical and surgical management
x.7.x	Exercise prescription and programming
x.8.x	Nutrition and weight management

x.9.x   Human behavior and counseling

x.10.x   Safety, injury prevention, and emergency procedures

x.11.x   Program administration, quality assurance, and outcome assessment

x.12.x   Clinical and medical considerations (ACSM Certified Personal Trainer[SM] only)

EXAMPLES BY LEVEL OF CERTIFICATION/CREDENTIAL

ACSM Certified Personal Trainer[SM] KSAs

1.1.10   Knowledge to describe the normal acute responses to cardiovascular exercise.

In this example, the practice area is *general population/core*; the content matter area is *exercise physiology and related exercise science*; and this KSA is the tenth KSA within this content matter area.

ACSM Certified Health Fitness Specialist KSAs

1.3.8   Skill in accurately measuring heart rate, blood pressure, and obtaining rating of perceived exertion (RPE) at rest and during exercise according to established guidelines.

In this example, the practice area is *general population/core*; the content matter area is *health appraisal, fitness, and clinical exercise testing*; and this KSA is the eighth KSA within this content matter area.

ACSM Certified Clinical Exercise Specialist KSAs[a]

1.7.17   Design strength and flexibility programs for individuals with cardiovascular, pulmonary, and/or metabolic diseases; the elderly; and children.

In this example, the practice area is *general population/core*; the content matter area is *exercise prescription and programming*; and this KSA is the seventeenth KSA within this content matter area. Furthermore, because this specific KSA appears in bold, it covers multiple practice areas and content areas.

ACSM Registered Clinical Exercise Physiologist® KSAs

7.6.1   List the drug classifications commonly used in the treatment of patients with a neoplastic, immunologic, and hematologic (NIH) disease, name common generic and brand-name drugs within each class, and explain the purposes, indications, major side effects, and the effects, if any, on the exercising individual.

The practice area is *neoplastic, immunologic, and hematologic*; the content matter area is *medical and surgical management*; and this KSA is the first KSA within this content matter area.

---

[a]*A special note about ACSM Certified Clinical Exercise Specialist KSAs*

Like the other certifications presented thus far, the ACSM Certified Clinical Exercise Specialist KSAs are categorized by content area. However, some CES KSAs cover multiple practices areas within each area of content. For example, several of them describe a specific topic with respect to both exercise testing and training, which are two distinct content areas. Rather than write out each separately (which would have greatly expanded the KSA list length), they have been listed under a single content area. When reviewing these KSAs, please note that KSAs in bold text cover multiple content areas. Each CES KSA begins with a 1 as the practice area. However, where appropriate, some KSAs mention specific patient populations (i.e., practice area). If a specific practice area is not mentioned within a given KSA, then it applies equally to each of the general population, cardiovascular, pulmonary, and metabolic practice areas. Note that "metabolic patients" are defined as those with at least one of the following: overweight or obese, diabetes (type I or II), or metabolic syndrome. Each KSA describes either a single or multiple knowledge (K), skill (S), or ability (A)—or a combination of K, S, or A—that an individual should have mastery of to be considered a competent ACSM Certified Clinical Exercise Specialist.

ACSM CERTIFIED PERSONAL TRAINER^{SM} KNOWLEDGE, SKILLS, AND ABILITIES (KSAs)

General Population/Core: Exercise Physiology and Related Exercise Science

1.1.1	Knowledge of the basic structures of bone, skeletal muscle, and connective tissue.
1.1.2	Knowledge of the basic anatomy of the cardiovascular system and respiratory system.
1.1.3	Knowledge of the definition of the following terms: inferior, superior, medial, lateral, supination, pronation, flexion, extension, adduction, abduction, hyperextension, rotation, circumduction, agonist, antagonist, and stabilizer.
1.1.4	Knowledge of the plane in which each muscle action occurs.
1.1.5	Knowledge of the interrelationships among center of gravity, base of support, balance, stability, and proper spinal alignment.
1.1.6	Knowledge of the following curvatures of the spine: lordosis, scoliosis, and kyphosis.
1.1.8	Knowledge of the biomechanical principles for the performance of common physical activities (e.g., walking, running, swimming, cycling, resistance training, yoga, Pilates, functional training).
1.1.9	Ability to distinguish between aerobic and anaerobic metabolism.
1.1.10	Knowledge to describe the normal acute responses to cardiovascular exercise.
1.1.11	Knowledge to describe the normal acute responses to resistance training.
1.1.12	Knowledge of the normal chronic physiologic adaptations associated with cardiovascular exercise.
1.1.13	Knowledge of the normal chronic physiologic adaptations associated with resistance training.
1.1.14	Knowledge of the physiologic principles related to warm-up and cool-down.
1.1.15	Knowledge of the common theories of muscle fatigue and delayed onset muscle soreness (DOMS).
1.1.16	Knowledge of the physiologic adaptations that occur at rest and during submaximal and maximal exercise following chronic aerobic and anaerobic exercise training.
1.1.17	Knowledge of the physiologic principles involved in promoting gains in muscular strength and endurance.
1.1.18	Knowledge of blood pressure responses associated with acute exercise, including changes in body position.
1.1.19	Knowledge of how the principle of specificity relates to the components of fitness.
1.1.20	Knowledge of the concept of detraining or reversibility of conditioning and its implications in fitness programs.
1.1.21	Knowledge of the physical and psychological signs of overtraining and to provide recommendations for these problems.
1.1.22	Knowledge of muscle actions, such as isotonic, isometric (static), isokinetic, concentric, eccentric.
1.1.23	Ability to identify the major muscles. Major muscles include, but are not limited to, the following: trapezius, pectoralis major, latissimus dorsi, biceps, triceps, rectus abdominis, internal and external obliques, erector spinae, gluteus maximus, quadriceps, hamstrings, adductors, abductors, and gastrocnemius.
1.1.24	Ability to identify the major bones. Major bones include, but are not limited to, the clavicle, scapula, sternum, humerus, carpals, ulna, radius, femur, fibula, tibia, and tarsals.
1.1.25	Ability to identify the various types of joints of the body (e.g., hinge, ball, and socket).

1.1.26   Knowledge of the primary action and joint range of motion for each major muscle group.

1.1.27   Ability to locate the anatomic landmarks for palpation of peripheral pulses.

1.1.28   Knowledge of the unique physiologic considerations of children, older adults, persons with diabetes (type 2), pregnant women, and persons who are overweight and/or obese.

1.1.29   Knowledge of the following related terms: hypertrophy, atrophy, and hyperplasia.

General Population/Core: Health Appraisal, Fitness, and Clinical Exercise Testing

1.3.1   Knowledge of and ability to discuss the physiologic basis of the major components of physical fitness: flexibility, cardiovascular fitness, muscular strength, muscular endurance, and body composition.

1.3.2   Knowledge of the components of a health/medical history.

1.3.3   Knowledge of the value of a medical clearance before exercise participation.

1.3.4   Knowledge of the categories of participants who should receive medical clearance before administration of an exercise test or participation in an exercise program.

1.3.5   Knowledge of relative and absolute contraindications to exercise testing or participation.

1.3.6   Knowledge of the limitations of informed consent and medical clearance.

1.3.7   Knowledge of the advantages/disadvantages and limitations of the various body composition techniques including, but not limited to, skinfolds, plethysmography (BOD POD®), bioelectrical impedance, infrared, dual-energy x-ray absorptiometry (DEXA), and circumference measurements.

1.3.8   Skill in accurately measuring heart rate and obtaining rating of perceived exertion (RPE) at rest and during exercise according to established guidelines.

1.3.9   Ability to locate body sites for circumference (girth) measurements.

1.3.10   Ability to obtain a basic health history and risk appraisal and to stratify risk in accordance with ACSM Guidelines.

1.3.11   Ability to explain and obtain informed consent.

1.3.13   Knowledge of preactivity fitness testing, including assessments of cardiovascular fitness, muscular strength, muscular endurance, flexibility, and body composition.

1.3.14   Knowledge of criteria for terminating a fitness evaluation and proper procedures to be followed after discontinuing such a test.

1.3.15   Knowledge of and ability to prepare for the initial client consultation.

1.3.16   Ability to recognize postural abnormalities that may affect exercise performance.

1.3.17   Skill in assessing body alignment.

General Population/Core: Exercise Prescription and Programming

1.7.1   Knowledge of the benefits and risks associated with exercise training and recommendations for exercise programming in children and adolescents.

1.7.2   Knowledge of the benefits and precautions associated with resistance and endurance training in older adults and recommendations for exercise programming.

1.7.3   Knowledge of specific leadership techniques appropriate for working with participants of all ages.

1.7.4   Knowledge of how to modify cardiovascular and resistance exercises based on age and physical condition.

1.7.5   Knowledge of and ability to describe the unique adaptations to exercise training with regard to strength, functional capacity, and motor skills.

1.7.6   Knowledge of common orthopedic and cardiovascular considerations for older participants and the ability to describe modifications in exercise prescription that are indicated.

1.7.7 Knowledge of selecting appropriate training modalities according to the age and functional capacity of the individual.

1.7.8 Knowledge of the recommended intensity, duration, frequency, and type of physical activity necessary for development of cardiorespiratory fitness in an apparently healthy population.

1.7.9 Knowledge to describe and the ability to safely demonstrate exercises designed to enhance muscular strength and/or endurance.

1.7.10 Knowledge of the principles of overload, specificity, and progression and how they relate to exercise programming.

1.7.11 Knowledge of how to conduct and the ability to teach/demonstrate exercises during a comprehensive session that would include pre-exercise evaluation, warm-up, aerobic exercise, cool-down, muscular fitness training, and flexibility exercise.

1.7.12 Knowledge of special precautions and modifications of exercise programming for participation at altitude, different ambient temperatures, humidity, and environmental pollution.

1.7.13 Knowledge of the importance and ability to record exercise sessions and performing periodic evaluations to assess changes in fitness status.

1.7.14 Knowledge of the advantages and disadvantages of implementation of interval, continuous, and circuit training programs.

1.7.15 Knowledge of the concept of activities of daily living (ADLs) and its importance in the overall health of the individual.

1.7.16 Knowledge of progressive adaptation in resistance training and its implications on program design and periodization.

1.7.17 Knowledge of interpersonal limitations when working with clients one on one.

1.7.19 Skill to teach and demonstrate appropriate modifications in specific exercises and make recommendations for exercise programming for the following groups: children, older adults, persons with diabetes (type 2), pregnant women, persons with arthritis, persons who are overweight and/or obese, and persons with chronic back pain.

1.7.20 Skill to teach and demonstrate appropriate exercises for improving range of motion of all major joints.

1.7.21 Skill in the use of various methods for establishing and monitoring levels of exercise intensity, including heart rate, RPE, and metabolic equivalents (METs).

1.7.22 Knowledge of and ability to apply methods used to monitor exercise intensity, including heart rate and rating of perceived exertion.

1.7.24 Ability to differentiate between the amount of physical activity required for health benefits and the amount of exercise required for fitness development.

1.7.25 Ability to determine training heart rates using two methods: percent of age-predicted maximum heart rate and heart rate reserve (Karvonen).

1.7.26 Ability to identify proper and improper technique in the use of resistive equipment, such as stability balls, weights, bands, resistance bars, and water exercise equipment.

1.7.27 Ability to identify proper and improper technique in the use of cardiovascular conditioning equipment (e.g., stair-climbers, stationary cycles, treadmills, and elliptical trainers).

1.7.28 Ability to teach a progression of exercises for all major muscle groups to improve muscular fitness.

1.7.29 Ability to modify exercises based on age and physical condition.

1.7.30 Ability to explain and implement exercise prescription guidelines for apparently healthy clients or those who have medical clearance to exercise.

1.7.31 Ability to adapt frequency, intensity, duration, mode, progression, level of supervision, and monitoring techniques in exercise programs for apparently healthy clients or those who have medical clearance to exercise.

1.7.34 Ability to evaluate, prescribe, and demonstrate appropriate flexibility exercises for all major muscle groups.

1.7.35   Ability to design training programs using interval, continuous, and circuit training programs.

1.7.36   Ability to describe the advantages and disadvantages of various types of commercial exercise equipment in developing cardiorespiratory and muscular fitness.

1.7.37   Ability to safely demonstrate a wide variety of conditioning exercises involving equipment, such as stability balls, BOSU® balls, elastic bands, medicine balls, and foam rollers.

1.7.38   Ability to safely demonstrate a wide range of resistance-training modalities, including variable resistance devices, dynamic constant external resistance devices, static resistance devices, and other resistance devices.

1.7.39   Ability to safely demonstrate a wide variety of conditioning exercises that promote improvements in agility, balance, coordination, reaction time, speed, and power.

1.7.40   Knowledge of training principles, such as progressive overload, variation, and specificity.

1.7.41   Knowledge of the Valsalva maneuver and the associated risks.

1.7.42   Knowledge of the appropriate repetitions, sets, volume, repetition maximum, and rest periods necessary for desired outcome goals.

1.7.43   Ability to safely demonstrate a wide variety of plyometric exercises and be able to determine when such exercises would be inappropriate to perform.

1.7.44   Ability to apply training principles so as to distinguish goals between an athlete and an individual exercising for general health.

1.7.45   Knowledge of periodization in exercise in aerobic and resistance-training program design.

General Population/Core: Nutrition and Weight Management

1.8.1   Knowledge of the role of carbohydrates, fats, and proteins as fuels.

1.8.2   Knowledge to define the following terms: obesity, overweight, percent fat, body mass index (BMI), lean body mass, anorexia nervosa, bulimia nervosa, and body fat distribution.

1.8.3   Knowledge of the relationship between body composition and health.

1.8.4   Knowledge of the effects of diet plus exercise, diet alone, and exercise alone as methods for modifying body composition.

1.8.5   Knowledge of the importance of an adequate daily energy intake for healthy weight management.

1.8.6   Knowledge of the importance of maintaining normal hydration before, during, and after exercise.

1.8.7   Knowledge and understanding of the current Dietary Guidelines for Americans, including the USDA Food Pyramid.

1.8.8   Knowledge of the female athlete triad.

1.8.9   Knowledge of the myths and consequences associated with inappropriate weight loss methods (e.g., saunas, vibrating belts, body wraps, electric simulators, sweat suits, fad diets).

1.8.10   Knowledge of the number of kilocalories in one gram of carbohydrate, fat, protein, and alcohol.

1.8.11   Knowledge of the number of kilocalories equivalent to losing one pound of body fat.

1.8.12   Knowledge of the guidelines for caloric intake for an individual desiring to lose or gain weight.

1.8.13   Knowledge of common ergogenic aids, the purported mechanism of action, and potential risks and/or benefits (e.g., anabolic steroids, caffeine, amino acids, vitamins, minerals, creatine monohydrate, adrostenedione, DHEA).

1.8.14   Ability to describe the health implications of variation in body-fat distribution patterns and the significance of the waist-to-hip ratio.

1.8.15   Ability to describe the health implications of commonly used herbs (e.g., echinacea, St. John's wort, ginseng).

General Population/Core: Human Behavior and Counseling

1.9.1   Knowledge of behavioral strategies to enhance exercise and health behavior change (e.g., reinforcement, goal setting, social support).

1.9.2   Knowledge of the stages of motivational readiness and effective strategies that support and facilitate behavioral change.

1.9.3   Knowledge of the three stages of learning: cognitive, associative, autonomous.

1.9.4   Knowledge of specific techniques to enhance motivation (e.g., posters, recognition, bulletin boards, games, competitions). Define extrinsic and intrinsic reinforcement and give examples of each.

1.9.5   Knowledge of the different types of learners (auditory, visual, kinesthetic) and how to apply teaching and training techniques to optimize a client's training session.

1.9.6   Knowledge of the types of feedback and ability to use communication skills to optimize a client's training session.

1.9.7   Knowledge of common obstacles that interfere with adherence to an exercise program and strategies to overcome these obstacles.

1.9.8   Ability to identify, clarify, and set behavioral and realistic goals with the client (i.e., SMART goals).

1.9.9   Knowledge of basic communication and coaching techniques that foster and facilitate behavioral changes.

1.9.10   Knowledge of various learning theories (e.g., motivation theory, attribution theory, transfer theory, retention theory, and goal theory).

1.9.11   Knowledge of attributes or characteristics necessary for effective teaching.

General Population/Core: Safety, Injury Prevention, and Emergency Procedures

1.10.1   Knowledge of and skill in obtaining basic life support, automated external defibrillators (AEDs), and cardiopulmonary resuscitation certification.

1.10.2   Knowledge of appropriate emergency procedures (i.e., telephone procedures, written emergency procedures, personnel responsibilities) in a health and fitness setting.

1.10.3   Knowledge of basic first-aid procedures for exercise-related injuries, such as bleeding, strains/sprains, fractures, and exercise intolerance (dizziness, syncope, heat injury).

1.10.4   Knowledge of basic precautions taken in an exercise setting to ensure participant safety.

1.10.5   Knowledge of the physical and physiologic signs and symptoms of overtraining.

1.10.6   Knowledge of the effects of temperature, humidity, altitude, and pollution on the physiologic response to exercise.

1.10.7   Knowledge of the following terms: shin splints, sprain, strain, tennis elbow, bursitis, stress fracture, tendonitis, patello-femoral pain syndrome, low back pain, plantar fasciitis, and rotator cuff tendonitis.

1.10.8   Knowledge of hypothetical concerns and potential risks that may be associated with the use of exercises such as straight-leg sit-ups, double leg raises, full squats, hurdler's stretch, yoga plow, forceful back hyperextension, and standing bent-over toe touch.

1.10.10 Knowledge of the Certified Personal Trainer's[SM] responsibilities, limitations, and the legal implications of carrying out emergency procedures.

1.10.11 Knowledge of potential musculoskeletal injuries (e.g., contusions, sprains, strains, fractures), cardiovascular/pulmonary complications (e.g., tachycardia, bradycardia, hypotension/hypertension, tachypnea), and metabolic abnormalities (e.g., fainting/syncope, hypoglycemia/hyperglycemia, hypothermia/hyperthermia).

1.10.12 Knowledge of the initial management and first-aid techniques associated with open wounds, musculoskeletal injuries, cardiovascular/pulmonary complications, and metabolic disorders.

1.10.13 Knowledge of the components of an equipment service plan/agreement and how it may be used to evaluate the condition of exercise equipment to reduce the potential risk of injury.

1.10.14 Knowledge of the legal implications of documented safety procedures, the use of incident documents, and ongoing safety training.

1.10.15 Skill in demonstrating appropriate emergency procedures during exercise testing and/or training.

1.10.16 Ability to identify the components that contribute to the maintenance of a safe exercise environment.

1.10.17 Ability to assist or spot a client in a safe and effective manner during resistance exercise.

General Population/Core: Program Administration, Quality Assurance, and Outcome Assessment

1.11.1 Knowledge of the Certified Personal Trainer's[SM] scope of practice and role in the administration/program management within a health/fitness facility.

1.11.2 Knowledge of and the ability to use the documentation required when a client shows abnormal signs or symptoms during an exercise session and should be referred to a physician.

1.11.3 Knowledge of professional liability and most common types of negligence seen in training environments.

1.11.4 Understanding of the practical and legal ramifications of the employee versus independent contractor classifications as they relate to the Certified Personal Trainer[SM].

1.11.5 Knowledge of appropriate professional responsibilities, practice standards, and ethics in relationships dealing with clients, employers, and other allied health/medical/fitness professionals.

1.11.6 Knowledge of the types of exercise programs available in the community and how these programs are appropriate for various populations.

1.11.7 Knowledge of and ability to implement effective, professional business practices and ethical promotion of personal training services.

1.11.8 Ability to develop a basic business plan, which includes establishing a budget, developing management policies, marketing, sales, and pricing.

General Population/Core: Clinical and Medical Considerations

1.12.1 Knowledge of cardiovascular, respiratory, metabolic, and musculoskeletal risk factors that may require further evaluation by medical or allied health professionals before participation in physical activity.

1.12.2 Knowledge of risk factors that may be favorably modified by physical activity habits.

1.12.3 Knowledge of the risk-factor concept of coronary artery disease (CAD) and the influence of heredity and lifestyle on the development of CAD.

1.12.4 Knowledge of how lifestyle factors—including nutrition, physical activity, and heredity—influence blood lipid and lipoprotein (i.e., cholesterol: high-density lipoprotein and low-density lipoprotein) profiles.

1.12.5 Knowledge of cardiovascular risk factors or conditions that may require consultation with medical personnel before testing or training, including inappropriate changes of resting or exercise heart rate and blood pressure; new onset discomfort in chest, neck, shoulder, or arm; changes in the pattern of discomfort during rest or exercise; fainting or dizzy spells; and claudication.

1.12.6   Knowledge of respiratory risk factors or conditions that may require consultation with medical personnel before testing or training, including asthma, exercise-induced bronchospasm, extreme breathlessness at rest or during exercise, bronchitis, and emphysema.

1.12.7   Knowledge of metabolic risk factors or conditions that may require consultation with medical personnel before testing or training, including body weight more than 20% above optimal, BMI >30, thyroid disease, diabetes or glucose intolerance, and hypoglycemia.

1.12.8   Knowledge of musculoskeletal risk factors or conditions that may require consultation with medical personnel before testing or training, including acute or chronic back pain, arthritis, osteoporosis, and joint inflammation.

1.12.10   Knowledge of common drugs from each of the following classes of medications and ability to describe their effects on exercise: antianginals, anticoagulants, antihypertensives, antiarrhythmics, bronchodilators, hypoglycemics, psychotropics, vasodilators, and over-the-counter medications such as pseudoephedrine.

1.12.11   Knowledge of the effects of the following substances on exercise: antihistamines, tranquilizers, alcohol, diet pills, cold tablets, caffeine, and nicotine.

ACSM CERTIFIED HEALTH FITNESS SPECIALIST KNOWLEDGE, SKILLS, AND ABILITIES (KSAs)

General Population/Core: Exercise Physiology and Related Exercise Science

1.1.1   Knowledge of the structures of bone, skeletal muscle, and connective tissues.

1.1.2   Knowledge of the anatomy and physiology of the cardiovascular system and pulmonary system.

1.1.3   Knowledge of the following muscle action terms: inferior, superior, medial, lateral, supination, pronation, flexion, extension, adduction, abduction, hyperextension, rotation, circumduction, agonist, antagonist, and stabilizer.

1.1.4   Knowledge of the plane in which each movement action occurs and the responsible muscles.

1.1.5   Knowledge of the interrelationships among center of gravity, base of support, balance, stability, posture, and proper spinal alignment.

1.1.6   Knowledge of the curvatures of the spine including lordosis, scoliosis, and kyphosis.

1.1.7   Knowledge of the stretch reflex and how it relates to flexibility.

1.1.8   Knowledge of biomechanical principles that underlie performance of the following activities: walking, jogging, running, swimming, cycling, weight lifting, and carrying or moving objects.

1.1.9   Ability to describe the systems for the production of energy.

1.1.10   Knowledge of the role of aerobic and anaerobic energy systems in the performance of various physical activities.

1.1.11   Knowledge of the following cardiorespiratory terms: ischemia, angina pectoris, tachycardia, bradycardia, arrhythmia, myocardial infarction, claudication, dyspnea, and hyperventilation.

1.1.12   Ability to describe normal cardiorespiratory responses to static and dynamic exercise in terms of heart rate, stroke volume, cardiac output, blood pressure, and oxygen consumption.

1.1.13   Knowledge of the heart rate, stroke volume, cardiac output, blood pressure, and oxygen consumption responses to exercise.

1.1.14   Knowledge of the anatomic and physiologic adaptations associated with strength training.

1.1.15   Knowledge of the physiologic principles related to warm-up and cool-down.

1.1.16   Knowledge of the common theories of muscle fatigue and delayed onset muscle soreness (DOMS).

1.1.17   Knowledge of the physiologic adaptations that occur at rest and during submaximal and maximal exercise following chronic aerobic and anaerobic exercise training.

1.1.18   Knowledge of the differences in cardiorespiratory response to acute graded exercise between conditioned and unconditioned individuals.

1.1.19   Knowledge of the structure and function of the skeletal muscle fiber.

1.1.20   Knowledge of the characteristics of fast- and slow-twitch muscle fibers.

1.1.21   Knowledge of the sliding filament theory of muscle contraction.

1.1.22   Knowledge of twitch, summation, and tetanus with respect to muscle contraction.

1.1.23   Knowledge of the principles involved in promoting gains in muscular strength and endurance.

1.1.24   Knowledge of muscle fatigue as it relates to mode, intensity, duration, and the accumulative effects of exercise.

1.1.26   Knowledge of the response of the following variables to acute static and dynamic exercise: heart rate, stroke volume, cardiac output, pulmonary ventilation, tidal volume, respiratory rate, and arteriovenous oxygen difference.

1.1.27   Knowledge of blood pressure responses associated with acute exercise, including changes in body position.

1.1.28   Knowledge of and ability to describe the implications of ventilatory threshold (anaerobic threshold) as it relates to exercise training and cardiorespiratory assessment.

1.1.29   Knowledge of and ability to describe the physiologic adaptations of the pulmonary system that occur at rest and during submaximal and maximal exercise following chronic aerobic and anaerobic training.

1.1.30   Knowledge of how each of the following differs from the normal condition: dyspnea, hypoxia, and hyperventilation.

1.1.31   Knowledge of how the principles of specificity and progressive overload relate to the components of exercise programming.

1.1.32   Knowledge of the concept of detraining or reversibility of conditioning and its implications in exercise programs.

1.1.33   Knowledge of the physical and psychological signs of overreaching/overtraining and to provide recommendations for these problems.

1.1.34   Knowledge of and ability to describe the changes that occur in maturation from childhood to adulthood for the following: skeletal muscle, bone, reaction time, coordination, posture, heat and cold tolerance, maximal oxygen consumption, strength, flexibility, body composition, resting and maximal heart rate, and resting and maximal blood pressure.

1.1.35   Knowledge of the effect of the aging process on the musculoskeletal and cardiovascular structure and function at rest, during exercise, and during recovery.

1.1.36   Knowledge of the following terms: progressive resistance, isotonic/isometric, concentric, eccentric, atrophy, hyperplasia, hypertrophy, sets, repetitions, plyometrics, Valsalva maneuver.

1.1.37   Knowledge of and skill to demonstrate exercises designed to enhance muscular strength and/or endurance of specific major muscle groups.

1.1.38   Knowledge of and skill to demonstrate exercises for enhancing musculoskeletal flexibility.

1.1.39   Ability to identify the major muscles. Major muscles include, but are not limited to, the following: trapezius, pectoralis major, latissimus dorsi, biceps, triceps, rectus abdominis, internal and external obliques, erector spinae, gluteus maximus, quadriceps, hamstrings, adductors, abductors, and gastrocnemius.

1.1.40   Ability to identify the major bones. Major bones include, but are not limited to, the clavicle, scapula, strernum, humerus, carpals, ulna, radius, femur, fibia, tibia, and tarsals.

1.1.41   Ability to identify the joints of the body.

1.1.42   Knowledge of the primary action and joint range of motion for each major muscle group.

1.1.43   Ability to locate the anatomic landmarks for palpation of peripheral pulses and blood pressure.

General Population/Core: Pathophysiology and Risk Factors

1.2.1   Knowledge of the physiologic and metabolic responses to exercise associated with chronic disease (heart disease, hypertension, diabetes mellitus, and pulmonary disease).

1.2.2   Knowledge of cardiovascular, pulmonary, metabolic, and musculoskeletal risk factors that may require further evaluation by medical or allied health professionals before participation in physical activity.

1.2.3   Knowledge of risk factors that may be favorably modified by physical activity habits.

1.2.4   Knowledge to define the following terms: total cholesterol (TC), high-density lipoprotein cholesterol (HDL-C), TC/HDL-C ratio, low-density lipoprotein cholesterol (LDL-C), triglycerides, hypertension, and atherosclerosis.

1.2.5   Knowledge of plasma cholesterol levels for adults as recommended by the National Cholesterol Education Program.

1.2.6   Knowledge of the risk-factor thresholds for ACSM risk stratification, which includes genetic and lifestyle factors related to the development of CAD.

1.2.7   Knowledge of the atherosclerotic process, the factors involved in its genesis and progression, and the potential role of exercise in treatment.

1.2.8   Knowledge of how lifestyle factors, including nutrition and physical activity, influence lipid and lipoprotein profiles.

General Population/Core: Health Appraisal, Fitness, and Clinical Exercise Testing

1.3.1   Knowledge of and ability to discuss the physiologic basis of the major components of physical fitness: flexibility, cardiovascular fitness, muscular strength, muscular endurance, and body composition.

1.3.2   Knowledge of the value of the health/medical history.

1.3.3   Knowledge of the value of a medical clearance before exercise participation.

1.3.4   Knowledge of and the ability to perform risk stratification and its implications toward medical clearance before administration of an exercise test or participation in an exercise program.

1.3.5   Knowledge of relative and absolute contraindications to exercise testing or participation.

1.3.6   Knowledge of the limitations of informed consent and medical clearance before exercise testing.

1.3.7   Knowledge of the advantages/disadvantages and limitations of the various body-composition techniques, including but not limited to, air displacement plethysmography (BOD POD®), dual-energy x-ray absorptiometry (DEXA), hydrostatic weighing, skinfolds, and bioelectrical impedence.

1.3.8   Skill in accurately measuring heart rate and blood pressure, and obtaining rating of perceived exertion (RPE) at rest and during exercise according to established guidelines.

1.3.9   Skill in measuring skinfold sites, skeletal diameters, and girth measurements used for estimating body composition.

1.3.10   Knowledge of calibration of a cycle ergometer and a motor-driven treadmill.

1.3.11   Ability to locate the brachial artery and correctly place the cuff and stethoscope in position for blood-pressure measurement.

1.3.12   Ability to locate common sites for measurement of skinfold thicknesses and circumferences (for determination of body composition and waist-hip ratio).

1.3.13   Ability to obtain a health history and risk appraisal that includes past and current medical history, family history of cardiac disease, orthopedic limitations, prescribed medications, activity patterns, nutritional habits, stress and anxiety levels, and smoking and alcohol use.

1.3.14   Ability to obtain informed consent.

1.3.15   Ability to explain the purpose and procedures and perform the monitoring (heart rate, RPE, and blood pressure) of clients before, during, and after cardiorespiratory fitness testing.

1.3.16   Ability to instruct participants in the use of equipment and test procedures.

1.3.17   Ability to explain purpose of testing, determine an appropriate submaximal or maximal protocol, and perform an assessment of cardiovascular fitness on the treadmill or the cycle ergometer.

1.3.18   Ability to describe the purpose of testing, determine appropriate protocols, and perform assessments of muscular strength, muscular endurance, and flexibility.

1.3.19   Ability to perform various techniques of assessing body composition.

1.3.20   Ability to analyze and interpret information obtained from the cardiorespiratory fitness test and the muscular strength and endurance, flexibility, and body-composition assessments for apparently healthy individuals and those with controlled chronic disease.

1.3.21   Ability to identify appropriate criteria for terminating a fitness evaluation and demonstrate proper procedures to be followed after discontinuing such a test.

1.3.22   Ability to modify protocols and procedures for cardiorespiratory fitness tests in children, adolescents, and older adults.

1.3.23   Ability to identify individuals for whom physician supervision is recommended during maximal and submaximal exercise testing.

General Population/Core: Electrocardiography and Diagnostic Techniques

1.4.1   Knowledge of how each of the following arrhythmias differs from the normal condition: premature atrial contractions and premature ventricular contractions.

1.4.3   Knowledge of the basic properties of cardiac muscle and the normal pathways of conduction in the heart.

General Population/Core: Patient Management and Medications

1.5.1   Knowledge of common drugs from each of the following classes of medications and ability to describe the principal action and the effects on exercise testing and prescription: antianginals, antihypertensives, antiarrhythmics, anticoagulants, bronchodilators, hypoglycemics, psychotropics, and vasodilators.

1.5.2   Knowledge of the effects of the following substances on the exercise response: antihistamines, tranquilizers, alcohol, diet pills, cold tablets, caffeine, and nicotine.

General Population/Core: Exercise Prescription and Programming

1.7.1   Knowledge of the relationship between the number of repetitions, intensity, number of sets, and rest with regard to strength training.

1.7.2   Knowledge of the benefits and precautions associated with exercise training in apparently healthy and controlled disease.

1.7.3   Knowledge of the benefits and precautions associated with exercise training across the life span (from youth to the elderly).

1.7.4   Knowledge of specific group exercise leadership techniques appropriate for working with participants of all ages.

1.7.5   Knowledge of how to select and/or modify appropriate exercise programs according to the age, functional capacity, and limitations of the individual.

1.7.6   Knowledge of the differences in the development of an exercise prescription for children, adolescents, and older participants.

1.7.7	Knowledge of and ability to describe the unique adaptations to exercise training in children, adolescents, and older participants with regard to strength, functional capacity, and motor skills.
1.7.8	Knowledge of common orthopedic and cardiovascular considerations for older participants and the ability to describe modifications in exercise prescription that are indicated.
1.7.10	Knowledge of the recommended intensity, duration, frequency, and type of physical activity necessary for development of cardiorespiratory fitness in an apparently healthy population.
1.7.11	Knowledge of and the ability to describe exercises designed to enhance muscular strength and/or endurance of specific major muscle groups.
1.7.12	Knowledge of the principles of overload, specificity, and progression and how they relate to exercise programming.
1.7.13	Knowledge of the various types of interval, continuous, and circuit training programs.
1.7.14	Knowledge of approximate METs for various sport, recreational, and work tasks.
1.7.15	Knowledge of the components incorporated into an exercise session and the proper sequence (i.e., pre-exercise evaluation, warm-up, aerobic stimulus phase, cool-down, muscular strength and/or endurance, and flexibility).
1.7.16	Knowledge of special precautions and modifications of exercise programming for participation at altitude, different ambient temperatures, humidity, and environmental pollution.
1.7.17	Knowledge of the importance of recording exercise sessions and performing periodic evaluations to assess changes in fitness status.
1.7.18	Knowledge of the advantages and disadvantages of implementation of interval, continuous, and circuit training programs.
1.7.19	Knowledge of the exercise programs that are available in the community and how these programs are appropriate for various populations.
1.7.20	Knowledge of and ability to describe activities of daily living (ADLs) and its importance in the overall health of the individual.
1.7.21	Skill to teach and demonstrate the components of an exercise session (i.e., warm-up, aerobic stimulus phase, cool-down, muscular strength/endurance, flexibility).
1.7.22	Skill to teach and demonstrate appropriate modifications in specific exercises for groups such as older adults, pregnant and postnatal women, obese persons, and persons with low back pain.
1.7.23	Skill to teach and demonstrate appropriate exercises for improving range of motion of all major joints.
1.7.24	Skill in the use of various methods for establishing and monitoring levels of exercise intensity, including heart rate, RPE, and oxygen cost.
1.7.25	Ability to identify and apply methods used to monitor exercise intensity, including heart rate and RPE.
1.7.26	Ability to describe modifications in exercise prescriptions for individuals with functional disabilities and musculoskeletal injuries.
1.7.27	Ability to differentiate between the amount of physical activity required for health benefits and/or for fitness development.
1.7.28	Knowledge of and ability to determine target heart rates using two methods: percent of age-predicted maximum heart rate and heart rate reserve (Karvonen).
1.7.29	Ability to identify proper and improper technique in the use of resistive equipment, such as stability balls, weights, bands, resistance bars, and water exercise equipment.
1.7.30	Ability to identify proper and improper technique in the use of cardiovascular conditioning equipment (e.g., stair-climbers, stationary cycles, treadmills, elliptical trainers, rowing machines).

1.7.31   Ability to teach a progression of exercises for all major muscle groups to improve muscular strength and endurance.

1.7.32   Ability to communicate appropriately with exercise participants during initial screening and exercise programming.

1.7.33   Ability to design, implement, and evaluate individualized and group exercise programs based on health history and physical fitness assessments.

1.7.34   Ability to modify exercises based on age, physical condition, and cognitive status.

1.7.35   Ability to apply energy cost, $\dot{V}O_2$, METs, and target heart rates to an exercise prescription.

1.7.36   Ability to convert between the U.S. and metric systems for length/height (inches to centimeters), weight (pounds to kilograms), and speed (miles per hour to meters per minute).

1.7.37   Ability to convert between absolute ($mL \cdot kg^{-1} \cdot min^{-1}$ or $L \cdot min^{-1}$) and relative ($mL \cdot kg^{-1} \cdot min^{-1}$, and/or METs) oxygen costs.

1.7.38   Ability to determine the energy cost for given exercise intensities during horizontal and graded walking and running stepping exercise, cycle ergometry, arm ergometry, and stepping.

1.7.39   Ability to prescribe exercise intensity based on $\dot{V}O_2$ data for different modes of exercise, including graded and horizontal running and walking, cycling, and stepping exercise.

1.7.40   Ability to explain and implement exercise prescription guidelines for apparently healthy clients, increased risk clients, and clients with controlled disease.

1.7.41   Ability to adapt frequency, intensity, duration, mode, progression, level of supervision, and monitoring techniques in exercise programs for patients with controlled chronic disease (e.g., heart disease, diabetes mellitus, obesity, hypertension), musculoskeletal problems (including fatigue), pregnancy and/or postpartum, and exercise-induced asthma.

1.7.42   Ability to design resistive exercise programs to increase or maintain muscular strength and/or endurance.

1.7.43   Ability to evaluate flexibility and prescribe appropriate flexibility exercises for all major muscle groups.

1.7.44   Ability to design training programs using interval, continuous, and circuit training programs.

1.7.45   Ability to describe the advantages and disadvantages of various commercial exercise equipment in developing cardiorespiratory fitness, muscular strength, and muscular endurance.

1.7.46   Ability to modify exercise programs based on age, physical condition, and current health status.

1.7.47   Ability to assess postural alignment and recommend appropriate exercise to meet individual needs and refer as necessary.

General Population/Core: Nutrition and Weight Management

1.8.1   Knowledge of the role of carbohydrates, fats, and proteins as fuels for aerobic and anaerobic metabolism.

1.8.2   Knowledge of the following terms: obesity, overweight, percent fat, BMI, lean body mass, anorexia nervosa, bulimia nervosa, metabolic syndrome, and body-fat distribution.

1.8.3   Knowledge of the relationship between body composition and health.

1.8.4   Knowledge of the effects of diet, exercise, and behavior modification as methods for modifying body composition.

1.8.5   Knowledge of the importance of an adequate daily energy intake for healthy weight management.

1.8.6   Knowledge of the difference between fat-soluble and water-soluble vitamins.

1.8.7   Knowledge of the importance of maintaining normal hydration before, during, and after exercise.

1.8.8   Knowledge of the USDA Food Pyramid and Dietary Guidelines for Americans.

1.8.9   Knowledge of the importance of calcium and iron in women's health.

1.8.10   Knowledge of the myths and consequences associated with inappropriate weight loss methods (e.g., fad diets, dietary supplements, overexercising, starvation diets).

1.8.11   Knowledge of the number of kilocalories in one gram of carbohydrate, fat, protein, and alcohol.

1.8.12   Knowledge of the number of kilocalories equivalent to losing one pound (0.45 kg) of body fat and the ability to prescribe appropriate amount of exercise to achieve weight-loss goals.

1.8.13   Knowledge of the guidelines for caloric intake for an individual desiring to lose or gain weight.

1.8.14   Knowledge of common nutritional ergogenic aids, the purported mechanism of action, and any risk and/or benefits (e.g., carbohydrates, protein/amino acids, vitamins, minerals, herbal products, creatine, steroids, caffeine).

1.8.15   Knowledge of nutritional factors related to the female athlete triad syndrome (i.e., eating disorders, menstrual cycle abnormalities, and osteoporosis).

1.8.16   Knowledge of the NIH consensus statement regarding health risks of obesity, Nutrition for Physical Fitness Position Paper of the American Dietetic Association, and the ACSM position stand on proper and improper weight loss programs.

1.8.17   Ability to describe the health implications of variation in body-fat distribution patterns and the significance of the waist-to-hip ratio.

1.8.18   Knowledge of the nutrition and exercise effects on blood glucose levels in diabetes.

General Population/Core: Human Behavior and Counseling

1.9.1   Knowledge of behavioral strategies to enhance exercise and health behavior change (e.g., reinforcement, goal setting, social support).

1.9.2   Knowledge of the important elements that should be included in each behavior-modification session.

1.9.3   Knowledge of specific techniques to enhance motivation (e.g., posters, recognition, bulletin boards, games, competitions).

1.9.4   Knowledge of extrinsic and intrinsic reinforcement and ability to give examples of each.

1.9.5   Knowledge of the stages of motivational readiness.

1.9.6   Knowledge of approaches that may assist less motivated clients to increase their physical activity.

1.9.7   Knowledge of signs and symptoms of mental health states (e.g., anxiety, depression, eating disorders) that may necessitate referral to a medical or mental health professional.

1.9.8   Knowledge of the potential symptoms and causal factors of test anxiety (i.e., performance, appraisal threat during exercise testing) and how it may affect physiologic responses to testing.

1.9.9   Ability to coach clients to set achievable goals and overcome obstacles through a variety of methods (e.g., in person, on phone, and on Internet).

General Population/Core: Safety, Injury Prevention, and Emergency Procedures

1.10.1   Knowledge of and skill in obtaining basic life support, first aid, cardiopulmonary resuscitation, and automated external defibrillator certifications.

1.10.2   Knowledge of appropriate emergency procedures (i.e., telephone procedures, written emergency procedures, personnel responsibilities) in a health and fitness setting.

1.10.3   Knowledge of and skill in performing basic first-aid procedures for exercise-related injuries, such as bleeding, strains/sprains, fractures, and exercise intolerance (dizziness, syncope, heat and cold injuries).

1.10.4   Knowledge of basic precautions taken in an exercise setting to ensure participant safety.

1.10.5   Knowledge of the physical and physiologic signs and symptoms of overtraining and the ability to modify a program to accommodate this condition.

1.10.6   Knowledge of the effects of temperature, humidity, altitude, and pollution on the physiologic response to exercise and the ability to modify the exercise prescription to accommodate for these environmental conditions.

1.10.7   Knowledge of the signs and symptoms of the following conditions: shin splints, sprain, strain, tennis elbow, bursitis, stress fracture, tendonitis, patellar femoral pain syndrome, low back pain, plantar fasciitis, and rotator cuff tendonitis; the ability to recommend exercises to prevent these injuries.

1.10.8   Knowledge of hypothetical concerns and potential risks that may be associated with the use of exercises such as straight-leg sit-ups, double leg raises, full squats, hurdler's stretch, yoga plow, forceful back hyperextension, and standing bent-over toe touch.

1.10.9   Knowledge of safety plans, emergency procedures, and first-aid techniques needed during fitness evaluations, exercise testing, and exercise training.

1.10.10   Knowledge of the Health Fitness Specialist's responsibilities and limitations, and the legal implications of carrying out emergency procedures.

1.10.11   Knowledge of potential musculoskeletal injuries (e.g., contusions, sprains, strains, fractures), cardiovascular/pulmonary complications (e.g., tachycardia, bradycardia, hypotension/hypertension, tachypnea), and metabolic abnormalities (e.g., fainting/syncope, hypoglycemia/hyperglycemia, hypothermia/hyperthermia).

1.10.12   Knowledge of the initial management and first-aid techniques associated with open wounds, musculoskeletal injuries, cardiovascular/pulmonary complications, and metabolic disorders.

1.10.13   Knowledge of the components of an equipment maintenance/repair program and how it may be used to evaluate the condition of exercise equipment to reduce the potential risk of injury.

1.10.14   Knowledge of the legal implications of documented safety procedures, the use of incident documents, and ongoing safety training documentation for the purposes of safety and risk management.

1.10.15   Skill to demonstrate exercises used for people with low back pain; neck, shoulder, elbow, wrist, hip, knee and/or ankle pain; and the ability to modify a program for people with these conditions.

1.10.16   Skill in demonstrating appropriate emergency procedures during exercise testing and/or training.

1.10.17   Ability to identify the components that contribute to the maintenance of a safe environment, including equipment operation and maintenance, proper sanitation, safety and maintenance of exercise areas, and overall facility maintenance.

1.10.18   Knowledge of basic ergonomics to address daily activities that may cause musculoskeletal problems in the workplace and the ability to recommend exercises to alleviate symptoms caused by repetitive movements.

General Population/Core: Program Administration, Quality Assurance, and Outcome Assessment

1.11.1   Knowledge of the Health Fitness Specialist's role in administration and program management within a health/fitness facility.

1.11.2   Knowledge of and the ability to use the documentation required when a client shows signs or symptoms during an exercise session and should be referred to a physician.

1.11.3   Knowledge of how to manage a fitness department (e.g., working within a budget, interviewing and training staff, scheduling, running staff meetings, staff development).

1.11.4   Knowledge of the importance of tracking and evaluating member retention.

1.11.6   Ability to administer fitness-related programs within established budgetary guidelines.

1.11.7   Ability to develop marketing materials for the purpose of promoting fitness-related programs.

1.11.8   Ability to create and maintain records pertaining to participant exercise adherence, retention, and goal setting.

1.11.9   Ability to develop and administer educational programs (e.g., lectures, workshops) and educational materials.

1.11.10   Knowledge of basic sales techniques to promote health, fitness, and wellness services.

1.11.11   Knowledge of networking techniques with other healthcare professionals for referral purposes.

1.11.12   Ability to provide and administer appropriate customer service.

1.11.13   Knowledge of the importance of tracking and evaluating health promotion program results.

Cardiovascular: Pathophysiology and Risk Factors

2.2.1   Knowledge of cardiovascular risk factors or conditions that may require consultation with medical personnel before testing or training, including inappropriate changes of resting or exercise heart rate and blood pressure; new onset discomfort in chest, neck, shoulder, or arm; changes in the pattern of discomfort during rest or exercise; fainting or dizzy spells; and claudication.

2.2.2   Knowledge of the pathophysiology of myocardial ischemia and infarction.

2.2.3   Knowledge of the pathophysiology of stroke, hypertension, and hyperlipidemia.

2.2.4   Knowledge of the effects of the above diseases and conditions on the cardiorespiratory responses at rest and during exercise.

Pulmonary: Pathophysiology and Risk Factors

3.2.1   Knowledge of pulmonary risk factors or conditions that may require consultation with medical personnel before testing or training, including asthma, exercise-induced asthma/bronchospasm, extreme breathlessness at rest or during exercise, bronchitis, and emphysema.

Metabolic: Pathophysiology and Risk Factors

4.2.1   Knowledge of metabolic risk factors or conditions that may require consultation with medical personnel before testing or training, including obesity, metabolic syndrome, thyroid disease, kidney disease, diabetes or glucose intolerance, and hypoglycemia.

Orthopedic/Musculoskeletal: Pathophysiology and Risk Factors

5.2.1   Knowledge of musculoskeletal risk factors or conditions that may require consultation with medical personnel before testing or training, including acute or chronic back pain, osteoarthritis, rheumatoid arthritis, osteoporosis, inflammation/pain, and low back pain.

Neuromuscular: Pathophysiology and Risk Factors

6.2.1   Knowledge of neuromuscular risk factors or conditions that may require consultation with medical personnel before testing or training, including spinal cord injuries and multiple sclerosis.

Immunologic: Pathophysiology and Risk Factors

7.2.1 Knowledge of immunologic risk factors or conditions that may require consultation with medical personnel before testing or training, including AIDS and cancer.

NOTE: The KSAs listed above for the ACSM Certified Health Fitness Specialist are the same KSAs for educational programs in Exercise Science seeking undergraduate (Bachelor's) academic accreditation through the CoAES. For more information, please visit www.coaes.org.

ACSM CERTIFIED CLINICAL EXERCISE SPECIALIST KNOWLEDGE, SKILLS, AND ABILITIES (KSAs)

General Population/Core: Exercise Physiology and Related Exercise Science

1.1.1 Describe and illustrate the normal cardiovascular anatomy.

1.1.2 Describe the physiologic effects of bed rest, and discuss the appropriate physical activities that might be used to counteract these changes.

1.1.3 Identify the cardiorespiratory responses associated with postural changes.

1.1.5 Identify the metabolic equivalent (MET) requirements of various occupational, household, sport/exercise, and leisure-time activities.

1.1.6 Demonstrate knowledge of the unique hemodynamic responses of arm versus leg exercise, combined arm and leg exercise, and of static versus dynamic exercise.

1.1.7 Define the determinants of myocardial oxygen consumption (i.e., heart rate $\times$ systolic blood pressure = double product OR rate-pressure product) and the effects of acute exercise and exercise training on those determinants.

1.1.8 Describe the methodology for measuring peak oxygen consumption ($\dot{V}O_{2peak}$).

1.1.9 Plot the normal resting and exercise values associated with increasing exercise intensity (and how they may differ for cardiac, pulmonary, and metabolic diseased populations) for the following: heart rate, stroke volume, cardiac output, double product, arteriovenous O_2 difference, O_2 consumption, systolic and diastolic blood pressure, minute ventilation, tidal volume, breathing frequency, Vd/Vt, $\dot{V}_E/\dot{V}O_2$, $\dot{V}_E/\dot{V}CO_2$, $FEV_{1.0}$, SaO_2, and blood glucose.

1.1.10 Discuss the effects of isometric exercise in individuals with cardiovascular, pulmonary, and/or metabolic diseases.

1.1.11 Demonstrate knowledge of acute and chronic adaptations to exercise for those with cardiovascular, pulmonary, and metabolic diseases.

1.1.12 Describe the effects of variation in environmental factors (e.g., temperature, humidity, altitude) for normal individuals and those with cardiovascular, pulmonary, and metabolic diseases.

1.1.13 Understand the hormonal (i.e., insulin, glucagon, epinephrine, norepinephrine, angiotensin, aldosterone, renin, erythropoieten) responses to acute and chronic exercise.

1.1.14 Identify normal and abnormal respiratory responses during rest and exercise as assessed during a pulmonary function test (i.e., FVC, MVV, $FEV_{1.0}$, flow volume loop).

General Population/Core: Pathophysiology and Risk Factors

1.2.1 Summarize the atherosclerotic process, including current hypotheses regarding onset and rate of progression and/or regression.

1.2.2 Compare and contrast the differences between typical, atypical, and vasospastic angina and how these may differ in specific subgroups (i.e., men, women, people with diabetes).

1.2.3 Describe the pathophysiology of the healing myocardium and the potential complications after acute myocardial infarction (MI) (remodeling, rupture).

1.2.5   Examine the role of lifestyle on cardiovascular risk factors, such as hypertension, blood lipids, glucose tolerance, and body weight.

1.2.6   Describe the lipoprotein classifications, and define their relationship to atherosclerosis.

1.2.7   Describe the resting and exercise cardiorespiratory and metabolic responses in those with pulmonary disease.

1.2.8   Describe the influence of exercise on cardiovascular, pulmonary, and metabolic risk factors.

1.2.11   Describe the cardiorespiratory and metabolic responses in myocardial dysfunction and ischemia at rest and during exercise.

1.2.12   Recognize and describe the pathophysiology of the differing severities (e.g., NYHA classification) of heart failure, including cardiac output, heart rate, blood pressure, cardiac dimensions, and basic echocardiography parameters (ejection fraction, wall motion, left ventricular dimension).

1.2.13   Recognize and describe the pathophysiology of diabetes mellitus (prediabetes, types 1 and 2, gestational), including blood glucose, Hb_{A1c}, insulin sensitivity, and the risk and affect on comorbid conditions.

1.2.14   Identify the contributing factors to metabolic syndrome, their pathologic sequelae, and their affect on the primary or secondary risk of cardiovascular disease.

1.2.15   Recognize the pathologic process that various risk factors contribute for the development of cardiac, pulmonary, and metabolic diseases (e.g., smoking, hypertension, abnormal blood lipid values, obesity, inactivity, sex, genetics, diabetes).

General Population/Core: Health Appraisal, Fitness, and Clinical Exercise Testing

1.3.1   Describe common procedures and apply knowledge of results from radionuclide imaging (e.g., thallium, technetium, sestamibi, tetrafosmin, single-photon emission computed tomography [SPECT]), stress echocardiography, and pharmacologic testing (e.g., dobutamine, adenosine, persantine).

1.3.2   Demonstrate knowledge of exercise testing procedures for various clinical populations, including those individuals with cardiovascular, pulmonary, and metabolic diseases in terms of exercise modality, protocol, physiologic measurements, and expected outcomes.

1.3.3   Describe anatomic landmarks as they relate to exercise testing and programming (e.g., electrode placement, blood pressure).

1.3.4   Locate and palpate anatomic landmarks of radial, brachial, carotid, femoral, popliteal, and tibialis arteries.

1.3.5   Select an appropriate test protocol according to the age, functional capacity, physical ability, and health status of the individual.

1.3.6   Identify individuals for whom physician supervision is recommended during maximal and submaximal exercise testing.

1.3.7   Conduct pre-exercise test procedures.

1.3.8   Describe basic equipment and facility requirements for exercise testing.

1.3.9   Instruct the test participant in the use of the RPE scale and other appropriate subjective rating scales, such as the dyspnea, pain, claudication, and angina scales.

1.3.11   Describe the importance of accurate and calibrated testing equipment (e.g., treadmill, ergometers, electrocardiograph [ECG], gas analysis systems, and sphygmomanometers) and demonstrate the ability to recognize and remediate equipment that is no longer properly calibrated.

1.3.12   Obtain and recognize normal and abnormal physiologic and subjective responses (e.g., symptoms, ECG, blood pressure, heart rate, RPE and other scales, oxygen saturation, and oxygen consumption) at appropriate intervals during the test.

1.3.15　Demonstrate the ability to provide testing procedures and protocol for children and the elderly with or without various clinical conditions.

1.3.16　Evaluate medical history and physical examination findings as they relate to health appraisal and exercise testing.

1.3.17　Accurately record and interpret right and left arm pre-exercise blood pressures in the supine and upright positions.

1.3.18　Describe and analyze the importance of the absolute and relative contraindications and test termination indicators of an exercise test.

1.3.19　Select and perform appropriate procedures and protocols for the exercise test, including modes of exercise, starting levels, increments of work, ramping versus incremental protocols, length of stages, and frequency of data collection.

1.3.20　Describe and conduct immediate postexercise procedures and various approaches to cool-down and recognize normal and abnormal responses.

1.3.21　Record, organize, perform, and interpret necessary calculations of test data.

1.3.22　Describe the differences in the physiologic responses to various modes of ergometry (e.g., treadmill, cycle and arm ergometers) as they relate to exercise testing and training.

1.3.23　Describe normal and abnormal chronotropic and inotropic responses to exercise testing and training.

1.3.24　Understand and apply pretest likelihood of CAD, the positive and negative predictive values of various types of stress tests (e.g., ECG only, stress echo, radionuclide), and the potential of false positive/negative and true positive/negative results.

1.3.25　Compare and contrast obstructive and restrictive lung diseases and their effect on exercise testing and training.

1.3.26　Identify orthopedic limitations (e.g., gout, foot drop, specific joint problems, amputation, prosthesis) as they relate to modifications of exercise testing and programming.

1.3.27　Identify basic neuromuscular disorders (e.g., Parkinson's disease, multiple sclerosis) as they relate to modifications of exercise testing and programming.

1.3.28　Describe the aerobic and anaerobic metabolic demands of exercise testing and training in individuals with cardiovascular, pulmonary, and/or metabolic diseases undergoing exercise testing or training.

1.3.29　Identify the variables measured during cardiopulmonary exercise testing (e.g., heart rate, blood pressure, rate of perceived exertion, ventilation, oxygen consumption, ventilatory threshold, pulmonary circulation) and their potential relationship to cardiovascular, pulmonary, and metabolic disease.

1.3.31　Understand the basic principle and methods of coronary calcium scoring using computed-tomography (CT) methods.

1.3.32　Recognize the emergence of new imaging techniques for the assessment of heart disease (e.g., CT angiography).

1.3.33　Recognize the value of heart and lung sounds in the assessment of patients with cardiovascular and/or pulmonary disease.

1.3.34　Demonstrate the ability to perform a six-minute walk test and appropriately use the results to assess prognosis, fitness, and/or improvement.

General Population/Core: Electrocardiography and Diagnostic Techniques

1.4.1　Summarize the purpose of coronary angiography.

1.4.2　Describe myocardial ischemia and identify ischemic indicators of various cardiovascular diagnostic tests.

1.4.3　Describe the differences between Q-wave and non-Q-wave infarction, and ST elevation (STEMI) and non-ST elevation myocardial infarction (non-STEMI).

1.4.4   Identify the ECG patterns at rest and responses to exercise in patients with pacemakers and implantable cardiac defibrillators (ICDs). In addition, recognize the ability of biventricular pacing and possibility of pacemaker malfunction (e.g., failure to sense and failure to pace).

1.4.5   Identify resting and exercise ECG changes associated with the following abnormalities: axis; bundle-branch blocks and bifascicular blocks; atrioventricular blocks; sinus bradycardia and tachycardia; sinus arrest; supraventricular premature contractions and tachycardia; ventricular premature contractions (including frequency, form, couplets, salvos, tachycardia); atrial flutter and fibrillation; ventricular fibrillation; myocardial ischemia, injury, and infarction.

1.4.6   Define the ECG criteria for initiating and/or terminating exercise testing or training.

1.4.7   Identify ECG changes that correspond to ischemia in various myocardial regions.

1.4.8   Describe potential causes and pathophysiology of various cardiac arrhythmias.

1.4.9   Identify potentially hazardous arrhythmias or conduction defects observed on the ECG at rest, during exercise, and recovery.

1.4.10 Describe the diagnostic and prognostic significance of ischemic ECG responses and arrhythmias at rest, during exercise, or recovery.

1.4.11 Identify resting and exercise ECG changes associated with cardiovascular disease, hypertensive heart disease, cardiac chamber enlargement, pericarditis, pulmonary disease, and metabolic disorders.

1.4.12 Administer and interpret basic resting spirometric tests and measures, including $FEV_{1.0}$, FVC, and MVV.

1.4.13 Locate the appropriate sites for the limb and chest leads for resting, standard, and exercise (Mason Likar) ECGs, as well as commonly used bipolar systems (e.g., CM-5).

1.4.14 Obtain and interpret a pre-exercise standard and modified (Mason-Likar) 12-lead ECG on a participant in the supine and upright position.

1.4.15 Demonstrate the ability to minimize ECG artifact.

1.4.16 Describe the diagnostic and prognostic implications of the exercise test ECG and hemodynamic responses.

1.4.17 Identify ECG changes that typically occur as a result of hyperventilation, electrolyte abnormalities, and drug therapy.

1.4.18 Identify the causes of false-positive and false-negative exercise ECG responses and methods for optimizing sensitivity and specificity.

1.4.19 Identify and describe the significance of ECG abnormalities in designing the exercise prescription and in making activity recommendations.

General Population/Core: Patient Management and Medications

1.5.2   Describe mechanisms and actions of medications that may affect exercise testing and prescription (i.e., β-blockers, nitrates, calcium channel blockers, digitalis, diuretics, vasodilators, antiarrhythmic agents, bronchodilators, antilipemics, psychotropics, nicotine, antihistamines, over-the-counter [OTC] cold medications, thyroid medications, alcohol, hypoglycemic agents, blood modifiers, pentoxifylline, antigout medications, and anorexiants/diet pills).

1.5.3   Recognize medications associated in the clinical setting, their indications for care, and their effects at rest and during exercise (i.e., β-blockers, nitrates, calcium channel blockers, digitalis, diuretics, vasodilators, anitarrhythmic agents, bronchodilators, antilipemics, psychotropics, nicotine, antihistamines, OTC cold medications, thyroid medications, alcohol, hypoglycemic agents, blood modifiers, pentoxifylline, antigout medications, and anorexiants/diet pills).

1.5.4   Recognize the use of herbal and nutritional supplements, OTC medications, homeopathic remedies, and other alternative therapies often used by patients with chronic diseases.

1.5.5   Practice disease/case management responsibilities, including daily follow-up concerning patient needs, signs and symptoms, physician appointments, and medication changes for patients with chronic diseases, including cardiovascular, pulmonary, and metabolic diseases; comorbid conditions; arthritis; osteoporosis; and renal dysfunction/transplant/dialysis.

1.5.6   Direct patients actively attempting to lose weight in a formal or informal setting using behavioral, diet, exercise, or surgical methods.

1.5.7   Manage patients on oxygen therapy as needed during exercise testing or training.

1.5.8   Recognize patient clinical need for referral to other (non-ES) allied health professionals (e.g., behavioralist, physical therapist, diabetes educator, nurse).

1.5.9   Recognize patients with chronic pain who may be in a chronic pain management treatment program and who may require special adaptations during exercise testing and training.

1.5.10   Recognize exercise testing and training needs of patients with joint replacement or prosthesis.

1.5.11   Address exercise testing and training needs of elderly and young patients.

1.5.12   Recognize treatment goals and guidelines for hypertension using the most recent JNC report and other relevant evidence-based guidelines.

1.5.13   Recognize treatment goals and guidelines for dyslipidemia using the most recent NCEP report and other relevant evidence-based guidelines.

1.5.14   Demonstrate the ability to perform pulse-oximetry and blood glucose evaluations and appropriately interpret the data in a given clinical situation.

1.5.15   Demonstrate the ability to assess for peripheral edema and other indicators of fluid retention and respond appropriately in a given clinical setting.

General Population/Core: Medical and Surgical Management

1.6.1   Describe percutaneous coronary interventions (PCI) and peripheral interventions as an alternative to medical management or bypass surgery.

1.6.2   Describe indications and limitations for medical management and interventional techniques in different subsets of individuals with CAD and peripheral arterial disease (PAD).

1.6.3   Identify risk, benefit, and unique management issues of patients with mechanical, prosthetic valve replacement and valve repair.

1.6.4   Describe and recognize bariatric surgery as a therapy for obesity.

1.6.5   Recognize external counterpulsation (ECP) as a method of treating severe, difficult-to-treat chest pain (i.e., angina).

General Population/Core: Exercise Prescription and Programming

1.7.2   Compare and contrast benefits and risks of exercise for individuals with risk factors for or established cardiovascular, pulmonary, and/or metabolic diseases.

1.7.3   Design appropriate exercise prescription in environmental extremes for those with cardiovascular, pulmonary, and metabolic diseases.

1.7.4   Design, implement, and supervise individualized exercise prescriptions for people with chronic disease and disabling conditions or for people who are young or elderly.

1.7.5   Design a supervised exercise program beginning at hospital discharge and continuing for up to six months for the following conditions: MI; angina: left ventricular assist device

(LVAD); congestive heart failure; PCI; coronary artery bypass graft (surgery) (CABG[S]); medical management of CAD; chronic pulmonary disease; weight management; diabetes; metabolic syndrome; and cardiac transplants.

1.7.6   Demonstrate knowledge of the concept of activities of daily living (ADLs) and its importance in the overall rehabilitation of the individual.

1.7.7   Prescribe exercise using nontraditional modalities (e.g., bench stepping, elastic bands, isodynamic exercise, water aerobics, yoga, tai chi) for individuals with cardiovascular, pulmonary, or metabolic diseases.

1.7.8   Demonstrate exercise equipment adaptations necessary for different age groups, physical abilities, and other potential contributing factors.

1.7.9   Identify patients who require a symptom-limited exercise test before exercise training.

1.7.10   Organize graded exercise tests and clinical data to counsel patients regarding issues such as ADL, return to work, and physical activity.

1.7.11   Describe relative and absolute contraindications to exercise training.

1.7.12   Identify characteristics that correlate or predict poor compliance to exercise programs and strategies to increase exercise adherence.

1.7.13   Describe the importance of warm-up and cool-down sessions with specific reference to angina and ischemic ECG changes, and for overall patient safety.

1.7.14   Identify and explain the mechanisms by which exercise may contribute to reducing disease risk or rehabilitating individuals with cardiovascular, pulmonary, and metabolic diseases.

1.7.15   Describe common gait, movement, and coordination abnormalities as they relate to exercise testing and programming.

1.7.16   Describe the principle of specificity as it relates to the mode of exercise testing and training.

1.7.17   Design strength and flexibility programs for individuals with cardiovascular, pulmonary, and/or metabolic diseases; the elderly; and children.

1.7.18   Determine appropriate testing and training modalities according to the age, functional capacity, physical ability, and health status of the individual.

1.7.19   Describe the indications and methods for ECG monitoring during exercise testing and training.

1.7.20   Discuss the appropriate use of static and dynamic resistance exercise for individuals with cardiovascular, pulmonary, and metabolic disease.

1.7.21   Demonstrate the ability to modify exercise testing and training to the limitations of PAD.

1.7.22   Design, describe, and demonstrate specific resistance exercises for major muscle groups for patients with cardiovascular, pulmonary, and metabolic diseases and conditions.

1.7.23   Identify procedures for pre-exercise assessment of blood glucose, determining safety for exercise, and avoidance of exercise-induced hypoglycemia in patients with diabetes. Manage postexercise hypoglycemia when it occurs.

General Population/Core: Nutrition and Weight Management

1.8.1   Describe and discuss dietary considerations for cardiovascular and pulmonary diseases, chronic heart failure, and diabetes that are recommended to minimize disease progression and optimize disease management.

1.8.2   Compare and contrast dietary practices used for weight reduction, and address the benefits, risks, and scientific support for each practice. Examples of dietary practices are high-protein/low-carbohydrate diets, Mediterranean diet, and low-fat diets, such as the American Heart Association recommended diet.

1.8.3   Calculate the effect of caloric intake and energy expenditure on weight management.

1.8.4   Describe the hypotheses related to diet, weight gain, and weight loss.

1.8.5   Demonstrate the ability to differentiate and educate patients between nutritionally sound diets versus fad diets and scientifically supported supplements and anecdotally supported supplements.

1.8.6   Differentiate among and understand the value of the various vegetarian diets (i.e., Ovo-lacto, vegan).

General Population/Core: Human Behavior and Counseling

1.9.1   List and apply behavioral strategies that apply to lifestyle modifications, such as exercise, diet, stress, and medication management.

1.9.2   Describe signs and symptoms of maladjustment and/or failure to cope during an illness crisis and/or personal adjustment crisis (e.g., job loss) that might prompt a psychological consult or referral to other professional services.

1.9.3   Describe the general principles of crisis management and factors influencing coping and learning in illness states.

1.9.4   Identify the psychological stages involved with the acceptance of death and dying and demonstrate the ability to recognize when it is necessary for a psychological consult or referral to a professional resource.

1.9.5   Recognize observable signs and symptoms of anxiety or depressive symptoms and the need for a psychiatric referral.

1.9.6   Describe the psychological issues to be confronted by the patient and by family members of patients who have cardiovascular or pulmonary disease or diseases of the metabolic syndrome.

1.9.7   Identify the psychological issues associated with an acute cardiac event versus those associated with chronic cardiac conditions.

1.9.8   Recognize and implement methods of stress management for patients with chronic disease.

1.9.9   Use common assessment tools to access behavioral change, such as the Transtheoretical Model.

1.9.10   Facilitate effective and contemporary motivational and behavior modification techniques to promote behavioral change.

1.9.11   Demonstrate the ability to conduct effective and informative group and individual education sessions directed at primary or secondary prevention of chronic disease.

General Population/Core: Safety, Injury Prevention, and Emergency Procedures

1.10.1   Respond appropriately to emergency situations (e.g., cardiac arrest, hypoglycemia and hyperglycemia; bronchospasm; sudden onset hypotension; severe hypertensive response; angina; serious cardiac arrhythmias; ICD discharge; transient ischemic attack [TIA] or stroke; MI) that might arise before, during, and after administration of an exercise test and/or exercise session.

1.10.2   List medications that should be available for emergency situations in exercise testing and training sessions.

1.10.3   Describe the emergency equipment and personnel that should be present in an exercise testing laboratory and rehabilitative exercise training setting.

1.10.4   Describe the appropriate procedures for maintaining emergency equipment and supplies.

1.10.5   Describe the effects of cardiovascular and pulmonary disease and the diseases of the metabolic syndrome on performance of and safety during exercise testing and training.

1.10.6   Stratify individuals with cardiovascular, pulmonary, and metabolic diseases, using appropriate risk-stratification methods and understanding the prognostic indicators for high-risk individuals.

1.10.7   Describe the process for developing and updating emergency policies and procedures (e.g., call 911, call code team, call medical director, transport and use defibrillator).

1.10.8   Be aware of the current CPR, AED, and ACLS standards to be able to assist with emergency situations.

General Population/Core: Program Administration, Quality Assurance, and Outcome Assessment

1.11.1   Discuss the role of outcome measures in chronic disease management programs, such as cardiovascular and pulmonary rehabilitation programs.

1.11.2   Identify and discuss various outcome measurements used in a cardiac or pulmonary rehabilitation program.

1.11.3   Use specific outcome collection instruments to collect outcome data in a cardiac or pulmonary rehabilitation program.

1.11.4   Understand the most recent cardiac and pulmonary rehabilitation Centers for Medicare Services (CMS) rules for patient enrollment and reimbursement (e.g., diagnostic current procedure terminology [CPT] codes, diagnostic related groups [DRG]).

ACSM REGISTERED CLINICAL EXERCISE PHYSIOLOGIST® KNOWLEDGE, SKILLS, AND ABILITIES (KSAs)

General Population/Core: Exercise Physiology and Related Exercise Science

1.1.1   Describe the acute responses to aerobic, resistance, and flexibility training on the function of the cardiovascular, respiratory, musculoskeletal, neuromuscular, metabolic, endocrine, and immune systems.

1.1.2   Describe the chronic effects of aerobic, resistance, and flexibility training on the structure and function of the cardiovascular, respiratory, musculoskeletal, neuromuscular, metabolic, endocrine, and immune systems.

1.1.3   Explain differences in typical values between sedentary and trained persons in those with chronic diseases for oxygen uptake, heart rate, mean arterial pressure, systolic and diastolic blood pressure, cardiac output, stroke volume, rate pressure product, minute ventilation, respiratory rate, and tidal volume at rest and during submaximal and maximal exercise.

1.1.4   Describe the physiologic determinants of $\dot{V}O_2$, $m\dot{V}O_2$, and mean arterial pressure and explain how these determinants may be altered with aerobic and resistance exercise training.

1.1.5   Describe appropriate modifications in the exercise prescription that are due to environmental conditions in individuals with chronic disease.

1.1.6   Explain the health benefits of a physically active lifestyle, the hazards of sedentary behavior, and summarize key recommendations of U.S. national reports of physical activity (e.g., U.S. Surgeon General, Institute of Medicine, ACSM, AHA).

1.1.7   Explain the physiologic adaptations to exercise training that may result in improvement in or maintenance of health, including cardiovascular, pulmonary, metabolic, orthopedic/musculoskeletal, neuromuscular, and immune system health.

1.1.8   Explain the mechanisms underlying the physiologic adaptations to aerobic and resistance training, including those resulting in changes in or maintenance of maximal and submaximal oxygen consumption, lactate and ventilatory (anaerobic) threshold, myocardial oxygen consumption, heart rate, blood pressure, ventilation (including ventilatory threshold), muscle structure, bioenergetics, and immune function.

1.1.9   Explain the physiologic effects of physical inactivity, including bed rest, and methods that may counteract these effects.

1.1.10   Recognize and respond to abnormal signs and symptoms during exercise.

General Population/Core: Pathophysiology and Risk Factors

1.2.1   Describe the epidemiology, pathophysiology, risk factors, and key clinical findings of cardiovascular, pulmonary, metabolic, orthopedic/musculoskeletal, neuromuscular, and NIH diseases.

General Population/Core: Health Appraisal, Fitness, and Clinical Exercise Testing

1.3.1   Conduct pretest procedures, including explaining test procedures, obtaining informed consent, obtaining a focused medical history, reviewing results of prior tests and physical exam, assessing disease-specific risk factors, and presenting concise information to other healthcare providers and third-party payers.

1.3.2   Conduct a brief physical examination including evaluation of peripheral edema, measuring blood pressure, peripheral pulses, respiratory rate, and ausculating heart and lung sounds.

1.3.3   Calibrate lab equipment used frequently in the practice of clinical exercise physiology (e.g., motorized/computerized treadmill, mechanical cycle ergometer and arm ergometer), electrocardiograph, spirometer, respiratory gas analyzer (metabolic cart).

1.3.4   Administer exercise tests consistent with U.S. nationally accepted standards for testing.

1.3.5   Evaluate contraindications to exercise testing.

1.3.6   Appropriately select and administer functional tests to measure individual outcomes and functional status, including the six-minute walk, Get Up and Go, Berg Balance Scale, and the Physical Performance Test.

1.3.8   Interpret the variables that may be assessed during clinical exercise testing, including maximal oxygen consumption, resting metabolic rate, ventilatory volumes and capacities, respiratory exchange ratio, ratings of perceived exertion and discomfort (chest pain, dyspnea, claudication), ECG, heart rate, blood pressure, rate pressure product, ventilatory (anaerobic) threshold, oxygen saturation, breathing reserve, muscular strength, muscular endurance, and other common measures employed for diagnosis and prognosis of disease.

1.3.9   Determine atrial and ventricular rate from rhythm strip and 12-lead ECG and explain the clinical significance of abnormal atrial or ventricular rate (e.g., tachycardia, bradycardia).

1.3.10   Identify ECG changes associated with drug therapy, electrolyte abnormalities, subendocardial and transmural ischemia, myocardial injury, and infarction, and explain the clinical significance of each.

1.3.11   Identify SA, AV, and bundle-branch blocks from a rhythm strip and 12-lead ECG, and explain the clinical significance of each.

1.3.12   Identify sinus, atrial, junctional, and ventricular dysrhythmias from a rhythm strip and 12-lead ECG, and explain the clinical significance of each.

1.3.14   Determine an individual's pretest and posttest probability of coronary heart disease, identify factors associated with test complications, and apply appropriate precautions to reduce risks to the individual.

1.3.16   Identify probable disease-specific endpoints for testing in an individual with cardiovascular, pulmonary, metabolic, orthopedic/musculoskeletal, neuromuscular, and NIH disease.

1.3.17   Select and employ appropriate techniques for preparation and measurement of ECG, heart rate, blood pressure, oxygen saturation, RPE, symptoms, expired gases, and other measures as needed before, during, and following exercise testing.

1.3.18   Select and administer appropriate exercise tests to evaluate functional capacity, strength, and flexibility in individuals with cardiovascular, pulmonary, metabolic, orthopedic/musculoskeletal, neuromuscular, and NIH disease.

1.3.19   Discuss strengths and limitations of various methods of measures and indices of body composition.

1.3.20   Appropriately select, apply, and interpret body-composition tests and indices.

1.3.21   Discuss pertinent test results with other healthcare professionals.

General Population/Core: Exercise Prescription and Programming

1.7.3   Determine the appropriate level of supervision and monitoring recommended for individuals with known disease based on disease-specific risk-stratification guidelines and current health status.

1.7.4   Develop, adapt, and supervise appropriate aerobic, resistance, and flexibility training for individuals with cardiovascular, pulmonary, metabolic, orthopedic/musculoskeletal, neuromuscular, and NIH disease.

1.7.6   Instruct individuals with cardiovascular, pulmonary, metabolic, orthopedic/musculoskeletal, neuromuscular, and NIH disease in techniques for performing physical activities safely and effectively in an unsupervised exercise setting.

1.7.7   Modify the exercise prescription or discontinue exercise based on individual symptoms, current health status, musculoskeletal limitations, and environmental considerations.

1.7.8   Extract and interpret clinical information needed for safe exercise management of individuals with cardiovascular, pulmonary, metabolic, orthopedic/musculoskeletal, neuromuscular, and NIH disease.

1.7.9   Evaluate individual outcomes from serial outcome data collected before, during, and after exercise interventions.

General Population/Core: Human Behavior and Counseling

1.9.1   Summarize contemporary theories of health behavior change, including social cognitive theory, theory of reasoned action, theory of planned behavior, transtheoretical model, and health belief model. Apply techniques to promote healthy behaviors, including physical activity.

1.9.2   Describe characteristics associated with poor adherence to exercise programs.

1.9.3   Describe the psychological issues associated with acute and chronic illness, such as anxiety, depression, social isolation, hostility, aggression, and suicidal ideation.

1.9.4   Counsel individuals with cardiovascular, pulmonary, metabolic, orthopedic/musculoskeletal, neuromuscular, and NIH disease on topics such as disease processes, treatments, diagnostic techniques, and lifestyle management.

1.9.6   Explain factors that may increase anxiety before or during exercise testing, and describe methods to reduce anxiety.

1.9.7   Recognize signs and symptoms of failure to cope during personal crises such as job loss, bereavement, and illness.

General Population/Core: Safety, Injury Prevention, and Emergency Procedures

1.10.1   List routine emergency equipment, drugs, and supplies present in an exercise testing laboratory and therapeutic exercise session area.

1.10.2   Provide immediate responses to emergencies, including basic cardiac life support, AED, activation of emergency medical services, and joint immobilization.

1.10.3   Verify operating status of emergency equipment, including defibrillator, laryngoscope, and oxygen.

1.10.4   Explain universal precautions procedures and apply as appropriate.

1.10.5   Develop and implement a plan for responding to emergencies.

1.10.6   Demonstrate knowledge of advanced cardiac life support procedures.

General Population/Core: Program Administration, Quality Assurance, and Outcome Assessment

1.11.1   Describe appropriate staffing for exercise testing and programming based on factors such as individual health status, facilities, and program goals.

1.11.2   List necessary equipment and supplies for exercise testing and programs.

1.11.3   Select, evaluate, and report treatment outcomes using individual-relevant results of tests and surveys.

1.11.4   Explain legal issues pertinent to healthcare delivery by licensed and nonlicensed healthcare professionals providing rehabilitative services and exercise testing and legal risk-management techniques.

1.11.5   Identify individuals requiring referral to a physician or allied health services such as physical therapy, dietary counseling, stress management, weight management, and psychological and social services.

1.11.6   Develop a plan for individual discharge from therapeutic exercise program, including community referrals.

Cardiovascular: Exercise Physiology and Related Exercise Science

2.1.2   Describe the potential benefits and hazards of aerobic, resistance, and flexibility training in individuals with cardiovascular diseases.

2.1.4   Explain how cardiovascular diseases may affect the physiologic responses to aerobic and resistance training.

2.1.5   Describe the immediate and long-term influence of medical therapies for cardiovascular diseases on the responses to aerobic and resistance training.

Cardiovascular: Pathophysiology and Risk Factors

2.2.1   Describe the epidemiology, pathophysiology, rate of progression of disease, risk factors, and key clinical findings of cardiovascular diseases.

2.2.2   Explain the ischemic cascade and its effect on myocardial function.

2.2.4   Explain methods of reducing risk in individuals with cardiovascular diseases.

Cardiovascular: Health Appraisal, Fitness, and Clinical Exercise Testing

2.3.1   Describe common techniques used to diagnose cardiovascular disease, including graded exercise testing, echocardiography, radionuclide imaging, angiography, pharmacologic testing, and biomarkers (e.g., troponin, CK), and explain the indications, limitations, risks, and normal and abnormal results for each.

2.3.2   Explain how cardiovascular disease may affect physical examination findings.

2.3.4   Recognize and respond to abnormal signs and symptoms—such as pain, peripheral edema, dyspnea, and fatigue—in individuals with cardiovascular diseases.

2.3.5   Conduct and interpret appropriate exercise testing methods for individuals with cardiovascular diseases.

Cardiovascular: Medical and Surgical Management

2.6.2   Explain the common medical and surgical treatments of cardiovascular diseases.

2.6.3   Apply key recommendations of current U.S. clinical practice guidelines for the prevention, treatment, and management of cardiovascular diseases (e.g., AHA, ACC, NHLBI).

2.6.4   List the commonly used drugs (generic and brand names) in the treatment of individuals with cardiovascular diseases, and explain the indications, mechanisms of actions, major side effects, and the effects on the exercising individual.

2.6.5   Explain how treatments for cardiovascular disease, including preventive care, may affect the rate of progression of disease.

Cardiovascular: Exercise Prescription and Programming

2.7.2   Design, adapt, and supervise an appropriate Exercise Prescription (e.g., aerobic, resistance, and flexibility training) for individuals with cardiovascular diseases.

2.7.4   Instruct an individual with cardiovascular disease in techniques for performing physical activities safely and effectively in an unsupervised setting.

2.7.5   Counsel individuals with cardiovascular disease on the proper uses of sublingual nitroglycerin.

Pulmonary (e.g., Obstructive and Restrictive Lung Diseases): Exercise Physiology and Related Exercise Science

3.1.1   Describe the potential benefits and hazards of aerobic, resistance, and flexibility training in individuals with pulmonary diseases.

3.1.2   Explain how pulmonary diseases may affect the physiologic responses to aerobic, resistance, and flexibility training.

3.1.3   Explain how scheduling of exercise relative to meals can affect dyspnea.

3.1.5   Describe the immediate and long-term influence of medical therapies for pulmonary diseases on the responses to aerobic, resistance, and flexibility training.

Pulmonary: Pathophysiology and Risk Factors

3.2.1   Describe the epidemiology, pathophysiology, rate of progression of disease, risk factors, and key clinical findings of pulmonary diseases.

3.2.3   Explain methods of reducing risk in individuals with pulmonary diseases.

Pulmonary: Health Appraisal, Fitness, and Clinical Exercise Testing

3.3.1   Explain how pulmonary disease may affect physical examination findings.

3.3.3   Demonstrate knowledge of lung volumes and capacities (e.g., tidal volume, residual volume, inspiratory volume, expiratory volume, total lung capacity, vital capacity, functional residual capacity, peak flow rate, diffusion capacity) and how they may differ between normals and individuals with pulmonary disease.

3.3.4   Recognize and respond to abnormal signs and symptoms to exercise in individuals with pulmonary diseases.

3.3.5   Describe common techniques and tests used to diagnose pulmonary diseases, and explain the indications, limitations, risks, and normal and abnormal results for each.

3.3.6   Conduct and interpret appropriate exercise testing methods for individuals with pulmonary diseases.

Pulmonary: Medical and Surgical Management

3.6.3   Explain how treatments for pulmonary disease, including preventive care, may affect the rate of progression of disease.

3.6.5   Explain the common medical and surgical treatments of pulmonary diseases.

3.6.6   List the commonly used drugs (generic and brand names) in the treatment of individuals with pulmonary diseases, and explain the indications, mechanisms of actions, major side effects, and the effects on the exercising individual.

3.6.7   Apply key recommendations of current U.S. clinical practice guidelines (e.g., ALA, NIH, NHLBI) for the prevention, treatment, and management of pulmonary diseases.

Pulmonary: Exercise Prescription and Programming

3.7.2   Design, adapt, and supervise an appropriate exercise prescription (e.g., aerobic, resistance, and flexibility training) for individuals with pulmonary diseases.

3.7.4   Instruct an individual with pulmonary diseases in proper breathing techniques and exercises and methods for performing physical activities safely and effectively.

3.7.5   Demonstrate knowledge of the use of supplemental oxygen during exercise and its influences on exercise tolerance.

Metabolic (e.g., Diabetes, Hyperlipidemia, Obesity, Frailty, Chronic Renal Failure, Metabolic Syndrome): Exercise Physiology and Related Exercise Science

4.1.1   Explain how metabolic diseases may affect aerobic endurance, muscular strength and endurance, flexibility, and balance.

4.1.2   Describe the immediate and long-term influence of medical therapies for metabolic diseases on the responses to aerobic, resistance, and flexibility training.

4.1.3   Describe the potential benefits and hazards of aerobic, resistance, and flexibility training in individuals with metabolic diseases.

Metabolic: Pathophysiology and Risk Factors

4.2.1   Describe the epidemiology, pathophysiology, rate of progression of disease, risk factors, and key clinical findings of metabolic diseases.

4.2.5   Describe the probable effects of dialysis treatment on exercise performance, functional capacity, and safety, and explain methods for preventing adverse effects.

4.2.6   Describe the probable effects of hypo/hyperglycemia on exercise performance, functional capacity, and safety, and explain methods for preventing adverse effects.

4.2.7   Explain methods of reducing risk in individuals with metabolic diseases.

Metabolic: Health Appraisal, Fitness, and Clinical Exercise Testing

4.3.1   Describe common techniques and tests used to diagnose metabolic diseases, and explain the indications, limitations, risks, and normal and abnormal results for each.

4.3.3   Explain appropriate techniques for monitoring blood glucose before, during, and after an exercise session.

4.3.4   Recognize and respond to abnormal signs and symptoms in individuals with metabolic diseases.

4.3.5   Conduct and interpret appropriate exercise testing methods for individuals with metabolic diseases.

Metabolic: Medical and Surgical Management

4.6.2   Apply key recommendations of current U.S. clinical practice guidelines (e.g., ADA, NIH, NHLBI) for the prevention, treatment, and management of metabolic diseases.

4.6.3   Explain the common medical and surgical treatments of metabolic diseases.

4.6.4   List the commonly used drugs (generic and brand names) in the treatment of individuals with metabolic diseases, and explain the indications, mechanisms of actions, major side effects, and the effects on the exercising individual.

4.6.5   Explain how treatments for metabolic diseases, including preventive care, may affect the rate of progression of disease.

Metabolic: Exercise Prescription and Programming

4.7.2   Design, adapt, and supervise an appropriate exercise prescription (e.g., aerobic, resistance, and flexibility training) for individuals with metabolic diseases.

4.7.4   Instruct individuals with metabolic diseases in techniques for performing physical activities safely and effectively in an unsupervised exercise setting.

4.7.5   Adapt the exercise prescription based on the functional limits and benefits of assistive devices (e.g., wheelchairs, crutches, and canes).

Orthopedic/Musculoskeletal (e.g., Low Back Pain, Osteoarthritis, Rheumatoid Arthritis, Osteoporosis, Amputations, Vertebral Disorders): Exercise Physiology and Related Exercise Science

5.1.1   Describe the potential benefits and hazards of aerobic, resistance, and flexibility training in individuals with orthopedic/musculoskeletal diseases.

5.1.4   Explain how orthopedic/musculoskeletal diseases may affect aerobic endurance, muscular strength and endurance, flexibility, balance, and agility.

5.1.5   Describe the immediate and long-term influence of medical therapies for orthopedic/musculoskeletal diseases on the responses to aerobic, resistance, and flexibility training.

Orthopedic/Musculoskeletal: Pathophysiology and Risk Factors

5.2.1   Describe the epidemiology, pathophysiology, risk factors, and key clinical findings of orthopedic/musculoskeletal diseases.

Orthopedic/Musculoskeletal: Health Appraisal, Fitness, and Clinical Exercise Testing

5.3.1   Recognize and respond to abnormal signs and symptoms to exercise in individuals with orthopedic/musculoskeletal diseases.

5.3.2   Describe common techniques and tests used to diagnose orthopedic/musculoskeletal diseases.

5.3.3   Conduct and interpret appropriate exercise testing methods for individuals with orthopedic/musculoskeletal diseases.

Orthopedic/Musculoskeletal: Medical and Surgical Management

5.6.1   List the commonly used drugs (generic and brand names) in the treatment of individuals with orthopedic/musculoskeletal diseases, and explain the indications, mechanisms of actions, major side effects, and the effects on the exercising individual.

5.6.2   Explain the common medical and surgical treatments of orthopedic/musculoskeletal diseases.

5.6.3   Apply key recommendations of current U.S. clinical practice guidelines (e.g., NIH, National Osteoporosis Foundation, Arthritis Foundation) for the prevention, treatment, and management of orthopedic/musculoskeletal diseases.

5.6.4   Explain how treatments for orthopedic/musculoskeletal disease may affect the rate of progression of disease.

Orthopedic/Musculoskeletal: Exercise Prescription and Programming

5.7.1   Explain exercise training concepts specific to industrial or occupational rehabilitation, which includes work hardening, work conditioning, work fitness, and job coaching.

5.7.2   Design, adapt, and supervise an appropriate exercise prescription (e.g., aerobic, resistance, and flexibility training) for individuals with orthopedic/musculoskeletal diseases.

5.7.3   Instruct an individual with orthopedic/musculoskeletal disease in techniques for performing physical activities safely and effectively in an unsupervised exercise setting.

5.7.4   Adapt the exercise prescription based on the functional limits and benefits of assistive devices (e.g., wheelchairs, crutches, and canes).

Neuromuscular (e.g., Multiple Sclerosis, Muscular Dystrophy and Other Myopathies, Alzheimer Disease, Parkinson Disease, Polio and Postpolio Syndrome, Stroke and Brain Injury, Cerebral Palsy, Peripheral Neuropathies): Exercise Physiology and Related Exercise Science

6.1.1   Describe the potential benefits and hazards of aerobic, resistance, and flexibility training in individuals with neuromuscular diseases.

6.1.4   Explain how neuromuscular diseases may affect aerobic endurance, muscular strength and endurance, flexibility, balance, and agility.

6.1.5   Describe the immediate and long-term influence of medical therapies for neuromuscular diseases on the responses to aerobic, resistance, and flexibility training.

Neuromuscular: Pathophysiology and Risk Factors

6.2.1   Describe the epidemiology, pathophysiology, risk factors, and key clinical findings of neuromuscular diseases.

Neuromuscular: Health Appraisal, Fitness, and Clinical Exercise Testing

6.3.1   Recognize and respond to abnormal signs and symptoms to exercise in individuals with neuromuscular diseases.

6.3.2   Describe common techniques and tests used to diagnose neuromuscular diseases.

6.3.3   Conduct and interpret appropriate exercise testing methods for individuals with neuromuscular diseases.

Neuromuscular: Medical and Surgical Management

6.6.1   Explain the common medical and surgical treatments of neuromuscular diseases.

6.6.2   List the commonly used drugs (generic and brand names) in the treatment of individuals with neuromuscular disease, and explain the indications, mechanisms of actions, major side effects, and the effects on the exercising individual.

6.6.3   Apply key recommendations of current U.S. clinical practice guidelines (e.g., NIH) for the prevention, treatment, and management of neuromuscular diseases.

6.6.4   Explain how treatments for neuromuscular disease may affect the rate of progression of disease.

Neuromuscular: Exercise Prescription and Programming

6.7.1   Adapt the exercise prescription based on the functional limits and benefits of assistive devices (e.g., wheelchairs, crutches, and canes).

6.7.3   Design, adapt, and supervise an appropriate exercise prescription (e.g., aerobic, resistance, and flexibility training) for individuals with neuromuscular diseases.

6.7.4   Instruct an individual with neuromuscular diseases in techniques for performing physical activities safely and effectively in an unsupervised exercise setting.

Neoplastic, Immunologic, and Hematologic (e.g., Cancer, Anemia, Bleeding Disorders, HIV, AIDS, Organ Transplant, Chronic Fatigue Syndrome, Fibromyalgia): Exercise Physiology and Related Exercise Science

7.1.1   Explain how NIH diseases may affect the physiologic responses to aerobic, resistance, and flexibility training.

7.1.2   Describe the immediate and long-term influence of medical therapies for NIH on the responses to aerobic, resistance, and flexibility training.

7.1.3   Describe the potential benefits and hazards of aerobic, resistance, and flexibility training in individuals with NIH diseases.

Neoplastic, Immunologic, and Hematologic: Pathophysiology and Risk Factors

7.2.1   Describe the epidemiology, pathophysiology, risk factors, and key clinical findings of NIH diseases.

Neoplastic, Immunologic, and Hematologic: Health Appraisal, Fitness, and Clinical Exercise Testing

7.3.1   Recognize and respond to abnormal signs and symptoms to exercise in individuals with NIH diseases.

7.3.2   Describe common techniques and tests used to diagnose NIH diseases.

7.3.3   Conduct and interpret appropriate exercise testing methods for individuals with NIH diseases.

Neoplastic, Immunologic, and Hematologic: Medical and Surgical Management

7.6.1   List the commonly used drugs (generic and brand names) in the treatment of individuals with NIH disease, and explain the indications, mechanisms of actions, major side effects, and the effects on the exercising individual.

7.6.2   Apply key recommendations of current U.S. clinical practice guidelines (e.g., ACS, NIH) for the prevention, treatment, and management of NIH diseases.

7.6.3   Explain the common medical and surgical treatments of NIH diseases.

7.6.4   Explain how treatments for NIH disease may affect the rate of progression of disease.

Neoplastic, Immunologic, and Hematologic: Exercise Prescription and Programming

7.7.1	Design, adapt, and supervise an appropriate exercise prescription (e.g., aerobic, resistance, and flexibility training) for individuals with NIH diseases.
7.7.4	Instruct an individual with NIH diseases in techniques for performing physical activities safely and effectively in an unsupervised exercise setting.

NOTE: The KSAs listed above for the ACSM Registered Clinical Exercise Physiologist® are the same KSAs for educational programs in clinical exercise physiology seeking graduate (master's degree) academic accreditation through the CoAES. For more information, please visit www.coaes.org.

Additional KSAs required (in addition to the ACSM Certified Health Fitness Specialist KSAs) for programs seeking academic accreditation in applied exercise physiology. The KSAs that follow, IN ADDITION TO the ACSM Certified Health Fitness Specialist KSAs above, represent the KSAs for educational programs in applied exercise physiology seeking graduate (master's degree) academic accreditation through the CoAES. For more information, please visit www.coaes.org.

General Population/Core: Exercise Physiology and Related Exercise Science

1.1.1	Ability to describe modifications in exercise prescription for individuals with functional disabilities and musculoskeletal injuries.
1.1.2	Ability to describe the relationship between biomechanical efficiency, oxygen cost of activity (economy), and performance of physical activity.
1.1.3	Knowledge of the muscular, cardiorespiratory, and metabolic responses to decreased exercise intensity.

General Population/Core: Pathophysiology and Risk Factors

1.2.1	Ability to define atherosclerosis, the factors causing it, and the interventions that may potentially delay or reverse the atherosclerotic process.
1.2.2	Ability to describe the causes of myocardial ischemia and infarction.
1.2.3	Ability to describe the pathophysiology of hypertension, obesity, hyperlipidemia, diabetes, chronic obstructive pulmonary diseases, arthritis, osteoporosis, chronic diseases, and immunosuppressive disease.
1.2.4	Ability to describe the effects of the above diseases and conditions on cardiorespiratory and metabolic function at rest and during exercise.

General Population/Core: Health Appraisal, Fitness, and Clinical Exercise Testing

1.3.1	Knowledge of the selection of an appropriate behavioral goal and the suggested method to evaluate goal achievement for each stage of change.
1.3.2	Knowledge of the use and value of the results of the fitness evaluation and exercise test for various populations.
1.3.3	Ability to design and implement a fitness testing/health appraisal program that includes, but is not limited to, staffing needs, physician interaction, documentation, equipment, marketing, and program evaluation.
1.3.4	Ability to recruit, train, and evaluate appropriate staff personnel for performing exercise tests, fitness evaluations, and health appraisals.

General Population/Core: Patient Management and Medications

1.5.1   Ability to identify and describe the principal action, mechanisms of action, and major side effects from each of the following classes of medications: antianginals, antihypertensives, antiarrhythmics, bronchodilators, hypoglycemics, psychotropics, and vasodilators.

General Population/Core: Human Behavior and Counseling

1.9.1   Knowledge of and ability to apply basic cognitive-behavioral intervention, such as shaping, goal setting, motivation, cueing, problem solving, reinforcement strategies, and self-monitoring.

1.9.2   Knowledge of the selection of an appropriate behavioral goal and the suggested method to evaluate goal achievement for each stage of change.

General Population/Core: Safety, Injury Prevention, and Emergency Procedures

1.10.1   Ability to identify the process to train the exercise staff in cardiopulmonary resuscitation.

1.10.2   Ability to design and evaluate emergency procedures for a preventive exercise program and an exercise testing facility.

1.10.3   Ability to train staff in safety procedures, risk-reduction strategies, and injury-care techniques.

1.10.4   Knowledge of the legal implications of documented safety procedures, the use of incident documents, and ongoing safety training.

General Population/Core: Program Administration, Quality Assurance, and Outcome Assessment

1.11.1   Ability to manage personnel effectively.

1.11.2   Ability to describe a management plan for the development of staff, continuing education, marketing and promotion, documentation, billing, facility management, and financial planning.

1.11.3   Ability to describe the decision-making process related to budgets, market analysis, program evaluation, facility management, staff allocation, and community development.

1.11.4   Ability to describe the development, evaluation, and revision of policies and procedures for programming and facility management.

1.11.5   Ability to describe how the computer can assist in data analysis, spreadsheet report development, and daily tracking of customer utilization.

1.11.6   Ability to define and describe the total quality management (TQM) and continuous quality improvement (CQI) approaches to management.

1.11.7   Ability to interpret applied research in the areas of exercise testing, exercise programming, and educational programs to maintain a comprehensive and current state-of-the-art program.

1.11.8   Ability to develop a risk factor screening program, including procedures, staff training, feedback, and follow-up.

1.11.9   Knowledge of administration, management, and supervision of personnel.

1.11.10   Ability to describe effective interviewing, hiring, and employee termination procedures.

1.11.11   Ability to describe and diagram an organizational chart and show the relationships between a health/fitness director, owner, medical advisor, and staff.

1.11.12	Knowledge of and ability to describe various staff training techniques.
1.11.13	Knowledge of and ability to describe performance reviews and their role in evaluating staff.
1.11.14	Knowledge of the legal obligations and problems involved in personnel management.
1.11.15	Knowledge of compensation, including wages, bonuses, incentive programs, and benefits.
1.11.16	Knowledge of methods for implementing a sales commission system.
1.11.17	Ability to describe the significance of a benefits program for staff and demonstrate an understanding in researching and selecting benefits.
1.11.18	Ability to write and implement thorough and legal job descriptions.
1.11.19	Knowledge of personnel time-management techniques.
1.11.20	Knowledge of administration, management, and development of a budget and of the financial aspects of a fitness center.
1.11.21	Knowledge of the principles of financial management.
1.11.22	Knowledge of basic accounting principles, such as accounts payable, accounts receivable, accrual, cash flow, assets, liabilities, and return on investment.
1.11.23	Ability to identify the various forms of a business enterprise, such as sole proprietorship, partnership, corporation, and S-corporation.
1.11.24	Knowledge of the procedures involved with developing, evaluating, revising, and updating capital and operating budgets.
1.11.25	Ability to manage expenses with the objective of maintaining a positive cash flow.
1.11.26	Ability to understand and analyze financial statements, including income statements, balance sheets, cash flows, budgets, and pro forma projections.
1.11.27	Knowledge of program-related break-even and cost/benefit analysis.
1.11.28	Knowledge of the importance of short-term and long-term planning.
1.11.29	Knowledge of the principles of marketing and sales.
1.11.30	Ability to identify the steps in the development, implementation, and evaluation of a marketing plan.
1.11.31	Knowledge of the components of a needs assessment/market analysis.
1.11.32	Knowledge of various sales techniques for prospective members.
1.11.33	Knowledge of techniques for advertising, marketing, promotion, and public relations.
1.11.34	Ability to describe the principles of developing and evaluating product and services, and establishing pricing.
1.11.35	Knowledge of the principles of day-to-day operation of a fitness center.
1.11.36	Knowledge of the principles of pricing and purchasing equipment and supplies.
1.11.37	Knowledge of facility layout and design.
1.11.38	Ability to establish and evaluate an equipment preventive maintenance and repair program.
1.11.39	Ability to describe a plan for implementing a housekeeping program.
1.11.40	Ability to identify and explain the operating policies for preventive exercise programs, including data analysis and reporting, confidentiality of records, relationships with healthcare providers, accident and injury reporting, and continuing education of participants.
1.11.41	Knowledge of the legal concepts of tort, negligence, liability, indemnification, standards of care, health regulations, consent, contract, confidentiality, malpractice, and the legal concerns regarding emergency procedures and informed consent.
1.11.42	Ability to implement capital improvements with minimal disruption of client or business needs.
1.11.43	Ability to coordinate the operations of various departments, including, but not limited to, the front desk, fitness, rehabilitation, maintenance and repair, day care, housekeeping, pool, and management.

1.11.44 Knowledge of management and principles of member service and communication.

1.11.45 Skills in effective techniques for communicating with staff, management, members, healthcare providers, potential customers, and vendors.

1.11.46 Knowledge of and ability to provide strong customer service.

1.11.47 Ability to develop and implement customer surveys.

1.11.48 Knowledge of the strategies for management conflict.

1.11.49 Knowledge of the principles of health promotion and ability to administer health-promotion programs.

1.11.50 Knowledge of health-promotion programs (e.g., nutrition and weight management, smoking cessation, stress management, back care, body mechanics, and substance abuse).

1.11.51 Knowledge of the specific and appropriate content and methods for creating a health-promotion program.

1.11.52 Knowledge of and ability to access resources for various programs and delivery systems.

1.11.53 Knowledge of the concepts of cost-effectiveness and cost-benefit as they relate to the evaluation of health-promotion programming.

1.11.54 Ability to describe the means and amounts by which health-promotion programs might increase productivity, reduce employee loss time, reduce healthcare costs, and improve profitability in the workplace.

Index

Page numbers in *italics* designate figures; page numbers followed by the letter "t" designate tables; page numbers followed by the letter "b" designate text boxes; *(see also)* designates related topics or more detailed subtopics